Orthopaedic Practice

Orthopaedic Practice

Edited by

P. M. Yeoman MA, MB, BChir, MD, FRCS
Emeritus Consultant Orthopaedic Surgeon, The Royal United Hospital and The Royal National Hospital for
Rheumatic Diseases NHS Trust, Bath, UK

and

D. M. Spengler MD
Chairman, Department of Orthopaedics and Rehabilitation, Vanderbilt University, Nashville, Tennessee, USA

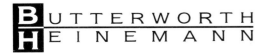

Butterworth-Heinemann
Linacre House, Jordan Hill, Oxford OX2 8DP
A division of Reed Educational & Professional Publishing Ltd

R A member of the Reed Elsevier plc group

OXFORD BOSTON JOHANNESBURG
MELBOURNE NEW DELHI SINGAPORE

First published 1996

British Library Cataloguing in Publication Data
Orthopaedic Practice
  I. Yeoman, Philip   II. Spengler, Dan M.
  617.3

ISBN 0 7506 1624 5

Library of Congress Cataloguing in Publication Data
Orthopaedic practice/edited by P. M. Yeoman and D. M. Spengler
    p. cm.
  Includes bibliographical references and index.
  ISBN 0-7506-1624-5
  1. Orthopedics.   I. Yeoman, P. M. (Philip M.) II. Spengler, Dan M.
  [DNLM: 1. Musculoskeletal Diseases—therapy. 2. Orthopedics—
methods.   WE 168 C9763 1995]
  RD731.C87 1995
  617.3—dc20   94-44573
                                              CIP

Printed in Great Britain by The Bath Press plc, Bath, Avon

Contents

Contributors

Barton, N. J. FRCS
Consultant Hand Surgeon, Nottingham
University Hospital and Harlow Wood
Orthopaedic Hospital, Civilian Consultant in
Hand Surgery to the Royal Air Force, UK

Baylink, D. J. MD
Jerry L. Pettis Veterans Hospital and Loma
Linda University, Loma Linda, California, USA

Bliss, P. MB FRCS JP
Emeritus Consultant Orthopaedic Surgeon,
Royal United Hospital and The Royal
National Hospital for Rheumatic Diseases,
Bath, UK

Bullimore, J. MB BS DMRT FRCR
Consultant Clinical Oncologist, Bristol
Oncology Centre, Bristol Royal Infirmary,
Bristol, UK

Catterall, A. MChir FRCS
Children's Unit, Royal National Orthopaedic
Hospital, London, UK

Cruz-Conde Delgado, R. MD
Head of Orthopaedic Department, Asepeyo
Orthopaedic Hospital, Coslada, Madrid, Spain

Denton, J. S.
Department of Orthopaedic Surgery,
University of Liverpool, Liverpool, UK

Dickson, R. A. MA ChM FRCS DSc
Professor of Orthopaedic Surgery, University
of Leeds, St James's Hospital, Leeds, UK

Dunkerley, D. R. FRCS
Consultant Orthopaedic and Hand Surgeon,
Royal United Hospital NHS Trust, Combe
Park, Bath, UK

Fitzgerald, R. H. Jr MD
Professor and Chairman, Wayne State
University, School of Medicine, Detroit, USA

Griffiths, W. E. G. FRCS Eng FRCS Ed
Consultant in Orthopaedics, Queen Alexandra
Hospital, Cosham, Portsmouth, UK

Grimer, R. J. FRCS FRCS Ed (Orth)
Consultant Orthopaedic Oncologist, The
Orthopaedic Oncology Service, The Royal
Orthopaedic Hospital, Northfield, Birmingham,
UK

Hall, G. MD FRCS
Consultant Orthopaedic Surgeon, West Dorset
Health Trust, Dorset, UK

Irving, Sir M. MD ChM FRCS
Professor of Surgery, University of
Manchester, Hope Hospital, Manchester, UK

Kenwright, J. MA MD FRCS
Nuffield Professor of Orthopaedic Surgery,
University of Oxford, Nuffield Orthopaedic
Centre, Headington, Oxford, UK

Kirkup, J. R. MA MD FRCS
Emeritus Consultant Orthopaedic Surgeon,
Royal National Hospital for Rheumatic
Diseases, Bath, UK

Little, R. A. PhD FRCPath FFAEM
Head MRC Trauma Group, Director North
Western Injury, Research Centre, University of
Manchester, Manchester, UK

Mariano-Menez, M. R. MD
Jerry L. Pettis Veterans Hospital and Loma
Linda University, Loma Linda, California,
USA

Marsh, D. MD FRCS
Senior Lecturer in Orthopaedics, University of
Manchester, Hope Hospital, Manchester, UK

Marti Gonzalez, J. C. MD
Unit of External Fixation, Asepeyo
Orthopaedic Hospital, Coslada, Madrid, Spain

Morrison, P. J. M. FRCS
Consultant Orthopaedic Surgeon, Royal
National Hospital for Rheumatic Diseases,
Bath, UK

Narakas, A. O. MD FRCS EngHon
(Deceased)
Associate Professor at the Medical School and
Consultant at the University Hospital of
Lausanne, Lausanne, Switzerland

Newman, J. H. MA MB BChir FRCS
Consultant Orthopaedic Surgeon, Bristol Royal
Infirmary and Avon Orthopaedic Centre,
Southmead, Bristol, UK

Pozo, J. L. MA FRCS
Consultant Orthopaedic Surgeon, Royal
United Hospital and The Royal National
Hospital for Rheumatic Diseases, Bath, UK

Price, R. R. PhD
Professor of Radiology, Director, Radiological
Sciences Division, Department of Radiology
and Radiological Sciences, Vanderbilt
University Medical Center, Nashville,
Tennessee, USA

Sandler, M. P. MD
Professor and Vice-Chairman, Radiology and
Radiological Sciences, Director of Nuclear
Science, Vanderbilt University Medical Center,
Nashville, Tennessee, USA

Semple, C. FRCS
Hand Surgeon, 79 Harley Street, London, UK

Sneath, R. S. FRCS
Consultant Orthopaedic Surgeon, Formerly
Director, The Orthopaedic Oncology Service,
The Royal Orthopaedic Hospital, Northfield,
Birmingham, UK

Spengler, D. M. MD
Chairman, Department of Orthopaedics and
Rehabilitation, Vanderbilt University,
Tennessee, USA

Swiontkowski, M. F. MD
Professor, Department of Orthopaedics,
University of Washington, Chief of
Orthopaedics, Harborview Medical Center,
Seattle, Washington, USA

Szalay, E. A. MD
Paediatric Orthopaedics and Scoliosis,
Beaumont Bone and Joint Clinic, Beaumont,
Texas, USA

Townsend, P. L. G. BSc FRCS(c) FRCS
Consultant Plastic Surgeon, Department of
Plastic and Reconstructive Surgery, Frenchay
Hospital, Bristol, UK

Wilkinson, J. A. BSc MCh FRCS
Senior Consultant Orthopaedic Surgeon
(Emeritus), Southampton University Hospitals
and The Lord Mayor Treloar Hospital, Alton,
UK

Wynn Jones, C. H. MBBS FRCS
Consultant Orthopaedic Surgeon, Hartshill
Orthopaedic Hospital, Stoke-on-Trent, UK

Wynn Parry, C. B. MBE MA DM FRCP
FRCS
Formerly Director of Rehabilitation, Royal
National Orthopaedic Hospitals, London and
Stanmore, UK

Yeoman, P. M. MD FRCS
Emeritus Consultant Orthopaedic Surgeon,
Royal United Hospital and The Royal
National Hospital for Rheumatic Diseases,
Bath, UK

Foreword

There are many problems in orthopaedic surgery 'upon which it is difficult to speak, and impossible to be silent'. Difficult to speak, because at this stage in our learning no one fully understands them; impossible to ignore, because they make up a large part of daily practice. The subjects discussed in this book are mainly those for which no complete solution has yet been found. The list of chapter headings might serve as a student's guide to areas in which research is most needed and most likely to prove rewarding.

Not that these subjects have been overlooked in the past. On the contrary, they have been the very stuff of orthopaedics ever since our speciality was born. There has hardly been a major orthopaedic meeting without papers on Perthes' disease and club foot, but the best protocol for the treatment of talipes is not yet agreed and doubts remain about the efficacy of any of the procedures devised for Perthes' disease. Similarly, in the field of traumatology, although there is consensus on how to treat many types of fracture, the challenge of the multiply injured patient is still debated. Our knowledge of these subjects, like the knowledge that underpins most surgery, has accrued over the years mainly from experience in the field and from retrospective analysis. Very little of it has resulted from prospective study or structured research. The time may now have come for surgeons to start to build on this vast and incoherent legacy by submitting their theories to better informed criticism and their practices to the test of controlled prospective trials. The 'difficult' subjects dealt with in this book might then become easier to write about.

Practising surgeons, however, cannot wait for the last word to be said. They need to make decisions here and now, and they will find in this collection of essays an authoritative review of our current understanding (and present ignorance) of several of the most testing areas in which they are called upon either to take action or, what is just as important, to withhold it.

John Goodfellow MS, FRCS
Sometime Consultant Surgeon,
Nuffield Orthopaedic Centre,
Oxford UK

Preface

The intention of this book entitled *Orthopaedic Practice* is to highlight many of the more difficult conditions which affect the musculo-skeletal system and not to encompass all orthopaedic disorders. Although our text is not a comprehensive volume we believe it will appeal to those houseofficers and registrars who seek knowledge to prepare for higher qualifications, or indeed to those consultants who are already in practice yet still searching for sound information.

A team of contributors from the USA, the UK, Spain and Switzerland were purposely selected because of their special knowledge and interest in their particular subject. Each chapter provides a reasoned account without entering into too many detailed operative techniques.

The chapters provide sufficient detail to allow acceptable discussion during Socratic/oral examinations and to provide selected references for further reading.

Where advances have been made, the specialists have risen to the challenge which is very evident in the chapters on shock, multiple injuries, scoliosis, nerve injuries and the fairly wide coverage on rheumatoid arthritis. Osteoporosis and mineral content of bone is one of the topics in the forefront of research today. In addition, the combined management of bone tumours is related to the team on the Bristol Bone Tumour panel.

Sadly, since the book was almost in the proof stage, we have to announce the death of Algy Narakas from Lausanne who was a great pioneer in the understanding of brachial plexus injuries. He was an international expert and ran a stimulating course each year which attracted surgeons from far and wide. His chapter is published almost unabridged and comes as a token of the high regard we had for him. The detail of his operative findings and the results of his surgery are remarkable and should be appreciated by all even if they had not the privilege of knowing him.

On a happier note we send congratulations to Miles Irving who received a knighthood in the recent Honours List for his great contribution to surgery in general.

We wish to thank all our contributors who have written memorable chapters in spite of difficulties; their forbearance is much appreciated. Finally we also wish to thank Susan Devlin at Butterworth-Heinemann for her help and guidance through some rough patches, and also Alison Duncan for her patience and efficient work at the editorial desk.

Philip M. Yeoman
Dan M. Spengler

1

Problem solving in orthopaedics

D. M. Spengler

Introduction

All of us in medicine realize the importance of rendering a precise and accurate diagnosis [1]. All too often, however, we falter and recommend a treatment approach which, although appropriate for our perceived diagnosis, may be seen to be unwarranted in light of the proper diagnosis. For example, many patients undergo surgical intervention for a lumbar disc herniation, when in fact many of these patients do not demonstrate a herniation at surgery [2]. Thus, for whatever reason, the preoperative assessment was faulty. The most common source of error is misinterpretation of the classic straight leg raising test [3]. Unless distracting signs are employed, symptom amplifiers will also appear to have positive straight leg raising signs, indicative of sciatic tension. Other possible causes for a faulty assessment include inappropriate intervention because of the prevalance of 'asymptomatic' extradural lesions on most imaging studies, including the computed tomographic scan, myelography and magnetic resonance imaging [4,5].

Numerous other sources of error in assessment of the musculoskeletal system could be described. Since many of these errors involve benign processes, the orthopaedist often dismisses an error of intervention as 'a rational attempt to help the patient with little downside risk.' Although a certain level of false negative explorations may be

very reasonable when treating patients for acute appendicitis, this is not the case in other instances. For example, an unwarranted surgical intervention for a benign process such as a lumbar disc herniation has been shown to result in a markedly decreased likelihood for a good outcome. This fact has been clearly demonstrated by Spangfort; patients who undergo lumbar spine surgery, but who have no evidence of a pathological process, have poorer outcomes than would be predicted by the natural history for the symptom complex [8].

These unfortunate clinical realities provide a strong incentive to develop a logical, consistent approach to clinical decision-making. Such an approach can range from the pragmatic algorithms developed by individual clinicians to sophisticated formal decision analysis strategies devised by theoreticians [5–7]. The main objectives for all organized approaches to this problem-solving process include: 1) to quantify uncertainty, 2) to select the most efficient and consistent approach to manage patients, and 3) to minimize risk and to optimize benefit or outcome [5–7].

This chapter will review some of the interesting and potentially useful data which are relevant to decision analysis. In addition, the author hopes to challenge orthopaedists to continue to design scientifically sound clinical studies to fill the many gaps in our knowledge, so that in the future we will improve our diagnostic and therapeutic accuracy with resultant improved outcomes for our patients.

Process of problem solving

Any process which analyses clinical judgement is inevitably complex. The traditional medical assessment described by Weed, which includes subjective, objective, assessment and plan (SOAP), can be used to summarize a clinical approach for the evaluation and treatment of patients. The subjective phase of this process begins with the medical history and review of the presenting complaint. This process requires a large data base. The sophisticated clinician probably recognizes important patterns of symptoms which will enhance both retention and recall of important information. Such knowledge is essential to recognize unusual presentations of common clinical entities, as well as to raise the index of suspicion for symptoms consistent with uncommonly encountered clinical entities, such as Gaucher's disease. The subjective evaluation merges into the objective phase in the physical examination. However, certain observations in the physical examination are definitely subjective. Consider the analysis of range of motion of the spine. The examiner determines that the patient can forward flex only 20°, clearly a marked restriction. Does this restriction of motion reflect a limitation imposed secondary to a pathological process, or does the limitation reflect a decrease in effort on the part of the patient to exaggerate symptoms? Such questions are not trivial. Indeed, they deal with a fundamental principle of medicine – proper diagnosis = proper treatment. Although this is a clear-cut example of 'subjective' information, we routinely use such data to assess impairment! [1].

Examples of objective measures which can be identified on the physical examination include the presence or absence of a reflex, circumferential atrophy of an extremity, deformity and Horner's syndrome. Presumably, the ideal physician considers the degree of subjectivity/objectivity of various data and prioritizes this information during data synthesis.

Following completion of the history and physical examination, the examiner next considers additional diagnostic studies to reaffirm or refute the tentative diagnosis. In most situations, the need for a particular diagnostic test is based on the likelihood of usefulness combined with the relative risk of the study. Thus, a physician would seldom recommend a lumbar myelogram for a patient who has had only mild low back pain for less than 24 hours. The same clinician, however, may well recommend an emergent myelogram in a patient who presents with a progressive neural deficit. Once laboratory data and relevant imaging studies have been reviewed, the differential diagnostic possibilities are again considered to determine the specific diagnosis. If the diagnosis can be validated by the data available to this point, treatment is instituted and an optimal outcome will probably result. If the diagnosis cannot be validated, additional, more invasive tests may be required (e.g., arteriography, myelography, biopsy).

Once all necessary studies have been obtained and the appropriate diagnosis has been formulated, many tasks remain before treatment is instituted. For example, the clinician will probably inform the patient of the diagnosis and the natural history of the pathological process. Both the short-term consequences and the long-term implications should be discussed. The risks or complications that may be encountered should also be reviewed. This communication with the patient and family is of primary importance to develop and maintain a good patient–physician relationship. Honesty is always the best policy. If you do not have the data available to accurately detail all implications, tell the patient, 'I do not know . . .' Often doctors have been advised not to say those four simple words, but rather to say 'idiopathic . . .', even though 'I don't know' is more honest. Once a pathological process or lack of such a process has been elucidated, the next task requires an appraisal of the goals and expectations of the patient. These goals are then integrated into the various treatment options available. Clearly, the patient must play a major role in this process. For example, if total hip replacement, hip arthrodesis, and extra-articular osteotomy comprise three viable alternatives for management, the orthopaedist should present these options and discuss the relative advantages and disadvantages with the patient. The patient will usually ask pertinent questions, followed by the inevitable 'What would you do, Doctor, if it were your hip?' This question, although perceptive, is usually not relevant unless the patient is close in age to the physician. The patient must be permitted adequate time to reflect and gather additional data, or to seek other consultations, before reaching a final decision. Treatment options must also take into account multiple factors, including the patient's age and gender as well as occupation and general health. In the field of orthopaedics, we are presently experiencing a technological frenzy. Many new surgical techniques and implants are being rapidly developed and implemented. Indeed, long-term outcomes for most of these approaches remain unknown. Although newer strategies may improve on previous failures in certain situations, in other conditions they may only increase the risk side of the risk–benefit ratio. Approaches which offer risk without any enhanced benefits must be eliminated from general application. If necessary, such approaches can be evaluated through proper prospective studies which include a comparable control group. Classic marketing objections to evaluations, such as '. . . this study would be unethical since my product is so good, etc., etc. . . .', must be dismissed as non-persuasive.

Background noise

Now that we have considered the general process used to solve clinical problems, we must consider factors which impede our ability to render a proper diagnosis and to proceed with treatment. The major problems can be divided into two categories: biological variation and inadequate data [5,6]. These problems must be considered throughout the entire decision analysis process, not just during the treatment phase. Thus, biological variation may affect the subjective (clinical history) portion of decision analysis as well as the plan (response to treatment).

We are all overwhelmed with data. How can I then suggest that inadequate data represent a major hurdle to proper patient evaluation and treatment? Easy: quantity does not reflect quality. Most of us receive every week five or more throw-away journals containing articles espousing the latest and greatest treatment approaches for most orthopaedic conditions. We also subscribe to several journals which may or may not submit to a rigorous peer review process. In addition, the lay press continuously subjects

our patients and us to reports of extraordinary medical progress which emphasize the successes, and downplay the risks or failures, of the treatment being presented. These articles usually represent marketing efforts rather than good science. Depending on the circulation of the journal in question, we will be certain to receive a large number of phone calls requesting the new 'super surg procedure' reported in the local 'Enquirer'. In these situations, an impatient and demanding public attempts to short circuit the complex problem-solving approach herein described through the 'aunt Minnie' logic scenario. The 'aunt Minnie' syndrome works in this way: 'I have the same symptoms as the patient in the magazine. "Super surg" worked for that person. Therefore, I need "super surg"!'

Likewise, the tremendous proliferation of the printed word through the publication of meeting abstracts, case reports and review articles creates significant background noise which may easily confuse us when we attempt to call into focus articles which relate to a specific problem. Deyo has persuasively shown that the vast majority of articles which deal with the common clinical phenomenon of low back pain are worthless [2]. Since all clinicians are not as thoughtful as Deyo, many may accept the written word as fact, and ignore the validity or reproducibility of the information presented.

Finally, most of us are constantly approached by sales representatives who offer us even more articles and advice attesting to the brilliant performance of their company's product in contrast to the miserable record of that of their competitor. Alas, a veritable minefield appears when we attempt to pursue additional knowledge. If we are not critical, we may attempt problem solving with an outmoded or insufficient data base. When such major deficiencies are present in our data base, the entire process of decision analysis becomes invalid.

Relevant data

Given the above problems which may adversely affect our desire to provide quality care for our patients, what should we do? Where should we turn? I hope to formulate data and challenges which may result in enhanced knowledge over the long term.

One of the most important characteristics of the ideal clinician is his or her unparalleled knowledge of the natural history for the clinical entity to be managed. If one has a good grasp of the outcome of a particular pathological process, one is in an excellent position to compare the natural history of the disorder with the course noted with newer treatment approaches, and thus to determine if an improved outcome results. One must be careful, however, to ensure that a different outcome is related to the different treatment approach. In addition, one must ascertain how well the new approach works over time. For example, assume that a manufacturer has developed a new widget to cure a common clinical symptom complex such as backache. The company then lines up several clinicians to evaluate the widget. Following an exhaustive 3 month study, the company reports on a major TV program that the widget cures low back pain in 70% of the patients who were treated and followed for this length of time. Moreover, the widget also permits the patient to be managed as an outpatient, eliminating the need for costly hospital admissions. Sounds good? Indeed, you would have to be extremely sceptical not to rush out and buy the widget. But sceptical you must be, or you will add to the ever burgeoning cost of health care.

If the performance of the widget is carefully evaluated, we quickly realize that a control group of patients treated for backache with untuned diathermy also responded with a 70% success rate. Moreover, with longer follow-up, we discover that 50% of the patients treated with the widget require additional hospitalization and treatment. Thus, the widget is not only ineffective, but fuels the increasing health care cost spiral in an upward direction. This is a hypothetical story, but one does not need to look very far to find widgets throughout our field. The important point is that as concerned physicians, we must critically analyse our approaches to patients and we must always insist on proper information to allow us to formulate logical conclusions. To do less is to abrogate the trust and responsibility which have been placed on us by our patients.

All of us can help meet the ongoing need for data. We must meticulously follow our patients so that we recognize early problems with our treatment approaches. We can then appropria-tely modify our strategies to decrease complications and optimize outcome. Only through the establishment of large multi-centre trials will we ever be able to fill in all of the gaps in knowledge, and thus be able to identify the ideal treatment approach for a specific patient! We must persevere – after all, that patient will some day be us.

Summary

This presentation has reviewed some of the more important aspects of clinical problem solving. We can all benefit by being thorough in our approach to the evaluation and treatment of patients. Approaches which have been validated and which are logically consistent should be emphasized. We must continually seek additional data to improve our ability to quantify human performance, which will help us to better understand biological variation. Finally, our biggest challenge will be to focus on objective outcome criteria to reaffirm that careful decision analysis does indeed make a positive difference in patient care.

References

1. AMA (1984) *Guides to the Evaluation of Permanent Impairment*. AMA, Chicago.
2. Deyo, R. A. (1983) Conservative therapy for low back pain: Distinguishing useful from useless therapy. *JAMA*, **250**, 1057–1062.
3. Hitselberger, W. and Witten, R. (1968) Abnormal myelograms in asymptomatic patients. *J. Neurosurg.*, **28**, 204–206.
4. Lippert, F. G. and Farmer, J. (1984) *Psychomotor Skills in Orthopaedic Surgery*. Williams and Wilkins, Baltimore.
5. Pauker, S. and Kassirer, J. (1987) Decision analysis. *N. Engl. J. Med.*, **316**, 250–258.
6. Pauker, S. and Kassirer, K. (1980) The threshold approach to clinical decision making. *N. Engl. J. Med.*, **302**, 1109–1117.
7. Sisson, J., Schoomaker, E. and Ross, J. (1976) Clinical decision analysis. *JAMA*, **236**, 1259–1263.
8. Spangfort, E., (1972) The lumbar disc herniation. *Acta Orthop. Scand. (Suppl.)*, **142**, 1–95.
9. Spengler, D. and Freeman, C. (1979) Patient selection for lumbar discectomy: An objective approach. *Spine*, **4**, 129–134.
10. Wiesel, S., Tsourmas, N., Feffer, H. *et al.* (1984) A study of CAT. *Spine*, **9**, 549–551.

2

Club foot

A. Catterall

Introduction

There are now many texts which deal with the problems of children born with club foot deformities. The majority of these deal comprehensively with the whole subject and explain the failures of previous series on the lack of a sufficiently radical operation to correct the deformity. Few, however, define in simple terms the deformities with which they are dealing or the indications for minor and major procedures during the course of treatment. Most authors recognize a postural deformity of good prognosis; but are there other forms of this condition for which minor surgery will produce a satisfactory outcome? Main et al. [1] and Green et al. [2] report

that a simple posterior release alone produced a satisfactory result in one-third of cases. Assessment must, therefore, be the major key to a solution of this condition and must be made with the knowledge of the way the normal foot moves in dorsiflexion together with the site of any fixed deformities which are to be found in the club foot. This chapter will not, therefore, deal with the topic in the standard way but will concentrate on a method of assessment made by a common language of 'Observer independent observations' and will define a protocol of treatment, the object of which is to convert a tendon or joint contracture into the resolving pattern of deformity.

Anatomy

A hypothesis of foot movement

In thinking about the way the normal foot moves, it is suggested that functionally the foot consists of a medial and lateral ray with a number of link mechanisms (Fig. 2.1). The medial ray consists of the talus, navicular, medial cuneiform and first metatarsal while below it the lateral ray consists of the calcaneum, cuboid and fifth metatarsal. Connecting these two rays are three link mechanisms. At the talo-calcaneal level there is the interosseous ligament which permits rotation of the talus on the calcaneum and therefore divergence of the medial and lateral rays. Anterior to this is a bony link mechanism comprising the

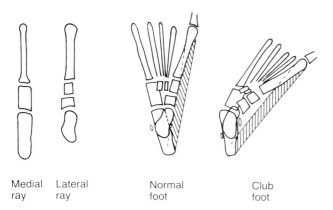

Medial Lateral   Normal   Club
ray   ray   foot   foot

Fig. 2.1 Drawing of the rays of the foot.

remaining bones of the tarsus stabilizing the two rays but allowing rotatory movement. Beyond this the middle metacarpals act as spacers connected anteriorly by the intermetatarsal ligament. This latter ligament should be looked on as a restraining check ligament to the normal spreading of the foot which would occur in inversion and eversion if such a ligament was absent. There is one other structure which links these two rays, namely the plantar fascia, which starting from the posterior surface of the lateral ray reaches forward to pass underneath the anterior end of the medial ray in an oblique direction. By doing so it maintains the medial arch. Being attached to the great toe, dorsiflexion of the M-P joint will depress the first metatarsal. The movements of inversion and eversion, pronation and supination are in essence rotatory with one ray moving over the other, and the movement limited by the natural tension in the three link mechanisms. In eversion a space forms between the navicular and cuboid and a tether in this region will hold the foot in supination, a position commonly encountered in the club foot.

Ossification centres

Not all the foot bones are fully ossified at birth and it is important to realize where the ossification centres within the individual bones lie, particularly in the talus and calcaneum. In the talus the centre lies in the anterior body and the neck. This means it will lie anterior to the tibia in full equinus (Fig. 2.2) and moves back to become parallel to the lower margin of the tibia as dorsiflexion proceeds. The centre for the calcaneum is centrally placed but square in shape and a globular appearance commonly seen in the club foot is a rotated, oblique view. The navicular is seldom ossified in the first few months of life but its position may be identified by extending the line of the first metatarsal proximally where it should cross the ossification in the talus. By contrast, the cuboid is normally ossified early in life and its position on the lateral ray is easily identified and assessed on plain radiographs.

The anatomy of the normal dorsiflexion in the infant child

From the position of full equinovarus the movement of dorsiflexion occurs mainly at two sites: the ankle and the subtaloid joint [3,4]. At the ankle joint there is a posterior movement of the talus on the tibia with the fibula and lateral malleolus rotating around its curved lateral border. For this movement to occur relaxation of the calf and Achilles tendon is required. At the subtaloid joint the calcaneum and lateral ray rotates under the talus and medial ray with the centre of rotation being the interosseous ligament. For this second phase of dorsiflexion to occur, relaxation of both the Achilles tendon and the tendon of the tibialis posterior is required. If dorsiflexion proceeds without relaxation of the tibialis posterior from the position of equinovarus the foot will reach a right angle (Fig. 2.3) but it will be noted that the lateral malleolus is remaining posterior and that the forefoot is seen in oblique rather than lateral projection. A lateral radiograph of the foot (Fig. 2.4b) in this position confirms the clinical appearances and shows a position very similar to the relapsed club foot in which a supination deformity is present. Release of the tendon of the tibialis posterior at this stage allows the second phase of dorsiflexion to proceed normally so that the forefoot is seen in lateral projection and the lateral malleolus moves forward to cover the anterior margin of the lateral border of the talus. A lateral radiograph

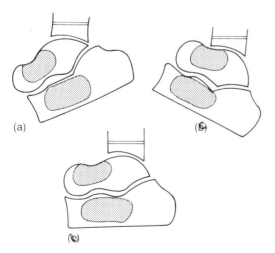

(a)   (b)

(c)

Fig. 2.2 Drawing of the ankle with the hind foot. (a) In plantar flexion. (b) Plantargrade position. (c) Dorsiflexion to show position of the ossification centres. Note that the talus moves forward on the calcaneum in plantarflexion and backwards in dorsiflexion.

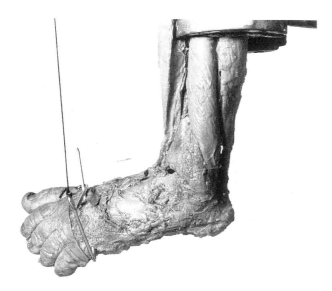

Fig. 2.3 Lateral view of an infant foot with the foot dorsiflexed but with tethering of the tibialis posterior (Fig. 2.4b).

(Fig. 2.4b) of the foot at this stage confirms the true nature of the process. The rotatory aspect of dorsiflexion is most easily observed with the fore-foot removed (Fig. 2.5a and b). In full equinus

the anterior portion of the body of the talus is forward out of the mortice and inclined downwards and medially with the calcaneum lying directly below it. In full dorsiflexion the body of the talus has moved backwards into the mortice and its direction now points laterally with the calcaneum lying lateral to it. It may be concluded that for every 10° of dorsiflexion from the position of full equinus 10° of external rotation of the

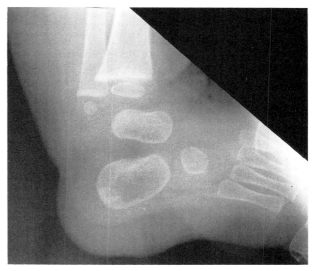

(b)

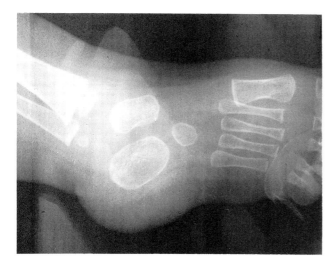

(a)

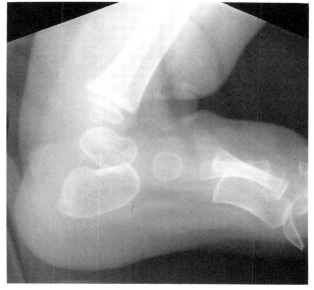

(c)

Fig. 2.4 Lateral radiographs of the infant foot in (a) full equinovarus. (b) dorsiflexion without relaxation of the tibialis posterior. (c) in full dorsiflexion. Note that in (b) the lateral malleolus is remaining posterior and the forefoot is seen in oblique projection.

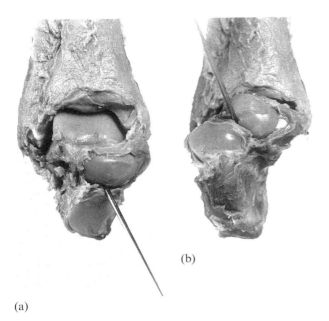

(b)

(a)

Fig. 2.5 Anterior view of the hind foot and tibia with the forefoot removed through the talo-navicular and calcaneo-cuboid joint. (a) Plantarflexion. (b) Dorsiflexion. Note the backward and rotatory movement of the talus. The calcaneum also rotates laterally on the interosseous ligament.

foot on the tibia occurs [3]. This means that if the foot is placed in full dorsiflexion without external rotation a spurious position is being produced.

Pathology

The untreated infant foot

In terms of the normal anatomy which has already been described there are a number of deformities present in the infant with a club foot deformity.

1. Investigations by Irani and Sherman [5], Carroll *et al.* [6], Bensahel *et al.* [7] and others have demonstrated that the neck of the talus is short and is more medially deviated than normal. The talus lies in equinus and the navicular articulates with the medial surface of the head, being itself tethered to the medial malleolus in a position of medial subluxation. The tissues between the navicular and medial malleolus have been shown to be abnormal and contain an excess of myofibrils and elastic fibres, allowing continuing contracture of this tissue to occur [8].

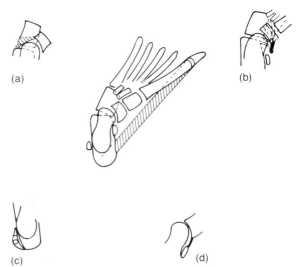

(a)

(b)

(c)

(d)

Fig. 2.6 The tethers of the club foot. (a) Antero-lateral, (b) distal attachment of tibialis posterior, (c) postero-lateral, (d) medial malleolus-navicular.

2. The calcaneum is normal in shape, but in full equinus. In this position the body of the talus moves forwards on the tibia and also on the calcaneum at the posterior talocalcaneo facet (Figs 2.2 and 2.7). There is adaptive shortening of the posterior capsule of the ankle, the Achilles tendon and lateral ligamentous structures. As a result, the body of the talus is displaced forwards out of the mortice and comes to lie so that its greatest vertical height is in front of the anterior part of the mortice. The talus, therefore, cannot move back into the mortice until this posterior space has been increased. In essence the talus is being driven forward out of the anterior aspect of the mortice as an orange pip (Figs 2.2, 2.4 and 2.7)

3. There is a medial subluxation of the cuboid on the calcaneum. In addition, a knot of tissue lying lateral to the head of the talus tethers the navicular to the calcaneum and cuboid, preventing independent movement of the medial and lateral rays of the foot (Figs 2.1 and 2.6a).

4. The tibialis posterior is abnormal [9]. The excursion of its muscle fibres is reduced and its attachment distal to the navicular to the cuboid, calcaneum and metatarsals is shortened. By contrast, the flexor digitorum and flexor hallucis are capable of normal movement in the majority of cases if they are progressively stretched. They are, however, functionally short. The long plantar

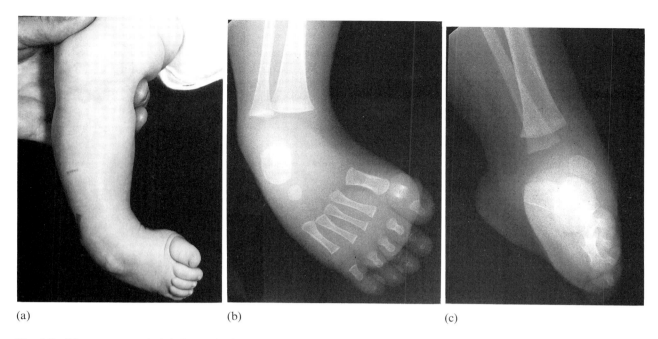

(a)   (b)   (c)

Fig. 2.7 The uncorrected club foot. (a) Photograph. (b) Lateral radiograph of the foot. (c) True lateral radiograph of the ankle. Note the anterior displacement of the talus outside the mortice and the cavus deformity of the forefoot.

ligament lying between the distal attachment of the tibialis posterior and peroneus longus is adaptably short, as is the plantar fascia. The effect of shortening of these tissues within the sole of the foot produces a cavus deformity and tethering of the medial and lateral rays at the level of the bony link mechanism. Scott *et al.* [3] have shown that tethering in this site reduces the ability of the foot to dorsiflex by preventing the second stage of rotation from occurring.

Late or relapsed cases

Following surgical release of the posterior, medial or more radical type, a number of secondary changes may be noted. These will depend on the severity of the surgical procedure, the duration of the remodelling and the presence of avascular necrosis in centres of ossification within the foot bones.

1. The talus. The neck of the talus remains short and points medially. In addition, the body of the talus loses height, particularly posteriorly, and becomes wedge shaped [10]. This results in an apparent equinus position of the talus and will

make the results of posterior release very unpredictable.

2. Fixed forefoot supination. Soft tissue tethering of the bony link mechanism has already been discussed. If this has not been corrected at the time of soft tissue release, apparent correction of the deformity can be achieved by a dorsolateral subluxation of the navicular on the talus. Such a correction elevates the first ray which can only be brought to the ground by eversion of the hind foot and flexion of the MP joints. This produces a dorsal bunion and prominence of the navicular which can be seen laterally in the region anterior to the ankle. Clinically, fixed forefoot supination is recognized by noting a prominence of the head of the first metatarsal dorsally, a hallux flexus and varus deformities of the lateral toes. In addition, there is a persisting subluxation of the calcaneo-cuboid joint with adaptive remodelling of the joint surface which will result in an incongruous joint if it is released. Calcaneo-cuboid fusion (Dilwyn-Evans procedure [11]) is required for such cases.

3. The talo-calcaneal joint. Radical release of the talo-calcaneal joint may result in a valgus subluxation with over-correction. This has been

documented by Fahrenbach *et al.* [12] and Ghali *et al.* [13], and in the majority of cases this valgus deformity compensates for forefoot supination.

Clinical assessment of the fixed deformities

Swann *et al.* [4] were the first to report the presence of a concealed external rotation deformity in a number of feet with a relapsed club foot deformity (Figs 2.8, 2.9 and 2.10). This concealed external rotation deformity demonstrated by palpation of the medial and lateral malleoli represents the end of the first phase of dorsiflexion where the second phase is blocked by the effect of tight tissues. In addition to the concealed external rotation deformity, a number of other fixed deformities may be present and concealed. Fixed equinus is masked by recurvatum in the knee and often recognized by a slight apparent valgus deformity in the knee (Figs 2.8 and 2.9). When the child stands this valgus is also associated with external rotation of the leg, confirming that it is compensating for deformity of the forefoot. Turning the knee and ankle forward reveals the full extent of the forefoot deformity. Fixed fore-

foot supination is best observed with the foot off the ground when with the heel in the neutral position there is a rotatory supination of the forefoot. When the child stands, however, the heel goes into valgus and the great toe flexes to compensate for the elevation of the first ray producing a dorsal bunion and a compensatory varus deformity of the lateral toes (Fig. 2.8). This deformity is seldom seen in the untreated foot. Where there has been previous extensive soft tissue release the supination deformity may be masked by fixed valgus in the hind foot secondary to lateral displacement of the calcaneum on the talus. The cardinal sign in such cases is fixed valgus of the hind foot with the heel outside the line of weight bearing when the child stands. Fixed cavus which has already been described in relation to the untreated foot may be observed and grossly exaggerated in the treated or relapsed foot (Figs 2.9 and 2.10).

A method of examination

With a working knowledge of the anatomy of dorsiflexion and where to find the concealed rota-

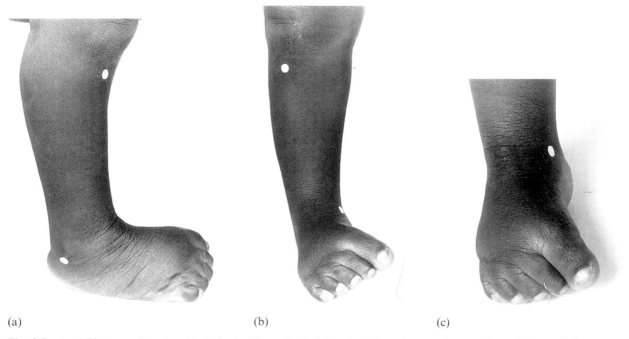

(a)   (b)   (c)

Fig. 2.8   (a–c) Photographs of a child's foot with residual deformity. Note the anterior position of the medial malleolus; posterior position of the lateral malleolus; and the external position of the leg and knee are shown. Fixed forefoot supination is also present with flexion of the great toe.

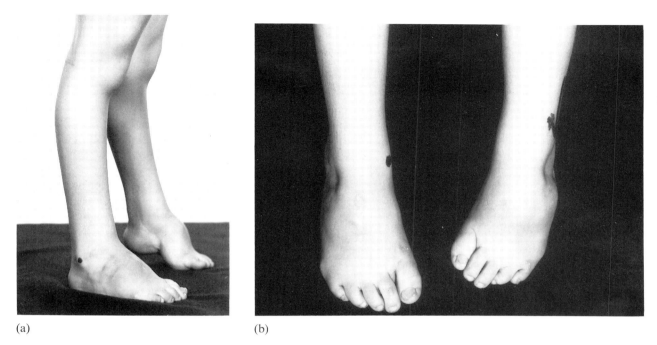

(a)   (b)

Fig. 2.9 (a,b) Clinical photograph of a child of 4 years with recurrent deformity. The external rotation of the hindfoot, recurvature of the knee is noted compensating and the fixed equinus is observed.

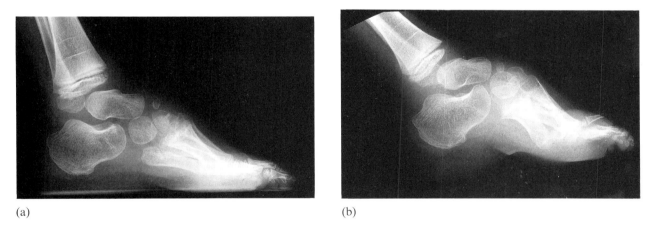

(a)   (b)

Fig. 2.10 Lateral radiographs of the child in Fig. 2.9. (a) As the child stands, (b) true lateral of the ankle. Note that the 'flat topped talus' in (a) became normal in (b) revealing the rotatory deformity present.

tory deformities it is now possible to establish a method of examination for a child, initially at presentation and subsequently at follow-up. Implicit in this method of examination must be the production of observations which are 'observer independent' (Table 2.1) [30,31]; these are signs which may be made without observer bias and provide a language for discussion of cases. They are therefore reproducible.

Assessment should begin with the child in general and only later proceed to the feet. Is there a generalized anomaly or a recognized syndrome (Tables 2.2 and 2.3)? Specific attention should be paid to the spine for evidence of spinal dysraphism which would suggest a neurological cause for the foot deformity. The hips must be carefully examined for instability in the neonatal period and for restriction of abduction in flexion in the

Table 2.1   The observer-independent observations

1. Fixed equinus
2. Lateral malleolus
   – position
   – mobility
3. Creases
   – medial
   – posterior
   – anterior
4. Foot
   – lateral border curved or straight?
   – correctable in equinus
5. Changes on dorsiflexion
6. Fixed forefoot deformity
   – cavus
   – supination

Table 2.2   Congenital syndromes with CTEV

Arthrogryposis multiplex congenita
Diastrophic dwarfism
Spina bifida and spinal dysraphism
Larsen syndrome

Table 2.3   General assessment of CTEV

1. Is there a congenital anomaly?
2. The spine
   – scoliosis?
   – dysraphism?
3. The hips – congenital dislocation?
4. Generalised joint laxity?

older child. Restricted hip movements may be associated with congenital dislocation of the hip but are also seen in children with a neurological deficit. It is convenient at this stage to note the general laxity of the joints, as if this is marked it is often associated with the problem of false correction during treatment.

Examination of the leg

Examination is now turned to the feet. In the baby, the feet should be examined with the hips and knees flexed in order to orientate the tibia. In the older child this is more easily assessed with the child sitting. The tibia is orientated by palpation of the tibial tubercle, and medial and lateral malleoli (Fig. 2.11a). Having identified the plane of the ankle joint and the orientation of the tibia, the head of the talus is now palpated (Fig. 2.11b) and the posterior tubercle of the calcaneum. This will establish the position of the hind foot and the presence of fixed equinus.

Having identified the position and orientation of the hind foot the foot should now be examined to establish the relationship of forefoot to hind foot. This is best achieved by observing the foot from below. The lateral border of the foot is either straight or curved (Fig. 2.11c). With the foot in full equinus and the tendons relaxed can the lateral border of the foot if curved be brought straight by gentle manipulation (Fig. 2.11d)? If this does occur the head of the talus should be palpated to see if it becomes covered by the navicular and the space between the navicular and medial malleolus felt to be sure that there is movement of the navicular away from the medial malleolus (Fig. 2.11e). The presence of these signs implies a mobile and reducible mid-tarsal joint.

Only at this stage should an attempt be made to dorsiflex the foot. As the normal foot dorsiflexes from the position of a full equinovarus three observations are recorded. The lateral malleolus moves forward, a gap appears between the navicular and the medial malleolus, and the posterior border of the ankle changes from bulbous to straight.

Failure of these signs to be present implies that normal dorsiflexion is not occurring and the point at which this block occurs is noted (Fig. 2.11f). On occasions the foot appears to reach the plantarflexed position but the shape of the heel does not change and a crease appears on the anterior aspect of the ankle. This foot is breaking in the mid-tarsal joint with the hind foot remaining in the plantargrade position, producing the so-called 'rocker bottom foot'. An X-ray taken of the foot in maximal dorsiflexion will confirm this. Finally, a general neurological examination is performed looking for evidence of neurological abnormality particularly in the lower limb.

Gait

Only after this detailed examination of the foot should the child be observed walking and run-

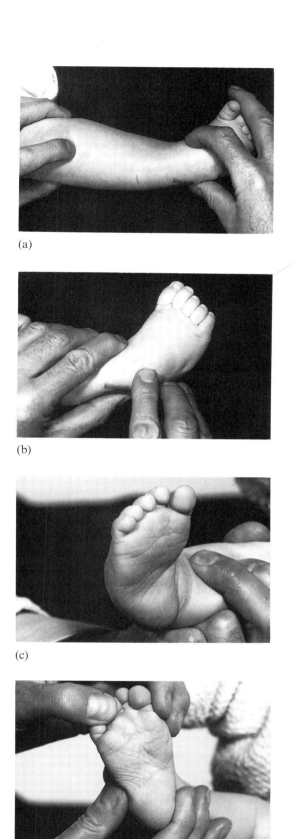

(a)

(b)

(c)

(d)

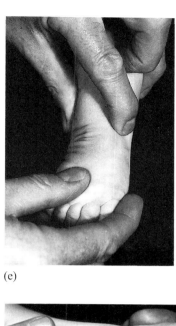

(e)

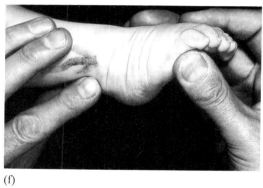

(f)

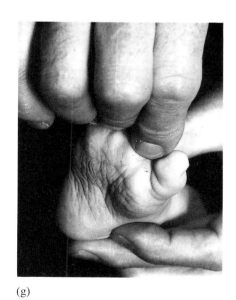

(g)

Fig. 2.11 (a–g) The stages of clinical examination.

Table 2.4   Reproduced with permission from *Clinical Orthopaedics*

Type of foot	Resolving pattern	Tendon contracture	Joint contracture	False correction
Observation				
Fixed equinus	No	Yes	Yes	Yes
Lateral malleolus				
– position	Anterior	Anterior	Posterior	Posterior
– mobility	Yes	Yes	No	Yes
Creases				
– posterior	No	Yes	Yes	Yes
– medial	No	No	Yes	No
– anterior	±	No	No	Yes
Lateral border				
– curved or straight	Straight	Curved	Curved	Rooker Bottom
– correctable	Yes	Yes	No	Yes
Cavus	No	±	Yes	No
Supination	No	No	±	No

ning. The position of the knee in walking will show the degree of the fixed or postural external rotation of the leg and the recurvatum describes the degree of concealed equinus. Commonly, the forefoot varus increases with exercise but will reduce as the child stands. Simple muscle testing will establish whether the child can stand on its toes and heels.

Conclusions

At the end of this examination which has included a careful assessment of any neurological deficit the clinician should be able to identify four types of foot deformity (Table 2.4); resolving pattern, tendon contracture, joint contracture and a false correction. The last variety is a form of tendon contracture and is an absolute indication for a posterior release in view of the hypermobility of the joints in the mid tarsal area. In a tendon contracture the hind foot remains locked by tightness of the tibialis posterior and Achilles tendon and tethering of the lateral malleolus; the forefoot is mobile with the foot in full equinus. Such a foot is suitable for a posterior release. The presence of fixed deformity in the forefoot will require a more extensive posterior

and medial release if all the tethers present are to be corrected.

Management

Traditionally, the primary management of the club foot deformity at birth is conservative by the use of manipulation and either plaster of Paris or strapping splintage. If the results of this primary management are, however, reviewed [13–15], it will be found that some form of operative procedure will be required during treatment in between 40% and 90% of cases (Table 2.5). With this high failure rate of primary treatment the question has to be asked as to whether this primary treatment does more harm than good.

Table 2.5

	No. of feet	Operations
Harrold *et al.* [14]	129	52
Lavaage *et al.* [15]	104	57
Ghali *et al.* [13]	$\frac{94}{327}$	$\frac{74}{183}$ (56%)

An additional factor in this consideration is the observation that when a child comes without previous treatment after the walking age, although the foot is still in the position of full equinovarus it is seldom stiff, being mobile within the position of deformity. It must be questioned, therefore, whether the stiffness commonly seen in the later stages of treatment is acquired as the result of inadequate treatment.

Few series consider the results of primary treatment in relation to the initial severity. Where this is done [14] three types of primary deformity may be recognized.

1. *A postural deformity*. Here the deformity is mild and the foot can be brought to the plantargrade position by gentle manipulation on the day of birth. Such a foot has no fixed deformity and corresponds to the resolving pattern in previous discussion. Such feet have a high incidence of bilateral involvement and are more common in girls (Table 2.6). Conservative treatment results in a 90% good overall result.

2. *Moderate deformity*. Harrold has defined this group as having 20 of either fixed varus or equinus at the time of primary assessment. Conservative therapy results in between 40% and 50% good results. This type corresponds to the tendon contracture of the previous discussion.

3. *Severe deformity*. This includes all the severe club foot deformities and Harrold has defined them as having more than 20° of fixed varus or equinus at primary presentation. Deep creases are usually found posteriorly and medially and a successful outcome with conservative treatment only occurs in approximately 10% of cases. These correspond to the joint contracture of the previous discussion. If such feet are left untreated at birth the fixed deformities remain unchanged but the foot which is commonly stiff at the time of initial presentation gradually loosens up and this mobilization may be encouraged by gentle manipulation.

It would be a conclusion of the preceding discussion that conservative treatment would undoubtedly be indicated in the postural or resolving type of foot, where the outcome is likely to be extremely satisfactory. In the moderate deformity because there is approximately a 50% chance of success, treatment should be undertaken but reviewed very objectively after a period of 2–3 weeks when if no improvement is occurring in the fixed deformities or particularly if the foot is becoming swollen it should be abandoned in favour of operative treatment which should be delayed until the swelling has resolved and mobility has returned to the foot. This commonly takes approximately 4–6 weeks.

It would, however, be a principle of management that, if the foot without fixed deformity does well in the long term, the object of treatment is to convert a 'joint or tendon contracture' into the 'resolving pattern' by release of the fixed deformities. The risk of inadequate conservative or operative treatment is damage to the cartilage anlage, leading to inevitable deformity of the tarsal bones in the long term.

Form of primary management

Traditionally, there have been two types of primary conservative treatment, in both the foot is manipulated and then splinted. Splintage will either be by plaster of Paris or by strapping (Robert Jones). If the object of treatment is to restore mobility to the foot and overcome fixed deformities, manipulation should be performed as many times a day as possible and this would be an obvious advantage of the splintage by strapping. However, in the newborn foot in which there is a lot of fixed deformity, strapping is often ineffective in holding a position until such time as the forefoot element of the deformity is corrected. In such feet it is the author's practice to

Table 2.6

Group	No.	Fixed deformity	Boys:Girls	Unilateral/ bilateral	Successful conservative treatment
I	49	0	18:21	36:13	89%
II	32	<20°	21:11	18:14	46%
III	48	>20°	34:14	32:16	10%

start correction with the foot in equinus with the use of serial plasters which are changed on a twice-a-week basis and then proceed to the use of strapping immobilization once the lateral border of the foot can be brought into the everted position. It is important when applying the serial plasters to be sure that the foot is locked in equinus so that a good stretch can be exerted on the tibialis posterior. As the foot is manipulated pressure is applied over the head of the talus to encourage reduction of the talo-navicular joint. This will have the effect of immobilizing the hindfoot and preventing a false correction from occurring as the result of a twist in the tibia.

Timing of surgical intervention

It is the author's practice to examine the feet on a weekly basis during the course of primary management but formally to assess them in relation to the observer independence signs at 3-weekly intervals. This allows an objective change in position to be noted. Failure of the foot to progress towards the resolving pattern is regarded as an indication for surgical treatment. Where the signs of a tendon contracture (Table 2.4) are observed a tendon release procedure with release of the posterior ankle capsule is indicated [17]. This operation should be regarded as an incident in continuing conservative treatment where a tendon contracture is converted to the resolving pattern. It is therefore undertaken during the course of primary management, and is best performed at approximately 6–8 weeks provided that adequate and competent anaesthesia is available for a child of this age. Where, however, the deformity is more marked and the signs of a joint contracture are present the timing of more radical surgery becomes difficult. There are many reports now in the literature of an early radical operation performed in the first few weeks of life [13,18,19].

The majority of these reports show good results but it is pertinent to ask whether the overall results deteriorate with time and are less likely to be successful if they are undertaken in a child who is perhaps 1 year of age. The reported literature is clear on this point; the results of radical procedure undertaken either in the first few weeks or at approximately 12 months of age are the same. An advantage of the later operation

is that the foot is bigger and the operation is technically more simple. It is therefore the author's practice to wait until the child is crawling and showing evidence of wishing to stand before proceeding to a radical soft tissue procedure correcting both the hindfoot and forefoot deformities at one operation.

Siting of incisions for soft tissue procedure

Traditionally the club foot has been approached through a postero-medial incision starting well above the ankle and following the line of the vessels around the medial aspect of the ankle and along the medial side of the foot [20]. Access to the tight medial structures is satisfactory but there is commonly a deep scar tethering the skin to the underlying calcaneum and Achilles tendon. This factor may contribute to recurrent deformity. Healing of the wound is not usually a problem. More recently a number of surgeons, including the author, have been using two incisions, one placed on the postero-lateral aspect of the hindfoot and a second on the medial side of the foot reaching from the calcaneum to the medial malleolus and down the line of the first metatarsal. The advantages of this two-fold incision are that better access is gained to the lateral tissues behind the ankle, particularly the lateral malleolus and its ligaments; in addition, there is an important intact medial skin bridge on the inner side of the ankle. This produces a better cosmetic result. The medially placed incision allows good access to all the tissues which are tight, particularly the plantar fascia.

More recently the Cincinnati incision has been introduced [21]. This incision is currently popular and allows very good access to the subtaloid joint which some surgeons consider to be the most important part of the progressive release [22,23]. It heals well provided that no undue reflection of the distal flaps has occurred. It will, however, be realized that in the majority of late cases the plantar fascia is tight and requires release and it is not uncommon, if a radical release is required for the tissues on the medial side of the ankle, for it to be slow to heal and become necrotic. This incision, however, remains a very useful one provided that there is no undue cavus, and allows good access to the medial, posterior and lateral aspects of the ankle and foot.

Concept of a progressive release of tethers

It has been concluded in the sections on the anatomy of dorsiflexion and pathology that there are a number of tethers, both ligamentous and tendinous which may contribute to the maintenance of the club foot deformity (Fig. 2.6). It has also been suggested that one of the objectives of treatment is to convert the tendon or joint contracture to the 'resolving pattern'. When this later state has been achieved conservative therapy, mainly by manipulation, would finally correct the deformity. In considering surgical correction of these deformities it is suggested that these tethers should be progressively released until an adequate correction has been obtained. In contrast to manipulative therapy, surgical release should start posteriorly by releasing the ankle and lateral structures and by doing so unlock the rotatory element of dorsiflexion. When a joint contracture is present the medial side of the foot should then be approached to release progressively the plantar fascia, the distal attachment of tibialis posterior together with the short and long plantar ligaments, and the talo-navicular joint and the lateral tether between the navicular, cuboid and calcaneum. This last tether will also involve opening the calcaneo-cuboid joint to correct any fixed deformity. Such a protocol of progressive release will not result in over correction as the pivot of rotation between the talus and calcaneum has not been seriously disrupted. Division of the interosseous ligament between the talus and calcaneum with the necessary release of the medial side of the talo-calcaneo joints is liable to lead to progressive subluxation, valgus deformity and the complications of over-correction which have already been eluded to. This is not to say that in some extremely stiff feet, such as those associated with arthrogryposis, such a release may not be necessary but its indications are extremely rare.

A long term review by Green and Lloyd-Roberts [2] have confirmed the observation that in one third of cases coming to surgical treatment only a posterior release was necessary for satisfactory long term results.

In the older child over the age of 4 years where there has been considerable remodelling, both the talo-navicular and calcaneo-cuboid joints are abnormal and radiography shows a fixed medial subluxation of the calcaneo-cuboid joint. In these circumstances a progressive release will not be satisfactory unless the alignment of the calcaneo-cuboid joint is improved. This may be achieved, either by excising the calcaneo-cuboid joint (Dilwyn Evans procedure [11] or alternatively by realigning the joint by removing a wedge from the lateral aspect of the calcaneum. Many surgeons now currently feel that a medial release is not necessary in the Dilwyn Evans procedure but it cannot be stressed too much that the principle of the operation is a medial release coupled with a realignment of the calcaneo-cuboid joint by arthrodesis. The reported results of this operation show good satisfactory long term results, although radiologically the correction is seldom complete. The feet retain good mobility [25,26].

Problem of over-correction

With the more radical procedures that have recently been developed [13,22,23] lateral displacement of the calcaneum may result. Although the deformity is apparently well corrected as the result of these procedures it will be realized from study of the anatomy that the tethers have not necessarily been released, particularly those under the tarsus and metatarsal areas. While in the short term this may not be a problem, in the longer term the valgus in the heel becomes fixed and will result in a painful unstable ankle which is particularly difficult to treat. Over-correction, therefore, must be avoided in the long term and there is no doubt that a supple foot even with mild deformity will be very little trouble in the long term.

Later residual deformity

Following the posterior and postero-medial releases a number of cases will present with a mobile foot which is passively correctable but in which posturally the child walks in varus and supination. Although in many cases this will resolve without further treatment [27], in others the deformity seems to persist. Clinical experience has shown that a tibialis anterior transfer from the medial to the lateral side of the foot is often beneficial in these circumstances [28]. Care must be undertaken in carrying out this procedure that it is not put in tight and great attention must be paid to the joint laxity of the child, as it is not unknown for over-correction to occur in follow-up with the whole foot being pulled into eversion and valgus. Prompt return of the tendon transplant to the mid-line is indicated in these cases.

A number of children, particularly with arthrogryposis, and after repeated surgery remain with stiff deformed feet often with marked equinus. These children are too young for bony operations such as triple arthrodesis but too rigid for soft tissue procedures. Talectomy, in these circumstances, will result in a plantargrade foot of greatly improved shape. The reported results [2,29] are satisfactory. When this operation is performed, it is important to remove a segment from the Achilles tendon and to remove completely the talus without damage to the navicular.

There remain a few children who reach the age of early adolescence with persisting residual deformity in which the heel and forefoot are inside the line of weight bearing and who walk, therefore, in varus taking excessive weight on the lateral border of the foot and often complaining of recurrent ankle instability. These children are well treated by triple arthrodesis, but it is to be hoped that with the present improving understanding of the nature of the club foot, this procedure will become progressively less necessary in the course of time. It remains, however, a useful procedure for the stiff foot with a residual deformity.

References

1. Main, B. J., Crider, R. J., Lloyd-Roberts, G. C., Swann, M. and Kamdar, B. A. (1977) The results of early operation in talipes equino-varus. *J. Bone Joint Surg.*, **59B**, 337–341.
2. Green, A. D. L., Fixsen, J. A. and Lloyd-Roberts, G. C. (1986) Talectomy for arthrogryposis multiplex congenita. *J. Bone Joint Surg.*, **68B**, 697–699.
3. Scott, W. A., Hoskings, S. W. and Catterall, A. (1984) Club foot. Observations on the surgical anatomy of dorsiflexion. *J. Bone Joint Surg.*, **66B**, 71–76.
4. Swann, M., Lloyd-Roberts, G. C. and Catterall, A. (1969) The anatomy of the uncorrected club foot. A study of rotational deformity. *J. Bone Joint Surg.*, **51B**, 263–269.
5. Irani, R. M. and Sherman, M. S. (1963) The pathological anatomy of the club foot. *J. Bone Joint Surg.*, **45A**, 45–52.
6. Carroll, N. C., McMurtry, R. and Leete, S. F. (1978) The patho-anatomy of the congenital club foot. *Orthop. Clin. North Am.*, **9**, 225.
7. Bensahel, H., Hugueria, P. and Thermar-Noel, C. (1983) Functional anatomy of the club foot. *J. Pediatr. Orthop.*, **3**, 191–196.
8. Roberts, J. M. (1985) Personal communication.
9. Handelsman, J. H. E. and Badalamento, M. E. (1981) Neuro-muscular studies in club foot. *J. Pediatr. Orthop.*, **1**, 23–32.
10. Hutchins, P. M., Forster, B. K., Paterson, D. C. and Cole, E. A. (1985) The long-term results of early surgical release in club foot. *J. Bone Joint Surg.*, **67B**, 791–799.
11. Evans, D. (1961) Relapsed club foot. Operative techniques and results in thirty feet. *J. Bone Joint Surg.*, **43B**, 722.
12. Fahrenbach, G. J., Kuchn, D. N. and Tachdjian, M. O. (1983) Occult subluxation of the subtaloid joint in club foot. *J. Pediatr. Orthop.*, **3**, 334–340.
13. Ghali, N. N., Smith, R. B., Clayden, A. D. and Silk, P. F. (1983) The results of pantalar reduction in the management of congenital talipes equinovarus. *J. Bone Joint Surg.*, **65B**, 1–7.
14. Harrold, A. J. and Walker, C. J. (1983) Treatment and prognosis in congenital club foot. *J. Bone Joint Surg.*, **65B**, 8–11.
15. Laaveg, S. I. and Ponseti, N. (1980) Long term results of treatment of congenital club foot. *J. Bone Joint Surg.*, **62A**, 23–31.
16. Kite, J. H. (1964) *The Club Foot*. Grune and Stratton, New York.
17. Williams, D. H., Grant, C. E. P. and Catterall, A. (1987) Postero-lateral release for resistant club foot: early clinical results. *J. Bone Joint Surg.*, **69B**, 155.
18. Pous, J. G. and Dimeglio, A. (1978) Neonatal surgery in club foot. *Orthop. Clin. North Am.*, **9**, 233–240.
19. Ryoppy, S. and Sairanen, H. (1983) Neonatal operation, treatment of club foot. *J. Bone Joint Surg.*, **65**, 320–325.
20. Turco, V. J. (1981) *Club Foot: (Current Problems in Orthopaedics)*. Churchill-Livingstone, New York, Edinburgh, London, Melbourne.
21. Crawford, A. H., Marxen, J. L. and Osterfeld, D. L. (1982) The Cincinnati incision. A comprehensive approach for surgical procedures of the foot and ankle in childhood. *J. Bone Joint Surg.*, **64A**, 1355-1358.
22. McKay, D. W. (1983) New concept of and approach to club foot treatment (Section III). *J. Pediatr. Orthop.*, **3**, 141–148.
23. Simons, G. W. (1985) Complete subtalar release in club feet. *J. Bone Joint Surg.*, **67A**, 1044–1055.

24. Green, A. D. L. and Lloyd-Roberts, G. C. (1985) The results of early posterior release in the resistant club foot. A long term review. *J. Bone Joint Surg.*, **67B**, 588–593.

25. Tayton, K. J. J. and Thompson, P. (1979) Relapsing club foot. Late results of delayed operation. *J. Bone Joint Surg.*, **61B**, 474–480.

26. Addison, A., Fixsen, J. A. and Lloyd-Roberts, G. C. (1983) A review of the Dilwyn-Evans type of collateral operation in severe club feet. *J. Bone Joint Surg.*, **65B**, 12–14.

27. Wynne-Davies, R. (1964) Club foot? A review of eighty-four cases after completion of treatment. *J. Bone Joint Surg.*, **46B**, 53.

28. Kernohan, J. G., Kavanagh, T. G., Fixsen, J. A. and Lloyd-Roberts, G. C. (1985) A long term review of tibialis anterior transfer in congenital club foot. *J. Bone Joint Surg.*, **67B**, 490.

29. Hsu, L. C. S., Jaffrey, D. and Leong, J. C. Y. (1986) Talectomy for club foot in arthrogryposis. *J. Bone Joint Surg.*, **68B**, 694–696.

30. Catherall, A. (1991) A method of assessment of the club foot. *Clinical Orthopaedics and Related Research*, **264**, 225–232.

31. Catherall, A. (1994) Early assessment and management of the club foot. In *Children's Orthopaedics and Fractures* (M. D. K. Bewson, J. A. Fixsen and M. F. Macnicol, eds), Edinburgh: Churchill Livingston.

3

The surgical treatment of congenital displacement of the hip joint

J. A. Wilkinson

In a consecutive series of 201 infants between 10 months and 3 years of age, a two-stage surgical programme has evolved over the past 20 years. At the time of initial reduction, any soft tissue impediment is removed before the joint is splinted in flexion and abduction for 6 months to stimulate any growth potential for bony congruity and stability. Then the child is allowed to extend and medially rotate both legs and also take full weight for a further 6 months. Any muscle imbalance, articular incongruity or instability developing during this trial period is corrected by the realignment of the bony components, 1 year following the initial reduction.

The response to this surgery has been under constant review up to skeletal maturity. This assessment is confined to the first 117 patients with 140 displaced hip joints, who were treated between 1965 and 1980. Factors that have complicated and influenced the outcome of treatment have been investigated and assessed.

Introduction

The assessment of conservative treatment in a similar series of infants [1] reveal that the commonest cause of failure was due to re-displacement of the hip, either during the period of splintage or later. This failure resulted from eccentric reduction of the femoral head, often combined with fragmentation of the proximal femoral epiphysis. Those patients with a family history of congenital displacement of the hip

(CDH) were prone to do badly and infants with genetic acetabular dysplasia also failed to respond to conservative treatment.

Ludloff [2] was the first to record dissatisfaction concerning the results of conservative treatment, 'because even some early cases treated expertly failed to respond'. He found that many hips redislocated once the plaster cast or splints were removed and he claimed that his anatomical dissections of dislocated hip joints revealed variations from the normal structure which were responsible for the failure of conservative treatment. They included the infolding of the limbus and the interposition of the capsule, which were thought to be more frequent hindrances to closed reduction and retention than previously believed and were best eliminated by open operation. Ludloff also described the contracture of the anterior capsule and felt this to be another cause of reluxation, advocating its incision at the time of arthrotomy through an antero-inferior approach to the intra-articular structures.

Putti [3] first advised gentle stretching of such capsular contractures using a portable splint or divaricator which imposed a gradual degree of abduction on both legs. He claimed that his method reduced 95% of CDH in patients under the age of 12 months, and produced a perfect functional result. Later on, traction was added to abduction by various authorities [4,5]. The same concept of atraumatic reduction of the dislocated hip in an infant was developed by Scott [6] using a horizontal frame which he claimed reduced the prevalence of epiphysitis to less than 10%. The

Wingfield frame became a popular appliance, but it had to be tailored to fit each individual which restricted its use to orthopaedic centres with appliance workshops. The management called for specialized nursing care and many children had to be sedated in the earlier stages. They were kept on their frames up to 2 months and even then it was sometimes necessary to apply cross-traction to bring the femoral head down to the level of the acetabulum so as to attain a satisfactory reduction.

Somerville [7] found that the majority of patients thus reduced required surgery to gain concentric reduction and this prevented re-dislocation. He used a restricted anterior arthrotomy on the dislocatable hip, the laxity of the capsular ligaments allowing him to displace the femoral head downward to reveal the limbus at the back of the joint. Following its excision, stable reduction was best maintained by splinting the hip in extension, abduction and medial rotation, but this had to be followed by a lateral rotation femoral osteotomy 6–9 weeks later to maintain reduction and sometimes the osteotomy had to be repeated to prevent the femoral head resubluxing out of the acetabulum.

Fergusson [8] revived Ludloff's approach as a primary surgical reduction without preoperative traction, as he felt the latter was responsible for the enlargement and inversion of the limbus. He also found it necessary to splint the hip in abduction, extension and medial rotation, being led to believe that the Lorenz position produced pathological changes in the splinted hip joint. He did not find that the ligamentum teres or the limbus were obstacles to his surgical reduction. Others using his technique have encountered recurrent instability after the removal of the splint and have found it necessary to perform either pelvic or femoral osteotomies to prevent any residual subluxation [9–11].

So it appears that there are three primary requirements to attain atraumatic and concentric reduction and stabilization of an established congenitally displaced hip joint in the infant.

1. A release of the contracture of the anteromedial capsule, either by gentle stretching or by surgical incision.
2. A restricted arthrotomy to excise any soft tissue impediment causing eccentric reduction, so preventing undue pressure on the acetabulum and femoral head.
3. A period of postoperative splinting in flexion and abduction maintains concentric reduction and stimulates reciprocal bone growth of the femoral head and acetabulum, lowering the risk of residual subluxation and dislocation when the child is freed.

Bony realignment is usually necessary and is best performed during the second or third year of life in the majority of patients as the pelvis is thicker and more stable at that stage. A year after reduction, there is usually radiological evidence of persistent acetabular dysplasia on the side of dislocation. This is sometimes associated with varying degrees of subluxation but rarely with redislocation.

Selection of patients

There were 251 established dislocations in infants aged from 10 months to 3 years and 60% were girls. They formed a consecutive series, 30%

Table 3.1   Number of infants presenting with established CDH between 1965 and 1985

Group	Year treated	Length of follow-up	Number of patients treated	Number of CDH	Percentage		
					Right	Left	Bilateral
A	1965–70	15 yrs +	21	25	20	56	24
B	1970–75	10–15 yrs	42	51	17	49	34
C	1975–80	5–10 yrs	54	64	24	48	28
D	1980–85	<5 yrs	84	111	29	23	49
	Totals		201	251			

being diagnosed in the first 2 months of life but failing to respond to early treatment; another 30% presented between 2 and 12 months, but 40% were not diagnosed until the second year of life [12] (see Table 3.1).

After the first 2 months, most displacements had become established or permanent. It was policy to delay treatment until the proximal femoral epiphysis had appeared radiologically, because this not only established the diagnosis, but also appeared to reduce the complications of epiphysitis in response to treatment. Similar observations have been made in other series [13].

In unilateral cases, the degree of acetabular development on the non-dislocated side, assessed by measuring the acetabular angle predicts the potential for spontaneous acetabular recovery on the side of dislocation [1].

On admission, careful examination was undertaken to exclude those infants with scars on the buttock caused by a previous septic arthritis [14], and also those with stigmata of spinal dysraphism including abnormal sacral hair distribution, local pigmentation and lipomata. Other signs of neuromuscular hypoplasia included calf wasting, calcaneo-valgus or cavus deformities of the foot and inequality of foot size. The presence and degree of familial joint laxity in both upper and lower limbs is significant especially in familial cases and may complicate treatment. It is important to question the parents repeatedly concerning any family history of CDH for when this is present, it gives a poor prognosis to the outcome of treatment and calls for greater vigilance at all stages of management.

Treatment

The child is first examined under general anaesthesia to assess whether the hip is reducible and also to detect any degree of adductor contracture. The latter can be released by tenotomy so that subsequent traction is applied directly to the capsular contracture without any hindrance. It is important to record the reducibility of the hip before and after tenotomy, and to assess the stability of reduction before and after the period of traction, when the hip is re-examined under anaesthesia. Most hips are found to be reducible but unstable at the beginning of treatment. Some may be irreducible, even after adductor teno-

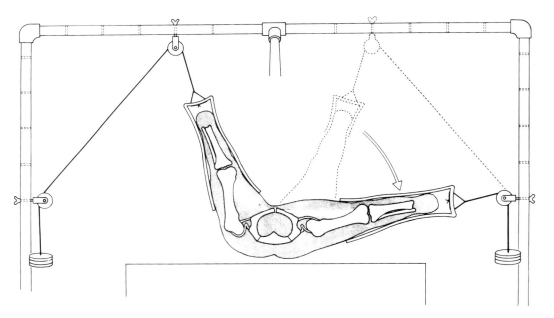

Fig. 3.1 Diagram of traction apparatus illustrating the two primary soft tissue impediments to reduction including infolding of the posterior capsule and a contracture of the anterior capsule. Correction of the latter allows eccentric reduction at the end of traction (previously published by Springer, [19]).

tomy, but this does not contraindicate traction as stretching of the capsular contracture often facilitates reduction (Fig. 3.1).

Traction

A simple form of balanced and vertical traction has been used over the past 20 years with a frame similar to the gallows frame [15], but wider to allow gradual abduction of both legs. The method is not unique as various forms of vertical traction have been used by others to reduce CDH [15–18]. The technique has been described [19] and has proved to be successful in the majority of infants providing a very low prevalence of femoral epiphysitis.

At the end of the 3- to 4-week traction period, the child is again examined under anaesthesia to assess the degree of initial reduction and the stability of the joint, the patients falling into three groups.

Group 1 comprised 15% of hips which reduced and proved to be non-dislocatable at the end of traction. If there was any doubt about the degree and stability of reduction, an arthrogram confirmed its concentricity (Fig. 3.2). If the hip was not dislocatable at the beginning of traction and remained stable at the end, the infants were allowed free without splinting but they were fol-

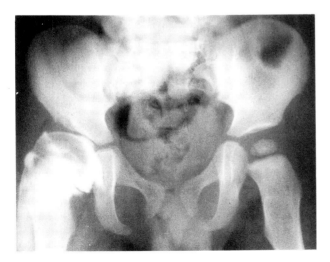

Fig. 3.2 Arthrogram of hip at the end of traction, stable reduction, the hip remaining non-dislocatable the arthrogram shows concentric reduction with no infolding of the limbus.

lowed up at regular intervals. Most recovered spontaneously, turning out to be cases of apparent displacement [20]. They have been excluded from the series.

If the hip was unstable at the beginning of traction, but stabilized during the treatment, the child was splinted in a Denis Browne harness for 6 months. The majority of these patients were found to have persistent radiological dysplasia a year after reduction and became candidates for pelvic osteotomy to stabilize the joint. At the time of surgery, the hip was explored and it was usual to find a small infolded limbus between the femoral head and the acetabulum. This impediment was extracted from the acetabulum and excised. These were genuine cases of CDH and have been included in the series.

Group 2 comprised 83% of hips that were unstable at the beginning of traction and remained so at the end, i.e. the hips were reducible but dislocatable. Arthrography showed that this was due to eccentric reduction and the impediment was a large infolded limbus between the femoral head and acetabulum. Pooling of the dye on the floor of the acetabulum confirmed the degree of eccentric reduction (Fig. 3.3). Posterior arthrotomy and excision of the limbus was preferred at this stage rather than providing a trial reduction; thus concentric reduction of the head was achieved and stabilized by the plication of the lax posterior capsule, before the hip was splinted in a Lorenz plaster with the thighs flexed above a right angle and abducted 70° (Fig. 3.4).

The child was sent home and 2 months later the plaster was replaced by a Denis Browne harness (Fig. 3.5) which was retained for a further 4 months, maintaining concentric reduction in flexion and neutral rotation. The child was allowed free at 6 months after reduction and quickly regained a normal standing posture and gait.

In bilateral hip displacement, when both hips remain dislocatable at the end of the traction, posterior arthrotomy was performed on each hip at the same time. The postoperative management was similar to that of unilateral cases.

Group 3 consisted of a very few cases that failed to reduce on vertical traction because of soft tissue impediment. In such cases, neither anterior nor posterior restricted arthrotomy should be attempted. It is better to undertake a formal surgical open reduction through an

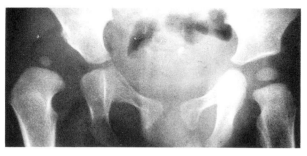

(a)

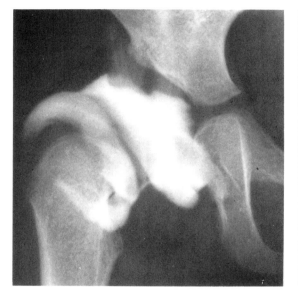
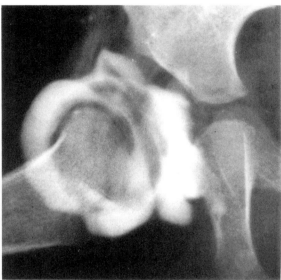

(b)

Fig. 3.3 (a) Right CDH presenting at 12 months with total displacement of femoral head into the upper and outer quadrant. (b) Arthrogram at the end of reduction revealing infolding of the limbus causing eccentric reduction of the femoral head. The hip was reducible but dislocatable and reduction was unstable due to the eccentricity of the femoral head.

anterolateral approach as described by Salter [21]. This allows an extensive incision of the capsule to provide unrestricted access to the acetabulum. It is usual to find a large circumferential limbus extending across the acetabulum, creating a total obstruction to the reduction of the femoral head. The ligamentum teres is usually intact and leads through a central hiatus in the limbus to the underlying bony acetabulum. Excision of the limbus reveals a bony acetabulum which is usually normal in size and depth, well able to accept a concentrically reduced femoral head. The hip is again splinted in a Lorenz plaster and the further care is as previously described.

Posterior arthrotomy

Should only be performed on hips that are dislocatable after the period of traction, as the aim is to reduce and stabilize the eccentrically reduced femoral head (group 2). It is unnecessary in patients whose hips are non-dislocatable at the end of traction, as the reduction is stable and it would also be difficult to displace the head out of the acetabulum to gain sufficient access to excise the limbus. It is important to proceed to posterior arthrotomy before any splints are applied to the child, as eccentric reduction can cause damage to both bony components. The posterior approach

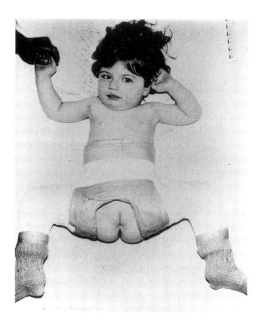

Fig. 3.4   Lorenz plaster (previously published by Springer, [19]).

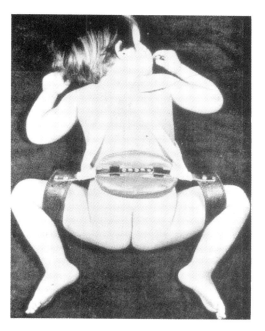

Fig. 3.5   Denis Browne harness (previously published by Springer, [19]).

has been developed to provide a direct access to the limbus which lies posteriorly. It provides an unimpeded view of the limbus allowing its complete excision, and also plication of the lax posterior capsule to stabilize the concentric reduction. It is not a major procedure and does not necessitate blood transfusion.

The child is placed in the lateral position with the affected hip upward and the affected leg is prepared and draped separately to allow free manipulation. The femoral head is reduced into the acetabulum and the hip is half flexed before making a 4-cm incision extending obliquely upward and backward above the tip of the greater trochanter. Splitting of the gluteus maximus reveals the posterior edge of the gluteus medius. This is retracted upward to reveal the gluteus minimus and piriformis tendon. These two structures are separated and stripped from the underlying capsule before being retracted superiorly and inferiorly, respectively. A blunt hook is placed under the tip of the greater trochanter to apply lateral traction and then the rim of the acetabulum can be felt deep to the posterior capsule.

An incision in the capsule, parallel, but 0.5 cm lateral to the rim of the acetabulum, releases any excess fluid in the joint. The incision is extended superiorly and inferiorly to allow the retractors to be placed within the joint. The blunt hook previously placed under the greater trochanter is replaced to retract the lateral edge of the capsule. The medial edge is incised at its mid-point at right angles to the previous incision to reveal the base of the limbus. Another blunt hook is introduced into the acetabulum around the free edge of the limbus to retract it out of the joint. It also defines the attachment of the limbus to the rim of the acetabulum, facilitating the complete excision along the limbus. The upper half is first detached and then the inferior part. Sometimes the limbus is adherent to the posterior articular surface of the acetabulum and has to be gently lifted off by blunt dissection. Occasionally, it is in two layers, the more superficial one lying free but the deeper one remaining adherent to the articular surface. Each layer has to be removed under direct vision. Never incise the capsule towards the base of the greater trochanter, as this will disrupt the arterial supply to the femoral head. Do not excise excess capsule, but reef the capsule by placing deep absorbable sutures well away from the edges; this reefing will take up the capsular hood and stabilize the reduction of the femoral head. It is not necessary to excise the ligamentum teres, as it never appears to obstruct reduction. Superficial sutures are placed in the fascia of the gluteus maximus, and the wound edges are closed with a subcuticular absorbable suture.

When both hips are dislocatable, one is explored and then the wound is sealed, before turning the child to perform the same procedure on the opposite side.

Postoperatively, the child is placed on the plaster frame in the supine position and both legs are flexed above a right angle and are allowed to abduct to their full extent. The lower legs are held in neutral rotation. It is necessary to test the reduction and stability of both hips before applying the wool and plaster and this must be done by the surgeon himself, as he is responsible for making sure that neither joint has redislocated. Failure to maintain reduction at this stage may have disastrous consequences, as the displaced femoral head becomes adherent to the capsular incision and makes further attempts at closed reduction impossible. Thus it is the most important step in the surgical management.

Postoperative radiographs confirm reduction (Fig. 3.6). The child is sent home and the plaster maintained for 8 weeks, allowing the capsular incision to heal and the joint to stabilize. It is then replaced with a Denis Browne abduction harness which will maintain reduction and also allow controlled movements to stimulate the develop-ment of the acetabulum and femoral head. It is retained for 4 months and then the child is allowed free to extend and medially rotate the thighs and weight bear on the leg. Within 4–6 weeks, the child is usually running around without a limp or any clinical evidence of previous displacement of the hip joint.

The initial response to gradual concentric reduction followed by 6 months of abduction splinting has to be assessed 1 year from the outset of treatment, as it is then decided whether to proceed to correct any residual incongruity of the bony components. At this stage, all but four of the 117 children in the series were walking normally and running without a limp. Two children redislocated one of their hips and two children developed abductor contractures producing apparent lengthening of the leg. The other children appeared quite normal and there was little evidence of stiffness of the affected joints.

Radiological assessment at 1 year from the onset of treatment was more critical. It confirmed the two redislocations which were due to extreme degrees of familial joint laxity, but there was evidence of residual subluxation or lateral drift in another 15 hips, i.e. 10% of the series. In five of these patients, the residual subluxation appeared to be due to a combination of genetic acetabular dysplasia and joint laxity, whereas 14 revealed no overt evidence to account for the instability.

In 10 of the hips, the femoral epiphysis lost some of its definition and appeared to undergo a mild degree of epiphysitis but there was no actual deformity or loss of epiphyseal height.

All the hips showed evidence of persistent acetabular dysplasia with increase of the acetabular angle above the normal standards of development (Fig, 3.7) [1]. Pelvic osteotomy was performed routinely 1 year following reduction as it was found that any delay tended to allow the

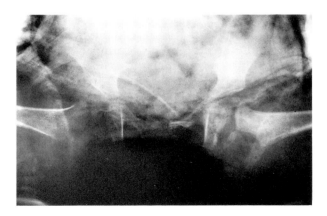

Fig. 3.6 Postoperative reduction, femoral head concentrically reduced following posterior arthrotomy. Patient in Lorenz plaster.

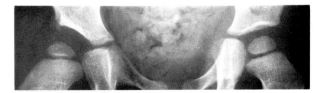

Fig. 3.7 Radiograph 1 year following posterior arthrotomy, right hip concentrically reduced but persistent acetabular dysplasia.

development of coxa magna and it was then difficult to obtain good acetabular cover following osteotomy.

Bony realignment (pelvic osteotomy)

In a previous assessment of the results of conservative treatment [1], 61% of the infants failed to respond adequately. Femoral head deformity, subluxation and in some cases redislocation, occurred because of severe degrees of epiphysitis secondary to traumatic manipulative reduction. Eccentric reduction also caused early subluxation and redislocation. In the 40% of patients whose hips were not damaged and were concentrically reduced, nearly half ended up with shallow hips (grade 2 and 3 results) which was thought at the time to be due to genetic acetabular dysplasia, especially in the unilateral cases.

In the present series, the above iatrogenic factors have almost been eliminated and concentricity of reduction has been attained by posterior arthrotomy and excision of the limbus. To improve on the 40% good results of conservative treatment, all the hip joints treated in this series have been subjected to routine pelvic osteotomy performed a year from reduction, i.e. after the child had been walking freely for 6 months. This period of freedom was found to be necessary, not only to ensure the normal development of femoral anteversion but also to observe the development of the femoral epiphysis following reduction.

As the child extended and medially rotated the hips following the removal of the abduction Denis Browne harness, taking full weight on the legs for the first time, the medial torsion placed on the proximal thirds of the femurs stimulated the development of the normal degree of femoral anteversion (approximately 30°). The postural torsion is normally transmitted to the acetabulum, but in previously dislocated hips the residual laxity of the capsular ligaments prevented this, resulting in a persistence of the primary acetabular retroversion. The combination of femoral anteversion and acetabular retroversion institutes the incongruity of the bony components with resulting instability (Fig. 3.8). Congruity of the bony components can be attained by either performing a lateral rotation femoral osteotomy or a pelvic osteotomy. The

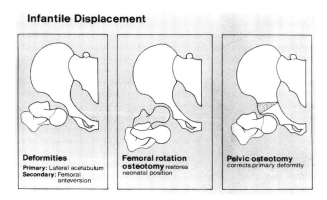

Infantile Displacement

Fig. 3.8 Diagrams demonstrating bony incongruity, combination of acetabular retroversion and femoral anteversion with correction by femoral osteotomy and pelvic osteotomy (previously published by Springer, [19]).

former retroverts the femur and allows it to become congruous with the acetabular retroversion, while the latter anteverts the acetabulum to accommodate the normal degree of femoral anteversion.

Pelvic (innominate) osteotomy has been preferred in this series for a number of functional and cosmetic reasons. The technique previously described [19] not only reorientates the retroverted acetabulum outward and forward to improve the cover of the femoral head, but it also decompresses the bony components of the articulation. This prevents any postoperative stiffness and the development of avascular necrosis (Fig. 3.9).

If posterior arthrotomy had not been performed at the time of reduction, as in the nondislocatable hip joints (group 1), the opportunity is taken to explore the hip at the time of pelvic osteotomy, as it does not add much to the operative procedure. It is usual to find a thin limbus infolded into the joint and it can be hooked out and excised. In cases of bilateral CDH, a second osteotomy is usually delayed for at least 4 months from the time of the initial pelvic osteotomy.

Postoperatively, a plaster spica is applied with both hips splinted in full extension with 20° of abduction and medial rotation. The latter is maintained on the side of dislocation by extending the plaster distal to the flexed knee joint. The cast is maintained for 6–8 weeks, a longer period being indicated if the capsule has been opened to explore the hip and plicate its lax capsule during which time the child can return home. At the end

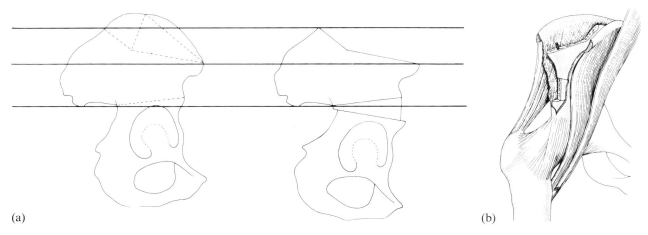

(a)

(b)

Fig. 3.9   Pelvic osteotomy. (a) Diagram showing excision of upper third of iliac crest. (b) drawing of pelvic osteotomy procedure (previously published by Springer, [19]).

of the 6–8 week period, the child is readmitted for removal of plaster, hydrotherapy and medial rotation exercises. The two fixation pins can be removed at that time.

Results

A yearly follow-up has been undertaken until the patients reach full skeletal maturity. When the families have moved away from the area, arrangements are made for the children to be assessed either locally or return for review (Table 3.2).

Each parent is given a booklet of instruction on the management and assessment and they are warned that the 10–14 year period is the most testing time for the children's hip joints. During this period, the last spurt of skeletal growth occurs and this coincides with the pre-puberty secretion of hormones which produces hormonal joint laxity in the girls. At this age period, loss of

Table 3.2   Results of surgery radiological results using modified Severin's classification

Group	Year treated	Length of follow-up	Number of hips treated	Results				
				Successes			Failures	
				1	2	3	4	5
A	1965–70	15 yrs +	25	Perfect	Minimal stigmata	Slight stigmata and dysplasia	Moderate stigmata	Residual subluxation
				12	5	4	4	
				68%		16%	16%	
B	1970–75	10–15 yrs	51	26	11	8	3	3
				72%		16%	12%	
C	1975–80	5–10 yrs	64	27	26	6	1	4
				83%		9%	8%	
D	1980–85	< 5 yrs	111	Not assessed for review				

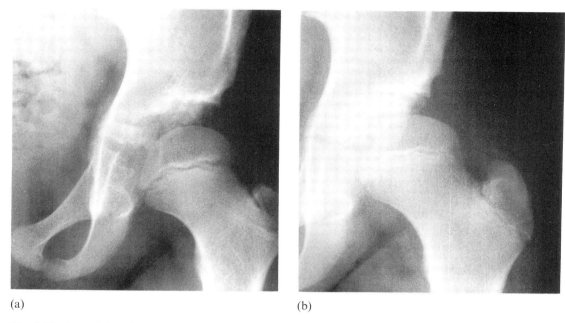

(a)   (b)

Fig. 3.10   Late deformity and subluxation of the hip. Result at (a) 6 years of age and (b) 12 years of age. Although the early result was good, the late result showed recurrence of subluxation and loss of epiphyseal height.

epiphyseal height or premature fusion of the physis with or without late subluxation of the hip joint, can occur (Fig. 3.10). Any tendency to subluxate, i.e. those in group 3 (9%), is aggravated by these two factors and it may be necessary to repeat the pelvic osteotomy at this stage.

Yet the majority of patients need no further surgery and they mature with minimal stigmata and no residual instability (Fig. 3.11).

A retrospective review of groups 4 and 5 (8% failures) has revealed that half were due to iatrogenic epiphysitis, usually the result of splinting in

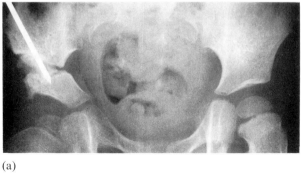

(a)

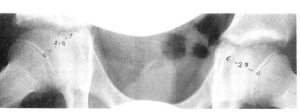

(c)

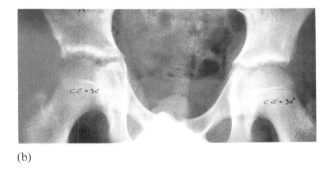

(b)

Fig. 3.11   Late good result from surgery.

the first 3 months of life, and sometimes to a combination of familial genetic factors. In the remaining half, there were no obvious causes for the failure to respond to treatment, but recent research has indicated that there may well be a muscle imbalance in these cases due to occult spinal dysraphism [22].

Discussion

From the very beginning of this surgical programme, it has been accepted that the persistence or establishment of congenital displacement of the hip beyond the first 10 months of life, is invariably due to the presence of an infolded limbus, or fold of posterior capsule, which has prevented spontaneous concentric reduction and recovery [7]. It has been confirmed that eccentric reduction of the femoral head is the commonest cause of redisplacement and epiphysitis following frame reduction, in a previous series treated conservatively. It is now accepted that a plaster cast or splints should never be applied to an infant before one is certain that the head is concentrically reduced in the acetabulum from the very outset of management [23]. It has been found from natural selection, that patients presenting for the first time in whom the radiographs reveal the presence of a femoral epiphysis within a displaced femoral head, respond much better to surgical management. This radiological sign not only confirms that diagnosis of total displacement of the hip joint, but it also indicates that a mature blood supply has developed in the proximal third of the femur. Experimental research has shown that the femoral head is more able to resist compression when the epiphysis occupies one third of the volume of the femoral head. This increases the resistance as compared to that offered by a purely cartilaginous head in the first 6 months of life [24].

It has been suggested previously that abduction on a vertical frame causes infolding of the limbus and its secondary hypertrophy [8], but this has been disproved in a small series of my patients who were simply placed on vertical traction and their legs were not abducted. In each case a limbus was found but the method was not continued, because the anterior capsular contracture was not stretched so effectively and limi-

tation of abduction of the hip persisted in these children.

Somerville [7] claimed to have few cases of epiphysitis in his series and the figures are comparable to the present series. In each the excision of the infolded limbus has been performed routinely on all dislocatable hips through a restricted surgical approach, before the application of splints and without any trial period of reduction. This low incidence of avascular necrosis common to both series (as compared to other series that have not included the routine excision of the limbus, i.e. the 15–30% prevalence reported by Salter, Kostuick and Dallas) is due to the concentricity of reduction and the stability of the hip joint. Truetta [25] pointed out that continuous severe pressure affects the growth by interference of the circulation adjacent to the growing cartilage. This could well explain the dire effect of an infolded limbus in the eccentrically reduced hip joint.

Posterior arthrotomy is preferred to the anterior approach described by Somerville, because it provides direct access to the limbus and allows adequate excision under direct vision and repair of the posterior capsule. It was once suggested that there was a risk to the capsular vessel which might cause an ischaemia of the femoral head, but Tucker [26] found this to be an erroneous view and this series has sustained his belief. Whenever anterior or anteromedial arthrotomy is performed, it is necessary to splint the legs in extension and medial rotation [2,7,8]. This position tends to wind up the capsule and so stabilize the reduction, whereas the Lorenz position relaxes the capsule. In this position, the stability of the femoral head is dependent upon the integrity of the anterior capsule which is intact if a posterior arthrotomy has been performed.

Summary

Thus, the first stage of surgical management is the concentric reduction of the hypoplastic femoral head into the primary acetabulum, involving minimal trauma and disturbance of its blood supply. The measure of the success of the manoeuvre is provided by the radiological appearance of the femoral head and the normal subsequent growth of both bony components.

Adductor tenotomy, controlled abduction with balanced traction on a vertical frame followed by posterior arthrotomy and excision of the limbus in 85% of the displaced hip joints, has proved to be an effective way of gaining concentricity of reduction. The Lorenz position has proved to be a very effective way of retaining concentric reduction over a period of 6 months. In view of the inherent tendency for persistent bony incongruity [27], osteotomy of the pelvis or femur is invariably necessary as a second stage procedure. Pelvic osteotomy has been preferred in this series as the incision leaves a lesser cosmetic blemish, whereas the osteotomy itself not only realigns the two bony components to produce a congrous articulation, but it can also be adjusted to decompress the hip joint and so prevent the late inhibition of epiphyseal growth which leads to permanent coxa plana in the adult hip.

References

1. Wilkinson, J. A. and Carter, C. O. (1960) Congenital dislocation of the hip. *J. Bone Joint Surg.*, **42B**, 652.
2. Ludloff, K. (1913) The open reduction of the congenital hip dislocation by an anterior incision. *Am. J. Surg.*, **10**, 438–454.
3. Putti, V. (1929) Early treatment of congenital dislocation of the hip. *J. Bone Joint Surg.*, **11**, 798–809.
4. Coonse, G. K. (1931) A simple modification of Perthes' splint for the early treatment of congenital dislocation of the hip. *J. Bone Joint Surg.*, **13**, 602.
5. Stewart, W. J. (1934) Further observations on the abduction-traction treatment of congenital dislocation of the hip. *J. Bone Joint Surg.*, **16**, 303.
6. Scott, J. C. (1953) Frame reduction in congenital dislocation of the hip. *J. Bone Joint Surg.*, **35B**, 372.
7. Somerville, E. W. (1953) Development of congenital dislocation of the hip. *J. Bone Joint Surg.*, **35B**, 363.
8. Fergusson, A. B. (1973) Primary open reduction of congenital dislocation of the hip using a median adductor approach. *J. Bone Joint Surg.*, **55A**, 671–689.
9. Tsuchiya, K. and Yamanda, K. (1978) Open reduction of congenital dislocation of the hip in infancy using Ludloff's approach. *Int. Orthop. (SICOT)*, **1**, 337.
10. Lehman, W. B. (1980) Early soft-tissue release in congenital dislocation of the hip. *Isr. J. Med. Sci.*, **16(4)**, 267.
11. Weinstein, S. L. (1980) The medical approach in congenital dislocation of the hip. *Isr. J. Med. Sci.*, **16(4)**, 272.
12. Catford, J. A., Bennet, G. C. and Wilkinson, J. A. (1982) Congenital dislocation: an increasing and still uncontrolled disability? *Br. Med. J.*, **285**, 1527.
13. Tonnis, D. (1982) *Congenital Hip Dislocation – Avascular Necrosis*. Thieme-Stratton, New York.
14. Fairbank, H. A. T. (1934) Congenital dislocation of the hip. *Cambridge University Medical Society Magazine*, **11**, 133.
15. Bryant, T. (1880) On the value of parallelism in the lower extremities in the treatment of hip disease and hip injuries with the best means of maintaining it. *Lancet*, **1**, 159.
16. Salter, R. B., Kostuick, J. and Dallas, S. (1969) Avascular necrosis of the femoral head as a complication of treatment for congenital dislocation of the hip in young children. *Can. J. Surg.*, **12**, 44.
17. Maw, H., Dorr, W. M., Henkel, L. and Lutsche, J. (1971) Open reduction of congenital dislocation of the hip by Ludloff's method. *J. Bone Joint Surg.*, **53A**, 1281–1288.
18. Lloyd-Roberts, G. C. (1971) *Orthopaedics in Infancy and Childhood*, 1st edn. Butterworths, London, p. 213.
19. Wilkinson, J. A. (1985) *Congenital Displacement of the Hip Joint*, Springer, Berlin.
20. Lloyd-Roberts, G. C. and Swann, M. (1966) Pitfalls in the management of congenital dislocation of the hip. *J. Bone Joint Surg.*, **48B(4)**, 666.
21. Salter, R. B. (1961) Innominate osteotomy in the treatment of congenital dislocation and subluxation of the hip. *J. Bone Joint Surg.*, **43B**, 518.
22. Wilkinson, J. A. and Sedgwick, E. M. (1988) Occult spinal dysraphism in established congenital dislocation of the hip. *J. Bone Joint Surg.*, **70B(5)**, 744.
23. Putti, V. (1933) Early treatment of congenital dislocation of the hip. *J. Bone Joint Surg.*, **15**, 16–21.
24. Hall, G. (1985) Personal communication.
25. Truetta, A. (1968) *Studies of the Development and Decay of the Human Frame*. Heinemann, London.
26. Tucker, F. R. (1949) Arterial supply to the femoral head and its clinical importance. *J. Bone Joint Surg.*, **31B**, 82.
27. Platt, H. (1953) Congenital dislocation of the hip. *J. Bone Joint Surg.*, **35B**, 339.

4

Orthopaedic management in spina bifida

E. A. Szalay

Introduction

The incidence of spina bifida is of the order of 1 in 2000 live births [1], making it one of the most common birth defects. Improved management has led to survival of most affected newborns, and a marked increase in adolescents and adults with spina bifida.

The first step in dealing with these children and their parents is realistic goal setting. Factors to be considered include level of neurological impairment, associated anomalies or other health problems, and intellectual and developmental achievements. Using these data, one seeks to maximize the individual potential of each child, without placing undue emphasis on unrealistic achievements. Mobility, activities of daily living, and cosmesis are important goals. Surgery should be prevented if possible; if surgery must be undertaken, hospitalization time and time out of school should be minimized by combining needed procedures into a single anaesthetic.

A myelodysplastic child should be enabled to achieve motor milestones at approximately the same age as does a neurologically normal child: sitting at approximately 6 months of age, standing at 10–12 months, and walking at 12–14 months. Limbs ideally should be free of deformity to allow shoeing and bracing, and appropriate assistive devices, such as corner chairs or standing frames, are provided when indicated.

Mobility

Ideal mobility is the ability to get from one place to another with minimum energy expenditure.

Most young children, regardless of level of neurological involvement, can be taught to 'walk' with braces and walker. Increasing body weight with age requires increased energy expenditure to 'walk' with braces. Many children with paralysis above the L4 level [2] cannot meet the long-term energy requirement for independent ambulation; for these children, ideal mobility is wheelchair ambulation. Our goal is to maximize function; a child in a wheelchair can keep pace with peers and may participate in sports, which cannot be done with braces and crutches.

None the less, ambulation, albeit short-term, is a goal for many children with spina bifida. Intellectual and motor development is encouraged if the child can be taught to stand and walk independently. The upright posture improves postural contractures such as equinus and knee flexion; weight-bearing encourages normal bone density and growth [3]. Most importantly, parents more readily accept the ambulatory limitation of their child if they feel that a reasonable attempt at ambulation has been made.

A number of factors influence ambulatory capability, and must be considered when setting long-range goals. Intelligence, balance, spatial orientation, and spasticity are partially determined by the status of the central neurological axis with respect to hydrocephalus and anomalies of the brain and spinal cord [4–10]; these problems may preclude ambulation even in children with excellent motor function. The level of neurological involvement is the next determining factor: long-term ambulation generally requires strong quadriceps and medial hamstring function, i.e. an L4 neurological level. Thirdly, fixed joint contractures must be addressed by stretching or by surgery to enable bracing; surgical risks must be weighed against long-term ambulatory potential. Last but not least, obesity is often a limiting factor, as many children with myelodysplasia become severely overweight.

Taking all these factors into consideration, emphasis must ultimately be placed on mobility rather than on ambulation *per se*. The concept of wheelchair mobility must be introduced early as a positive rather than a negative potential in those children who are likely to be unsuccessful at long-term community ambulation. Wheelchairs should be provided early for long-distance, independent mobility to those children capable of only household ambulation.

Role of the orthopaedic surgeon

In the perinatal period, the orthopaedic surgeon conducts a careful motor examination, preferably when the child is awake and vigorously active, to establish a baseline for voluntary muscular function. This allows early parental education regarding prognosis, ambulatory potential, and expected problems (Table 4.1) [11]. Stretching exercises and positioning suggestions may be offered. Radiographs of the spine are examined for congenital anomalies other than spina bifida. If congenital scoliosis or kyphosis

is noted, its implications are explained to the parents, and plans for careful follow-up are made. The presence or absence of hip dislocations is noted and discussed with parents, along with whether or not treatment is contemplated. The care of anaesthetic skin, the need for long-term weight consciousness, and the importance of neurosurgical and urological care are communicated to the family.

As the child grows, examinations are repeated at appropriate intervals and are compared to the baseline examination, to update prognosis and to watch for neurological deterioration, development of scoliosis, or limb deformity.

Neurological deterioration may take the form of increasing spasticity, loss of motor levels, or change in bowel or bladder control. Shunt malfunction, hydromyelia, diastematomyelia and cord tethering are all potentially treatable causes of neurological deterioration; a high index of suspicion must be maintained to prevent functional loss in an already compromised individual [12].

Sixty to 100% of children with spina bifida develop scoliosis [13] and the orthopaedist must monitor the child carefully for its presence. Its diagnosis and management will be discussed in a later section.

Limb deformity such as congenital club foot and acquired postural or spastic contractures is

Table 4.1 **Prediction of functional outcome based on neurological level**

Highest functional level	Lower extremity function	Anticipated mobility	Expected problems
Thoracic	No voluntary L.E. motors	Childhood ambulation difficult with HKAFOS; wheelchair by adolescence	'Frog' contracture of hips; poor trunk control; scoliosis/kyphosis
High lumbar (L1–L3)	Functioning hip flexors and adductors	Ambulation in childhood with KAFOS; wheelchair by adolescence	Hip flexion/adduction contracture, knee extension contracture; hip dislocation; lordosis/scoliosis
Low lumbar (L4–L5)	Functioning quadriceps and medial hamstrings; may have tibialis anterior	May be long-term ambulators; require AFOS	Hip subluxation/dislocation; lower extremity torsional problems; calcaneus deformity of feet
Sacral	All muscles function except foot intrinsics	Independent ambulation, usually with no bracing	

noted, and decisions regarding management are made. Cosmetic considerations such as the ability to wear shoes, the desirability or practicality of bracing, and functional expectations are weighed against the physiological and psychological risks of surgical correction.

Lastly, the orthopaedist must coordinate physical and occupational therapy and prescribe and oversee orthotic and mobility aids.

Orthotics

Bracing can stabilize weak joints, help prevent postural contractures, and provide lower extremity and trunk stability to allow independent upper extremity activity. Bracing cannot correct fixed joint deformities nor increase the energy available for ambulation. Braces are hot and encumbering, and make dressing and toileting difficult. Ill-fitting braces may cause pressure sores in insensate skin. For these reasons, the decision to brace and the type of braces must be individualized for each patient.

Orthotics can be fabricated of plastic or of metal. Polypropylene braces can conform exactly to a deformed limb, and are useful in providing total contact to distribute weight and to decrease pressure concentration. They are cosmetically more acceptable because the child can vary shoe wear. However, the plastic braces are hot and often not sturdy enough for a very heavy child.

Metal braces are stronger, cooler, and more appropriate for a heavy child or adolescent. They may be attached to 'space shoes' if plantar ulcers are a problem. The metal uprights and attachment to unsightly 'orthopaedic' shoes make them less cosmetically desirable.

Principles of bracing in spina bifida

In children with neurological levels above L3, the parapodium [3], or standing frame, provides stable support to enable upright positioning of the child from 10 to 18 months old. This encourages head control, allows independent bimanual activity and helps the child develop confidence in the upright position. Some parapodia can be modified for swivel gait as the child gains confidence, or the child may then be fitted for ambulatory braces.

In all but the child with a very low neurological level, children most often benefit by a process of progressive brace weaning. They begin ambulation with a hip-knee-ankle-foot orthosis, i.e. a long leg brace with pelvic band, locked hips, and locked knees. The child then learns progressive control of joints, beginning with a toddler's walker and a swivel or swing-to gait with the hips locked. When this is mastered, the hips are unlocked and reciprocal gait is learned; the pelvic band may then be discarded. If quadriceps strength is sufficient, the child may then unlock the knee hinges, and the thigh pieces are removed when good knee control is achieved. This weaning process allows progressive learning of ambulation, and control of each joint is achieved independently. The type of final bracing is determined by the level of paralysis, with an upper lumbar level child requiring long leg braces, while a lower lumbar level child may wear short leg braces.

The hip

Myelodysplastic hip problems can result from positional contractures, muscle imbalance, or spasticity; establishing the aetiology of the deformity aids in treatment decision making.

Children with very high level or thoracic paralysis often develop a positional 'frog leg' deformity due to the tendency of the flail hip to fall into abduction when the child lies supine or prone. In children with neurological levels of L1 to L4, unopposed hip flexors and adductors commonly produce a flexion/adduction contracture which may progress to subluxation or dislocation. Hydrocephalus, central nervous system injury, or anomaly may cause spasticity; the spastic myelodysplastic hip may assume any of the deformities seen in a child with cerebral palsy.

Whether or not to treat the myelodysplastic posterior hip dislocation remains quite controversial. A dislocated hip in a child with spina bifida is usually not painful and does not prevent bracing or ambulation [14]. The surgical reconstruction of the dislocated hip is extensive, and redislocations have been noted postoperatively in as many as 45% [15]. For these reasons, treatment of the dislocated hip is not indicated in the child with a very high level of paralysis, or if other factors render the child a poor candidate for long-term ambulation.

In the child with excellent long-term ambulatory potential, such as a child with L4 function or below and no spasticity, surgical treatment of the dislocated hip may be considered.

A unilateral hip dislocation poses additional problems. In the ambulatory child, it produces an apparent limb length discrepancy. In the wheelchair-ambulatory child, the role of unilateral hip dislocation in the production of pelvic obliquity and scoliosis has not been clearly defined [16,17]. It has not been shown that treatment of a subluxating or dislocating hip will affect the development of scoliosis.

If, considering these factors, treatment is elected, early soft tissue releases (hip flexors and adductors) may be combined with prolonged night-time bracing in extension and abduction. The Sharrard iliopsoas transfer has been used to balance the hip musculature; some authors feel this procedure has a place in the treatment of the L4 level myelodysplastic. Others, however, feel that iliopsoas tenotomy achieves much the same end with significantly lower surgical morbidity [18].

In the older child with more significant subluxation or frank dislocation, bony procedures may be needed. The 'developmental' dislocation is often not marked by the severe acetabular dysplasia seen in congenital dislocation, and a varus femoral osteotomy may be sufficient to maintain reduction. If the acetabulum is deficient, the Chiari innominate osteotomy provides posterior as well as superior coverage.

Very rarely, spasticity may produce an extension contracture of the hip which results in loss of sitting ability and may progress to anterior hip dislocation. Treatment is indicated to prevent loss of sitting ability, and requires soft tissue release with occasional femoral shortening [19].

The knee

Knee deformities are also grouped as to aetiology as positional, due to muscle imbalance, or to spasticity.

A flexion contracture can result from prolonged sitting or crawling. In spastic children it may result from hamstring spasticity.

A knee flexion contracture may be an acceptable deformity in a wheelchair-ambulatory individual; in the ambulatory child, this contracture makes bracing difficult and decreases quadriceps efficiency. If treatment is elected, stretching and/ or soft tissue release may address the mild contracture. Radical soft tissue release is needed for the severe deformity [20]. If the soft tissue release is limited by tightness of neurovascular structures or if bony derotation is desired, an extension/ shortening/derotational osteotomy of the femur or tibia may significantly facilitate bracing and ambulation.

A rigid extension contracture of the knee may be seen in the child with an L3 neurological level due to strong quadriceps opposite flail hamstring muscles. The extended position of the knee is a braceable position – surgical release should only be considered if problems with wheelchair sitting or other positioning are encountered. A V-Y quadricepsplasty [20] may occasionally be indicated in the ambulatory child; quadriceps release and even patellectomy may be needed to achieve sufficient flexion for sitting in the non-ambulatory child.

Intoeing

A number of problems can cause intoeing in the myelodysplastic. Femoral anteversion, spasticity resulting in a gait similar to that seen in cerebral palsy, hamstring imbalance (functioning medial hamstrings while lateral hamstrings are flail), internal tibial torsion and foot deformities can all result in intoeing [21]. One must identify the aetiology of the intoeing so that orthotic or surgical correction can be appropriately directed. Adductor and/or hamstring release may be indicated; for bony deformities, femoral or tibial osteotomies may provide cosmetic or functional improvement that results in a more efficient gait.

Twister cables applied to braces have been used in the past and are seen to improve the gait in some children, at the expense of increased energy consumption and increased encumbrance. As energy limitation and encumbrance by braces are causes of ambulatory failure, twister cables are not advocated.

Out-toeing

The foot normally dorsiflexes during the swing phase to allow ground clearance; where dorsiflexion is limited, as in paralysis, or even when a fixed-ankle orthosis or cast is worn, a patient often externally rotates the limb to facilitate ground clearance. Other causes of externally rotated gait in myelodysplasia include external tibial torsion or a plano-valgus foot from heelcord contracture or peroneal spasticity.

External tibial torsion is often seen with increased femoral anteversion, and may be associated in myelodysplasia with a valgus ankle joint [19]. Orthotic fitting becomes difficult, and pressure sores on the medial malleolus may occur. The torsion may be treated by supramalleolar osteotomy with simultaneous correction of the angular deformity of the ankle. Isolated ankle valgus is addressed in the ambulatory child by medial physeal stapling or hemiepiphysiodesis at an appropriate age to allow correction of the deformity by subsequent growth.

Limb length discrepancy

Limb length discrepancy is seen in the child with a unilateral hip dislocation, pelvic asymmetry, and especially in the child with an asymmetrical or unilateral paralysis. Careful attention is paid to this problem, with the goal being symmetry at skeletal maturity if the child is projected to be a long-term ambulator. It must be emphasized that limb length symmetry is only of importance if the child is projected to be a community ambulator at skeletal maturity.

Serial measurements of limb length are monitored, with epiphysiodesis or limb lengthening performed at an appropriate skeletal age. Shoe lifts in the face of an asymmetric pelvis or a subluxated hip may be seen to worsen the pelvic asymmetry while improving the gait only cosmetically.

Children with myelodysplasia often have advanced bone age and overall short stature; this must be considered when timing limb equalization procedures.

Foot deformity

Foot deformities are seen in almost two-thirds of children with myelodysplasia [22]. Feet must be plantigrade if bracing and ambulation are to be accomplished. Children whose ambulatory potential is poor often benefit psychologically and socially if foot deformities are corrected to allow normal footwear.

Deformities may be either congenital or acquired secondary to muscle imbalance or spasticity. The aetiology of the foot deformity must be defined if treatment is to be successful and recurrence avoided.

Congenital foot deformities include clubfoot and vertical talus. These are often severe in nature, resembling the arthrogrypotic foot. Serial casting is attempted by some to partially correct the deformity and minimize skin tightness at surgery. The author, however, does not employ serial casting in a rigid, insensate foot in which surgery is inevitable. Occasionally, a percutaneous heelcord tenotomy is performed, followed by several weeks of casting. In the minimally deformed foot, this may suffice to enable shoewear and significantly improve cosmesis.

If surgical correction is needed, a complete release is performed in the same manner as for a similar deformity in the nonparalytic foot. In contrast to the neurologically normal foot, however, unopposed tendons are not repaired. Talectomy may be required in the severely deformed foot or in the older child. One must beware of anomalous vascularity or sympathetic dysvascularity, and must be prepared for skin grafting if closure is difficult after correction of a severe deformity.

Deformities may result from muscle imbalance. Examples of these include the calcaneus deformity from a functioning tibialis anterior in a child who lacks triceps surae function, as seen in an L4 or L5 neurological level. The calcaneus gait can produce disastrous ulcerations as a result of weight-bearing on the point of the heel.

The treatment of foot deformities resulting from muscle imbalance is to balance the foot by removing or transferring the unopposed muscular influence. For the calcaneus deformity in the above example, treatment consists of tibialis anterior tenotomy with subsequent bracing, or transfer of the tibialis anterior to the heelcord [23].

The third cause of foot deformity in myelodysplasia and often the most difficult to treat is spasticity; deformities resulting from myelodysplastic spasticity resemble those found in cerebral palsy. Tenotomy may be performed, or muscle-balancing surgery may be cautiously attempted.

Increasing spasticity or development of foot deformity such as cavus may indicate a tethered cord or other central nervous system lesion. Before the foot deformity is addressed, the central nervous system must be assessed.

Spinal deformity

Patients with spina bifida develop scoliosis in from 60 to 100% of cases [13]. A distinction must be made between congenital and so-called 'developmental' or 'paralytic' curvatures.

Congenital curves result from malformations of the vertebrae aside from the dysraphism, and all newborns should be radiographically screened for such anomalies. If anomalies are noted, the spine is carefully observed for curve progression. As in congenital scoliosis without myelodysplasia, spinal fusion is performed as soon as curve progression is documented, even if that be at less than 1 year of age. Early posterior fusion alone may be performed in nondysraphic segments; in dysraphic areas anterior fusion or hemiepiphysiodesis is needed. A high index of suspicion is maintained for the existence of diastematomyelia and other cord anomalies in any patient with congenital anomalies [5], and myelographic computed tomography or magnetic resonance imaging should be undertaken to determine cord anatomy [12].

The 'developmental' or 'paralytic' scoliosis is an entirely different entity. The child is straight at birth and has no anomalies of the vertebral bodies, except the posterior bony dysraphism. The mechanisms for production of 'developmental' scoliosis are not well explained, as curves are often well above the level of the myelomeningocele. The literature suggests a strong correlation between this type of scoliosis and hydrocephalus or spinal cord anomalies such as syringomyelia and tethered spinal cord [8,24–28]; these lesions should be sought through diagnostic imaging.

The treatment for noncongenital scoliosis in spina bifida is generally surgical. Bracing may be used in the very young child as a temporizing measure, but the natural history of such curves is generally one of progression. When surgery is undertaken, better results are obtained with anterior spinal fusion with release and grafting or anterior instrumentation, followed by posterior fusion and segmental instrumentation [29–31]. When fusion to the pelvis is desired [31], the Galveston technique of intrailiac rod passage has proved useful. This is a major undertaking in these individuals, and carries a high complication rate [32], but these curves often become severe, and spinal stabilization provides prevention of further progression and pulmonary compromise while improving sitting balance and cosmesis.

A far more ominous problem is seen in the congenital kyphosis observed with very high level neurological lesions and high posterior defects. As neurosurgical care improves the survival rate of more severely involved infants, this problem occurs with greater frequency. Surgical correction in the young child is often unsuccessful and deformity recurs [33]; most successful results are obtained in the older child (8–12 years old) by resection of the apex and lordotic segment followed by rigid internal stabilization [31].

Fractures

Disuse and osteopenia in the nonambulatory or braced patient predisposes bone to fracture. Particularly vulnerable is the postoperative patient in whom cast immobilization has been used. Fractures in children with spina bifida often occur in insensate limbs, making diagnosis difficult. Children may present appearing slightly ill and mildly febrile, with a swollen, hot extremity. Significant sequelae from fracture may occur, such as fat embolism, pulmonary embolism, or hypovolemia from fracture bleeding.

Younger children may develop physeal changes from repeated microtrauma to the physis. This so-called 'Charcot physis' must be distinguished from neoplasm or other growth disturbance. Identification of the problem suggests protection of the physis to allow healing [34].

A high index of suspicion for fracture must be maintained for children with spina bifida. Postoperative casting should be minimized, with casts designed to permit early standing and weight-bearing.

Conclusion

Myelodysplasia is a multi-system disease, and its orthopaedic care cannot be divorced from that of the pediatrician, neurosurgeon, urologist, and physical and occupational therapists. All must work together to maximize function and minimize deformity.

The orthopaedic care of myelodysplasia begins at birth by determination of neurological level and a search for congenital spinal anomalies or other congenital defects. Education of the parents begins by outlining expected ambulatory potential and predicting deformities that may be anticipated due to muscle imbalance.

As the child grows, developmental milestones are assisted by sitting or balance devices and bracing as indicated. Long-term mobility is achieved by bracing or by the use of a wheelchair. The child is not pressured to accomplish unrealistic goals, but is enabled to achieve his or her full individual functional capacity.

References

1. McLaughlin, J. *et al.* (1984) Management of the fetus and newborn with neural tube defects. *J. Perinatol.*, **4**, 3–11.
2. Waters, R. L. and Lunsford, B. R. (1985) Energy cost of paraplegic locomotion. *J. Bone Joint Surg.*, **67A**, 1245–1250.
3. Menelaus, M. B. (1980) *The Orthopaedic Management of Spina Bifida Cystica*, ed 2. Churchill Livingstone, Edinburgh.
4. Brown, H. P. (1978) Management of spinal deformity in myelomeningocele. *Orthop. Clin. North Am.*, **9**, 391–402.
5. Winter, R. B., Haven, J. J., Moe, J. H. and Lagaard, S. M. (1974) Diastematomyelia and congenital spine deformities. *J. Bone Joint Surg.*, **56A**, 27–39.
6. Mazur, J. A. *et al.* (1986) The significance of spasticity in the upper and lower extremities in myelomeningocele. *J. Bone Joint Surg.*, **68B**, 213–217.
7. McLone, D. G. and Naidich, T. (1985) Spinal dysraphism: experimental and clinical. In *The Tethered Spinal Cord* (ed. R. N. N. Holzman), Thieme-Stratton, New York, pp. 14–28.
8. Park, T. S., Cail, W. S., Maggio, W. M. and Mitchell, D. C. (1985) Progressive spasticity and scoliosis in children with myelomeningocele. *J. Neurosurg.*, **62**, 367–375.
9. Venes, J. L., Black, K. and Latack, J. T. (1986) Preoperative evaluation and surgical management of the Arnold–Chiari malformation. *J. Neurosurg.*, **64**, 363–370.
10. Williams, B. (1979) Orthopaedic features in the presentation of syringomyelia. *J. Bone Joint Surg.*, **61B**, 314–323.
11. Szalay, E. A. (1987) Orthopaedic management of the lower extremities in spina bifida, in Griffin, M. D., *Instructional Course Lectures XXXVI*, American Academy of Orthopedic Surgeons, Chicago.
12. Szalay, E. A., Roach, J. W., Smith, H. *et al.* (1987) Magnetic resonance imaging of the spinal cord in spinal dysraphisms. *J. Pediatr. Orthop.*, **7**, 541–545.
13. Mackel, J. L. and Lindseth, R. E. (1975) Scoliosis in myelodysplasia. *J. Bone Joint Surg.*, **57A**, 1031.
14. Barden, H. (1975) Myelodysplastics: fate of those followed for twenty years or more. *J. Bone Joint Surg.*, **57A**, 643–647.
15. Bazih, J. and Gross, R. H. (1981) Hip surgery in the lumbar level myelomeningocele patient. *J. Pediatr. Orthop.*, **1**, 405–411.
16. Kahanovitz, N. and Duncan, J. W. (1981) The role of scoliosis and pelvic obliquity in functional disability in myelomeningocele. *Spine*, **6**, 494–497.
17. Stillwell, A. and Menelaus, M. B. (1983) Walking ability in mature patients with spina bifida. *J. Pediatr.*, **3**, 184–190.
18. Breed, A. L. and Healy, P. M. (1982) The mid-lumbar myelomeningocele hip: Mechanisms of dislocation and treatment. *J. Pediatr. Orthop.*, **2**, 15–24.
19. Szalay, E. A., Roach, J. W., Wenger, D. *et al.* (1986) Extension-abduction contracture of the spastic hip. *J. Pediatr. Orthop.*, **6**, 1–6.
20. Dias, L. S., Jasty, M. J. and Collins, P. (1984) Rotational deformities of the lower limb in myelomeningocele. *J. Bone Joint Surg.*, **66A**, 215–223.
21. Dias, L. S. (1985) Valgus deformity of the ankle joint: pathogenesis of fibular shortening. *J. Pediatr. Orthop.*, **5**, 176–180.
22. Duckworth, T. (1982) Management of the feet in spinal dysraphism and myelodysplasia. In *Disorders of the Foot* (ed. M. J. Jahss), Saunders, Philadelphia.
23. Banta, J. V. and Sutherland Wyatt, M. (1981) Anterior tibial transfer to the os calcis with achilles tenodesis for calcaneal deformity in myelomeningocele. *J. Pediatr. Orthop.*, **1**, 125–131.
24. Emery, J. L. (1986) The cervical cord of children with meningomyelocele. *Spine*, **11**, 318–321.
25. Hall, P. V., Campbell, R. L. and Kalsbeck, J. E. (1975) Meningomyelocele and progressive hydromyelia. *Neurosurgery*, **43**, 457–463.
26. Hall, P. V., Lindseth, R. E., Campbell, R. L. and Kalsbeck, J. E. (1976) Myelodysplasia and developmental scoliosis: a manifestation of syringomyelia. *Spine*, **1**, 48–56.

27. Hall, P. V., Lindseth, R. E., Campbell, R. L. *et al.* (1979) Scoliosis and hydrocephalus in myelocele patients. *J. Neurosurg.*, **50**, 174–178.

28. Sherk, H. H., Charney, E., Pasquariello, P. D. *et al.* (1986) Hydrocephalus, cervical cord lesions, and spinal deformity. *Spine*, **11**, 340–342.

29. Osebold, W. R., Mayfield, J. K., Winter, R. B. and Moe, J. H. (1982) Surgical treatment of paralytic scoliosis associated with myelomeningocele. *J. Bone Joint Surg.*, **64A**, 841–856.

30. Mayfield, J. K. (1981) Severe spine deformity in myelodysplasia and sacral agenesis. *Spine*, **6**, 498–509.

31. Allan, B. L. and Ferguson, R. L. (1979) The operative treatment of myelomeningocele spinal deformity. *Orthop. Clin. North Am.*, **10**, 845–862.

32. Sriram, K., Bobechko, W. E. and Hall, J. E. (1972) Surgical management of spinal deformities in spina bifida. *J. Bone Joint Surg.*, **54B**, 666–676.

33. Christoffersen, M. R. and Brooks, A. L. (1985) Excision and wire fixation of congenital rigid kyphosis in myelomeningocele children. *J. Pediatr. Orthop.*, **5**, 691–696.

34. Wenger, D. R., Jeffcoat, B. T. and Herring, J. A. (1980) The guarded prognosis of physeal injury in paraplegic children. *J. Bone Joint Surg.*, **62A**, 241–246.

5

Perthes' disease

G. Hall

We are at times painfully aware of the fact that there are many symptoms which we readily recognise in our clinical observations to which we can assign no cause, and it is also an undoubted fact that there are many conditions, even which exist today, of which we are ignorant, simply from our neglect to observe, or again, from faulty deduction even from good observation.
Alfred T. Legg [1]

Introduction

The statement made by Legg over half a century ago can equally apply today to the understanding of the condition which partly bears his eponym.

Although there has been a great deal of research and speculation, no significant advances in the understanding of Perthes' disease has occurred and the condition remains an enigma. The cause remains unknown; the prognosis is difficult to determine and the influence of treatment impossible to establish.

It now seems certain that Perthes' disease is the result of a series of vascular insults to the immature femoral head [2,3], and that these changes are most likely to occur in children with certain morphological changes first described by Burwell [4]. Once established, the outcome of the condition is variable and there are differing published views as to the natural history of the disease. Ratliff [5] has reviewed 34 cases of the condition and has suggested that in the long term only one in three cases obtain a good end result. Using a different method of assessment Eaton [6]

claims 61% of his cases achieved good results in adult life. This suggests that the prognosis of Perthes' disease is usually benign.

Similarly, when trying to establish the influence of treatment on the outcome of the disease, differing reports are obtained from the literature. Brotherton and McKibben [7] have suggested that traction in abduction can improve the prognosis, while Lloyd-Roberts [8] maintains that an osteotomy below the hip has a similar effect.

It is therefore very difficult for clinicians dealing with this condition to have a clear understanding of the natural history of the disease, and the possible influence of treatment on the outcome.

An attempt has been made to resolve this dilemma by reviewing a large series of children with Perthes' disease treated in Wessex over the last 50 years.

Patients and methods

One hundred and nine cases of Perthes' disease have been reviewed in an attempt to establish the natural history of the condition as well as the possible value of various prognostic features. All of the children in this review were treated in Wessex, either at the Bath and Wessex Orthopaedic Hospital or the Lord Mayor Orthopaedic Hospital, Alton, Hampshire. The original hospital records and radiographs were studied and a clinical and radiographic review performed on the patient in adult life. The average length of review from onset of the disease is 34 years (range 8–57).

End result

It is vital when comparing two differing forms of treatment that the outcome of the treatment is expressed in the same way. Many papers have been written where the outcome of the disease has been assessed before skeletal maturity, and obviously as children have such a growth potential it is foolhardy to be dogmatic about the outcome. The later in life that the review is performed the greater its value, and Ratliff [5] has suggested a method of assessing the outcome of Perthes' disease which is both clinical and radiographic, and is weighted heavily towards the clinical picture.

Assessment in adult life

The results obtained using the Ratliff method of assessment showed that the majority of hips (71.3%) had good results, being totally free of pain and functionally without impairment with a concentric hip free of degeneration on the radiograph. The average age of the patient when reviewed was 42 years. Only 10.6% of cases had poor end results in adult life assessed by this method, and four of the 109 hips reviewed had required surgery for pain relief.

At healing of the disease

A good result from Perthes' disease is obviously a hip that functions well throughout life without premature degeneration. It is of course helpful when attempting to evaluate the effect of treatment on the outcome of the disease to make an assessment of the result at an earlier stage.

In this review a radiographic assessment of the result was also made when the disease had healed, but before skeletal maturity. The shape of the healed femoral head was determined using the concentricity of Mose and also a visual assessment of the result was made using the method described by Catterall [9]. The cases were

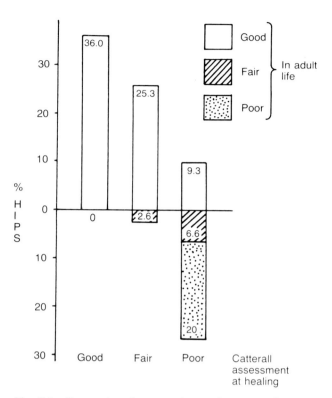

Fig. 5.1 Comparison between the result measured at healing of the disease with the actual result in adult life.

then assessed in adult life using the methods described by Ratliff, and also using the concentricity of Mose [10] on the adult radiograph. Comparison of these results suggests that a considerable improvement occurs in adult life (Fig. 5.1).

This improvement can also be seen by measuring the concentricity of Mose both at healing and on the adult radiograph. When the concentricity of Mose was measured at healing of the disease, 24.4% of hips had less than 2 mm of flattening and yet in adult life 54.2% of hips showed good concentricity with less than 2 mm of flattening.

The epiphyseal quotient is the ratio of epiphyseal height and width expressed as a percentage of the normal hip and gives an indication of the degree of flattening of the femoral head. This quotient has been used as an assessment of the result of Perthes' disease at healing of the disease and is thought to give a reasonable indication of the likely end result in adult life. In fact, only one

The 'head height'

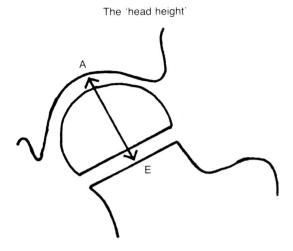

Fig. 5.2   The head height was measured from the acetabular roof to the epiphyseal plate.

hip in this review, with a quotient above 60%, had a poor result in adult life. However, 8.6% of hips with a severely flattened epiphysis with a quotient of 60% or less achieved a good result in adult life. The degree of distortion of the femoral head therefore does seem to be a fairly good indicator of the likely long term result of the disease.

A more accurate assessment of the outcome can, however, be gained by measuring the 'head height' (Fig. 5.2). This height probably represents the cartilaginous anlage of the hip and can be determined by measuring the distance between the acetabulum and the epiphyseal plate on both the affected and normal sides. When this height is related to the end result, it is seen quite clearly (Fig. 5.3) that those cases in which collapse of the cartilaginous anlage did not occur all achieved a good result. It is therefore apparent that any assessment of the likely end result which is not based upon the overall shape and position of the cartilaginous anlage of the hip will give a misleading impression of the prognosis.

Prognostic factors of Perthes' disease

Since the first descriptions of Perthes', attempts have been made to establish at an early stage the likely outcome. Legg described a 'cocked hat' appearance of the epiphysis and tried to relate it

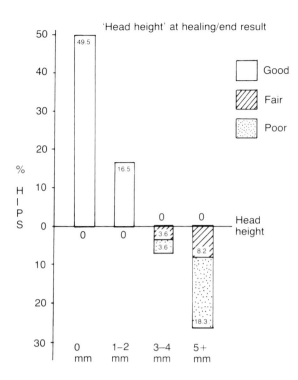

'Head height' at healing/end result

Fig. 5.3   The measurement of the head height on the initial radiograph is of great importance in determining the end result. A difference of more than 2 mm in head height always has a poor result.

to the end result. The features which may influence the possible outcome of the disease can be divided into radiographic and non-radiographic.

Non-radiographic features

In this review it would seem that the mode of onset, severity and duration of symptoms do not influence the end result. It has been suggested that girls have a worse prognosis than boys. In this review the ratio of girls to boys was as expected, approximately 1:4, and in fact there was no appreciable difference in the end result between girls and boys. It has been recognized that the child's age at the onset of the condition has a profound influence on the outcome, and that after the age of 8 years the outlook worsens. In this review a similar pattern emerges and children presenting after the age of 8 years have a relatively high proportion (88%) of unsatisfactory results (Fig. 5.4).

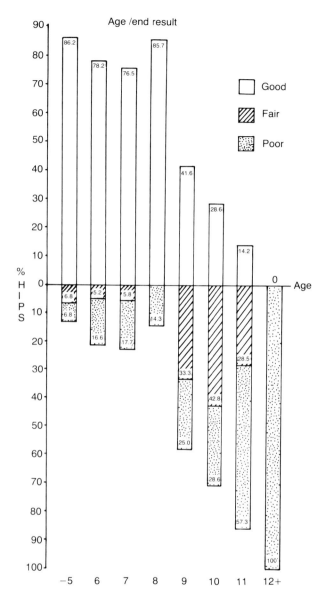

Fig. 5.4 The influence of age on the outcome of the disease.

Radiographic features

The diagnosis of Perthes' disease is entirely radiographic. Fragmentation, alteration in the density and shape of the hips' ossific nucleus as well as other specific radiographic changes characterize the disease. There have been several attempts in the past to establish from the initial radiograph various features which may guide the clinician to the likely outcome. The degree of involvement of

the ossific nucleus would seem to vary from case to case and it has been shown by Katz [11] and also by Catterall that the outcome is partly related to this. Not surprisingly, the children with more involvement of the femoral head tend to have a worse end result than those with a lesser degree of involvement. In this review there was a

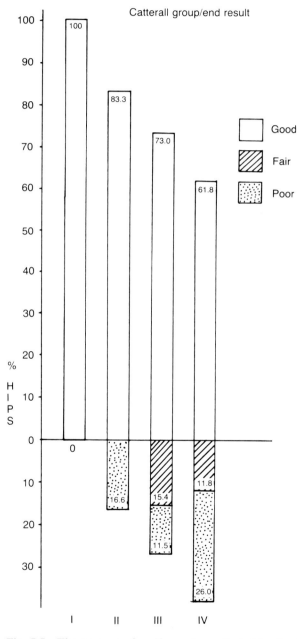

Fig. 5.5 The amount of ossific nucleus affected by the disease as defined by the Catterall group has a slight influence on the outcome.

progressive decline in the proportion of good results occurring in adult life with increasing involvement of the ossific nucleus (Fig. 5.5). Children with minor involvement of the ossific nucleus (Catterall groups 1 and 2) tended to fare better than those with whole head involvement, but even in the group of children with whole head involvement nearly half had satisfactory results in adult life.

The discrepancy between the results in this review and those of Catterall must be partially attributable to the difference in assessing the result. Catterall's group of children was assessed at healing of the disease, and as shown earlier, a considerable improvement can occur as the child matures.

'Head at risk' signs

Catterall has also described five features seen on the radiograph which are thought to help judge the outcome. He has termed these the 'Head at risk' sign, and suggested that when seen on the initial radiograph, the prognosis was poor.

Subluxation of the hip is one of the 'at risk' signs, and is described by Catterall in this context as an increase of medial joint space of more than 2 mm when compared to the normal side. Sixty-seven per cent of hips exhibited an increase of medial joint space of more than 2 mm on the initial radiograph, and of these 70% achieved good results in adult life. An increased medial joint space, therefore, is not a very accurate way of determining the likely end result and other ways of assessing subluxation of the hip should be considered.

A joint is subluxed when there is lack of apposition of the joint surfaces. In the hip this can be determined either by measuring directly the percentage of head uncovered by the acetabulum, or the centre edge angle of Wiberg. A reasonable estimate of the degree of subluxation can also be obtained by observing Shenton's line. These methods of assessment of subluxation give a more accurate means of determining the end result, and certainly the more profound the subluxation the worse was the outcome in adult life. The hips with an obvious break in Shenton's line on the initial radiograph generally tended to have poor end results, with only 25% achieving a good result. Similarly, in those hips which exhibited more than 20% uncovering of the hip, only 25% achieved a good end result.

The other 'at risk' signs are calcification seen laterally to the growth plate, a reaction in the metaphyseal region of the hip, a horizontally placed growth plate and the presence of a Gage sign.

Although Gage [12] first described his sign as a prominence of the contour of the superior aspect of the femoral neck, it has widely become used to denote an angular type defect in the lateral epiphyses which is not seen on the unaffected side. The individual merits of the 'at risk' signs are of doubtful significance and only the Gage sign is of any statistical significance as a prognostic indicator. Of the 109 hips reviewed, however, all but five however, showed one or more of the 'at risk' signs. Nine hips exhibited all five 'at risk' signs and of these four achieved a good end result in adult life. These results would tend to suggest that if treatment is based on the 'at risk' concept alone, half or more of the affected hips would be treated unnecessarily as they will probably achieve a good end result without intervention.

Femoral head shape

As a poor end result of Perthes' disease is usually associated with a mis-shapen femoral head, it would seem reasonable to attempt to predict this deformation in shape at an early stage.

A direct measurement of the affected ossific nucleus can be made and related to the unaffected side. This ratio can be expressed as a percentage (the epiphyseal quotient) and related to the end result. This measurement of the deformation of the ossific nucleus gives a more accurate indication of the outcome than the other prognostic features noted (Fig. 5.6). It is curious to note, however, that a number of hips show quite severe flattening of the ossific nucleus and still achieve a satisfactory outcome in adult life.

The structure of the developing hip in a child is, of course, not entirely bony in origin. Presumably deformation of the cartilaginous anlage can also occur in Perthes' disease. The shape, size and position of this cartilaginous anlage can be outlined by arthrography of the joint and, this can on occasion demonstrate that the ossific nucleus has collapsed leaving a relatively intact cartilaginous anlage. A reasonable estimate of the

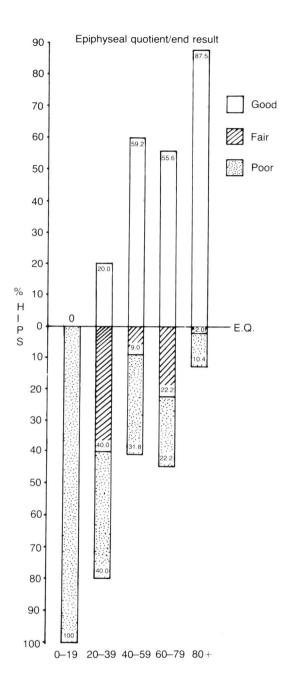

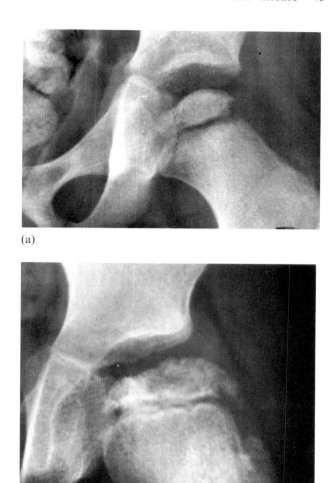

(a)

(b)

Fig. 5.7 Apparent increase in superior joint surface produced by collapse of the ossific nucleus without cartilagenous collapse.

Fig. 5.6 The epiphyseal quotient is a fairly reliable indicator of the outcome.

shape of the anlage can be obtained by measurement of the distance between the acetabulum and the femoral epiphysis. In some cases of Perthes' disease it appears that there is an apparent increase in the superior joint space after collapse of the ossific nucleus and yet in other cases there is

no such increase (Fig. 5.7) When the distance between the acetabulum and epiphyseal line is compared to the unaffected side and related to the end result it would appear that this is a very effective means of judging the outcome. Ninety-three per cent of cases exhibited loss of head height on the original radiographs, and all of the cases had an unsatisfactory result. Of the 84 cases who exhibited no loss of head height on the original radiograph, 93% achieved a good result in adult life. The group of children who showed

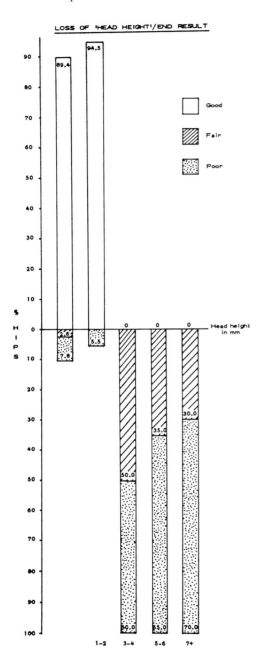

Fig. 5.8 The measurement of the head height on the initial radiograph is of great importance in determining the end result. A difference of more than 2 mm in head height always has a poor result.

indicator of the likely outcome of the disease. Unsatisfactory results only occurred in this review in the children whose hips exhibited distortion of the cartilaginous anlage. When the shape of the hip anlage was maintained throughout the disease process, the outcome was always good (Fig. 5.8).

Effect of treatment

The children in this review were all treated after the diagnosis of Perthes' disease was made by a period of recumbency and straight Pugh type traction until signs of healing of the femoral head occurred. None of the patients in this review appeared to have suffered from the irritable hip syndrome prior to their admission for Perthes' disease.

To assess the possible effect of treatment on the outcome of the disease it is interesting to compare the results of this series of patients with other groups treated in differing ways. This of course has obvious pitfalls. It is important that the results are assessed in a similar way and at a similar stage of the condition, and that the severity and age at onset of the disease are taken into account.

Catterall has reported a group of 54 children who were untreated and found that 31% had good results, 28% fair and 41% poor results. These results are directly comparable with the results in this review where 36% had good results when assessed at healing of the disease. This would suggest that simple traction without containment has very little effect on the outcome. Some further evidence that traction alone has little benefit on the outcome of the disease can be gained by studying whether those patients in whom treatment was delayed by a significant time tended to have a worse outcome than those in whom treatment was started at the onset of symptoms. Although this is a crude assessment in that patients had symptoms for at least 6 months before treatment started, this delay in instituting treatment did not seem adversely to affect the outcome of the condition.

The possible effect of containment can be judged by comparing the results of this review with those of Brotherton and McKibben [6]. In their series, children were treated by abduction traction, and therefore any benefit to be derived

no collapse on the original radiograph and yet did not achieve a satisfactory result all developed loss of head height on subsequent radiographs. It would therefore seem that the measurement of the shape of the cartilaginous anlage is the best from abduction should be apparent. The assessment of the Brotherton and McKibben review is the same as this review, and therefore a fair comparison can be made. It would seem that there is little if any benefit to be derived from the addition of abduction to traction.

This review would suggest that by and large Perthes' is a fairly benign condition and simple traction would not seem to influence the outcome.

Pathogenesis of head collapse

Quite clearly, the outcome of Perthes' disease is determined by the degree of deformation of the cartilaginous anlage which occurs during the course of the disease. The two factors which have been shown to influence the degree of distortion of the femoral head are: the age of the child at onset of the disease and the degree of involvement of the ossific nucleus. There is no evidence to suggest that the older child suffers from a more severe form of the condition and it is therefore likely that the deformity of the femoral head is related directly to the maturity of the child.

As the child's hip develops, there is alteration in the relative proportion of cartilage to bone. At birth the femoral anlage is totally cartilaginous, the ossific nucleus develops in the centre of this anlage and grows at a proportionally higher rate than the cartilaginous hip. By the age of 6 years the ossific nucleus occupies 30% of the femoral head and by 12 years of age the proportion of bone in the developing hip is 80%. As Perthes' disease appears to be entirely a condition affecting the developing nucleus, it is not surprising that the relative proportion of the hip occupied by ossific nucleus influences the mechanical strength of that developing hip.

In the younger child the majority of the affected hip is in fact cartilaginous: it therefore can withstand the mechanical deforming factors and deformation does not occur. At a later stage in development when the ossific nucleus occupies more of the hip, avascularity of that nucleus will produce a more pronounced effect on the ability of that hip to withstand deformation and subsequently collapse of that hip will occur (Fig. 5.9). It would appear that the critical level of development of the hip is when approximately 50% of the hip is ossific, which occurs at approximately 8 years of age. It is easy to understand why an ossific nucleus only partially affected by the disease can withstand deformation more than one with whole head involvement.

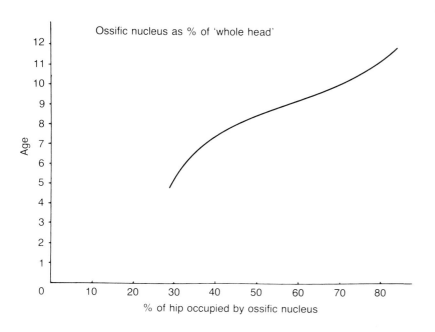

Fig. 5.9 Diagram shows how the proportion of bone in the hip increases with age.

Load testing of immature pig hips

To test this hypothesis, load testing experiments were performed on the hips of freshly killed piglets. Like the human hip, the hip of the piglet develops from a cartilaginous anlage with an increasing proportion of ossific nucleus as the pig matures.

Compression loading was performed on hips of varying maturity, and the degree of deformation produced by a given load noted. The experiments were repeated on hips of differing degrees of maturity after their ossific nuclei had been removed.

The results of these simple load testing experiments showed that the immature totally cartilaginous hip deforms quite readily under load. Once the ossific nucleus develops, however, the strength of the hip increases dramatically. When the ossific nucleus is removed from the developing hip the load/deformation characteristics change considerably. A hip which is mainly cartilaginous can withstand removal of its ossific nucleus without unduly affecting its load characteristics. However, when the hip's ossific nucleus is larger, removal of that ossific nucleus has a profound effect on the load bearing capacity of that hip. The load bearing characteristics of the developing hip appear to alter dramatically at the critical level when 50% of the hip is ossific nucleus.

It is interesting to relate the experimental findings with the clinical review. At the age of 8 years, approximately 50% of the child's hip is composed of the ossific nucleus. This relates well with the experimental evidence found in the piglets' hips.

When the end result is equated to the relative size of the ossific nucleus rather than the child's age it becomes apparent that the size of the ossific nucleus determines the outcome.

It would therefore seem that the outcome of Perthes' disease is directly related to the size and proportion of the ossific nucleus affected by the disease, and that the size of the ossific nucleus is determined by the skeletal maturity of the child.

Conclusions

For more than 70 years clinicians have advocated treatment of children suffering from Perthes'

disease. A review of the literature has failed to substantiate that treatment either by weight relief or containment has any effect on the outcome of the condition. Therefore the basic question must be asked: should Perthes' disease be treated?

This review has confirmed that the overall outcome of Perthes' disease is generally satisfactory. Only four hips in this review have required surgery in adult life for pain relief. The average age of the patient when this surgical intervention took place was 38 years. With the success of modern treatment of osteoarthrosis of the hip again it is difficult to justify the treatment of children with Perthes' disease, and it would therefore seem reasonable to restrict any attempts at treatment to those cases in which a poor outcome can be predicted with certainty.

References

1. Legg, A. T. (1910) *Boston Medical Journal*, **162**, 202–204.
2. McKibben, B. and Ralis, Z. (1974) Pathological changes in a case of Perthes' disease. *J. Bone Joint Surg.*, **56B**, 438.
3. Kemp, H. B. S. (1973) Perthes' disease with an experimental and clinical study. *Ann. R. Coll. Surg.*, **52**, 18.
4. Burwell, G. *et al.* (1978) Perthes' disease. An anthropometric study. *J. Bone Joint Surg.*, **60B**, 461.
5. Ratliff, A. H. C. (1977) Perthes' disease – study of sixteen patients followed up for 40 years. *J. Bone Joint Surg.*, **59B**, 248.
6. Eaton, G. O. (1967) Long term results of treatment of coxa-plana. *J. Bone Joint Surg.*, **49**, 1031.
7. Brotherton, B. J. and McKibben, B. (1978) Perthes' disease treated by prolonged recumbency and head containment. *J. Bone Joint Surg.*, **59B**, 8.
8. Lloyd-Roberts, G. C. *et al.* (1978) A controlled study of the indication for and the results of femoral osteotomy in Perthes' disease. *J. Bone Joint Surg.*, **58B**, 31.
9. Catterall, A. (1971) The natural history of Perthes' disease. *J. Bone Joint Surg.*, **53B**, 37.
10. Mose, K. (1964) *Legg–Calvé–Perthes' Disease*. Universitets for Laget, Arthus.
11. Katz, J. F. (1967) Conservative treatment of Legg–Calvé–Perthes' disease. *J. Bone Joint Surg.*, **49A 6**, 1043.
12. Gage, H. C. (1933) A possible early sign of Perthes' disease. *Br. J. Radiol.*, **6**, 295.

6

Slipped upper femoral epiphysis

W. E. G. Griffiths

The condition of slipped upper femoral epiphysis (SUFE) was first described by Ambroise Paré in 1572. Also known as epiphysiolysis or adolescent coxa vara, it may be defined as posterior displacement of the femoral capital epiphysis in otherwise normal adolescents.

In the Portsmouth Health District, UK, a population of approximately 530 000 produced 65 new cases of SUFE in the 13 years from July 1973 to July 1986, that is, an average of approximately one case per 106 000 population per year. Of these cases 48 were male (75%) and 14 were bilateral at presentation (21.5%). The males ranged from 8 years 2 months to 17 years 8 months in age, an average of 14 years 4 months. The females ranged from 8 years 6 months to 17 years 9 months, an average of 12 years 7 months.

Of the 79 hips 45 were mild or early slips (58%) and the remainder were sufficiently severe to merit surgical reconstruction of the relationship between head and neck of femur, in order to eliminate deformity and reduce the risk of osteo-arthritis in later life.

The management of mild degrees of slippage is now generally agreed by most authorities to consist of internal fixation *in situ* with slender steel pins. Conservative treatment alone has been abandoned as a result of complications such as chondrolysis after immobilization in plaster spica, or increasing slippage while on traction. A bone graft may be used instead of steel pins, but this guarantees the fusion of the growth plate prematurely.

The management of cases of severe degrees of slippage has, throughout several decades of spectacular advance in most other problem areas of orthopaedics, continued to present a challenge almost unique in its ability to stimulate controversy. Insidious in onset, often with minimal symptoms and signs, the average interval between onset and diagnosis is approximately 5 months, by which time the radiological changes may be far advanced, and *in situ* pinning no longer acceptable. Different schools advocate different methods of management, including manipulative reduction with or without traction, hip spica, or surgery, while surgical reconstruction can be achieved in different ways, including correction at the site of slippage through the physis, or at the base of the neck of the femur, or through the trochanteric region. A cortico-cancellous bone graft may be used to stabilize and fuse the growth plate in the slipped position without attempting reduction; and there are advocates of pinning *in situ* even for the more severe slips in the hope of remodelling taking place, though the evidence for this lacks substance. Aggressive surgical treatment carries an increased risk of the dreaded complication of avascular necrosis of the capital epiphysis, while chondrolysis may follow any treatment, or no treatment at all.

Blood supply to the capital epiphysis

A rational appraisal of this controversial subject must begin with a study of the blood supply to the adolescent capital epiphysis. Trueta [1] traced the developing stages through which the blood supply passes, from embryo to adult: in the adolescent phase the blood supply is mainly from the lateral epiphyseal vessels, themselves derived from the medial circumflex artery, with some variable anastomosis from the ligamentum teres. No vessels cross the growth plate itself at this stage. Green [2] emphasized the importance of the vessels carried up the postero-inferior aspect of the neck of the femur in the retinacula of Weitbrecht. Blood from these vessels enters the periphery of the capital epiphysis, bypassing the epiphyseal plate.

Direction of slippage

From radiographic observation, the direction of slippage appears to have three elements, the caput moving posteriorly, medially, and into internal rotation with respect to the neck of femur, and for many years this tri-plane concept governed the principle of surgical reconstruction. However, M. J. Griffith [3] argued that the tri-plane idea is unnecessarily complicated, and from morphological studies on cadaveric specimens he showed quite clearly that the epiphyseal plate can be represented by part of the surface of an imaginary cylinder, whose axis exists at an angle of 65° to the femoral shaft, in the trochanteric region, in the plane of anteversion (Fig. 6.1a). As

the epiphysis slips, it moves in a purely posterior direction about this curved surface. On the AP radiograph the head of the femur sinks over the horizon like the setting sun, and the loss of height of the capital epiphysis compared to the normal side may be the only early radiological sign. The appearance of medial or even lateral displacement can then be produced simply by taking further radiographs in positions of internal and external rotation; lack of understanding of this simple principle has in the past led to confusion in presenting and interpreting results of manipulative 'reduction'. In practice, three methods are commonly used to take lateral radiographs of the upper end of femur.

   (i) Frog lateral: an AP projection of the pelvis, with both thighs semiflexed, 45° abducted, and externally rotated to the maximum.
   (ii) 'Shoot through' lateral of the affected hip is taken with the patient supine and the other hip flexed up out of the way: the plate is tucked above the iliac crest.
   (iii) The 'turn over' view, with the patient supine and the pelvis tilted up on the unaffected side, the affected leg is partly flexed and externally rotated.

One or more of these views may be unobtainable if the patient is in severe discomfort, or if both hips are severely affected. The last method is probably the most reliable for routine use.

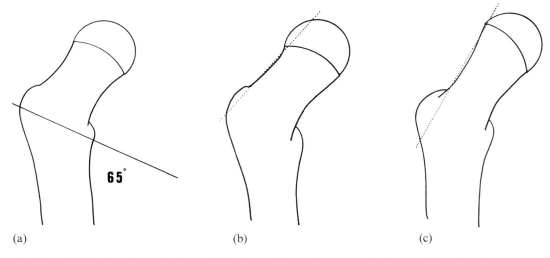

(a)   (b)   (c)

Fig. 6.1   (a) Showing the axis about which the epiphysis slips, posteriorly away from the observer. (b) Trethowan's line negative. (c) Trethowan's line positive.

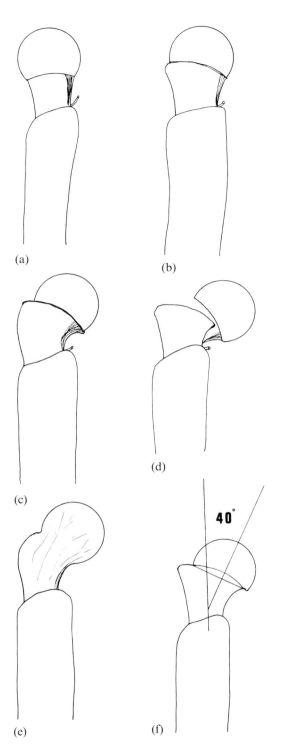

Fig. 6.2 (a) Normal lateral aspect of upper end of femur. (b) Early chronic slip, epiphyseal plate open: type 1. (c) Severe chronic slip, epiphyseal plate open: type 3. (d) Acute on chronic slip: type 2. (e) Severe chronic slip, epiphyseal plate closed: type 4. (f) To show the angle of slippage.

Pathological changes

As the caput advances posteriorly it strips up the periosteum on the posterior aspect of the femoral neck, laying down a curving beak of new bone formation (Fig. 6.2a, b). The exposed anterior margin of the neck (Fig. 6.2b, c) will tend to remodel away after an interval, although a nubbin of bone can lead to a mechanical blockage in flexion and abduction. If slippage accelerates, tearing will occur at the junction of the anterior periosteum of the neck with the hyaline cartilage of the receding caput, leading to haemarthrosis and increased pain. Acute separation of head and neck may follow a minor force such as stepping off the kerb (Fig. 6.2d) presenting clinically in the same way as a subcapital fracture, with severe pain and complete loss of function. More commonly, slow chronic slippage continues over many months resulting in severe remodelling of the femoral neck.

Slippage of any appreciable severity tends to be followed by premature fusion (Fig. 6.2e), though this is unpredictable and does not always happen. In cases of unilateral disease the normal hip continues to grow, but in most cases the resulting discrepancy in leg length is very small because little growth potential is left, the capital epiphysis contributes much less than the lower epiphysis of the femur, and the neck of the femur is at an angle to the vertical.

Microscopically, the epiphyseal plate consists of four layers of cells: the resting layer of cartilage cells adjacent to the epiphysis, the proliferating layer, the hypertrophied layer, and the zone of provisional calcification adjacent to metaphyseal bone. During slippage, cleavage occurs through the hypertrophied layer.

Aetiology

Harris [4] observed that there was a tendency for SUFE to occur in adolescents of heavy build and immature secondary sexual characteristics, the 'adiposo-genital' syndrome, and also in a second, smaller group of rapidly growing, tall thin individuals. It was known that anterior pituitary growth hormone stimulated the proliferative layer, leading to a thicker growth plate, less resistant to shearing force, while oestrogen, and to a lesser extent testosterone, inhibited the anterior pituitary production of growth hormone. He suggested that an imbalance in the ratio between these two sets of hormones in adolescence would therefore predispose to SUFE. In the adiposo-genital syndrome there is a deficiency of sex hormone and in the tall thin cases an excess of growth hormone. He supported this experimentally by measuring the resistance to shear force in the upper tibial epiphysis of the rat, showing that it could be increased by oestrogen, and reduced by growth hormone. Further evidence from clinical assessment of hormone levels in patients with SUFE is, however, lacking, and this would appear to be a ripe field for future investigation.

We have already defined SUFE as occurring in otherwise normal children, but it is worth recording that it may also occur as part of the manifestation of a variety of disorders, including hypopituitarism, hypothyroidism, also treated hypothyroidism resulting in a growth spurt, hyperparathyroidism, renal osteodystrophy, rickets, Morquio's disease, multiple epiphyseal dysplasia, achondroplasia, or after sepsis or radiotherapy.

Clinical features

SUFE presents mainly between the ages of 10 and 16, females younger than males, as a problem of pain in the groin or knee, and limp. Pain may be non-existent, or slight, or vary in intensity over a period of many months. It cannot be said too often that obscure knee pain in an adolescent should alert the clinician to the possibility of hip disease, but in practice the diagnosis is frequently delayed, and there is nearly always a radiograph of the knee in the envelope. Pain is only severe when acute separation supervenes.

Only about half the cases exhibit the typical overweight, sexually immature physique or are very tall and thin; the remainder vary as normal children do.

Trendelenburg test is positive except in early chronic slippage. The gait is striking, with the foot on the affected side held in external rotation, and even in early cases, fixed external rotation of the hip shows up in flexion, as the posteriorly displaced epiphysis sits more comfortable in the obliquely facing acetabulum in external rotation when the hip is flexed. Wasting of the buttock

and thigh will occur in time. The incidence of bilateral disease is in general thought to be about 35%, though figures vary in many different reports. There will be less than this at initial presentation, as the second side may slip later. This figure will also clearly be reduced if prophylactic pinning is done.

Radiographic diagnosis of the early chronic slip may be easily overlooked on AP projection only, as the only definite sign is loss of height of the capital epiphysis compared to the other side (if that is normal), as the caput recedes over the horizon of the neck. The epiphyseal plate may appear broader because of its geometric tilt. Trethowan's line is useful but not absolutely reliable as a few degrees of retroversion will negate it (Fig. 6.1b, c).

Classification

Dunn and Angel [5] emphasized that a clear and practical classification is essential if reliable comparisons between different methods of treatment are to be used, and suggested the following.

  (i) Acute traumatic. These cases are rare, involving violent trauma to mainly younger children with previously normal hips; there is no preexisting break. These are really separate from the syndrome of SUFE.
 (ii) Type 1. Chronic slip, early (Fig. 6.2b). There is no universally accepted method of differentiating between mild (early) slippage and severe slippage, the threshold being variously taken as 1 cm or 1/3 diameter, or 40° backwards angulation using the head/shaft angle or head/neck angle (Fig. 6.2f).
(iii) Type 2. Acute on chronic slip (Fig. 6.2d). In this situation an epiphysis which has already slipped sufficiently to create an identifiable beak on lateral radiograph, undergoes a further sudden movement, losing its adhesion to the metaphysis. The tone of the hip flexors and abductors and short external rotators produces proximal displacement of the femur, with external rotation and shortening clinically, accompanied by acute pain. On lateral radiograph the caput lies on the side of the femoral neck, with point contact between the beak and the concave aspect of the head. The periosteum is torn anteriorly, and stripped posteriorly from the femoral neck. Adaptive shortening of the retinacular vessels takes place within hours rather than days.

(iv) Type 3. Severe chronic slip, growth plate open (Fig. 6.2c). As this develops over a period of months, the epiphysis slips backwards and downwards, slowly stripping up the posterior periosteum which lays down a gradually increasing beak of new bone, thereby remodelling the shape of the metaphysis. The uncovered anterior margin will eventually remodel away, though this process lags behind and often leaves a protuberant bony nubbin. Severe deformity of the femoral neck will eventually result, again with shortening, fixed external rotation and limited flexion and limp, though not necessarily pain.

(v) Type 4. Severe chronic slip, growth plate closed (Fig. 6.2e). Metaphyseal vessels now cross the growth plate remnant to anastomose with capital vessels, and on no account must these anastomoses be disrupted. Any surgical reconstruction *must* now take place away from the head/neck junction.

Management

Acute traumatic slip demands emergency treatment for severe pain. Manipulative reduction (open if necessary) and internal fixation must be done as soon as anaesthesia is safe, as in the normal trauma situation. The risk of damage to the capital blood supply at the time of injury is

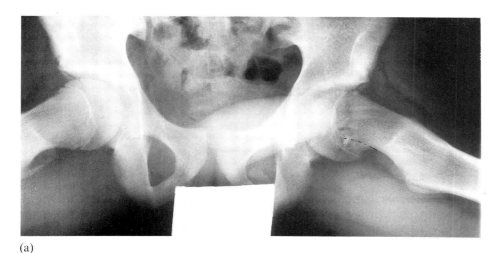

(a)

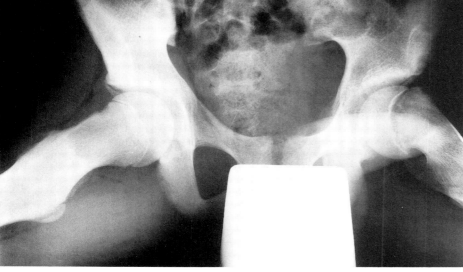

(b)

Fig. 6.3 (a) This male patient aged 16 years 8 months was admitted with moderately severe chronic slip of the left upper femoral epiphysis measuring 34° on January 4th 1982, but suffered increased pain, deformity and limitation of movement over the next 4 days while in bed on skin traction awaiting surgery. (b) The same patient on January 8th: a previously borderline case had now become unquestionably severe, with slippage measuring 52°. Open replacement was necessary.

great, delay will only increase it, and the best chance for a viable head lies in swift reduction and secure fixation.

Type 1. Early chronic slip. Conservative treatment is dangerous: traction in bed does not truly relieve the hip joint from compressive forces, so increased slippage is still possible (Fig. 6.3). Immobilization in a plaster spica leads to a high incidence of chondrolysis.

Internal fixation *in situ*, that is to say without reduction, using slender steel pins, is now generally agreed to be the treatment of choice, except by those who prefer epiphysiodesis (see type 3). A large bore nail such as Smith–Peterson should not be used as the dense cancellous bone of the caput will not accept it readily, and displacement or vascular damage may occur.

Of the various designs of slender pins, the Crawford Adams (Fig. 6.4a) is the most suitable for this purpose, with a 2 mm steel shank, and a built-up threaded section to grip the outer cortex. Beyond the thread the pin ends in a triangular section for ease of insertion and removal using a long slender triangular chuck in an ordinary hand drill. Four pins introduced under image intensifier control are sufficient to stabilize an early chronic slip. For moderately severe slips not bad enough for reconstruction, it is wise to begin drilling the outer cortex of the femur well anterior to the mid-lateral line and aim posteriorly so as to penetrate the middle of the epiphysis.

There is some controversy regarding the question of prophylactic pinning of the unslipped hip on the other side. As the risk of bilateral disease is of the order of 35%, the author prefers to pin the unslipped side in all cases except those close to maturity. From past personal experience, patients cannot be relied upon to report early symptoms which may in any case be minimal. The morbidity of prophylactic pinning carefully done is extremely small. Radiography of the good hip every 4 months has its advocates but that too is not free from morbidity. The risk of bilateral disease is increased in patients of Negro or Polynesian race, or heavy build, or if the triradiate cartilage is still open. Pins should be removed 6 months after radiological evidence of closure of epiphysis. Occasionally pins require replacing with larger ones as the epiphysis grows off the proximal ends of the pins.

Type 2 acute on chronic. Debate continues whether manipulation to reduce severe displacement should be done in every case, or sometimes, or never.

Many reports fail to differentiate between severe chronic and acute on chronic slips, but from the experience of operating upon both types it is plain that manipulation of a purely chronic slip must never be done. Anything short of brute force will not shift a chronic slip (at operation a broad curved gouge is necessary to lever the head and neck apart), and if the head did shift, the effect on its blood supply would be disastrous.

In cases of acute on chronic slip, on the other hand, by definition there is loss of cohesion between head and neck, and a gentle manipulation has at least a chance of improving the relationship, exactly as in a subcapital fracture in

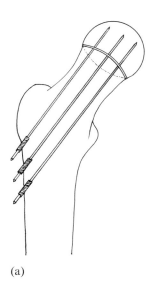
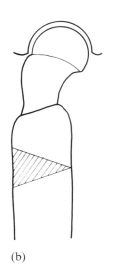
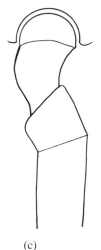

Fig. 6.4 (a) Crawford Adams pins internally fixing an early slip *in situ*: only three pins shown. (b) Trochanteric osteotomy: removal of an anteriorly based wedge from the trochanteric region, with closure of the wedge leading to (c) restoration of the capital epiphysis comfortably into the acetabulum.

(a)   (b)   (c)

an elderly patient. Certainly early closed reduction followed by pinning in anatomical position can lead to perfect restoration of hip function and development. In the ideal situation, reduction within hours of the acute episode, and only in the presence of minimal beak formation, would appear to carry only a small risk of damage to the retinacular vessels.

This risk would clearly increase:

(i) in the presence of a large beak;
(ii) after the passage of enough time following the acute episode to allow adaptive shortening of the soft tissues carrying the retinacular vessels, say 24 hours (N.B. some authorities define 'acute' slip so as to include any case within 3 weeks of an acute episode).
(iii) if over-reduction takes place, even momentarily.

It has been stated that there is no such thing as gentle manipulation of the retinacular vessels, and great care must be taken to avoid the trap of misreading radiographs taken in different degrees of rotation which, as have been clearly shown, can mimic reduction.

In practice it is rare to be presented with the ideal combination of circumstances favourable to closed reduction, the usual problem being delay between the moment of acute slippage, and either diagnosis, or availability of operating facilities. Probably after 24 hours, and certainly after 48 hours manipulation should not be done.

Acute on chronic slippage implies a degree of slipping already too great for pinning *in situ*, so if manipulation fails or only partly succeeds, surgical restoration of anatomy must now be contemplated, with the following options available.

(i) Allow the acute slip to stabilize in its presenting position, or partly reduced, either by immobilization or temporary internal fixation with pins. Prolonged immobilization would lead to a risk of chondrolysis, but the epiphysis will stabilize in quite a short time, say 3 weeks. This can then be followed by (ii).
(ii) elective trochanteric osteotomy, which carries little if any risk to the capital vascular supply. (Basal cervical osteotomy is also done, for the same reason but this is much less popular.) The object is to restore the caput neatly into the acetabulum by removing a wedge based anteriorly (Griffith [3]) or antero-laterally (Southwick [6]). No further growth or remodelling will take place but some length will be gained by

geometrical realignment. Viewed from the lateral aspect a somewhat Z-shaped upper end of femur results, and the critics of this line of treatment would say that perfect restoration of anatomy is never achieved, the abduction mechanism is permanently misaligned and progression to early osteoarthritis, say by the 4th decade, is a common sequel. The misshapen upper end of femur then leads to technical problems with total hip replacement. Avascular necrosis, however, is practically eliminated: the surgeon will not have to face early failures (Fig. 6.4b, c).

(iii) Open replacement; an intracapsular procedure variously referred to as cuneiform osteotomy, trapezoid osteotomy or cervical osteotomy has the attraction of restoring as accurately as possible the head/neck relationship at the site of the lesion itself, and is done immediately after diagnosis, without preliminary traction or spica. The anterior approach to the joint can be used [7] but a lateral approach detaching the greater trochanter is better, allowing visualization of the anterior, lateral, and posterior aspects of the femoral neck. The greater trochanter is detached extracapsularly, and after the capsule is opened, great care is taken not to disrupt the continuity of the retinacular vessels running up the back of the femoral neck from the capsular reflection at its base.

The head of the femur is levered gently off the neck (Fig. 6.5a) and the exposed end of the metaphysis trimmed carefully so as to remove a wedge or trapezium (viewed from lateral aspect) of bone, plus the beak of new bone. Bleeding back should be demonstrated by curetting the concave inner aspect of the epiphysis at this stage, showing that it is still viable.

The minimum amount of trimming of bone is done to allow easy reduction of the neck against the head without tension in the retinacular vessels. Dunn [5] recommends 20° valgus alignment rather than square reduction. Five Crawford Adams pins are used to fix the reduction (Figs 6.5b, c, 6.6a, b, c) and one or two screws to replace the greater trochanter. Postoperatively, the leg is maintained on light skin traction allowing supervised movements for 4 weeks, followed by partial weight bearing for a further 8 weeks. If avascular necrosis supervenes, the changes will be apparent, clinically and on radiography, within 6 months. In Dunn's series of 73 open replacements, nine out of 24 cases of acute on chronic slip went on to avascular necrosis, but only two of these were complete, and seven partial (segmental or mottling only).

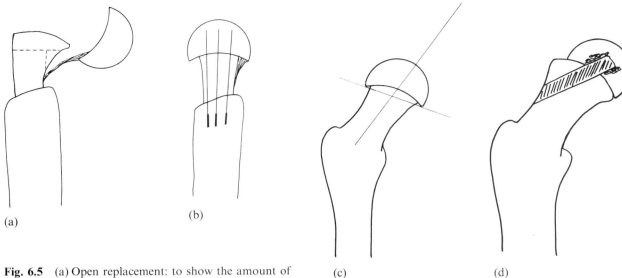

(a)   (b)

(c)   (d)

Fig. 6.5   (a) Open replacement: to show the amount of bone requiring removal at open replacement, including the beak, so as to allow reduction of head and neck without tension in the retinacular vessels. (b) Reduction and fixation achieved, square on the lateral view. (c) Up to 20° valgus is preferred on AP projection. (d) Epiphysiodesis.

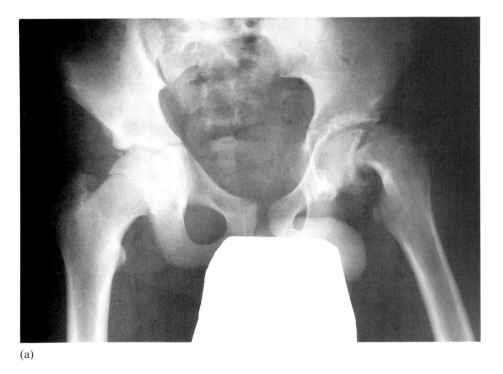

(a)

Fig. 6.6   (a) A severe case of acute on chronic left SUFE in a male aged 14 years 1 month: preoperative radiograph. (b) After open replacement. The greater trochanter has been refixed distally in order to tense the abductors. (c) Twelve months postoperatively, an excellent result, clinically and radiologically. The other side has been pinned prophylactically.

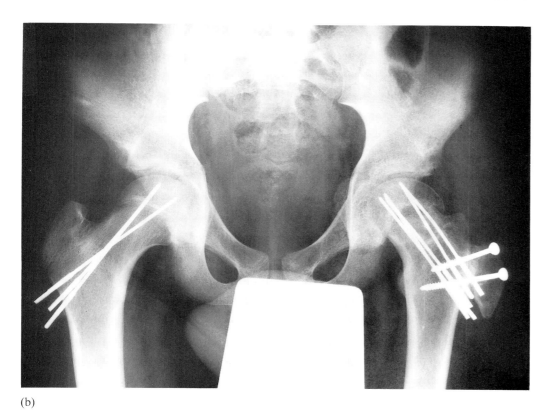

(b)

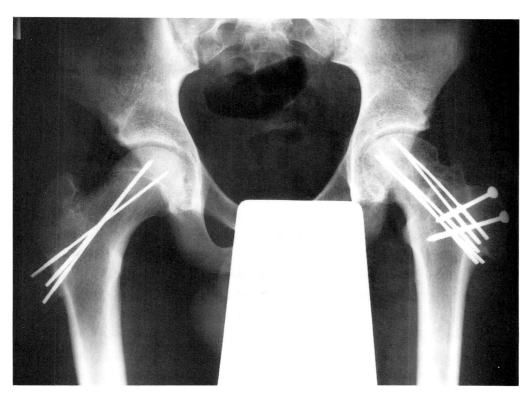

(c)

Type 3. Severe chronic slip, growth plate open. The author prefers a simple and reliable method of measuring backward angulation on the lateral radiograph, taking the axis of the femoral neck from the line of the original anterior cortex, ignoring the beak (Fig. 6.2f). The angle is measured between this line and the line bisecting the epiphysis. Severe chronic slip is defined as being over 40° of backward angulation.

Manipulation of a pure chronic slip without an

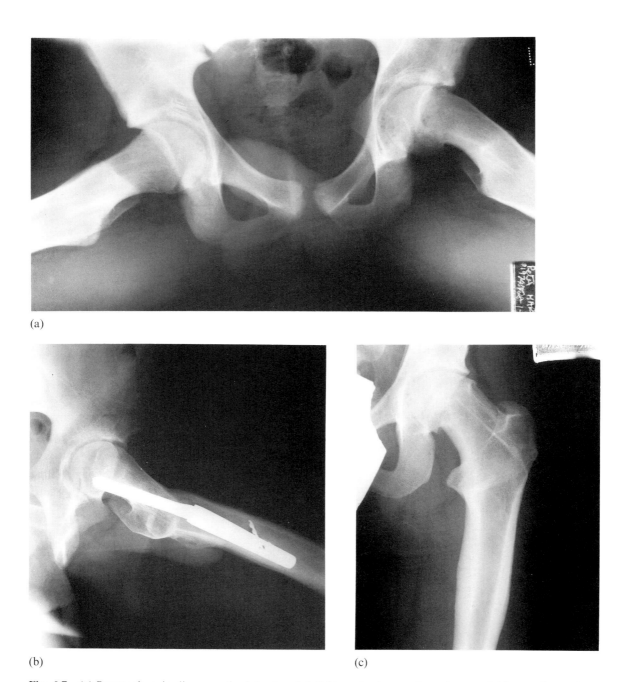

(a)

(b)   (c)

Fig. 6.7   (a) Severe chronic slip, growth plate closed, left hip only, in a male patient aged 15 years 5 months. (b) After trochanteric osteotomy, closing an anteriorly based wedge. (c) The appearance 3 years later. There is some flattening of the superior surface of the head of femur, and early osteophyte formation.

acute episode has no place, and the options now are as follows:

(i) Stabilization by pins *in situ*, with no attempt to restore the anatomical relationship, allowing remodelling to take place with further growth. This course has been advocated, but it is difficult to see how this can work for very severe slips which will remain very limited by fixed external rotation and surely progress to early osteoarthritis. The younger child should however have greater remodelling powers.

Simple stabilization in this way carries practically no risk of avascular necrosis, though chondrolysis has been reported.

(ii) Trochanteric osteotomy as above. Preliminary stabilization by pins, or traction etc., is not necessary.

(iii) Basal cervical osteotomy.

(iv) Open replacement, as above. In the absence of acute separation the capital epiphysis will need to be levered off the metaphyseal surface of the neck using a broad curved gouge.

(v) Epiphysiodesis (Heyman–Herndon procedure [8], Fig. 6.5d). This consists of stabilizing the slipped epiphysis with a cortico-cancellous bone peg and chips which act as internal fixation plus graft, rapidly uniting the femoral head and neck. This is accompanied where necessary by a 'nubbinectomy' to reduce mechanical blockage to abduction and flexion. The risk of avascular necrosis is practically non-existent, but no attempt is made to restore normal anatomy [9].

Dunn [5] (1/40) and Fish [7] (0/36) separately reported a very low incidence of avascular necrosis after open replacement for severe chronic (type 3) slip, and therefore this would seem the operation of choice as normal anatomy is most nearly restored.

Type 4. Severe slip, growth plate closed. The metaphyseal vessels now contribute the main source of blood supply to the head, crossing the growth plate remnant, and if surgical reconstruction is felt to be necessary on grounds of deformity, limited movement or exceptionally pain, or to improve the prognosis for the longevity of the joint, it must now be done at a level away from the head/neck junction, to avoid jeopardizing these vessels. Osteotomy in the trochanteric region is usually done with the aim of restoring the head of femur comfortably into the acetabulum (Figs 6.4b, c, 6.7a, b, c).

In summary, the surgeon faced with a case of severe SUFE must first decide which type of slip he is dealing with, and then has a choice of options. Each option has its potential penalties; of the surgical procedures described only pinning *in situ* is straightforward; the others are all difficult technical procedures requiring attention to detail and special training.

Major complications

Avascular necrosis

Severe radiological collapse of the femoral head results in shortening, limited movement, limp, and wasting of thigh and buttock with a positive Trendelenburg test. Pain however, is conspicuous by its absence in the majority of cases, and if the temptation to perform arthrodesis can be resisted, a pseudarthrosis gradually appears with a wide and very useful joint space (Fig. 6.8). Walking without a stick is eventually possible, limp is reduced by a heel raise, and reasonable function for many years may ensue. There is no contraindication to total joint replacement later in life.

Chondrolysis

Also known as acute necrosis of cartilage.

This complication is uncommon, except in Negroes and Polynesians. It may follow any mode of treatment, or no treatment at all, and may be uni- or bilateral. It is manifested by a uniform loss of joint space radiologically, and progressive stiffness clinically, sometimes leading to severe deformity in flexion and adduction.

The aetiology is obscure: cartilage nutrition through synovial fluid is probably interfered with by immobilization in some way.

Microscopically, hyaline cartilage is replaced by fibrocartilage in a thin irregular layer, with normal bone beneath, at least to begin with: atrophy may follow. Dense intracapsular adhesions are formed and the capsule itself becomes inflamed and thickened up to 2.5 cm. Synovium practically disappears. In some less severe cases, gradual recovery takes place. There is no known effective treatment leading to recovery of normal hyaline cartilage. Manipulation under anaesthesia can improve the range of motion: sometimes osteotomy is necessary to reduce fixed deformity.

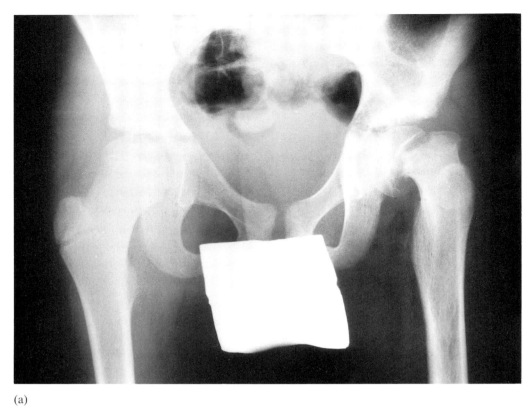

(a)

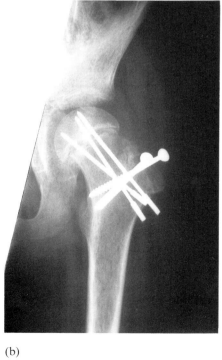

(b)

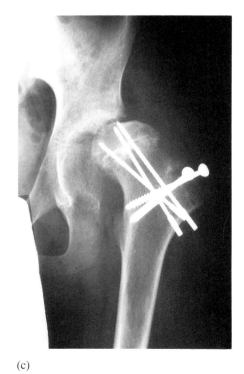

(c)

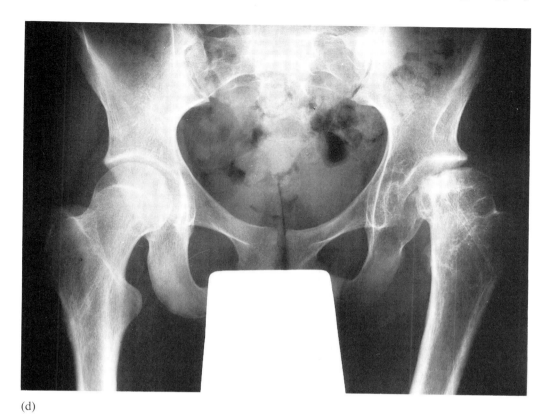

(d)

Fig. 6.8 (a) A case of acute on chronic displacement in a male aged 11 years 2 months, treated by open replacement. (b) Excellent reduction was achieved, but, (c) within 6 months, avascular necrosis of the capital epiphysis was obvious; subluxation is also occurring. (d) The eventual result, with 4 cm shortening, flexion to 90°, no pain, positive Trendelenburg (6 years later).

Osteoarthritis

Murray and Duncan [10] pointed out that many cases of 'idiopathic' osteoarthritis presenting in middle life on closer scrutiny can be seen to exhibit a minor degree of old slipped epiphysis, deduced from the shape of the head and neck of femur on radiography. They felt that athletic activity in adolescence might be a factor in the aetiology of such cases. Less commonly, the aetiology is obvious and the osteoarthritis severe (Fig. 6.9).

Jerre [11] in reviewing a large series, found that in addition to the cases of bilateral slip already diagnosed in adolescence, there were many undisclosed cases of minor slippage which came to light at review many years later: of 30 such cases, 18 had evidence of degenerative change on radiography at an average age of 37 years, though without symptoms at that time.

Dunn and Angel [5] described the articular cartilage of the femoral head as being thicker at its zenith than at its periphery, and suggested this might account for early degeneration if anatomy is not accurately restored, as weight is then borne on the thinner peripheral cartilage.

Osteoarthritis may follow, sooner or later, any of the surgical procedures described above, which all aim to minimize the deviation from the normal head/neck anatomical relationship, and it is reasonable to suppose that the greater the deviation, the worse the prognosis. Severe cases usually culminate in total hip replacement.

At the present time, the following questions remain open to debate.

1. Exactly where should one pitch the threshold of

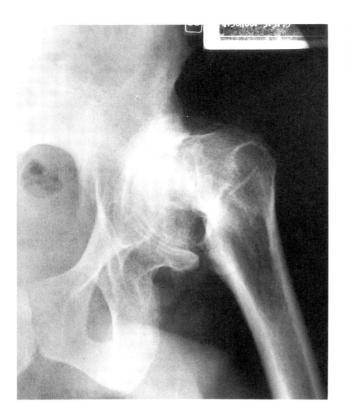

Fig. 6.9   This man presented at the age of 37 years with a history of slowly increasing limp, pain, stiffness and deformity of the left hip dating back to his teens. Osteoarthritis was severe, and the aetiology in this case was obvious. Total hip replacement was necessary.

severity, between cases suitable for pinning *in situ*, and those in which surgical reconstruction should be done.

2. In acute slippage, when, if ever, should manipulation be attempted.
3. Should surgical reconstruction be carried out at the level of the physis or base of the neck or trochanteric region?
4. Which method carries the greatest risk to the greater number?
5. What should be done for acute on chronic slip with severe displacement?

Open replacement most nearly restores anatomy at the level of the lesion, and has been shown to be safe in cases of severe chronic slip. In acute on chronic slips, especially those with severe displacement of up to 90° backward angulation, clearly something must be done to effect at least partial reduction before fixation is achieved. Open replacement carries a risk of avascular necrosis of the order of 20–25%. It has been suggested that the blood supply to the capital epiphysis may already be irreversibly damaged in the process of acute slippage in some cases. A pre-operative bone scan might clarify this point,

but reduced uptake in the capital epiphysis can be obscured by increased activity in the beak of new bone.

Trochanteric osteotomy carries virtually no risk of avascular necrosis, but the proponents of open replacement through the physis would argue that it is better to produce a near normal head/neck relationship with an excellent long term prognosis for the great majority, accepting a small number of early failures some of which will require further surgery, than to do a procedure which is relatively safer in the short term, but which condemns many of its recipients to osteoarthritis at an early age, with the prospect of difficult revision surgery in view of the deformity of the upper femur.

There is a lack of long term prospective reviews of properly classified series which might eventually give answers to these questions.

Acknowledgement

I should like to thank Mr R. J. McLean **ABIPP** of the Department of Medical Photography,

Queen Alexandra Hospital, Portsmouth, for his help in producing the illustration and photographs.

References

1. Trueta, J. (1957) The normal vascular anatomy of the human femoral head during growth. *J. Bone Joint Surg.*, **39B (2)**, 358–394.
2. Green, W. T. (1945) Slipping of the upper femoral epiphysis. Diagnostic and therapeutic considerations. *Arch. Surg.*, **50**, 19–33.
3. Griffith, M. J. (1976) Slipping of the capital femoral epiphysis. *A. R. Coll. Surg. Engl.*, **58**, 34–42.
4. Harris, W. R. (1950) The endocrine basis for slipping of the upper femoral epiphysis. *J. Bone Joint Surg.*, **32B**, 5–11.
5. Dunn, D. M., and Angel, J. C. (1978) Replacement of the femoral head by open operation in severe adolescent slipping of the upper femoral epiphysis. *J. Bone Joint Surg.*, **60B (3)**, 394–403.
6. Southwick, W. O. (1967) Osteotomy through the lesser trochanter for slipped capital femoral epiphysis. *J. Bone Joint Surg.*, **49A**, 807–835.
7. Fish, J. B. (1984) Cuneiform osteotomy of the femoral neck in the treatment of slipped capital femoral epiphysis. *J. Bone Joint Surg.*, **66A**, 1153–1168.
8. Herndon, C. H., Heyman, C. H. *et al.* (1963) Treatment of slipped capital femoral epiphysis by epiphysiodesis and osteoplasty of the femoral neck. *J. Bone Joint Surg.*, **45A**, 999–1012.
9. Melby, A., Hoyt, W. A. and Weiner, D. S. (1980) Treatment of chronic slipped capital femoral epiphysis by bone graft epiphyseodesis. *J. Bone Joint Surg.*, **62A**, 119–125.
10. Murray, R. O. and Duncan, C. (1971) Athletic activity in adolescence as an aetiological factor in degenerative hip disease. *J. Bone Joint Surg.*, **53B (3)**, 406–409.
11. Jerre, T. (1950) A study in slipped femoral epiphysis. *Acta Orthop. Scand.* **Suppl.**, **6**.

7

Spinal deformities

R. A. Dickson

Basic principles

In order to understand the treatment of spinal deformities it is important to have a clear appreciation of basic principles. 'Spinal deformities' has its own language as regards terminology and classification and much of the vocabulary is confusing if not meaningless. The aetiology of spinal deformities is perhaps the most important basic principle to grasp, as knowledge of this explains much about the natural history of spinal deformities. Then, before considering individual types of spinal deformity an overall management strategy is a necessity.

Terminology

Scoliosis is defined as a lateral curvature of the spine, a curvature in the coronal plane. This is an unsatisfactory definition as few, if any, scolioses exist solely in the coronal plane. The great majority are associated with axial rotation and thus the deformity also involves the sagittal plane. Moreover, vertebral shape in the transverse plane is also asymmetrical.

Kyphosis and lordosis are terms describing spinal shape in the sagittal plane only. Kyphosis refers to a curvature of the spine convex backwards (the posterior elements form the curve convexity), while lordosis describes a spinal curvature convex anteriorly (the vertebral bodies form the curve convexity). The terms 'structural' and 'non-structural' are applied to spinal de-

formities in an effort to distinguish those that are important from those that are not [1]. Unfortunately, the terms 'structural' and 'non-structural' do not describe any of the important distinguishing features (Fig. 7.1). A structural scoliosis, for example, is defined as a lateral curvature of the spine with rotation [1] and even this definition does not provide the information required. A structural scoliosis is important because it involves the spine primarily and has progression potential with spinal growth. It would be better termed 'primary' or 'progressive'. In contradistinction, a non-structural scoliosis is defined as a lateral curvature only, i.e. without rotation [1], but this again does not describe its important features. A non-structural scoliosis is not an intrinsic problem of the spine or its supporting mechanisms but occurs for some other reason, e.g. leg length inequality tilting the pelvis, or painful paraspinal muscle spasm accompanying a disc derangement. Moreover, these non-structural curves have no progression potential of their own and thus the term 'secondary' or 'non-progressive' would be infinitely preferable.

Scolioses are described according to the side of the convexity of the curve and where the apex of the curve is located. Thus right thoracic or left lumbar conveniently and quickly assigns a curve to a particular pattern. If the apex of the curve is T12 or L1 then it is referred to as thoraco-lumbar. If there is more than one curve in the spine, e.g. a combination of right thoracic and left lumbar curves, then this is called a double curve. If there

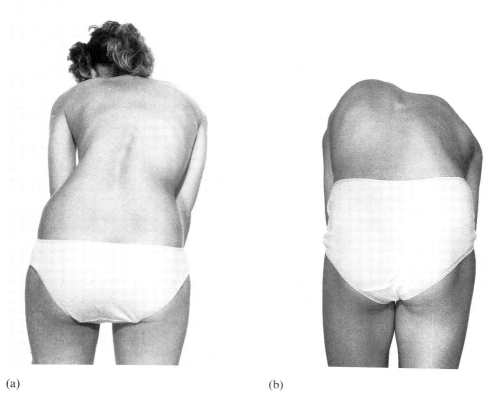

(a)   (b)

Fig. 7.1 (a) Non-structural scoliosis in a girl with an adolescent disc protrusion. There is a lateral curvature without rotation. (b) Structural scoliosis in a girl with idiopathic scoliosis. There is a marked rotational prominence.

are more than two curves then the expression 'multiple curve pattern' is applied.

The Cobb method of measurement is universally used to register radiographically the size of the deformity [2]. On an AP film lines are drawn parallel with the upper border of the upper end vertebra (the vertebra above the apex which is maximally tilted into the curve concavity) and along the lower border of the lower end-vertebra (the vertebra below the apex which is maximally tilted into the curve concavity) and these two lines are produced until they intersect. The angle subtended is referred to as the Cobb angle of the curve. While this may be a quick and easy method of estimating curve size, it is notoriously misleading. The bigger a curve becomes the more it is rotated away from the coronal plane of the patient such that the AP view progressively underestimates the true size of the deformity. Therefore a curve of 60° is much more than twice as bad as a curve of 30° and, similarly, a curve

that has been corrected surgically from 60° to 30° has achieved a much greater than 50% correction. Thus Cobb angle data cannot be handled in an arithmetic way by deriving percentage changes or means. Yet every article published about scoliosis with reference to curve size derives a mean Cobb angle which is quite inadmissible.

If the deformity is a kyphosis, existing solely in the sagittal plane, then the Cobb angle is a very reasonable method of measurement. Because of the rotation accompanying structural scoliosis, other measurements of deformity size are more relevant. From the AP radiograph the amount of apical rotation can be measured by the method of Pedriolle [3] and this is accurate for curves with a Cobb angle not much in excess of 60°. Because of the difficulty in obtaining a satisfactory radiographic measure of the size of the overall deformity, much attention has recently been focused on measurement of surface shape and there are a number of methods available including the sophisticated integrated shape imaging system (ISIS). In practice, the angle of trunk inclination (ATI) can be easily measured with a simple inclinometer [4]. Because it is body shape that requires correction in the great majority of cases coming to surgery, then it is important that some measure of surface shape be routinely used.

Classification

The basic classification proposed by the Scoliosis Research Society is simple and short [1]. The classification comprises idiopathic deformities, congenital deformities, neuromuscular deformities, deformities in association with neurofibromatosis, mesenchymal disorders (heritable disorders of connective tissue, mucopolysaccharidoses and skeletal dysplasias), trauma, infection and tumours. The classification is not strictly of spinal deformities, except idiopathic, but of the associated conditions. Table 7.1 shows the classification in more detail. While of descriptive use, it misleads into believing that there is something different about the deformities of, say, neurofibromatosis and osteogenesis imperfecta. This of course is not so, the deformities are the same, it is the conditions which differ.

Pathogenesis

Once the pathogenesis of idiopathic scoliosis is appreciated [5] it is not difficult to understand why spinal deformities are particularly prevalent when there is some associated condition as listed above in the classification. Indeed the aetiology of idiopathic scoliosis has been known for more than a century [6], but these published works have received scant attention and a seemingly enormous advantage of the development of X-rays has done more to confuse than to assist this issue by highlighting the lateral curvature component of the deformity. Thus X-rays have reduced down to two dimensions a deformity which is clearly happening in three. Accordingly, although for no obvious reason, most workers have sought to try and find something different between the convex and concave sides of a scoliosis without thinking about rotation. In the

belief, and belief only, that our normal healthy, and usually pretty, teenage girls with idiopathic scoliosis have subclinical muscular dystrophy, poliomyelitis, or other as yet unnamed neuro-

Table 7.1   Aetiological classification of spinal deformities: primary, progressive or structural deformities

A. Idiopathic deformities
  1. Idiopathic scoliosis
    a. Early onset
    b. Late onset
  2. Idiopathic kyphosis
    a. Type I – classical Sheuermann's disease
    b. Type II – 'apprentice's spine'

B. Congenital deformities
  1. Bone deformities
    a. Scoliosis (1) Failure of formation
    b. Kyphosis (2) Failure of segmentation
    c. Lordosis (3) Mixed
  2. Cord deformities
    a. Myelodysplasia scoliosis
    b. Myelodysplasia kyphosis
    c. Myelodysplasia lordosis

C. Neuromuscular deformities
  1. Cerebral palsy
  2. Poliomyelitis
  3. True 'neuromuscular disorders'

D. Deformities in association with neurofibromatosis
  1. Dystrophic deformities
  2. Idiopathic-type deformities

E. Mesenchymal deformities
  1. Heritable disorders of connective tissue
  2. Mucopolysaccharidoses
  3. Bone dysplasias
  4. Metabolic bone disease
  5. Endocrine disorders

F. Traumatic deformities
  1. Vertebral
  2. Extravertebral

G. Deformity due to infection
  1. Pyogenic infection
  2. Tuberculosis

H. Deformity due to tumours
  1. Intradural tumours
  2. Syringomyelia
  3. Paravertebral childhood tumours
  4. Primary extradural tumours
  5. Metastatic spinal disease

I. Miscellaneous conditions

muscular condition, the quest has been for some neuromuscular difference between right and left sides. This work has encompassed electro-encephalography, equilibrial function, and electromyography at one end of the spectrum to the structure and ultrastructure of the paraspinal muscles and the spinal cord at the other [7]. These investigations have shown that some evidence of abnormality can be demonstrated in some patients with idiopathic scoliosis, generally those with bigger curves, but not all patients, and indeed in many controls with straight backs. Thus these changes cannot be considered aetiological because if they were to be so then all patients with idiopathic scoliosis should have evidence of the abnormality. The correct inference from these studies is that such changes as have been demonstrated might be considered factors favouring progression of an established idiopathic deformity. Indeed it would be quite reasonable to imagine that if there was some subtle alteration in a spinal balance mechanism then the spine would be less able to resist buckling deformation.

Many studies, such as those concerned with electromyography or the structure of the paraspinal muscles, have demonstrated that whatever changes have been shown are secondary to the presence of the curve. This again is not surprising in the presence of a significant deformity of the axial skeleton. Moreover, none of these workers has produced any evidence of how a structural spinal deformity can be caused by, for example, a bit of equilibrial dysfunction.

Proponents of neuromuscular factors in the aetiology of idiopathic scoliosis have conveniently ignored the extensive literature on this subject dating from the beginning of the nineteenth century. The classic work of Adams in 1865 [6], and indeed other workers before him, indicated that the primary lesion of idiopathic scoliosis was a lordosis at the curve apex. Adams stated that 'lordosis plus rotation equals lateral flexion'. This statement was the result of his clinical observations as well as his dissections of individuals with idiopathic scoliosis. It was abundantly clear to him that once a lordosis developed in the thoracic spine, which should normally be kyphotic, then with both growth and forward flexion it would readily buckle round to the side to produce the appearances of a lateral curvature of the spine.

This lordosis theory can be readily confirmed by two simple observations. First, the PA radiograph of any patient with any form of structural scoliosis shows a lateral curvature of the spine with rotation such that the posterior elements lie in the curve concavity while the anterior vertebral bodies twist into the curve convexity (Fig. 7.2). As Roaf later pointed out, a line conjoining the tips of the spinous processes will thus pursue a shorter distance through the curve than a line conjoining the middle of the anterior bodies. The back of the spine is therefore shorter than the front and this elementary geometrical point confirms that every structural scoliosis, including the idiopathic variety, is lordotic. Second, it is a standard clinical observation since the time of Adams that the rotational deformity is much less obvious in the erect position than leaning forward. This is why the forward bending position is used in scoliosis clinics as well as in the field for epidemiological purposes. On forward flexion the over long front of the spine is forced to buckle to the side in order to be accommodated. The deformity of kypho-scoliosis does not therefore exist [5] and, as Steindler later pointed out [8], 'kyphosis is a condition which counteracts and not facilitates the presence of a lateral spinal curvature.'

If, however, the coronal and sagittal planes of the patient, and not the rotated deformity, are selected for X-ray purposes then both the PA and lateral views will therefore be oblique views of the apical region (the obliquity being dependent upon the degree of apical rotation). Stagnara demonstrated that by turning the patient or X-ray beam according to the amount of apical rotation a true PA view of the apex could be obtained and in this line of projection the deformity was maximal [9]. He referred to this as the 'plan d'election'. More importantly, if a true lateral view of the curve apex is obtained (90° to the plan d'election) then every structural scoliosis can be demonstrated to be lordotic over the apical three or four vertebral bodies (Fig. 7.3a). In Leeds we have now taken true planar views of more than 300 patients with idiopathic thoracic scoliosis and have also studied sagittal profile in the areas above and below the curve apex. The apical three or four vertebrae are always lordotic and this lordosis is at bone level, the disc height not contributing to spinal shape.

The appearances on the true lateral view are

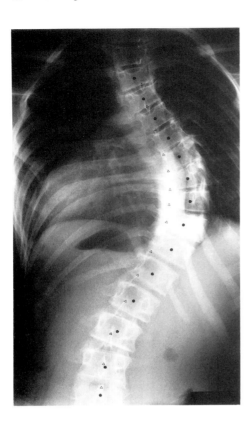

Fig. 7.2 PA radiograph of an idiopathic thoracic scoliosis. The tips of the spinous processes have been marked with hollow triangles and the centre of the anterior bodies with black dots. Therefore a line drawn through the curve along the posterior elements can be seen to be shorter than a line drawn down the vertebral bodies. The back of the spine is shorter than the front in every structural scoliosis and these deformities are therefore lordotic.

exactly the opposite of the other idiopathic deformity of childhood, Scheuermann's kyphosis (Fig. 7.3b). In the former the vertebral bodies are wedged, with anterior height being greater than posterior and any Schmorl node formation and end-plate irregularity being sited posteriorly. In Scheuermann's kyphosis, however, the bodies are wedged kyphotically with anterior height being reduced in comparison to posterior and any Schmorl's nodes or end-plate irregularity more anteriorly. Thus both idiopathic thoracic scoliosis and Scheuermann's kyphosis are principally concerned with shape in the sagittal plane over the three or four apical vertebrae. All that matters now is the position of this apical region in relationship to the axis of spinal column rotation, which normally passes anterior to the thoracic kyphosis and posterior to the cervical and lumbar lordoses. As the thoracic spine is normally kyphotic and lies behind this axis then it is under tension and will not therefore buckle to the side under the influence of either growth or forward flexion. Any excessive degree of thoracic kyphosis, as in Scheuermann's disease, puts the

thoracic kyphosis even further behind this axis while any degree of flattening of the thoracic spine brings the vertebral bodies closer to the buckling point. In the presence of a frank lordosis, as occurs in idiopathic scoliosis, then the front of the thoracic bodies at the curve apex lies anterior to the axis of spinal column rotation and on growth and forward flexion must mechanically buckle to the side to be accommodated.

These changes in the sagittal plane are not as gross as might be considered. The normal thoracic kyphosis extends from D3 to D10 (the upper and lower most thoracic vertebrae belonging to the cervical and lumbar lordoses, respectively). If we say that the degree of normal thoracic kyphosis from D3 to D 10 is of the order of 24° (this figure being selected for arithmetic ease principally) then the eight thoracic vertebrae between D3 and D10 would normally be kyphotically wedged by some 3° or so. Scheuermann's disease is diagnosed radiographically by three consecutive thoracic vertebrae being wedged by 5° or more [10]. Thus normal sagittal spine shape only has to increase over three vertebrae by 2° to be

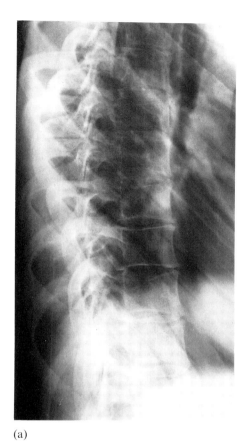 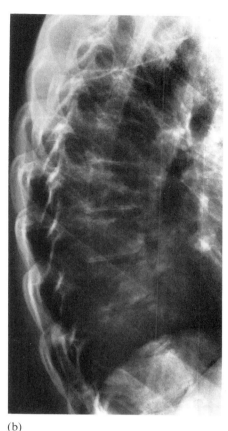

(a)　　　　　　　　　　　　　　　(b)

Fig. 7.3 (a) True lateral of the apex of an idiopathic thoracic curve showing lordotic vertebrae. (b) Lateral radiograph of the apex of idiopathic thoracic hyperkyphosis (Scheuermann's disease) which is the opposite deformity in the sagittal plane to idiopathic scoliosis.

diagnosed as Scheuermann's disease. Reciprocally, reduction of the normal thoracic kyphosis by just over 3° will produce an area of lordosis, the patient then developing idiopathic scoliosis.

Meanwhile children and adolescents are growing in three dimensions at the same time and it is an established fact that the normal thoracic kyphosis of late childhood flattens during early adolescence while again increasing just before maturity [11]. If the thoracic kyphosis flattens excessively during early adolescence and becomes frankly lordotic then the patient develops idiopathic scoliosis, a condition typically presenting in early adolescence [5]. On the other hand, if the patient's thoracic kyphosis becomes increased beyond the norm during later adolescence then the patient develops Scheuermann's disease, a condition characteristically appearing within 2 years of maturity. Both idiopathic scoliosis and Scheuermann's disease occur in otherwise entirely normal healthy children, occur at the same site with the D8–9 region being principally

affected, have a similar familial trend and community prevalence rate [10]. The familial trend has nothing whatever to do with a 'gene for idiopathic scoliosis or Scheuermann's disease' but reflects the familial trend in sagittal spine profile which has already been demonstrated in anthropometric studies. It is therefore quite unnecessary and indeed illogical to propose a primary neuromuscular cause.

However, should the neuromuscular balance mechanisms of the spine be in any way deficient then progression of this unstable deformity will be favoured. It is well known that in early onset idiopathic scoliosis the great majority of children have resolving curves. These children are characterized by being of normal birth weight, normotonic, and of normal neurological development scores. By contrast, the less common infantile malignant idiopathic progressive curve, while having exactly the same lordo-scoliotic deformity, is characteristically found in low birth weight, floppy, hypotonic babies with low neurological development scores [12]. In this situation progression of the deformity is strongly enhanced. Thus, as regards idiopathic deformities, they are divisible into two primordial types – lordosis (which buckles to the side to produce a secondary scoliotic deformity) and kyphosis (a deformity which is rotationally stable and stays in the sagittal plane). True sagittal plane views of the vertebrae above and below the apical region of an idiopathic scoliosis demonstrate that these vertebrae are truly kyphotic. Indeed this can be clearly seen on the PA radiograph of the patient (Fig. 7.2). Vertebral rotation, with the posterior elements being directed towards the curve concavity, persists into the upper and lower compensatory curves. If the scoliosis was of the typical right thoracic variety then above and below the apical region the compensatory curves are convex to the left, while the posterior elements are still rotated towards the left. This implies that

these areas of so-called 'compensatory scoliosis' are indeed asymmetric kyphoses restoring three dimensional spinal balance. In the infantile idiopathic malignant progressive curve the asymmetric kyphosis above the area of buckled lordosis can progress in its own right to produce a combination of deformities of angular kyphosis above and buckled lordosis below (Fig. 7.4).

Meanwhile in the patient with Scheuermann's kyphosis this area of deformity is balanced by lordoses above and below. The hyperlordosis below the apex of a Scheuermann's kyphosis may then buckle to the side to produce a secondary scoliotic deformity, as in idiopathic scoliosis. This accounts for why more than 60% of patients with Scheuermann's kyphosis have evidence of idiopathic scoliosis four or five segments below the apex of their kyphosis [13] (Fig. 7.5). It would be nonsensical to talk about two different pathological processes four or five vertebrae apart in an

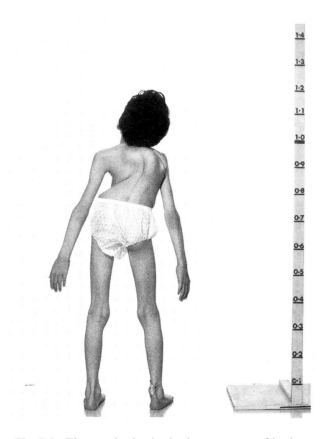

Fig. 7.4   The angular kyphosis above an area of lordoscoliosis is typical of the child with infantile progressive scoliosis.

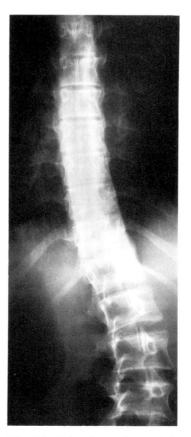

Fig. 7.5   PA spine radiograph in a case of Scheuermann's thoracic hyperkyphosis showing the associated lordoscoliosis in the lumbar region.

otherwise normal, healthy adolescent [5]. The idiopathic scoliosis below the Scheuermann's kyphosis seldom, however, achieves clinical significance. This is because the deformity of Scheuermann's kyphosis does not develop until much closer to skeletal maturity and because the area of kyphosis, so close to the area of buckled lordosis, protects from significant rotation.

The above analysis of idiopathic spinal deformities would reduce the average engineer to a state of boredom. He would readily confirm that his beam, or more strictly speaking cantilever, can in fact only fail in one of two ways – simple angular collapse (kyphosis) or beam buckling (lordo-scoliosis) [14]. He would also say that not only the development but also the subsequent behaviour of these two primordial deformity types is governed by elementary mechanical principles. This is where the rest of the aetiological classification of spinal deformities comes in. As regards beam buckling, this is governed by Euler's law and of the various parameters incorporated in this law some are more obviously relevant to spinal deformities.

If there is intrinsic weakness of the cantilever or, in this case spinal column, then beam buckling is facilitated. At bone level this weakness occurs in Von Recklinghausen's disease with its typical dystrophic vertebral form, osteogenesis imperfecta, the mucopolysaccharidoses, and skeletal dysplasias. Although the structural scoliosis in Von Recklinghausen's disease is of the same lordo-scoliotic type as seen in the idiopathic patient, the usually sharp, angular, dystrophic vertebral shape in association with an earlier onset deformity and more progressive one testifies to nothing more than the principles of Euler's law. Similarly in brittle bone disease, the worse the degree of the underlying condition, the more prevalent and progressive the spinal deformity associated with it. At soft tissue level, intrinsic spinal load is increased by soft tissue weakness of the cantilever or spinal column. Thus in Marfan's syndrome, homocystinuria, and Ehlers–Danlos syndrome, buckled lordo-scolioses are both more prevalent and progressive than in the idiopathic patient. At neuromuscular level, again Euler's law has to be obeyed. Patients with cerebral palsy, poliomyelitis, and the true neuromuscular conditions of childhood (e.g. the peripheral neuropathies, Friedreich's ataxia, and the muscular dystrophies) all have a higher prevalence rate and progression potential of buckled lordo-scolioses; the more severe the neuromuscular failure the more prevalent and progressive the spinal deformity. These neuromuscular deformities are generally long C-shaped collapsing deformities extending through the thoraco-lumbar region down to an oblique pelvis. Here the lumbar lordosis is often exaggerated as a part of the primary condition and once asymmetric paraspinal muscle action is applied then the deformity readily buckles (Fig. 7.6).

Simple angular collapse implies true material failure, either of the anterior column under compression, as in trauma, tumours, or infection, or the posterior elements under tension, as in flexion injuries of the spine, or post-laminectomy. As with the idiopathic counterpart, these deformities are behind the axis of spinal column rotation and do not rotate. In the trauma patient with para-

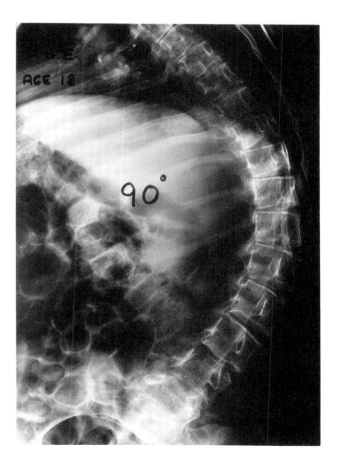

Fig. 7.6 The long c-shaped lordo-scoliosis with associated pelvic obliquity typical of the neuromuscular deformity.

lysis there is often an area of angular kyphosis where the bony injury occurred and below this an area of collapsing paralytic lordo-scoliosis secondary to neuromuscular failure in the region of a primary lordosis. If, however, paralysis is superimposed on an area of the spine which is primarily kyphotic, such as occurs with the congenital kyphosis of myelomeningocele, then the thoraco-lumbar spine is protected from buckling because the spine is behind the axis of spinal column rotation. Thus in the spina bifida kyphosis patient the spine remains in the sagittal plane (Fig, 7.7).

It can therefore be seen from the pathogenesis of idiopathic and other types of spinal deformity that these deformities can, and indeed must, be explicable on the basis of simple mechanical principles. Superimposed upon this is the biology of the situation and the more severe the underlying condition, the more its effect will be on increasing the intrinsic load to the spine. Meanwhile the idiopathic deformity, whose prevalence rate and progression potential is least obvious, must still obey Euler's law. The longer the cantilever or spinal column the more the centre of it will buckle, and it is interesting to note that patients with idiopathic scoliosis are marginally but significantly taller than their straight-backed counterparts [15]. Whether this merely implies a period of accelerated growth, the spine is still obeying Euler's law. Another important factor in this law is that the bigger the deformity the more likely it will be to progress. Thus a deformity of 40° is more progressive than a deformity of 20° on purely mechanical terms.

There are therefore two primordial types of spinal deformity – lordosis and kyphosis. The former can buckle to the side to produce the appearances of a structural scoliosis, while the latter remains in the sagittal plane. These two principal deformity types are seen throughout the classification of spinal deformities where the local biological situation dictates the severity of the mechanical response.

Management strategy

It is important to have an overall management strategy to which only detail needs to be added for the particular case or condition. There are four principal factors in this strategy – curve size, progression potential, the presence of paralysis, and the underlying condition.

Curve size

For centuries it has been recognized that the bigger the curve the more likely is the risk of subsequent cardiopulmonary dysfunction. Studies of untreated scoliosis patients have shown two to three times higher mortality and morbidity rates, as well as significant social and psychological impairment, with curves at the more severe end of the spectrum [16]. A figure of 60° has been bandied about as a threshold for thoracic curves at or above which it has been deemed necessary to prescribe surgical treatment in order to mitigate the future pulmonary consequences. This strategy, based upon curve size alone, is totally incorrect. The patients who form the basis of these long term studies were a hotchpotch of diagnoses, although usually idiopathic,

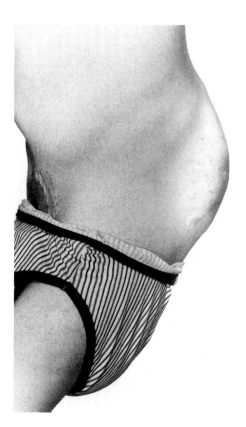

Fig. 7.7   The congenital lumbar kyphosis of myelomeningocele.

and had a very wide range of curve sizes. What was ignored in these studies was the age of onset of the curve. Clearly, all other things being equal, a curve of 130° must have started earlier than a curve of say 65°. The correct inference from these studies is that it is age of onset that matters rather than the actual curve size. Indeed in Nachemson's study he was able to identify a group of patients whose curves definitely started early in adolescence and these patients showed no differences whatever as regards organic ill health from control date [16].

More importantly Reid, the principal pathologist at the Brompton Hospital in London, had already performed autopsy studies on children with scoliosis who had died from other reasons and found that provided the curve was not considerable, not more than 60°, during the phase in which the pulmonary alveoli are developing, up to the age of 5, then there was no risk of severe pulmonary dysfunction no matter what size the curve ultimately achieved [17]. This largely ignored work has been recently confirmed by Branthwaite who surveyed all of Zorab's cases in the Brompton Hospital. She clearly demonstrated that late onset thoracic scoliosis, beyond the age of 5 years, was not associated with any risk of cardiopulmonary dysfunction in the future, while the much less common early onset progressive case, with an appreciable curve size during the phase of pulmonary alveolar development, was accountable for all the mortality and morbidity in thoracic scoliosis. It is therefore only necessary to consider two types of scoliosis – early onset and late onset. The former is a matter of great concern to organic ill health, while the latter is solely a question of deformity. Of course, the bigger the deformity, the more unfair life is to patients, with lower marriage rates, higher divorce rates, lower numbers of children per marriage, higher psychiatric consultation rates, and higher suicide rates, but this must be clearly demarcated from true organic ill health.

The majority of patients coming to surgical treatment are of the late onset variety and thus what matters is the deformity and what the patient and family's assessment of it is. If the deformity is deemed acceptable by the patient and family, and not by the surgeon whose opinion of somebody else's deformity is quite irrelevant, then preservation of acceptability is the aim. If, on the other hand, the deformity is

deemed unacceptable then treatment should be directed towards making it acceptable again. The management strategy for late onset scoliosis, as regards curve size, is therefore straightforward. If the deformity is acceptable then this would be the place for conservative treatment so that the deformity would never become unacceptable during growth. Thus far, bracing has been the mainstay of conservative treatment, although the French have used serial casts as an alternative and there has been some dabbling with electrospinal stimulation. The first popular brace was the Milwaukee brace [18] developed, not for the idiopathic patient, but for the poliomyelitis patient whose spine required support postoperatively. With the end of the great poliomyelitis epidemics the Milwaukee brace was soon used for idiopathic curves as a conservative measure. Although it enjoyed popularity for more than 2 decades, proponents never challenged its efficacy against untreated controls. There was therefore no scientific evidence that it either corrected the deformity or prevented its progression. A recent trial, albeit of a small number of patients, showed that there was no significant difference in the progression rates whether the brace was worn or not [19], while a recent study from Oxford showed that, even in the most apparently compliant patients, the brace was only worn for less than 20% of the time that it should have been. Meanwhile natural history studies have demonstrated that many fewer curves than formerly thought actually progress. For 30° curves in early adolescence one-third progress, one-third stay the same, and one-third actually improve somewhat. Against these natural history figures there is no evidence that either Milwaukee (or Boston) bracing is effective. Similarly, electro-spinal stimulation is ineffective and that has also been demonstrated by a controlled study [20].

It is not difficult to appreciate why the deformity of lordo-scoliosis cannot be treated non-operatively [21]. The opposite deformity of kyphosis, being a uniplanar deformity in the sagittal plane, requires extension and a patient with Scheuermann's disease can rapidly reduce their kyphosis wearing an extension brace or cast. This is because the deformity is rotationally stable. If, therefore, kyphosis requires extension then the opposite deformity of lordosis requires flexion and that is when it is rotationally unstable, buckling out to the side to enhance the rib

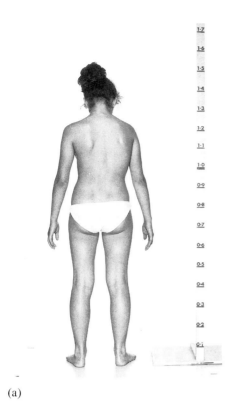

(a)

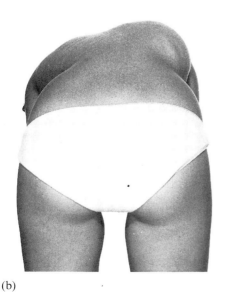

(b)

Fig. 7.8 (a, b) Erect and forward bending views of a girl
with idiopathic thoracic scoliosis showing that the
rotational prominence is enhanced on forward bending.

hump (Fig.7.8). It might, however, be conceived
that imprisoning a patient in some form of erect
orthosis or cast would at least minimize the
number of flexion cycles during the day and thus
attenuate progression but there is no evidence
that this is so. If the curve is going to get worse
then it will do so whether it is surrounded by a
brace or not.

Another common misunderstanding is the
duration of spinal growth. It has been assumed
that the spine stops growing at the same time as
the extremities and pelvis [22]. This would be at
about 15 years in girls and between 16 and 17
years in boys. As a result, inspection of the status
of ossification of the vertebral ring apophyses or
the iliac crest apophysis is used as an assessment
of adolescent growth and fusion is believed to
imply the attainment of spinal maturity.
Anatomists in previous centuries, have however
clearly shown that the vertebral end-plate epiphyses, not the ring apophyses which have
nothing whatever to do with spinal growth, do
not fuse on average until the 25th year [23]. This
does not mean that the spine grows inches
between 15 and 25 but that change of shape is still
possible until these end-plate epiphyses fuse.
While this may not have very much import to the
straight spine, it may be crucial for the deformed
spine whose buckling tendency will continue to
be accommodated until the middle of the third
decade. It is not therefore surprising to find evidence that curves continue to deteriorate until the
mid-20s although suppositions concerning the
effect of pregnancy have been shown to be erroneous. Thus, even if a conservative treatment
measure could be devised which prevented progression, it would have to be prescribed for a time
period not commensurate with patient com-
pliance. No 10-year-old girl would be prepared to
wear a contraption 23 hours a day for 15 years.

If the deformity is acceptable at presentation
then the patient should be observed at intervals
during the phase of spinal growth in order to
determine what the future has in store. The
majority will stay the same or regress and thus no
treatment will ever be required. The minority will
progress, but only some of them will progress
sufficiently to achieve unacceptability. These require surgical treatment.

For those that present with an unacceptable
deformity then correction is inherent in the
management strategy. This is the place of oper-

Spinal deformities 75

ative treatment. The earliest corrections were obtained pre-operatively using a localizer or turn-buckle cast but in the 1950s Harrington instrumentation was developed [24]. This system of distraction on the concave side combined with compression on the convex side was introduced for the poliomyelitis patient without fusion, but the metalwork rapidly failed without biological support. It was soon used for the idiopathic patient and although considerable spinal stability was achieved, such that the previously high pseudarthrosis rate was considerably reduced, the degree of correction was no better than that achieved by former casting methods. This is because the method of correction is by distraction at the top and bottom of the curve and cannot be expected to have any influence over the rotational disposition of the curve apex (Fig. 7.9). The rib hump therefore remained essentially unchanged.

The addition of wires attached to the posterior elements of the spine and tightened round the longitudinal metalwork enabled the apical region to be influenced, but the direction of pull was necessarily sideways [25]. Although the Cobb angle over the apical region was seen to be improved, there was no alteration of the rotational prominence because the metalwork was pulling behind the axis of spinal column rotation. Indeed in some cases rotation was made worse, while in others some cosmetic improvement occurred as a result of the rib hump being pulled more closely towards the midline. Like Harrington instrumentation, this technique of sublaminar wiring was developed for the poliomyelitis spine but soon found its greatest usage in the idiopathic case. In February 1982 in Leeds, following several years of clinical, mechanical, radiological, and animal experimentation [5], a technique was developed whereby the rib hump could be appreciably reduced by derotation. A longitudinal Harrington distraction rod was bent into 20° of kyphosis and segmental wires under the concave laminae were then tightened. The direction of the pull of these wires was thus more backwards than sideways so that the concave side was elevated and the convex side reciprocally depressed with a reduction in the rotational prominence (Fig. 7.10). As a result, there was not only an enhanced correction in the coronal plane but an average 50% correction of the rotational disposition of the apical vertebra [26]. Then, 1 year later, Cotrel

and Dubousset developed a similar system of derotation and thoracic kyphosis restoration by bending a longitudinal rod favouring the lateral curvature and then rotating it round 90° into the sagittal plane with the spine attached to it (Fig. 7.11). The addition of a convex rod, slightly less bent, applied downward pressure on the convex side. For mild, flexible curves only a 40% derotation was achieved [27]. None the less, it is the rotational prominence with which the majority of patients present and which in turn these patients wish corrected and these are the only two methods which will do so.

Then in the 1960s Dwyer, in Australia, developed his system of anterior spinal instrumentation, this time for the idiopathic thoracolumbar or lumbar curve [28]. Screws are passed transversely through the vertebral bodies from convex to concave sides and then a braided metal cable is passed through holes in the screw heads. Using a special cable tightener, followed by crimping the screw heads over the cable, the convex side was shortened and correction facilitated by excision of the intervertebral discs in the curve. Good corrections were observed in the coronal plane but the complication rate was high. More recently this instrumentation has been upgraded by Zielke and the German instrument school [29]. The metalwork is superior but the technique and results similar. Although popularized for the idiopathic case these instrumentation systems are more often used for paralytic thoraco-lumbar and lumbar curves with pelvic obliquity, as a preliminary first stage (Fig. 7.12).

The method by which all of these instrumentation techniques achieve a correction is by taking up the natural flexibility of the curve. If a curve measures say 60° standing and 30° on side bending or under maximum traction then the instrumentation will correct the curve down to 30° but seldom any further. The bigger a curve gets the more rigid it becomes and flexibility correspondingly reduces. Thus for the more severe and less flexible curve little is achieved by instrumentation alone. In order to enter this rigid phase spinal traction was devised so that before the instrumentation stage as much pre-operative correction as possible was obtained. Unfortunately there is no evidence that any form of traction enters this rigid phase, and one study comparing Cotrel dynamic traction versus localizer casting versus halo-pelvic traction showed

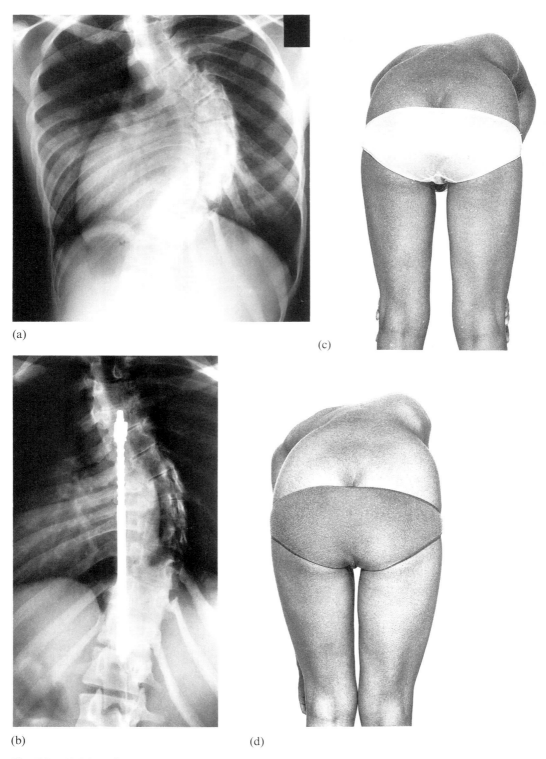

Fig. 7.9 (a) PA radiograph of an idiopathic thoracic scoliosis before surgery. (b) PA radiograph after Harrington distraction instrumentation and fusion showing a seemingly good correction. (c) Forward bending view of this girl before surgery. (d) Forward bending view 2 years after surgery showing no change whatever in the rotational prominence with which she presented.

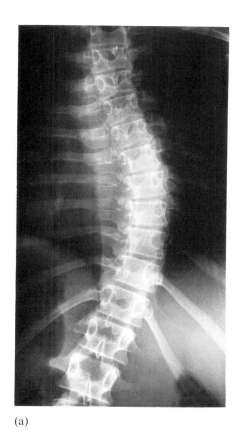

(a)

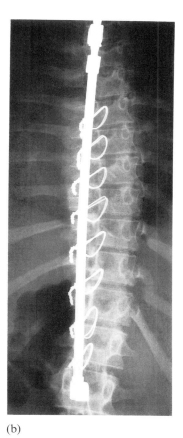

(b)

Fig. 7.10 The Leeds procedure – segmental derotation combined with thoracic kyphosis recreation. (a) PA radiograph of an idiopathic thoracic curve before surgery. (b) PA radiograph after the Leeds procedure. (c) Forward bending view showing the obvious rib hump before surgery. (d) Forward bending view 2 years after surgery showing an almost complete correction of the rotational element of the deformity.

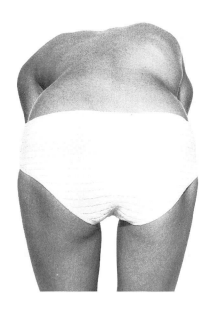

(c)

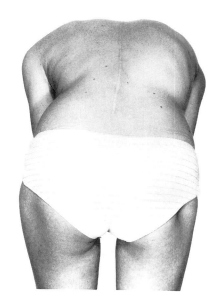

(d)

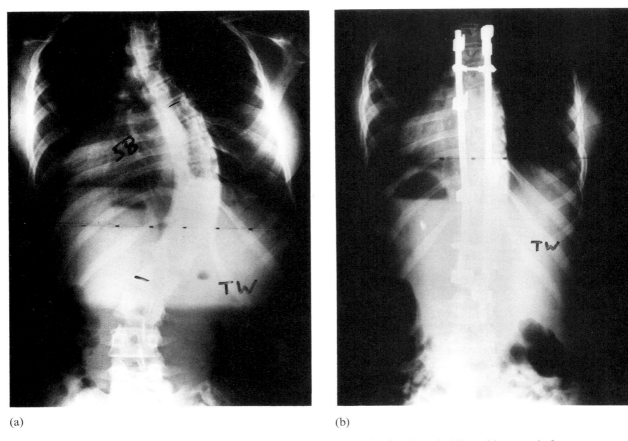

(a)   (b)

Fig. 7.11   Cotrel–Dubousset (CD) instrumentation. (a) PA radiograph of a thoracic idiopathic curve before surgery. (b) PA radiograph after surgery. The improved rib symmetry indicates appreciable derotation.

no significant differences with none of the treatment modalities able to enter the rigid phase [30].

The only effective way to enter this phase is by surgical intervention [26]. For curves that are not excessive, but are beyond a one posterior instrumentation stage, flexibility can be achieved by way of a preliminary soft tissue release. As the back of the spine is shorter than the front and is therefore the compression side, it would appear logical to release the relatively tighter posterior soft tissue structures, but this would lead to unacceptable lengthening of the curve with an increased risk of tension paralysis. The soft tissue release should therefore be performed anteriorly by way of multiple discectomies of the apical region. Then in the second posterior instrumentation stage, the same instrumentation procedure as is performed for the more mild and flexible curve, there is room for the over long front of the spine to be pulled through without causing undue

lengthening (Fig. 7.13). Moreover, and very importantly, along with the discs are removed the vertebral growing end-plates so that the front of the spine will not overgrow in the future.

For the most severe and rigid curves, of whatever aetiology, even anterior discectomy is insufficient. The only satisfactory solution to this problem of straightening a rigid, bent pipe which contains the vital spinal cord is to shorten the apex of the pipe itself. This is achieved by way of two stage wedge resection, a technique devised and popularized by Leatherman [31]. When rigid congenital curves were first dealt with it was by way of either one stage hemivertebrectomy or by opening wedge osteotomy. The complication rate, and in particular the paralysis rate, was unacceptably high because too much surgery was done at one sitting, shortening was not a feature of the procedure, and there was little stability available as Harrington instrumentation had not

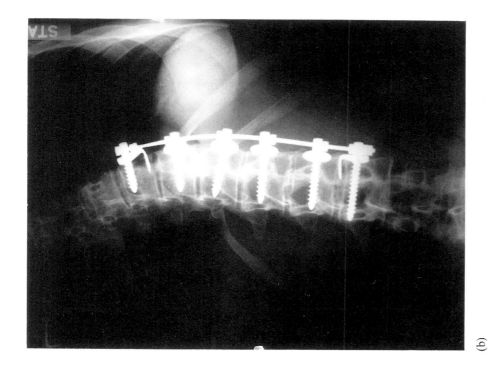

(b)

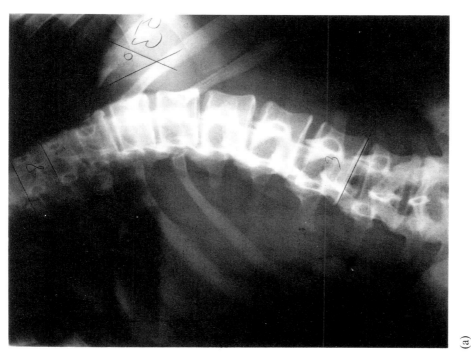

(a)

Fig. 7.12 The Zielke procedure. (a) PA radiograph of a thoraco-lumbar idiopathic curve before surgery. (b) PA radiograph after anterior segmental Zielke instrumentation showing a good correction.

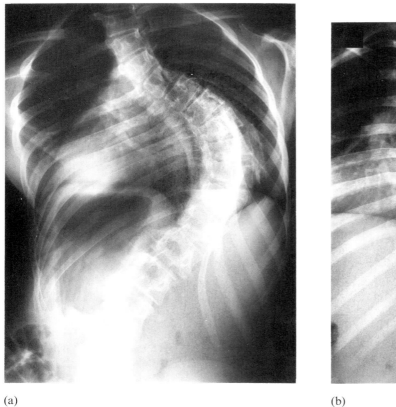

(a)

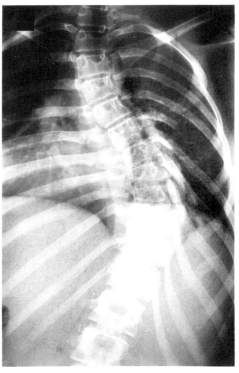

(b)

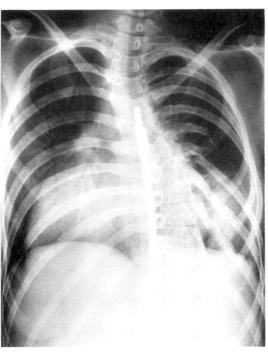

(c)

Fig. 7.13   Two stage anterior and posterior Leeds procedure. (a) PA radiograph of a severe thoracic idiopathic scoliosis before surgery. (b) PA radiograph a few days after anterior multiple discectomy. The deformity has collapsed into itself spontaneously without instrumental correction. (c) PA radiograph just after second stage posterior Leeds instrumentation showing further improvement but the great majority of the correction has occurred between stages spontaneously.

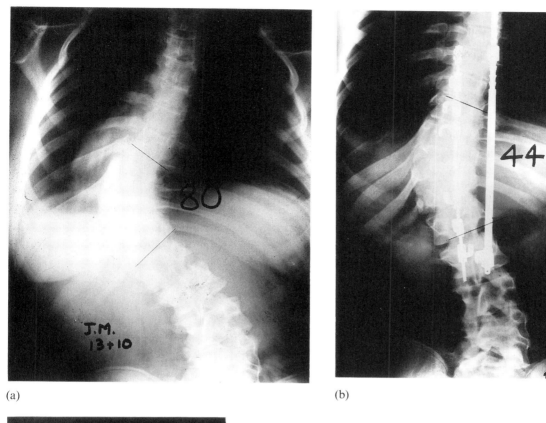

(a)

(b)

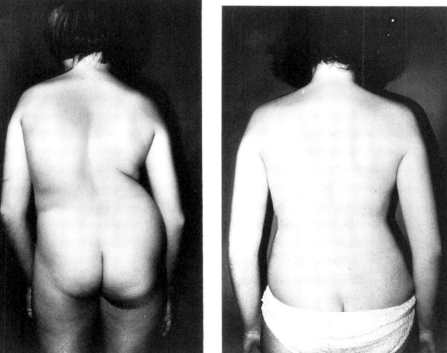

(c)

(d)

Fig. 7.14 Leatherman's two stage closing wedge osteotomy and fusion for severe rigid curves. (a) PA radiograph of a severe lower thoracic curve before surgery. (b) PA radiograph postoperatively. (c) Back view of this girl before surgery showing a severe deformity. (d) Back view 2 years after surgery showing no appreciable torso asymmetry. Radiographs say little about surface shape.

yet been devised. Two stage wedge resection fulfils these criteria and in the first stage the anterior vertebral body, which is always wedge shaped in three dimensions, is resected. In the second stage the posterior elements are resected to complete the wedge excision. Then a Harrington compression system is applied to the convex side and tightened so that the wedge is closed. Only then is a distraction rod inserted on the concave side to aid stability and to gain some correction in the upper and lower compensatory curves (Fig. 7.14). This procedure has stood the test of time and is the safest way of dealing with a severe rigid curve. It is always far better to plan two stages, although this means more surgery for the patient, than to take on too big and rigid curves by means of one instrumentation stage only.

The early onset curve is undoubtedly the most difficult to treat. Fortunately more than 90% of early onset idiopathic curves resolve spontaneously, but those that do not are as progressive as their congenital and Von Recklinghausen's counterparts. If the rib vertebra angle difference is in excess of 20° or rises on sequential measurements, particularly in the low birth weight hypotonic baby, then action must be taken immediately. Serial EDF casting has been shown to convert curves with all the hallmarks of progression into resolving or static ones [12]. This is infinitely preferable to having to tackle these curves surgically at such an early age. Unfortunately many do not present until curve size is excessive, and so of course is rigidity, in which case a preliminary anterior stage is very often necessary.

Progression potential

During the phase of spinal growth, i.e. the first 25 years of life, spinal deformities have progression potential. Thus for curves which have been seen to progress during the phase of observation, or those which have been corrected surgically, it is necessary to prevent subsequent progression with growth. This is the place for spinal fusion operations. At the beginning of this century when spinal fusion was first carried out it was performed posteriorly principally for the convenience of the surgeon. It was not, however, clear at that time that the essential lesion of structural

scoliosis is an apical lordosis [5] and thus posterior fusion would not appear to be the most logical solution to progression potential. It is rather akin to performing a postero-medial fusion for talipes equinovarus instead of the postero-medial release which is obviously to be preferred. None the less, the great majority of patients being treated were adolescents with idiopathic curves whose growth velocity was waning and for whom posterior fusion did appear to stop or minimize progression subsequently. With the development of Harrington instrumentation it became standard practice to correct the curve with the instrumentation and at the same sitting perform a posterior spinal fusion in order to prevent progression. Long term studies of this procedure have demonstrated that, despite an initial correction due to the instrumentation, the fusion of the over short back of the spine does lead in most cases to subsequent further buckling so that 2 or 3 years from surgery the deformity is very much the same as that pre-operatively.

The younger the child in whom posterior fusion is performed the greater is the risk of tethering the back of the spine in bone and thus allowing the anterior bodies, which are already overgrowing, to buckle round to the side (Fig. 7.15). Thus purely posterior fusion for young patients is positively harmful [32] and for early onset curves the spine must be fused front and back in order to both attenuate spinal growth locally and stabilize the deformity from progression. The opinion is still widely held that as soon as an early onset curve has demonstrated progression it should be forthwith dealt with by posterior fusion, but long term studies of this approach testify to its harmful effect. The strategy as regards progression potential is therefore simple. If the curve is late onset it can be held by a posterior fusion, but only reliably so if the thoracic kyphosis is recreated during the instrumentation procedure so that the spine is now put in its right position in relationship to the axis of spinal column rotation [26]. For young patients with progressive curves the spine must be fused front and back. Furthermore, for curves of greater progression potential than idiopathic ones, e.g. those in Von Recklinghausen's disease or the heritable disorders of connective tissue, posterior fusion is never sufficient to mitigate progression and an anterior fusion should always be performed.

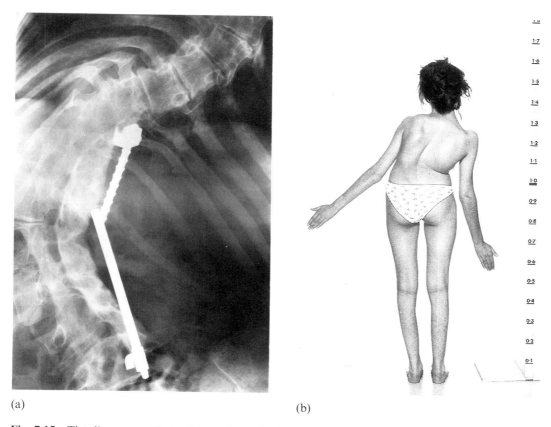

(a)   (b)

Fig. 7.15 The disastrous effects of posterior tethering fusion on the young spine. (a) & (b) PA radiograph and appearance in the erect position showing an idiopathic lumbar scoliosis with a tethered posterior fusion, a broken rod, and almost 90° of apical rotation.

The presence of paralysis

There are two important factors here – the presence of a neuromuscular condition, or the presence of a structure which may itself induce paralysis. For the typical paralytic lordo-scoliosis with pelvic obliquity it has become quite clear that the spine cannot be reliably propped up by posterior instrumentation and fusion alone. Anterior instrumentation and fusion should always be insisted upon as a preliminary first stage. Moreover, the indications for operating on the paralytic spine have also become quite clear. It was generally accepted that if either walking potential or sitting stability were being jeopardized by the presence of the scoliosis then surgery was indicated. However, Lonstein, when he looked at the results of surgery in more than 100 cases of cerebral palsy scoliosis, showed the futility and harm of operating on the walking patient [33]. The great majority of these patients do require a mobile lumbar hyper-lordosis in order to walk at all to counter gluteal muscle weakness. If the lumbar spine is then flattened and made rigid as a result of surgery, many of these patients, who still had walking potential were rendered wheelchair bound. Therefore the only indication for operating on the paralytic spine with pelvic obliquity is loss of sitting stability. If the patient is unable to sit in a wheelchair without the use of their arms for support then the spine should be stabilized surgically which will liberate the hands for prehensile function.

It is important to be aware of conditions associated with a high risk of paralysis by way of natural history or treatment. There is a high incidence of spinal dysraphism in patients with

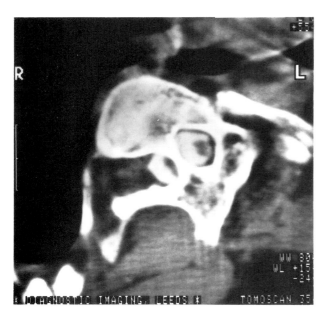

Fig. 7.16   CT myelogram showing a diastematomyelia, a bony spur splitting the cord.

congenital spine deformities and thus all patients should be assessed pre-operatively by way of spinal cord imaging (Fig. 7.16). Should the cord be cleaved by a diastematomyelia, or compressed locally by an intradural lipoma, or be associated with a tethered filum terminale then surgical treatment is extremely dangerous without the offending structure being removed by way of a preliminary laminectomy. In any event the spinal deformity must always be shortened during straightening in these rigid deformities [31].

If the patient with the seemingly typical idiopathic deformity is troubled by spinal pain, particularly at night, then this should raise suspicion of spinal tumour. Some will be found on technetium bone scanning to have an osteoid osteoma/osteoblastoma, but others will be shown by spinal cord imaging to be associated with an intradural neoplasm or syrinx. This latter group are particularly important. Spinal cord tissue is already embarrassed by the space occupying lesion and if this is not recognized and the spine is corrected by way of distraction instrumentation the paralysis rate is in excess of 50%. Such spines should therefore be dealt with neurosurgically and then stabilized by spinal fusion but no attempt at correction of the deformity should be made.

The underlying condition

Under no circumstances should the spinal deformity be divorced from the underlying condition. In patients with Duchenne dystrophy, homocystinuria, Ehlers–Danlos syndrome, and many other conditions associated with a spinal deformity there are matters of much greater import to the patient than the spinal deformity. Although most patients with Duchenne dystrophy develop a significant paralytic scoliosis while sitting in their wheelchair, death is inevitable from an underlying cardiomyopathic or pulmonary event by the end of their teens. While it may seem beneficial for these patients to have a stable spine during their terminal years the mortality rate of 10% from simple posterior spinal instrumentation and fusion is unacceptable.

Patients who demonstrate generalized ligament laxity and have features of the Marfan's syndrome should be very carefully assessed by clinical experts in this field. If the patient has true Marfan's syndrome, or a forme fruste thereof, then surgery is not contraindicated. If, however,

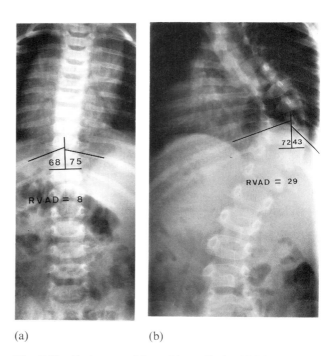

(a)   (b)

Fig. 7.17   Early onset idiopathic scoliosis. (a) PA radiograph of a resolving curve with a small Cobb angle and small/rib vertebra angle difference (RVAD). (b) PA radiograph of a progressive infantile curve with a large Cobb angle and RVAD.

the patient has homocystinuria then intra-vascular coagulation is very prevalent following surgical intervention such that the mortality is unacceptable high. Similarly if the patient has the type of Ehlers–Danlos syndrome which is associated with blood vessel fragility then excessive haemorrhage during surgical intervention is the rule rather than the exception. Again the mortality rate is too high to contemplate surgical intervention here.

Although these conditions are nowhere near as common as idiopathic scoliosis, knowledge of the important aspects of the underlying condition is crucial to the appreciation of when and when not to operate. With so many powerful weapons in our surgical armamentarium the most important decision a surgeon can reach is when not to operate.

Types of spinal deformity

Idiopathic deformities

Idiopathic scoliosis

Early onset idiopathic scoliosis

The much more common resolving form is differentiated from the progressive form by clinical and radiographic examination (Fig. 7.17). The resolving variety is found in normal birth weight healthy looking babies whose deformities are completely correctible during side bending over the examiner's knee. Curve size is modest and the rib-vertebra angle difference (RVAD) less than 20°. The progressive variety occurs in low birth weight floppy babies with rigid deformities which show no correction on side-bending. Curve size is greater and the RVAD is in excess of 20°. Both types share the same body moulding features of plagiocephaly, plagiopelvy, bat ear, and sometimes a torticollis [12]. This is attributable to lateral decubitus cot positioning, whereas prone cot positioning seems to prevent such moulding. The moulding features are more obvious in the progressive case.

Resolving scoliosis merely requires serial observation to ensure regression although the rotational prominence is often the last clinical feature to disappear, sometimes taking as long as 10 years. Progressive curves require immediate

treatment by way of serial EDF casting and this can be performed under very light general anaesthesia [12]. The cast is changed every 3 or 4 months according to the growth of the child. By this means some are converted to 'resolvers', but some remain static and may form the template for subsequent progression during adolescence. Although it is traditional to apply a spinal brace after, say, 2 years of casting there is no evidence that this alters the natural history of the condition. Clearly, the static curves may require surgical treatment for progression during adolescence. For those who present too late for effective cast treatment, or for those who fail to respond to cast treatment, surgical intervention is necessary. If the deformity is acceptable then anterior and posterior spinal fusion should be performed. If the deformity is unacceptable then correction is necessary. Moderate curves with some flexibility respond well to multiple anterior discectomy followed by posterior spinal fusion with Harrington instrumentation, trying as far as possible to create some degree of thoracic kyphosis [26]. For those with the most rigid curves there is no substitute for two stage wedge resection [31].

Late onset idiopathic scoliosis

If the deformity is acceptable then preservation of acceptability is the aim. Unfortunately no non-operative method alters the natural course of this form of scoliosis and thus a period of observation is necessary [21]. Should the deformity be unacceptable, or achieve unacceptability during observation, then surgical correction is necessary. It should be emphasized that unacceptability is a matter for the patient and family and not for the orthopaedic surgeon. Obviously if the patient is young with the curve progressing during observation then the surgeon can advise the parents that the deformity may finish up two or three times as bad as it is at present and this may influence in favour of early surgical intervention. However, if the patient is beyond skeletal maturity, or indeed in their early twenties, then progression potential is generally insignificant. Surgical intervention, therefore, is a matter solely for the patient and family to decide upon.

Thoracic curves should be dealt with by recreation of the thoracic kyphosis and in Leeds we favour a kyphotic distraction rod using sublaminar wires on the concave side to derotate [26] (Figs 7.10 and 7.13). If the convex rib prominence appears obvious following instrumentation then further correction of the rib hump can be achieved by dividing the apical ribs just beyond the transverse processes and tucking the lateral end under the medial. This is a minor procedure and is performed subperiosteally and extrapleurally. It adds little to the operative time and postoperative discomfort is minimized by infiltrating bupivacaine into, or cryoprobing, the local intercostal nerves. Posterior spinal fusion out to the tips of the transverse processes is then performed and homograft cancellous bank bone laid into the bed. It is quite unnecessary to remove bone from the patient's pelvis which adds to the scarring, operative time, blood loss, and postoperative discomfort.

It is preferable to perform this, and all other types of, instrumentation under continuous spinal cord monitoring and a 50% change in amplitude or latency demands an immediate 'wake-up' test to ensure that the spinal cord is not jeopardized by tension. The use of a combination of Harrington distraction instrumentation with sublaminar wiring is associated with a higher neurological complication rate but this is not due to the sublaminar position of the wires but rather what is done with them. If the Harrington rod is first maximally distracted before the wires are tightened then the spinal deformity is made rigid under tension. The wires will then almost certainly not be able to bring the spine in contact with the rod but more important the bony spine will be further lengthened, thus incurring the risk of paralysis. The correct method of performing this procedure is therefore to distract the rod sufficiently to engage the hooks only. Then the sublaminar wires are tightened. Further distraction is then only permissible when all the wires are tight and the spine is in contact with the rod throughout [26]. It is usually found that the rod will not distract any further after the wires have been tightened. It is therefore attention to operative detail in relationship to an understanding of the three dimensional nature of the deformity of structural scoliosis which minimizes neurological complication rather than having to rely on spinal cord monitoring or the 'wake-up' test.

It is probably unnecessary to support the spine postoperatively when there is a combination of rods and sublaminar wires, but in Leeds we prefer to apply a lightweight zippable polyurethane (Neofract) support for the first 6 months. For those who have undergone convex rib division we apply a Cotrel EDF cast with a pull strap over the rib prominence for the first 6 weeks until these iatrogenic rib fractures unite. This allows the rib hump to be favourably influenced until rib union.

Thoraco-lumbar and lumbar idiopathic curves require much thought before surgical intervention. Long term studies of these lower curves when dealt with by posterior spinal instrumentation and fusion have demonstrated a high incidence of the ugly flat back deformity with spinal pain, presumably from overloading the lower lumbar discs. This is in many situations a worse deformity than the patient had preoperatively. In Leeds we would endorse Nachemson's view that lumbar curves should not be operated upon and that a mobile lumbar spine, albeit deformed, is better than a straighter, flatter, rigid one [34]. Thoraco-lumbar curves can be managed by anterior Dwyer or Zielke instrumentation because it is not necessary to incorporate so many vertebrae in the fusion. None the less, some degree of flattening of the upper lumbar spine will occur. For double structural curves with a thoracic and thoraco-lumbar/lumbar component the same strictures apply. The lower curve should not be operated upon but, as is often the case, it is the thoracic component with its rib hump that is the more significant. This should be dealt with as for a single thoracic curve leaving a mobile, albeit somewhat deformed, lower spine. For a thoracic double structural curve, with two apices, one at D3 and one at D8/9, it is important that the rod crosses the spine to be inserted on the upper concave side of the upper curve. In this situation it is advisable not to use sublaminar wires but to perform convex rib division of the lower curve.

It is therefore thoracic curves with their associated rib hump which are most suitable for surgery. One stage posterior instrumentation and fusion is satisfactory for curves that are relatively mild and flexible but bigger curves, i.e. those with a Cobb angle between 65° and 90° do require anterior multiple discectomy in order to allow some flexibility and shortening [14,26]. For curves in excess of 90° or those which have undergone a previous fusion, there is no substitute for the safety and correctibility of two stage wedge resection [31] (Fig. 7.14).

Idiopathic kyphosis

This is the opposite deformity to idiopathic scoliosis and there are two types. Type I occurs in the thoracic region at the T8–9 level during late adolescence and is much the more common. Type II (apprentice's spine) occurs in the thoracolumbar or upper lumbar regions and is thought to be an epiphyseal response to strenuous activity.

Type II presents as a result of lumbar spine pain and the deformity is never considerable. By contrast, Type I presents with an increased thoracic kyphosis and local discomfort. On physical examination the deformity is rigid and this differ-

entiates it from postural round back deformity. Radiographs demonstrate the opposite lesion to idiopathic scoliosis with an increased kyphotic wedging over the apical three vertebrae. There is often a mild idiopathic scoliosis four or five segments below the apex of the kyphosis and this is due to the compensatory lordosis buckling to the side [13]. Treatment is nearly always conservative and any form of extension orthosis or cast leads to a rapid correction of this rotationally stable deformity (Fig. 7.18). Because spinal maturity does not occur until the middle of the third decade, conservative treatment should always be prescribed up to this age. Only if the deformity is excessive in the older individual should surgery be considered. Anterior multiple discectomy with interbody and strut grafting followed by a second stage posterior instrumentation using rectangular segmental instrumentation is required to correct and stabilise

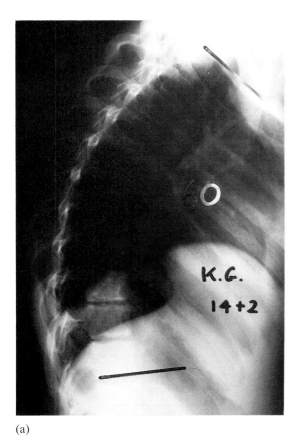

(a)

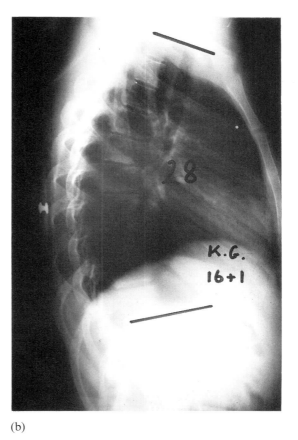

(b)

Fig. 7.18   Extension brace treatment for thoracic Scheuermann's disease. (a) Before treatment showing 60° of kyphosis. (b) After a year's extension bracing showing a more than 50% correction.

these deformities and this is not inconsiderable surgery while achieving a less than 50% correction of the degree of kyphosis. The real indication for surgery is the rare case with such a severe degree of kyphosis as to be jeopardizing neurological function in which case anterior dural decompression is additionally required in the first stage.

Congenital deformities

Congenital bony deformities

The offending congenital anomaly is either a failure of formation (hemivertebra) or a failure or segmentation (bar). There are two principal deformity types according to direction – scoliosis or kyphosis. If the hemivertebra or bar is on one side of the spine (unilateral) then a scoliosis develops, whereas if the growth discrepancy occurs in the sagittal plane an angular kyphosis develops. The progression potential is worst when there is a bar on one side and a hemivertebra on the other, there being no growth plates on one side of the spine and too many on the other. Thus prognosis can be estimated according to the nature of the underlying anomaly [35]. Solitary hemivertebrae do not give rise to a significant progressive deformity and occurs solely in the coronal plane (the only true progressive scoliosis). If the hemivertebra occur in the lower lumbar region in the presence of a sacral tilt towards the side of the hemivertebra (a bad lumbo-sacral offshoot) then a progressive list can develop which can produce an ugly deformity (Fig. 7.19). By contrast, unilateral bars affect the back of the spine as well and thus the typical structural lordo-scoliosis is produced which progresses both by way of growth asymmetry and mechanical buckling. A rotational prominence is thus generated [14] (Fig. 7.20).

In the sagittal plane kyphoses usually occur at the thoraco-lumbar region. Anterior bars seldom produce a kyphosis of significance but the dorsal hemivertebra (anterior failure of formation) is notorious in producing an angular progressive kyphosis with neurological signs.

The intradural anomalies of spinal dysraphism are common in association with a congenital spine deformity and should be excluded by myelography, CT, or both. In addition, there is also a high prevalence rate of urinary anomalies and these should be assessed routinely by intravenous urography.

Treatment is a question of either progression potential or the presence of neurological signs. A thoracic or thoraco-lumbar hemivertebra requires observation only and the less segmented the hemivertebra the less is the progression potential and therefore the likelihood of the need for treatment [35]. Failures of segmentation are dangerous in terms of progression potential and while they should also be observed with the passage of time surgical intervention is frequently required. If the deformity is acceptable then preservation of acceptability is the aim and for this anterior and posterior fusion is required. If the deformity is unacceptable then the only safe solution to this problem is by way of two stage wedge resection of the curve apex [31]. For the lower lumbar/lumbo-sacral hemivertebra no action is required if the sacrum is horizontal. In the pres-

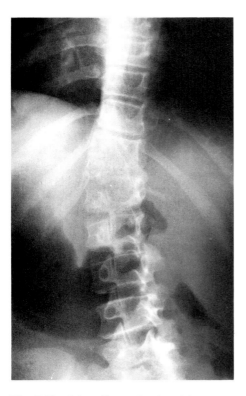

Fig. 7.19 PA radiograph of a girl with a lumbo-sacral hemivertebra on the right tilting the lumbar spine to the left. A T11–12 hemivertebra on the left helps to restore balance.

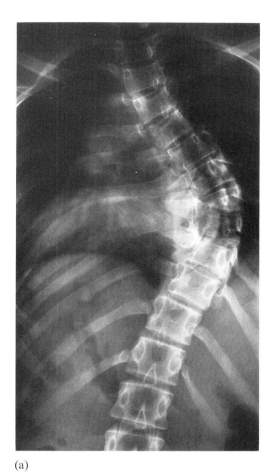

(a)

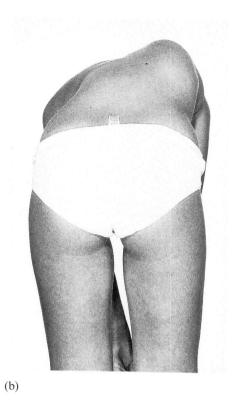

(b)

Fig. 7.20 (a) PA radiograph of a girl with a congenital thoracic scoliosis due to a unilateral unsegmented bar. (b) Forward bending view of this girl showing the significant rotational prominence associated with this lordo-scoliosis.

ence of an offshoot progression is inevitable and an early fusion does protect against progression. Because of the difficulties of anterior fusion in the lumbo-sacral region a posterior fusion suffices. For those presenting with an unacceptable deformity two stage hemivertebra resection is required [31]. In the second stage the lumbar lordosis must be maintained by contoured posterior metalwork and the entire structural curve should be fused. There is a considerable danger of L5 nerve root damage during hemivertebra removal and thus prophylactic fusion while the deformity is still acceptable is to be preferred.

Kyphoses should not be treated for cosmetic reasons only. The dorsal hemivertebra with the sinister neurological effects must be watched carefully (Fig. 7.21). There is a definite place for prophylactic anterior and posterior fusion for the progressive case. If neurological signs are already present (leg weakness, hyperreflexia, and clonus) then the spinal canal must be decompressed anteriorly by removal of the offending hemivertebra followed by anterior strut grafting 31]. The problem is pressure from the front and thus laminectomy is not only futile but positively harmful by way of removing the integrity of the posterior column.

If an intradural tethering structure is present then there is usually cutaneous evidence (tuft of hair, naevus, dimple, or sinus) and the patient may have already presented with either incomplete control of micturition or an attenuated lower limb, often with an associated club foot deformity. Opinion varies concerning the need for treatment but a consensus opinion would be to remove the offending structure by way of laminectomy to deter neurological deterioration in the future. If corrective surgery is contemplated on a congenital spinal deformity in the presence of an intradural tethering lesion, then the tether should be removed by a preliminary laminectomy [31].

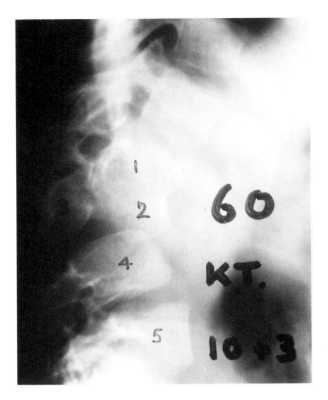

Fig. 7.21   Lateral radiograph showing a congenital dorsal hemivertebra. Cord compression commonly ensues.

Congenital cord deformities

These represent the spina bifida syndrome where there is evidence of myelodysplasia and neurological dysfunction. The more severe the neurological dysfunction the more the likelihood of a significant collapsing lordo-scoliosis with pelvic obliquity. This is difficult surgery with potentially serious complications (pseudarthrosis and sepsis being the most relevant). The walkers should not be treated lest a rigid and flat lumbar spine militates against ambulation. It is the wheelchair sitter who is losing sitting stability that merits surgical intervention and this must be in the nature of both anterior and posterior instrumentation and fusion [14] (Fig. 7.22).

Forty percent of progressive scolioses in the spina bifida syndrome are due to congenital bony anomalies in the thoraco-lumbar region with a relatively straight lumbar spine below. These should be dealt with by two stage wedge resection of the curve apex, again for sitting stability reasons [14].

Ten percent of deformities in association with myelodysplasia are lumbar kyphoses (the congenital lumbar kyphosis of myelomeningocele). The problem here is of kyphotic vertebral wedging at the curve apex, present since birth, associated with anterior soft tissue contracture (annulae fibrosi), anterior longitudinal ligament, diaphragmatic crura, iliac psoas, and even the anterior abdominal wall. Again treatment is for sitting stability that is being lost. Two-stage surgery is again required and in the first stage a thorough anterior division of all tight structures is required, followed by second stage posterior instrumentation and fusion [36] (Fig. 7.23).

Neuromuscular deformities

Cerebral palsy, poliomyelitis, and the true neuromuscular disorders of childhood (spinal muscular atrophy; the peripheral neuropathies, Friedreich's ataxia, and arthrogryposis; the muscular dystrophies) are all associated with a tendency towards a paralytic thoraco-lumbar collapsing scoliosis with pelvic obliquity. The prevalence rate and progression potential of these deformities correlates well with the degree of neuromuscular deficiency. Thus a scoliosis of significance occurs in 75% of patients with Friedreich's ataxia but only 10% of patients with the peripheral neuropathies. Similarly, the early onset (Werdnig–Hoffman) spinal muscular atrophy is notorious in comparison with the later onset (Kugelberg–Welander) variety. The underlying condition is also important. The more severe the neurological dysfunction in the cerebral palsy patient, the greater the degree of mental impairment, such that these children are often not able to capitalize on treatment programmes. The more severe the condition (e.g. Werdnig–Hoffman spinal muscular atrophy or Duchenne dystrophy) the shorter the life expectancy and while surgery may be clearly indicated for spinal reasons this must be balanced against the future for the child. By contrast, the congenital myopathy varieties of muscular dystrophy are stable and non-progressive conditions but surgery is often poorly tolerated because of cardiac and pulmonary dysfunction. All these matters must be taken into consideration before a decision is reached in favour of surgical intervention [14].

As for other paralytic spinal deformities it is

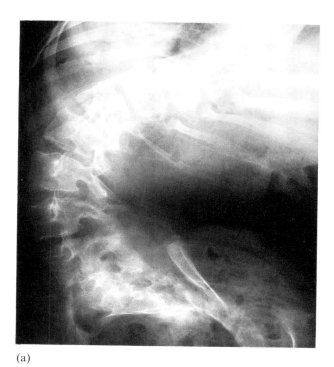

(a)

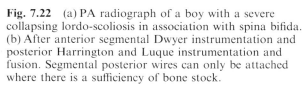

Fig. 7.22 (a) PA radiograph of a boy with a severe collapsing lordo-scoliosis in association with spina bifida. (b) After anterior segmental Dwyer instrumentation and posterior Harrington and Luque instrumentation and fusion. Segmental posterior wires can only be attached where there is a sufficiency of bone stock.

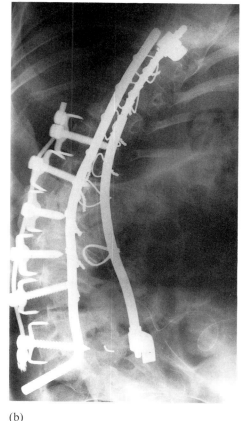

(b)

injudicious to contemplate surgery on the walker. A feature of the progressive types of neuromuscular condition is increasing gluteal muscle weakness with the development of a compensatory functional lumbar hyperlordosis above. If this is flattened or made rigid the patient is promptly converted from being a walker to a wheelchair patient [33]. Thus, again, surgery is principally indicated for the wheelchair patient who is losing sitting stability. Both anterior and posterior instrumentation and fusion is wherever possible to be preferred, but in conditions associated with cardiac and pulmonary dysfunction anterior surgery is usually contraindicated. Segmental spinal instrumentation combined with fusion may be strong enough to support the less severe and more flexible deformity, but these have not yet manifested themselves by way of loss of sitting stability. This surgery must therefore be regarded as prophylactic rather than immediately therapeutic and has to be balanced by a high

mortality rate combined with high morbidity rate involving preoperative tracheostomy in many severe cases [14].

Deformities associated with neurofibromatosis

Von Recklinghausen's disease is an autosomal dominant condition but at least 50% of cases are spontaneous mutations. The diagnosis is made by the presence of any two of the following clinical features – a positive family history, a positive nodule biopsy, six café au lait spots, and multiple nodules. The condition affects all components of the musculoskeletal system but the spine is most commonly involved, in more than 50% of cases. There is, however, a spectrum of spinal involvement which mirrors the degree of severity of the condition. At one end of the spectrum the spine appears clinically and radiographically normal while at the other there is evidence of severe dystrophic change with attenu-

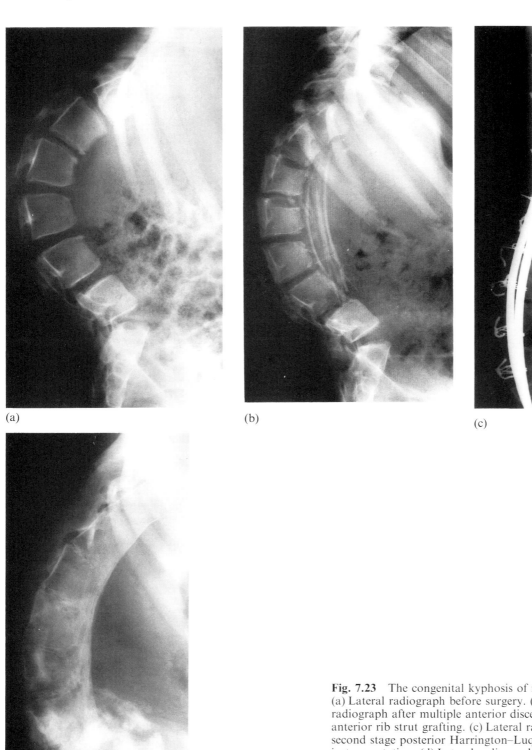

(a)

(b)

(c)

(d)

Fig. 7.23 The congenital kyphosis of myelomeningocele. (a) Lateral radiograph before surgery. (b) Lateral radiograph after multiple anterior discectomy and anterior rib strut grafting. (c) Lateral radiograph after second stage posterior Harrington–Luque instrumentation. (d) Lateral radiograph 5 years after surgery. The instrumentation was removed because of prominence under the skin. A solid spinal fusion has resulted except at the lumbo-sacral area where there is a hypertrophic non-union which was fortunately stable. The lumbo-sacral region is difficult to fuse in this condition.

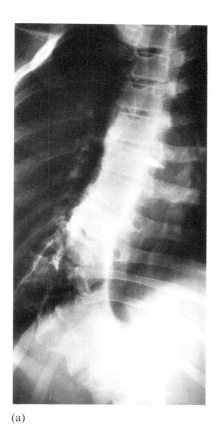

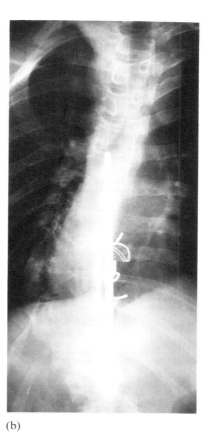

(a)   (b)

Fig. 7.24   (a) PA radiograph of a lower thoracic curve in association with Von Recklinghausen's disease. (b) After two stage anterior and posterior fusion showing a solid spine with some improvement. Even prevention of progression is an achievement in this unpredictable condition.

ated ribs, enlarged intervertebral foramina, and scalloped vertebrae. The prevalence rate and progression potential of spinal deformities reflect the degree of dystrophic change. At the mild end of the spectrum children have deformities indistinguishable from idiopathic ones and are treated accordingly. At the severe end of the spectrum, however, early onset, severely progressive, short angular curves are the rule rather than the exception. As in the idiopathic deformity, there are two types – buckling lordo-scolioses or kyphoses – and both may be present in the same spine, although several segments apart. The obviously dystrophic early onset curve will progress and if the deformity is still acceptable then anterior and posterior fusion should be prescribed to halt progression and thus to obviate the cardio-pulmonary consequences of these progressive early onset curves. All too frequently patients do not present until the deformity is severe and again two stage surgery is necessary with preliminary anterior soft tissue release or apical

wedge resection according to the degree of severity [14] (Fig. 7.24).

Kyphoses are much less common than generally considered because of failure to appreciate that most deformities which appear kyphotic are in reality severely buckled lordo-scolioses. None the less, pure kyphoses do exist and in dystrophic spines have a severe progression potential with a strong likelihood of neurological dysfunction. Prophylactic anterior and posterior fusion should be prescribed for the early deformity but in the presence of neurological signs anterior decompression and strut grafting is essential [14]. The cervical spine is not uncommonly involved and deformities here should be promptly fused front and back lest neurological signs develop which are extremely hazardous if not impossible to treat satisfactorily. Occasionally neurological signs arise from intraspinal neurofibromata but are much less commonly encountered than generally considered. Laminectomy followed by tumour removal is the treatment of choice.

Mesenchymal deformities

Here there is a wide spectrum of underlying conditions including the heritable disorders of connective tissue, the mucopolysaccharidoses and the skeletal dysplasias.

The heritable disorders of connective tissue comprise osteogenesis imperfecta, Marfan's syndrome, homocystinuria, and the Ehlers–Danlos syndrome. Osteogenesis imperfecta is a group of disorders arising from inherited defects in collagen synthesis, with the common feature of bone fragility. Cases at the most severe end of the spectrum are not compatible with longevity and it is the milder forms which come to clinical attention as regards the spine, the changes in which are indistinguishable from those in juvenile osteoporosis with multiple compression fractures and biconcave vertebrae. Anterior chest wall deformities are also common. As in Von Recklinghausen's disease the prevalence rate and progression potential of spinal deformities correlates well with the severity of the underlying condition, and in those with the type I mild tarda form scoliosis is not common, whereas those with the type II severe congenita form invariably have a spinal deformity. Again these deformities are of two types – lordo-scolioses or kyphoses (Fig. 7.25) and the indications for surgical intervention are not easy to define [14]. Posterior instrumentation and fusion has an extremely bad record, with high pseudarthrosis and other complication rates. Sublaminar wires are tolerated poorly because of weak bone and Harrington hooks often have to be supported by methyl methacrylate cement. For a severe early onset life threatening case two stage wedge resection is probably the best treatment.

Marfan's syndrome with its arachnodactyly, dislocated lenses, aortic dilatation and skeletal problem is associated with a scoliosis in about 50% of cases. Attention must be paid to the very delicate heart and great vessel status, but experience shows that this has not been a problem in spinal surgery. Treatment of the spinal deformities in association with Marfan's syndrome is along the same lines as that recommended for idiopathic scoliosis at the same site.

Homocystinuria is similar to Marfan's syndrome but mental impairment is common in the majority. The danger to surgery here is vascular damage leading to thrombosis in both arterial

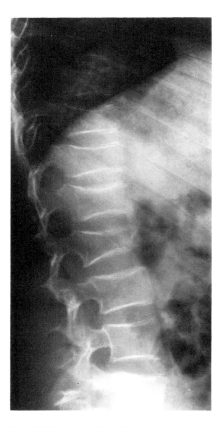

Fig. 7.25   Lateral radiograph showing a smooth kyphosis with platyspondyly typical of brittle bone disease.

and venous systems. The pattern of scoliosis is similar to that encountered in Marfan's syndrome but because of the thrombotic risk surgical treatment should be withheld. The Ehlers–Danlos syndrome of fragile, bruisable skin with loose-jointedness is also associated with the same type of spinal deformity. Biochemical advances have delineated several different types of this syndrome and it is essential to ensure that vessel friability is not a feature of the particular type of Ehlers–Danlos syndrome otherwise surgical treatment is most definitely contraindicated because of the haemorrhagic risk [14].

The mucopolysaccharidoses are skeletal disorders due to a failure of normal breakdown of complex carbohydrates which accumulate in tissue and appear in the urine. There is a range of severity with the Hurler syndrome, fatal before the age of 10 years, the milder Hunter syndrome with survival through to the second or third decades, the Morquio syndrome and the

Maroteaux–Lamy syndrome with moderate longevity. The Morquio syndrome is most commonly encountered and there are skeletal deformities in association with short-trunked dwarfism but intelligence is normal. Death occurs from cardiorespiratory dysfunction or spinal cord compression. It is the latter which is the real worry in patients with the Morquio syndrome and can occur from a progressive thoraco-lumbar kyphosis, or atlanto-axial instability as a result of a deficient odontoid (Fig. 7.26). The thoraco-lumbar kyphosis can respond to extension bracing and this should certainly be prescribed first. Should neurological signs develop then anterior resection of the bullet-shaped apical vertebra, followed by strut grafting, should be performed [14]. Because of the high incidence of neurological problems from atlanto-axial instability, many experienced surgeons recommend prophylactic fusion as soon as the patient is encountered.

The skeletal dysplasias represent a wide variety of conditions with disordered development and growth in some part of the skeleton. Some are common, but most are rare, and classification is generally by the skeletal site involved, e.g. epi-

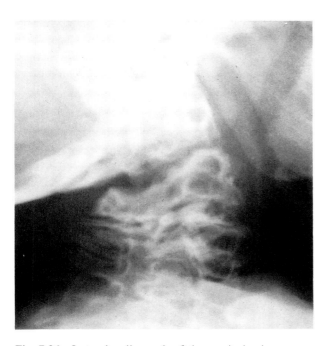

Fig. 7.26 Lateral radiograph of the cervical spine showing the typical odontoid aplasia of Morquio's syndrome.

physis, metaphysis, or spine [37]. The same two primordial types of spinal deformity can occur, i.e. lordo-scoliosis or kyphosis, but it is the latter which is the more common [14].

In multiple epiphyseal dysplasia, one of the more common types, in addition to hip, knee, and elbow epiphyseal dysplasia the spine is not severely involved, but most children have a thoracic kyphosis similar to Scheuermann's disease. The autosomal dominant achondroplasia has two important spinal features—spinal stenosis and a thoraco-lumbar kyphosis—both of which can give rise to neurological problems. A thoraco-lumbar kyphosis is the rule and develops early due to a thoraco-lumbar bullet shaped vertebra. More than 90% resolve spontaneously with growth and there is therefore no urgent therapeutic need. For the uncommon patient with a progressive kyphosis and neurological deterioration there is no substitute for anterior decompression and strut grafting. Although the entire spine is affected in achondroplasia the lumbar region most commonly produces symptoms and often requires decompressive laminectomy. Fortunately most patients have reached maturity by the time this posterior de-stabilizing procedure is required. In the adolescent, however, there is a real risk of producing a kyphosis by laminectomy such that prophylactic segmental rectangular support with fusion should be performed at the same time (Fig. 7.27).

The spondylo-epiphyseal dysplasias have both disordered epiphyseal growth and flattened vertebrae. The X-linked tarda variety is characterized by flat vertebrae which are humped posteriorly and this differentiates from multiple epiphyseal dysplasia and the Morquio syndrome. Kyphosis is common but scoliosis rare. Extension bracing can be effective but there is sometimes local instability at the site of the bullet-shaped vertebra in which case anterior strut grafting is required. The rare, but severe, congenita variety has irregular platyspondyly and a Scheuermann's-type kyphosis. Treatment is similar. In diastrophic dysplasia there are three spinal problems – odontoid hypoplasia, cervical kyphosis, and a structural scoliosis. Odontoid hypoplasia gives rise to atlanto-axial stability which frequently requires reduction, halo-cast stabilization and posterior fusion. Cervical kyphosis is more neurologically worrying and if progression is observed anterior and posterior

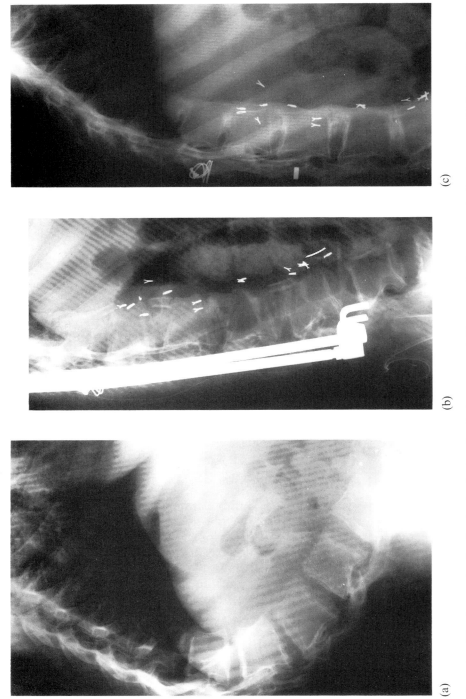

Fig. 7.27 The thoraco-lumbar kyphosis of achondroplasia compounded by posterior decompressive laminectomy. (a) Lateral radiograph showing a severe thoraco-lumbar kyphosis. (b) After two stage anterior and posterior fusion. (c) Three years after surgery showing a solid fusion with a gratifying correction.

(a)

(b)

(c)

fusion should be prescribed. A significant structural scoliosis is not a constant finding but is present in about 50% of cases. It is uncommon, however, for these scolioses to be severe. They should be dealt with as for any progressive scoliosis in association with a dystrophic bone situation – anterior and posterior fusion for milder curves, and two stage wedge resection for the more severe categories [14]. Spina bifida in the cervical or lumbar region, or both, is the rule in diastrophic dysplasia and if distraction instrumentation is contemplated CT myelography is essential to exclude spinal cord tether in these sites.

Included in the mesenchymal disorders are some metabolic conditions and it is probably true that rickets is the commonest cause of scoliosis worldwide. The deformity is indistinguishable from idiopathic scoliosis but the more severe the rachitic problem the earlier the onset and the more progressive the curve. Treatment is similar to the idiopathic counterpart.

Deformities due to trauma

These can be either spinal or extraspinal, with the former being much more common. Most spinal injuries are of the vertical loading with flexion variety, so typically characterized by Holdsworth. The anterior column fails under compression, while the posterior column fails under tension, and the axis of the injury is somewhere in between. The more anterior the axis, the more the spinal cord will be behind it and therefore vulnerable to tension insult. There are two principal spinal deformities resulting from spinal injuries of this nature – a kyphosis at the level of the bony injury and a lordo-scoliosis below in those who suffer a neurological insult [14] (Fig. 7.28). The progressive kyphosis is probably underestimated in its prevalence and generally results from inadequate initial management of the bony injury. It is debatable, however, whether this forms an indication for initial surgical stabilization as experienced spinal injuries centres show that the great majority of the acute kyphoses can be reduced and stabilized by hyperextension conservative treatment. The same can be said for injuries which are deemed radiographically 'unstable'. The only absolute indications for the fixation of a spinal fracture initially are three [38]

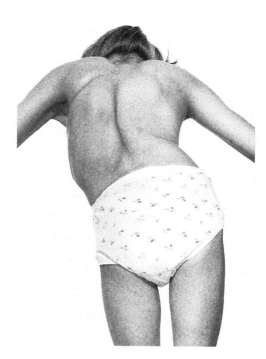

Fig. 7.28 Back view of a young girl with a progressive lordo-scoliosis secondary to a spinal cord tumour with radiotherapy.

– when there is total loss of spinal continuity at the level of injury (i.e. total dislocation), in the presence of multiple injuries, and in the presence of a significant head injury. In the former situation no conservative measure can reliably realign the spine. For the patient with multiple injuries the spine should be stabilized surgically lest treatment of other injuries and the nursing thereof impairs spinal stability. The patient with a severe head injury often goes through a phase of considerable cerebral irritability and an unstable spinal injury will not tolerate such vigorous body movements. None the less, there is an epidemic of early fixation of spinal fractures for which there is no clinical or scientific justification. Certainly there is no evidence whatever that the neurological situation is improved by any form of surgical intervention.

There is, however, perhaps due to orthopaedic surgeons not learning the lessons from spinal injuries centres, a rising prevalence rate of progressive and often painful local kyphosis. This can be most distressing to the patient and spinal stabilization should be performed. As in all kyphoses, the spine must be stabilized anteriorly using a strong cortico-cancellous strut graft.

Despite the fact that the great majority of spinal injuries are in effect acute kyphoses, laminectomy is still far too commonly performed. This destabilizes the spine by removing the integrity of the posterior column while doing nothing for the spinal cord pressure which, of course, is at the front. What is the inevitable result is progressive kyphosis often with its own neurological trouble in the future. Again anterior strut grafting is the treatment of choice with anterior dural decompression for the patient whose neurological signs are deteriorating.

In the child, what may appear simply to be an acute flexion spinal injury, without any neurological signs, frequently represents a Salter–Harris type V growth plate injury. Progressive kyphosis during growth is therefore not uncommon and must be watched for in the immature [14]. Any tendency towards progression should be countered by an anterior and posterior spinal fusion. If there has been lateral end-plate pressure then a true scoliosis can occur, but this is uncommon.

The higher the level of the spinal cord lesion following trauma the greater the potential for deformity as well as widespread spasticity. In children, the younger the child the more the tendency toward a progressive deformity. If the spinal cord damage is at the level of T12 or below there is no spinal deformity, but if the neurological lesion is at T10 or above then a progressive collapsing lordo-scoliosis is the rule. If this is impinging upon sitting stability then it should be dealt with by anterior and posterior spinal instrumentation and fusion as for any paralytic spine deformity.

Extraspinal causes of deformities due to trauma are much less common. Decades ago empyemas following pneumonia before the antibiotic era often gave rise to long, but relatively mild, spinal curvatures due to fibrotic pleural thickening, while thoracoplasty in relation to pulmonary tuberculosis also produced a relatively mild deformity. There does, however, appear to be an increasing prevalence rate of idiopathic-type scoliosis in association with thoracotomy, either for a cardiac problem or for a tracheo-oesophageal fistula. The deformities should be dealt with as for their idiopathic counterpart.

Rarely, retroperitoneal fibrosis, either idiopathic or as a result of trauma, or following the insertion of the old fashioned theco-peritoneal shunt for hydrocephalus, can give rise to a progressive and rigid lumbar hyperlordosis by way of soft tissue tether.

Deformities due to infection

Two-thirds of spinal infections are pyogenic and one-third tuberculous, and in both types there is potential for progressive deformity. Infection commences in the vascular end-plates which, untreated, show evidence of destruction along with the intervening disc. The majority of pyogenic infections are due to the *Staphylococcus aureus* and respond to anti-staphylococcal antibiotic therapy along with symptomatic treatment. Only in the florid case with abscess formation or neurological impairment is surgical treatment indicated and this is in the form of anterior decompression and strut grafting. Even untreated, pyogenic infections seldom produce a significant kyphosis.

Tuberculous spinal disease is, however, more insidious and produces a more significant local deformity with the gibbus being diagnostic. Treatment is contentious. The Medical Research Council, as a result of their controlled trials and other studies over the past 2 decades, preach that any degree of severity of tuberculous spinal disease can be managed by anti-tuberculous chemotherapy alone and they recognize no role for surgical intervention. This conservative approach also encompasses total tuberculous paralysis. Against this view is that of Hodgson [39] and other anterior spinal surgical experts. If there is abscess formation or neurological impairment then anterior surgical decompression and excision of all diseased tissue followed by strut grafting is not only therapeutic but curative (Fig. 7.29). Such treatment is only applicable where such anterior surgical expertise is available. None the less, as a result of anterior surgical intervention, the sinister progressive kyphosis is obviated. Once established and progressive it is very difficult to treat satisfactorily. Anterior decompression is only indicated for the subsequent development of neurological impairment but the anterior decompression is difficult to perform and is very dangerous, with many of these

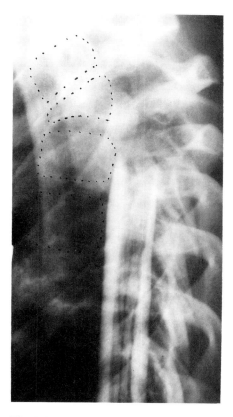

Fig. 7.29 Lateral myelogram of the upper thoracic spine showing an angular kyphosis with a block to the passage of dye in tuberculous spinal disease.

patients having a rigid chest and little pulmonary reserve. Accordingly, treatment should be reserved for the patient with frank neurological deterioration. This is more commonly encountered in children where even anterior surgical decompression and strut grafting cannot be expected to completely prevent progression of the kyphosis as the end-plates are involved in the fusion process.

Deformities due to tumours

As with infections, it is the anterior column which fails under compression with extradural tumours. However intradural tumours, and syringomyelia, as well as the paravertebral tumours of childhood, can produce spinal deformities. Any patient presenting with a seemingly idiopathic deformity but accompanied by pain, particularly at night, should be considered as having an intradural tumour or syringomyelia until proven otherwise (Fig. 7.30). The diagnosis is clinched by spinal cord imaging. While meningiomas and neurofibromas are the commonest intradural tumours in adults, it is malignant astrocytomas and neuroblastomas which are prevalent in children. Many of the latter present very late and are considered as having other conditions such as poliomyelitis, muscular dystrophy, or postural torticollis before the diagnosis is eventually made. Surprisingly, the prognosis is not bad and with surgical removal, even though it is often incomplete, followed by radiotherapy and chemotherapy the survival rate is in excess of 50%.

The problem for spinal stability is as the result of either the laminectomy approach for these lesions or the subsequent radiotherapy. The radiation changes to the vertebrae are usually minimal, although some degree of platyspondyly and a thoraco-lumbar kyphosis are not uncommon. If more than 5000 rad have been administered there is a rising prevalence rate of radiation myelopathy which can itself produce a paralytic curve due to spinal cord embarrassment. It is, however, the necessary laminectomy, which may have to be widespread, as an approach to the extirpation of these intradural tumours, which can produce in the immature a very progressive kyphosis. If the facet joints have not been sacrificed then a long rounded kyphosis, similar to Scheuermann's disease, develops and this may respond to extension brace treatment. With removal of the facet joints an angular kyphosis develops and this may produce its own neurological signs in the future. Should this occur, then anterior decompression and strut grafting must be performed.

The paravertebral tumours, Wilms' tumour and neuroblastoma, produce their deformities by way of local irradiation and these are seldom considerable.

Extradural tumours inevitably produce a local kyphosis, even in the lumbar region, as the line of the centre of gravity of the body passes anterior to the body of L4. Although these can occur in childhood, with Ewing's sarcoma, the malignant lymphomas, aneurysmal bone cyst, and eosinophilic granuloma, the majority are metastatic problems in the adult. The importance of these kyphoses is two fold – local pain and the poten-

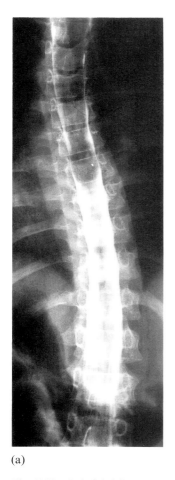

(a)

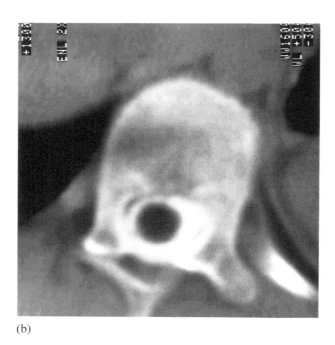

(b)

Fig. 7.30   Painful 'idiopathic' scoliosis in association with syringomyelia. (a) PA myelogram showing the deformity and the widened canal. (b) CT myelogram showing the typical appearance of a syrinx.

tial for neurological impairment. Both can be extremely distressing to the patient with metastatic disease. The great majority will, however, succumb within a matter of months, but those with breast or prostatic lesions can have some longevity. It is these patients to whom therapy should be particularly addressed. If the metastasis is solitary and painful or the source of a neurological insult, then anterior vertebral body excision followed by strut grafting is indicated. In these patients it is advisable to add posterior stabilization and fusion using rectangular segmental wiring. Although the prognosis is clearly limited it is most undignified and distressing for the patient to perish in a prolonged paraplegic state and thus surgery should always be prescribed where indicated [14] (Fig. 7.31).

Other spinal deformities

Some spinal deformities do not belong to any of the above categories and these can be encountered in both children and adults. In children idiopathic-type deformities are more prevalent with congenital heart disease, ocular and visual problems (blind children, ophthalmoplegia, and congenital strabismus) and in association with congenital anomalies of the upper extremity. These should be treated as for their idiopathic counterpart. A mild spinal deformity is also prevalent in juvenile chronic arthritis but these are nearly always non-structural, and thus non-progressive.

In the adult spinal deformities occur as a result of Paget's disease, ankylosing spondylitis, and

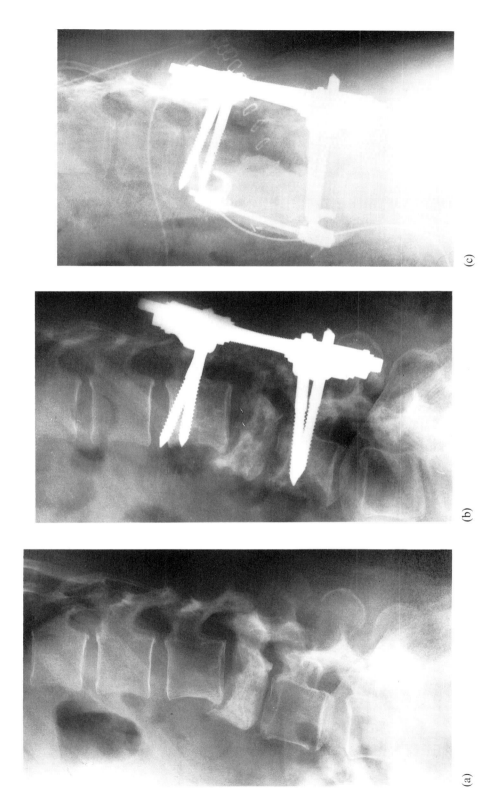

(a)

(b)

(c)

Fig. 7.31 Metastatic spinal disease with intractable pain and progressive paraparesis. (a) Lateral radiograph of a woman with breast cancer with a metastatic deposit in L3. (b) Lateral radiograph after first stage posterior transpedicular fixation using the A0 fixateur interne. (c) Lateral radiograph after second stage anterior dural decompression, the resultant gap being replaced with methyl methacrylate cement and a Harrington compression system operating in distraction mode.

osteoporosis or osteomalacia. In Paget's disease the vertebrae and pelvis are the commonest sites of skeletal involvement. Multiple vertebral involvement can cause a kyphotic deformity with pain and even neurological compression. Neurological embarrassment generally occurs as a result of vertebral collapse, which should therefore be dealt with by anterior decompression and strut grafting. However, there is a vascular steal syndrome whereby a vertebra magna can take blood preferentially so that the spinal cord vascularity is jeopardized. This steal syndrome can respond to diphosphonates or calcitonin.

Patients with ankylosing spondylitis, particularly of the more aggressive variety, can develop a progressive spinal kyphosis. This is most common in the thoraco-lumbar region, but also can occur in the cervico-thoracic area and it is most important to differentiate the true site of the deformity. If the kyphosis has progressed to the extent where the patient cannot see forward then osteotomy is indicated. If the area of kyphosis is thoraco-lumbar then the site of osteotomy is at the L2–3 level, just below the conus where the spinal canal is capacious. If however the area of maximum kyphosis is in the cervico-thoracic region then osteotomy at the C7–T1 level is necessary lest the spine be unbalanced. Many patients have concomitant hip disease and much of their kyphosis can be apparent due to a flexion contracture of the hip joints. In this situation total hip replacement should be prescribed before any considerations of spinal osteomy.

Spinal osteotomy is dangerous in the an-

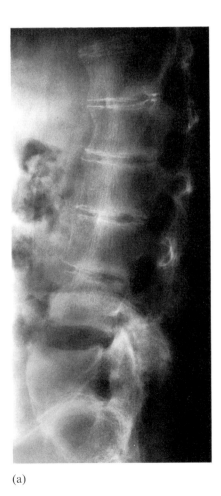

(a)

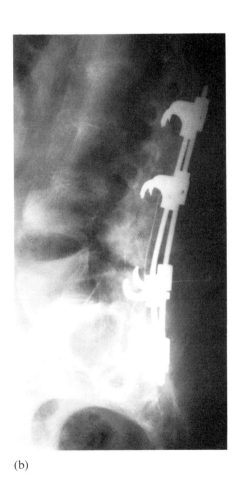

(b)

Fig. 7.32 (a) Lateral radiograph of the lumbar spine in a man with ankylosing spondylitis with a spontaneous pseudarthrosis at the L4/5 level. (b) Lateral radiograph after extension osteotomy at the site of the pseudarthrosis.

kylosing spondylitis patient and every series of any size reports anaesthetic problems, vascular problems from stretching or tearing of the aorta or its branches, and neurological impairment. Certainly anaesthesia is hazardous and often requires a preliminary tracheostomy. Patients should not be placed prone for surgery as this markedly hinders any form of access to the airway in case of emergency. For the patient with a cervico-thoracic kyphosis osteotomy is performed in the sitting position, under local anaesthesia, by the method of Simmons. For a thoraco-lumbar kyphosis the patient should be treated in the lateral decubitus position. Both techniques employ removal of a wedge of bone based posteriorly and apical at intervertebral foraminal level. In the thoraco-lumbar region the technique of McMaster is recommended whereby the posterior wedge is closed by double Harrington compression systems [40] (Fig. 7.32). This obviates the sudden correction achieved by a sudden manual pressure.

There are two other areas of spinal interest in the ankylosing spondylitis patient – spontaneous pseudarthroses and traumatic fractures. It is not uncommon in the spine which appears to be fused from top to bottom to have an area of instability due to a spontaneous pseudarthrosis (an area of the spine which has not completely ossified). These are potentially dangerous and represent a point of maximum mobility during spinal stress. Patients often present as a result of local pain or even neurological deterioration and spinal fixation and fusion is urgently required. Similarly, patients with true traumatic fractures of their ankylosed spine have the same neurological vulnerability. Conservative treatment is not adequate, as these patients can sustain severe neurological or even complete damage by standard nursing care. Fixation is urgently required.

There is a vogue for applying instrumentation to any spine and the osteoporotic/osteomalacic spine is no exception. Segmental instrumentation is increasingly prescribed for the kyphosis, often painful, of these elderly female patients. Certainly this condition is difficult to treat and these generally lightweight ladies do not tolerate at all well an orthosis of the sufficiency required to either abolish their pain or prevent progression of their kyphotic deformity. None the less, the application of segmental instrumentation throughout the whole thoraco-lumbar spine must be

viewed with considerable suspicion and this highlights, par excellence, the concept of knowing when and when not to operate.

References

1. Goldstein, L. A. and Waugh, T. R. (1973) Classification and terminology of scoliosis. *Clin. Orthop.*, **93**, 10–22
2. Cobb, J. R. (1948) Outline for the study of scoliosis. *American Academy of Orthopaedic Surgeons Instructional Course Lectures*, **5**, 261.
3. Perdriolle, R. (1979) *La scoliose – son etude tridimensionnelle*. Maloine, Paris.
4. Bunnell, W. P. (1984) An objective criterion for scoliosis screening. *J. Bone Joint Surg.*, **66A**, 1381–1387.
5. Dickson, R. A., Lawton, J. O., Archer, I. A. and Butt, W. P. (1984) The pathogenesis of idiopathic scoliosis. Biplanar spinal asymmetry. *J. Bone Joint Surg.*, **66B**, 8–15.
6. Adams, W. (1865) *Lectures on the Pathology and Treatment of Lateral and Other Forms of Curvature of the Spine*. J. Churchill & Sons, London.
7. Zorab, P. A. (ed.) (1974) *Scoliosis and Muscle*. William Heinemann Medical Books Ltd., London.
8. Steindler, A. (1929) *Diseases and Deformities of the Spine and Thorax*. C. V. Mosby, St Louis.
9. de Peloux, J., Fauchet, R., Faucon, B. and B. Stagnara, P. (1965) Le plan d'election pour l'examen radiologique des cypho-scolioses. *Rev. Chir. Orthop.*, **51**, 517–524.
10. Sorensen, K. H. (1964) *Scheuermann's Kyphosis. Clinical Appearances. Radiograph, Aetiology and Prognosis*. Munksgaard, Copenhagen.
11. Willner, S. and Johnsson, B. (1983) Thoracic kyphosis and lumbar lordosis during the growth period in boys and girls. *Acta Pediatr. Scand.*, **72**, 873–878.
12. Mehta, M. H. and Morel, G. (1979) The non-operative treatment of infantile idiopathic scoliosis. In *Scoliosis*. Proceedings of the Sixth Symposium (eds P. A. Zorab and O. Siegler). Academic Press, London, pp. 71–84.
13. Deacon, P., Berkin, C. R. and Dickson, R. A. (1985) Combined idiopathic kyphosis and scoliosis: an analysis of the lateral spine curvature associated with Scheuermann's disease. *J. Bone Joint Surg.*, **67B**, 189–192.
14. Leatherman, K. D. and Dickson, R. A. (1987) *Management of Spinal Deformities*. Wright, Bristol.
15. Archer, I. A. and Dickson, R. A. (1985) Stature

and idiopathic scoliosis. A prospective study. *J. Bone Joint Surg.*, **67B**, 185–188.

16. Nachemson, A. (1986) A long term follow up study of non-treated scoliosis. *Acta Orthop. Scand.*, **39**, 466–476.

17. Reid, L. (1971) Lung growth. In *Scoliosis and Growth* (ed. P. A. Zorab), Proceedings of a Third Symposium. Churchill Livingstone, Edinburgh.

18. Blount, W. P. and Moe, J. H. (1973) *The Milwaukee Brace*. Williams and Wilkins, Baltimore.

19. Miller, J. A., Nachemson, A. L. and Schultz, A. B. (1984) Effectiveness of braces in mild idiopathic scoliosis. *Spine*, **9**, 632–635.

20. Bradford, D. S., Tanguy, A. and Vanselow, J. (1983) Surface electrical stimulation in the treatment of idiopathic scoliosis: preliminary results in 30 patients. *Spine*, **8**, 757–764.

21. Dickson, R. A. (1985) Conservative treatment for idiopathic scoliosis. *J. Bone Joint Surg.*, **67B**, 176–181.

22. Risser, J. C. (1958) The iliac apophysis, an invaluable sign in the management of scoliosis. *Clin. Orthop.*, **11**, 111–119.

23. Deacon, P. and Dickson, R. A., Spinal growth. *J. Bone Joint Surg.* (in press).

24. Harrington, P. R. (1962) Treatment of scoliosis. Correction and internal fixation by spine instrumentation. *J. Bone Joint Surg.*, **44A**, 519–610.

25. Luque, E. R. (1982) The anatomic basis and development of segmental spinal instrumentation. *Spine*, **7**, 256–259.

26. Archer, I. A., Deacon, P. and Dickson, R. A. (1986) Idiopathic scoliosis in Leeds – a management philosophy. *J. Bone Joint Surg.*, **68B**, 670.

27. Dubousset, J., Graf, H., Miladi, L. and Cotrel, Y. (1986) Spinal and thoracic derotation with CD instrumentation. *Orthop. Trans.*, **10 (1)**, 36.

28. Dwyer, A. F., Newton, N. C. and Sherwood A. A. (1969) An anterior approach to scoliosis: a preliminary report. *Clin. Orthop.*, **62**, 192–202.

29. Griss, P., Harms, J. and Zielke, K. (1984) Ventral derotation spondylodesis (VDS). In *Management of Spinal Deformities* (eds R. A. Dickson and D. S. Bradford), Butterworths International Medical Reviews, London, pp. 193–236.

30. Edgar, M. A., Chapman, R. H. and Glasgow, M. M. S. (1982) Pre-operative correction in adolescent idiopathic scoliosis. *J. Bone Joint Surg.*, **64B**, 530–535.

31. Leatherman, K. D. and Dickson, R. A. (1979) Two-stage corrective surgery for congenital deformities of the spine. *J. Bone Joint Surg.*, **61B**, 324–328.

32. McMaster, M. J. and MacNicol, M. F. (1979) The management of progressive infantile idiopathic scoliosis. *J. Bone Joint Surg.*, **61B**, 36–42.

33. Lonstein, J. E. and Akbarnia, B. A. (1983) Operative treatment of spinal deformities in patients with cerebral palsy or mental retardation. *J. Bone Joint Surg.*, **65A**, 43–55.

34. Nachemson, A. (1987) Personal communication.

35. McMaster, M. J. and Ohtsuka, K. (1982) The natural history of congenital scoliosis. A study of 251 patients. *J. Bone Joint Surg.*, **64A**, 1128–1147.

36. Leatherman, K. D. and Dickson, R. A. (1978) Congenital kyphosis in myelomeningocele. Vertebral body resection and posterior spine fusion. *Spine*, **3**, 222–226.

37. Fairbank, T. (1951) *An Atlas of General Affections of the Skeleton*. Williams and Wilkins, Baltimore.

38. Gaines, R. W. and Humphreys, W. G. (1984) A plea for judgement in management of thoracolumbar fractures and fracture-dislocations. *Clin. Orthop.*, **189**, 36–42.

39. Hodgson, A. R. and Stock, F. E. (1960) Anterior spine fusion for the treatment of tuberculosis of the spine. *J. Bone Joint Surg.*, **42A**, 295–310.

40. McMaster, M. J. (1985) A technique for lumbar spinal osteotomy in ankylosing spondylitis. *J. Bone Joint Surg.*, **67B**, 204–210.

8

Lengthening of limbs by the Ilizarov method

R. Cruz-Conde Delgado and J. C. Marti Gonzalez

Ilizarov's external fixator was originally described in Kurgan, Siberia (USSR), in 1951 by Gavril Abramovich Ilizarov. The official title given by the Ministry of Health of the USSR was 'compression-distraction apparatus' [3,4], to encompass the idea of simultaneous or alternate distraction and compression which could be applied to a bone segment. The apparatus (Fig. 8.1) was developed at the Experimental and Clinical Institute of Scientific, Orthopaedic and Traumatic Studies (Kniiekot) in Kurgan, but introduced to the West in 1981 by ASAMI (the Italian Association for the study and application of the Ilizarov technique) [3,4].

It is basically a circular external fixator (Fig. 8.2) but also a complex system built with a limited number of parts yet able to provide a versatile construction capable of between 700 and 800 different combinations. As an external fixation device, it depends simply on the introduction of crossed Kirschner wires into the bone and fixed under tension to a ring, which in turn is secured to rods. A second ring is attached in a similar manner, thus allowing compression or distraction; additional forces of angulation or rotation can be applied by the use of multiple rings and crossed wires [3,4,15].

Osteogenesis

Ilizarov considered that his method not only allowed lengthening of a limb but induced new bone formation. Indeed, experimental evidence revealed that osteogenesis appeared to be stimulated by a combination of distracting forces on the periosteum and stability between the bone segments. Preservation of the blood supply is vital and is very dependent on the rate of length-

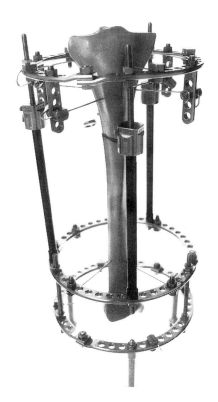

Fig. 8.1 Ilizarov's fixator for tibial lengthening with telescopic rods and corticotomy at the proximal end.

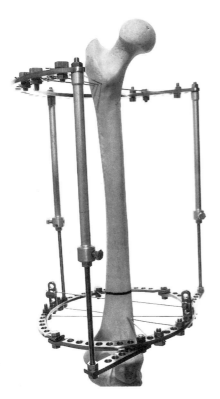

Fig. 8.2 Ilizarov's fixator for femoral lengthening with original set. (The site of corticotomy is marked with a black ring at the distal end.)

ening; and this also applies not only to the blood vessels but to all the surrounding connective tissue structures [15,16].

Stability

Perhaps the effect of weight bearing and exercise for the limb is another important factor in stimulating osteogenesis [3,4,15]; and the apparatus provides sufficient stability and strength to withstand full weight bearing. Initially the device was applied by inserting cross wires at either ends of the diaphysis but better stability is achieved by a four-level assembly; two in the proximal and two in the distal metaphysis.

Rate of lengthening

The studies carried out at the Kurgan Institute by Ilizarov were conducted in seven separate series

under varying conditions of stability, tension and rate of lengthening. They confirmed that the optimum rate of lengthening for osteogenesis was 1 mm per day, divided into 0.25 mm every 6 hours. These experiments, carried out on dogs, revealed that by increasing the rate to 1.5–2.0 mm per day caused thrombosis in the capillary vessels and subsequent necrosis in the regenerating bone; conversely, a slower rate of lengthening allowed early consolidation of new bone and prevented any distraction [4,16].

Preservation of blood supply to bone

The Ilizarov method tries to prevent any serious damage to the local blood vessels by (1) a delicate but accurate division of the cortical bone [3,4], (2) closed osteoclasis of the cancellous or medullary bone using minimal force and (3) minimal damage to the periosteum and surrounding tissues [2,3,4,10].

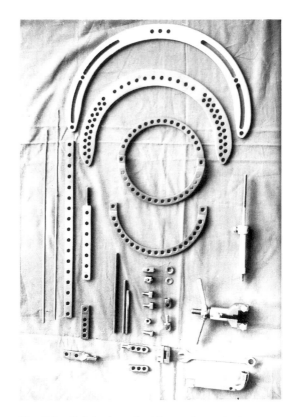

Fig. 8.3   Original set for Ilizarov's method.

Indications

Limb lengthening has been confined in the past to those limbs with acquired shortening due to trauma, poliomyelitis and infection causing arrest of growth. Recently there has been increasing interest in lengthening congenital short limbs due to achondroplasia, osteodystrophy, various forms of dwarfism, congenital shortening of the femur and agenesis of the long bones [2,6,7,8,9,17,21].

The apparatus

The component parts of the Ilizarov apparatus are illustrated (Fig. 8.3), and are translated from Russian with the help of the Italian (ASAMI) catalogue. There are two sets: (1) for bone anchorage and (2) for linkage [2,6,7,8,9,17,21].

Bone anchorage

(a) *Kirschner wires* in diameters of 1.5 and 1.8 mm with either three cutting edges for insertion into metaphysial bone or two cutting edges (bayonet) for penetration of the harder diaphysial cortex. This latter cutting edge is designed to reduce heat generated in their insertion into bone. They may support loads of up to 300 kg yet also provide some elasticity.
(b) *Tensor* is an essential component to be applied to the Kirschner wires so that they receive the correct tension. It is calibrated in kg [3,4].

Linkage

(a) Rings, half-rings and arches. They have many drill holes in various sites and angles to allow a wide choice of insertion of the Kirschner wires, and there are various sizes to accommodate the size of the limb.
(b) Bolts and clamps for securing the Kirschner wires to the rings and arches. They have drill holes and grooves to adapt to the position of the wires, rings and arches (Fig. 8.4) [3,4].

Rods

Threaded so that one complete turn equals 1 mm. There are various lengths from 60 to 200 mm.

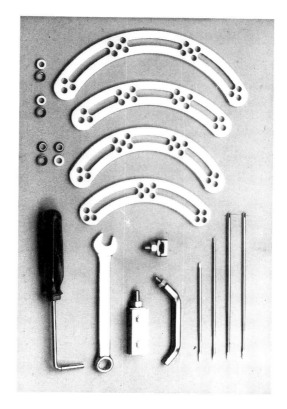

Fig. 8.4 Femoral set modified by Italian ASAMI.

Perforated for the Kirschner wires but only used for fractures.

Grooved for a more versatile fixation and again only used for fractures.

The Italian ASAMI has modified the original telescopic rods, as can be seen in Fig. 8.5, designed for monitoring the distraction as they are marked in millimetres and automatically lock at each quarter turn [3,4].

Preparation and maintenance

Before embarking on any application all the components must be checked. Sterilization can be carried out in a traditional autoclave; the use of gas (ethylene oxide) is preferred as it is less likely to affect the metal. Similarly, iodine and other corrosive materials should be avoided. It can be stored after cleaning with glycol [4].

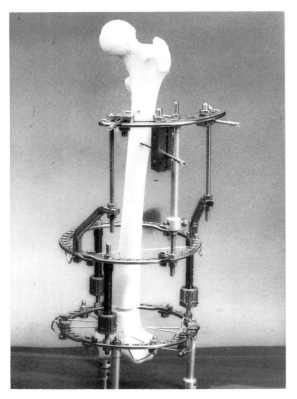

Fig. 8.5   Ilizarov's fixator modified by Italian ASAMI for femoral lengthening with telescopic rods and corticotomy at the distal end.

Application

The insertion of the wires and the construction of the external fixator may appear to be simple but unless the basic principles are carefully adopted complications may arise and ruin the result [4].

Insertion of the Kirschner wires

This requires a knowledge of the immediate important anatomical structures so that they can be avoided [24]. A low revolution drill is important in order to avoid any unnecessary burns to the skin and bone and the temperature can be reduced by frequent stops and irrigation with an antiseptic solution or saline. The wires should be inserted perpendicular to the long axis of the bone and the second wire should cross as near 90° as possible in order to achieve sound mechanical stability. Finally, the skin and soft tissues should not be subjected to undue stress particularly near the joints because walking must be encouraged. The site of the wires in flexion and extension of the joints must not produce tension in these important soft tissues. When the wires are being inserted via the anterior aspect of the limb, the adjacent joint should be kept in flexion and vice versa [3,4].

Choice of rings

The size of the ring is determined by the maximum diameter of the limb but a clearance of at least 2.0 cm is necessary in order to avoid any pressure necrosis in the skin if there is any swelling of the limb during treatment [3,4,10].

Tension of the wires

This is a fundamental requirement so that the strength and elasticity of the apparatus is achieved. The optimum tension lies between 100 and 110 kg and should be tested at intervals. Excessive tension will reduce the elastic property of the steel and may result in a bad fixation [3,4].

Fixation of the rings

This is achieved by attaching three telescopic or threaded rods so that they lie in the long axis of the bone and form the pattern of an equilateral triangle. This is not always as easy as it sounds because different sized rings may have been used but a perpendicular system can be worked out by use of some of the accessory fixation components [3,4,10].

Technique

The first stage is the assembly of the apparatus and the pattern depends on the bone which has to be lengthened.

Fig. 8.6   (a–d) Bilateral tibial lengthening of 14 cm in an 11-year-old boy with achondroplasia (total period of treatment: 10 months). (a) Preoperative radiograph of lower limbs. (b) Immediate postoperative radiograph. (c) One and 3 months postoperative radiographs during lengthening. (d) Final result.

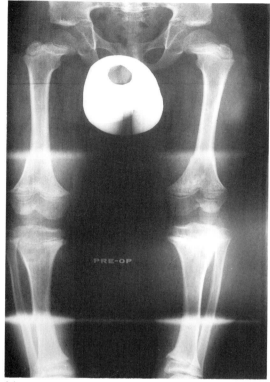

(a)

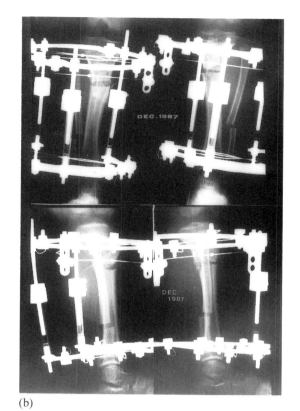

(b)

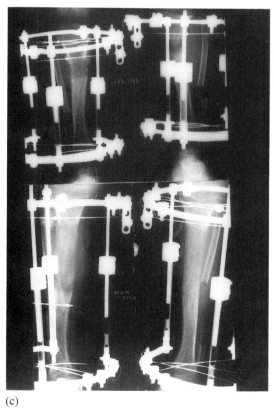

(c)

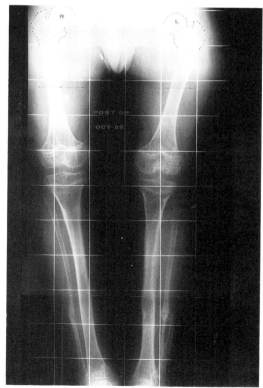

(d)

The *tibia* is the easiest of the bones to lengthen because it is not surrounded by bulky muscles and it is comparatively superficial [6,14,19]. A more ambitious programme of lengthening can be planned for the tibia compared with other long bones (Fig. 8.6a, b, c, d).

In the *proximal end* two rings are usually required, but one ring and a third or supplementary wire through the anterior cortex may be sufficient. This will tend to control the tendency of anterior bowing which may occur if it has been necessary to perform an anterior division of the cortex in the proximal metaphysis. One of the wires must pass through the head of the fibula in order to prevent dislocation of the superior tibio-fibular joint during lengthening [14].

In the *distal end*, one ring should be at the level of the junction between the middle and distal thirds, and the second is usually a half-ring placed on the anterior surface to allow access to the Achilles tendon which may require lengthening. A tenotomy is usually performed by the authors when they consider it necessary but a prophylactic tenotomy is described. This half-ring is placed in the distal metaphysis and one wire should penetrate both the tibia and the fibula just above the syndesmosis which should prevent any proximal migration of the lateral malleolus and any subsequent valgus deformity of the ankle and foot [19].

An *osteotomy of the fibula* is carried out through a small incision in the distal third of the leg.

Corticotomy, or division of the cortex, is performed at the junction between the metaphysis and the diaphysis. If extensive lengthening is planned, for example in achondroplasia, a double corticotomy is performed in the proximal and distal halves of the bone [5,12,13,14,21,25].

The *femur* requires a different assembly because of the problems involved and dangers of introducing wires through the proximal thigh. The Italian (ASAMI) team have designed an anchorage system using threaded pins which are inserted in different planes and then joined to an arch at the level of the greater trochanter. This arch is joined to two distally placed rings by using angled rods, thus providing an uniform force surrounding the femur and soft tissues (Fig. 8.7a, b, c) [4].

Corticotomy is performed just below the lesser trochanter which is preferable to the distal but

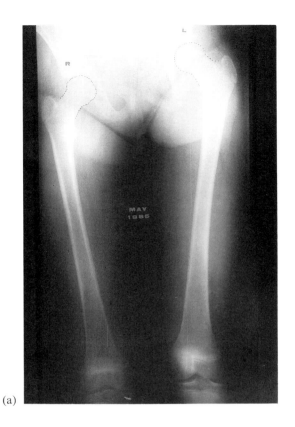

(a)

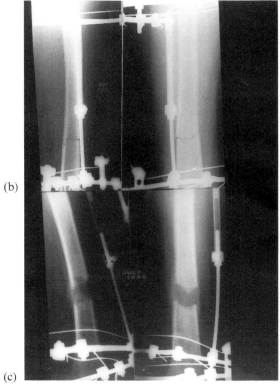

(b)

(c)

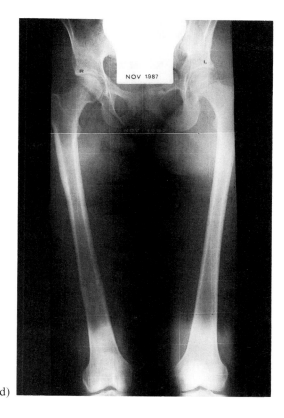

(d)

Fig. 8.7 (a–d) Femoral lengthening of 4 cm in a 14-year-old girl with idiopathic right femoral shortening (total period of treatment: 5 months). (a) Preoperative radiograph of lower limbs. (b) Corticotomy and (c) 2 months postoperative radiograph. (d) Two and a half years after lengthening (R) femur.

more accessible metaphysis where there is a danger of producing stiffness of the knee joint.

The *humerus* requires a two half-ring assembly; one in the proximal and the other in the distal third [9].

Corticotomy is performed in the proximal third.

Corticotomy

This technique is important and unique to the Ilizarov method and implies division of the cortical bone but with sparing of the cancellous or medullary bone and most of the surrounding periosteum [19]. The bone is finally broken by osteoclasis.

The tibia, for example, is approached by an incision 1.5 cm in length at the level of the proximal metaphysis and just below the tubercle. A very small and thin osteotome, 1.0 cm wide, is used to divide the periosteum which is carefully elevated on the antero-medial and lateral surfaces. The anterior crest of the tibia is cut to a depth of 5 mm using the small osteotome and mallet. The cortex on the antero-medial and lateral surfaces is also divided by lifting or depressing the handle of the osteotome, and this can all be performed through the 1.5 cm skin incision. The postero-medial cortex is divided in the same way. Finally, a force is applied to the bone by internally rotating the proximal and externally rotating the distal part until the bone breaks. The rotation is advised in this manner in order to prevent damage to the external popliteal nerve [23]. Radiographic control is made after the osteoclasis by using an image intensifier or conventional films in order to check the position of the divided bone. The lengthening rods are then applied. When a double level of lengthening is planned the central segment of bone has to be secured by an intermediate ring and wires in the bone.

Postoperative management

For 3 days the patient remains in bed with the limb elevated (the arm supported on pillows). Active exercises can be encouraged but are restricted by pain.

On the fourth day, walking and weight bearing is encouraged using crutches but preferably ordinary walking sticks.

On the fifth day, distraction starts at the rate of 0.25 mm every 6 hours.

On the eighth day, the patient may return home with instructions how to proceed with the distraction. Walking is to be encouraged.

On the tenth day, the patient is checked as an out-patient and radiographs are taken of the osteotomy site.

Physiotherapy may be required in order to encourage the patient to move the joints and to regain confidence in walking. If the femur has been lengthened it is unwise for the knee to be actively flexed more than 30° because further flexion may increase the tension on the ilio-tibial tract, which in turn may cause posterior subluxation of the knee.

Care of the wounds

The patient may have a shower every day and the entry and exit wounds of the wires need to be cleaned with soap and water. If any minor sepsis occurs it will usually clear up by applying an antiseptic solution; any obvious purulent discharge may require systemic antibiotic cover after taking a swab and culture assessment. If the local infection fails to clear up it may be necessary to replace the affected Kirschner wire in another site nearby.

Dismantling the apparatus

Osteogenesis and consolidation of the lengthened segment of bone will depend on the age of the patient and the distance that the bone has been lengthened. When the correct distance has been achieved and there is radiographic evidence of new bone filling the entire gap then the distraction nuts may be loosened. This will mean that the bone will be taking weight but not all the external stress. The apparatus can be removed when there is sound evidence of consolidated new bone (Fig. 8.8a, b) but activity will have to be restricted for at least 6 months.

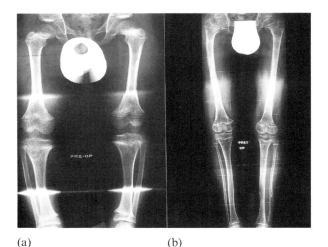

(a)   (b)

Fig. 8.8 The same patient as Fig. 8.6. (a) Preoperative radiograph of lower limbs. (b) At the end of treatment: both tibia and femur have been lengthened; total lengthening = 29 cm.

Complications

Generally there were few complications and they could be divided into three groups: (1) soft tissues, (2) bone and (3) apparatus [22].

Soft tissues

Skin may split occasionally when the lengthening exceeds 3.0 cm but it heals quickly without causing any problems. The main concern was pin-track infection which was fairly common, and minor infection occurred in 30% but cleared up after cleaning with an antiseptic solution. In 10% there was more persistent infection which responded to systemic antibiotic cover; two pins had to be repositioned. Slackening of tension in the pins was the main cause of skin irritation and local sepsis.

Pressure necrosis occurred on two occasions and in both the supporting rings were too small and failed to accommodate the swelling and increased circumference of the limb.

Nerve damage occurred twice. The external popliteal nerve was stretched, which caused paresis of the dorsi-flexors of the foot. It was perhaps due to over-ambitious lengthening of the tibia and fibula but both recovered within 9 months.

Arterial injuries did not occur in this series. Swelling of the limb was not uncommon and occurred in 70% of femoral and 30% of tibial lengthening which has to be borne in mind when planning the size of component. The swelling was not a permanent problem and tended to resolve either as a result of walking or after the apparatus had been removed at the conclusion of the lengthening procedure.

Contractures. An equinus contracture of the foot was not uncommon but most resolved as a result of physiotherapy and weight bearing during the lengthening phase. A persistent flexion contracture or worse, a posterior subluxation, at the knee can be a serious problem and should be avoided. It is caused by a combination of tight hamstring muscles, a tight ilio-tibial band, a persistent tendency to hold the knee flexed beyond 30° and the inherent tendency of the tibia to displace posteriorly when the joint is held in a flexed position. The authors have overcome this problem by insisting on a course of physiotherapy after the apparatus has been dismantled and by restricting the range of flexion to 30° during the lengthening phase. There were no permanent contractures of the joints in this series [22].

Bone

Infection occurred in one patient as a result of pin-track sepsis. The localized area of osteomyelitis resolved after the pin track had been changed and the affected area curretted.

Delayed bone production occurred in one patient who had trophic changes in the limb. This delayed consolidation of the lengthened segment and a cancellous bone graft was required, but eventually sound union was achieved.

Malalignment of the malleoli at the ankle will result if the distal end of the fibular diaphysis is not transfixed satisfactorily by the distal pin. Failure to secure the fibula will cause proximal migration of the lateral malleolus and this occurred in one patient. It was a difficult problem to overcome and it required a complicated osteotomy because the tibia had been lengthened by 14 cm.

Apparatus

Metal fatigue, fracture and loosening of nuts and bolts are all possibilities but unlikely if the apparatus has been constructed correctly. Loss of tension in the pins has been mentioned already and this has to be checked not only at the time of application but also at 3-weekly intervals during the lengthening phase.

The patients

A total of 121 bones were lengthened in this series from Asepeyo Hospital in Madrid (tibia, 74 cases and femur, 47 cases). Congenital abnormalities provided the largest source including idiopathic causes, achondroplasia, Turner's syndrome, congenital hypoplasia and fibular agenesis. Achondroplasia played a relatively large part in this group. The maximum increase in length of the tibia was 17.5 cm.

Acquired conditions were caused either by

trauma or infection. Again the tibia was the most commonly lengthened bone.

The time required to obtain the desired increase in length did not vary between the categories, and it was calculated at the rate of 1.0 month per 1.0 cm for patients under 10 years old and 1.5 months per centimetre for those older than 10 years.

Most patients were standing on the third day and walking on the fifth day.

The average time in hospital was 7 days.

Discussion

The method of limb lengthening as described originally by Ilizarov has been tried in Asepeyo Hospital and this chapter has hopefully confirmed the success which was claimed by the original author. There is no doubt that once the components of the apparatus have been mastered and the rules of its application are followed the variety of conditions which can be treated are enormous. It is fairly obvious that the acquired problems are more amenable to lengthening than the congenital, where soft tissues have not the advantage of genetic programming for normal bone growth. Nevertheless, the method can be adapted to more or less any long bone and Ilizarov has applied it successfully to feet.

The advantage that this method has over previous methods must include (a) the minimal operative exposure, (b) the minute division of periosteum, (c) the delicate division of cortical bone and preservation of vital structures such as blood vessels. Finally, the experience of using this method has not caused any serious complications but it has achieved a fair measure of success with a minimal stay in hospital and generally a painless experience. The patients are able to walk on the fifth day and do not find it difficult to master the technique of lengthening their limb at home.

References and further reading

1. Badelou, O. (1988) La technique d'Ilizarov chez l'enfant avec un fixateur externe radio transparent. *Rev. Chir. Orthop.*, **T.74 Sup. II**, 237–240.
2. Beguiristain, J. L., Oniaifo, A. and Cañadell, J. (1979) Consideraciones sobre nuestra experiencia en elongacion de femur y tibia, segun el metodo de Wagner. *Rev. Ortop y Traum.*, **23**, 227–230.

3. Bianchi-Maiocchi, A., Benedetti, G. B., Catagui, M., Cattaneo, R., Tentoni, L. and Villa, A. (1983) *Introduzione Alla Conoscenza Delle Metodiche d'Ilizarov in Ortopedia e Traumatologia.* Medi Surgical Video, Milano.

4. Bianchi-Maiocchi, A., Catagui, M., Cattaneo, R., Tentoni, L. and Villa, A. (1985) *L'Osteosintesi Transossea Secondo G. A. Ilizarov.* Medi Surgical Video, Milano.

5. Cañadell, J. and De Pablos, J. (1985) Breaking Bony Bridges by Physeal Distraction: A New Therapeutic Approach. *Int. Orthop. S.I.C.O.T.*, **9**, 223–229.

6. Catagni, M. A. and Villa, A. (1988) *Allungamento di Gamba Secondo la Metodica di G. A. Ilizarov.* Medi Surgical Video, Milano.

7. Cattaneo, R. (1985) Traitement des pseudo-arthroses diaphysaires – septiques ou non septiques selon la methode d'Ilizarov en compression monofocale. *Rev. Chir. Orthop.*, **T-71**, 223–229.

8. Cattaneo, R. (1986) Traitement des inegalites du femur par la methode d'Ilizarov. *Rev. Chir. Orthop.*, **T-72**, 203–209.

9. Cattaneo, R. (1986) Application de la methode d'Ilizarov dans l'allongement de l'humerus. *Rev. Chir. Orthop.*, **T-72**, 203–209.

10. Forum sur la Methode d'Ilizarov. *Rev. Chir. Orthop.*, **T-73, Sup. II**, 29–70.

11. Cattaneo, R. (1988) La methode d'Ilizarov dans le traitement des grandes déviations axiales des membres. *Rev. Chir. Orthop.*, **T-74, Sup. II**, 237–240.

12. De Bastiani, G. B., Aldegheri, R., Renzi-Brivio, L. and Trivela, G. (1986) Limb lengthening by distraction of the epiphyseal plate. *J. Bone Joint Surg.*, **68-B; 4**, 545–549.

13. De Bastiani, G. B., Aldegheri, R., Renzi-Brivio, L. and Trivela, G. (1986) Chondrodiastasis: controlled symmetrical distraction of the epiphyseal plate. *J. Bone Joint Surg.*, **68-B: 4**, 551–556.

14. De Pablos, J., Villas, C. and Cañadell, J. (1986) Bone lengthening by physeal distraction: an experimental study. *Int. Orthop.*, **10**, 163–170.

15. Ilizarov, G. A. (1981) Personal comunication. XII Italian A.O. Club Convention Bellagio, Italia.

16. Ilizarov, G. A. and Y Soybelman, L. M. (1969) Some clinical and experimental data on the bloodless lengthening of lower limbs. *Exp. Chir. Anest.*, **4**, 27–32.

17. Ilizarov, G. A. (1986) L'Osteossintesi Transossea Nelle Fractura e Pseuddartrosi Dell' Avambracio. Medi Surgical Video., Milano.

18. Lazo, J., Aguilar, F., Mozo, F., Gonzalez, R., Baquerizo, A. and Lazo, J. M. (1980) Biocompresion: un principio diferente en el tratamiento de fracturas. *Rev. Ortop. Traum.*, **24 1B**, 1–12.

19. Lee, D. Y., Choi, I. H., Chung, C. Y. *et al.* (1994) Experience with lengthening by the Ilizarov Technique. *Orthopaedics International*, **2(4)**, 349–359.

20. Mendoza, J. L. (1949) *Algunas Consideraciones y Experiencias Sobre Distraccion Osea. El Cálculo Matematico en la Reduccion de las Fracturas.* Comunicacion Primeras Jornadas Ortopedicas de la S.E.C.O.T. Julio, Bilbao.

21. Monticelli, G. and Spinelli, R. (1981) Limb lengthening by epiphyseal distraction. *Int. Orthop.* **5**, 85–90.

22. Paley, D. (1987) Hinges: theoretical aspects. *Abstracts from the International Conferences on the Ilizarov Techniques for Management of Difficult Skeletal Problems.* Hospital for Joint Diseases, New York, 1–3 Nov.

23. Paley, D. (1988) Current techniques of limb lengthening *J. Pediatr. Orthop.*, **8**, 73–92.

24. Pous J., Ruano, D. and Suso, S. (1988) *Atlas Anatomotopografico de las Extremidades y Fijacion Externa Anular* (ed. S. A. Jims), Barcelona.

25. Wagner, H. (1971) *Operative Beinverlangerung.* **42**, 260–266.

9

The multiply injured patient with musculoskeletal injuries

M. F. Swiontkowski

High velocity trauma is the number one cause of death in the 18 to 38-year age group worldwide. In the USA alone, loss of income due to death and disability resulting from high velocity trauma totals 75 billion dollars annually [1]. This is an economic loss of staggering proportions. The goal of all governmental agencies responsible for health care decisions must be to minimize mortality and maximize return to function in this large, productive segment of the population. In this light, difficult decisions must be made regarding funding of research into injury prevention and trauma management, and legislation must be passed which is designed to minimize road traffic accident morbidity and mortality. Within the health care system, much effort has recently been directed toward optimizing the care of the polytrauma victim to speed return of these individuals to productive life. These efforts must continue for the foreseeable future because of the enormous impact of this problem on the individual and society.

Philosophy

In the care of the multiply injured individual, the treatment of complex injuries in multiple organ systems demands a team approach. The team must be able to evaluate the patient swiftly, be willing to discuss the effect of the management of one problem on another and be able to arrive at decisions quickly in regard to performing life-saving procedures.

Every team must have a final decision-maker, the captain. In the case of the polytrauma patient, this should be the individual most experienced in performing procedures to maintain the airway, manage shock from multiple causes, manage emergent situations affecting cardiac output (i.e. cardiac tamponade or injury to the great vessels), diagnose and treat intrathoracic or intra-abdominal haemorrhage, and make appropriate decisions regarding the early management of central nervous system and extremity trauma. In most settings in the western world, this will be the general surgeon with an interest and background in the care of the multiply injured patient. This need not be the case, however, as a neurological, urological, or musculoskeletal trauma surgeon with the same qualifications may be the critical decision-making individual in some settings, especially in more rural areas. At a minimum, the definitive care setting must have adequate laboratory facilities to perform quick and accurate haematological and blood chemistry determinations, arterial blood gas analysis, and alcohol and drug screens, and to provide emergent blood product support services. The facility must have a radiological suite to provide high quality plain radiographs of the spine, abdomen, chest, pelvis, and extremities, as well as emergent angiography and computed tomography services. An operating room must be staffed and ready 24 hours a day to manage emergency chest, abdominal, head, pelvic, and extremity trauma. The hospital administration must be willing to support these services, expensive as they are, to deliver high quality care to the multiply injured patient. Equally important, the team captain must have the support of surgical specialists available to him or her at any hour. These individuals must be familiar with the problems unique to the multiply injured patient and be willing to work together to optimize the patient's recovery – that is, they must be 'team players'.

Transport

The multiply injured patient must reach the definitive care setting in a timely fashion. He or she must be appropriately cared for during extrication and transport to avoid a preventable death due to airway obstruction, and shock treatment should be initiated. The ambulance crews of the 1950s and 1960s who simply threw the individual into the back of the vehicle and drove to the nearest hospital have, for the most part, been replaced by skilled Emergency Medical Technicians (EMTs). The EMTs are generally affiliated with fire departments within the hospital and are dispatched by local emergency operators to reported accidents. The EMT is generally well trained in the initial management of the multiply injured patient, and arrives at the scene in a well-equipped vehicle which has the equipment needed for extrication, special support, airway management, vital sign monitoring, i.v. solutions administration, cardiac arrest management, and fracture splintage. Increasingly, the EMT may arrive in a similarly-equipped helicopter.

There exists a degree of controversy as to the function of the EMT in the United States today. On one side is the 'scoop and run' philosophy, which holds that EMTs should swiftly and safely extricate the patient with spinal precautions and place the victim on a backboard [2]. The airway should be cleared and if spontaneous respirations are occurring, the individual should be placed in the vehicle and transported to the definitive care unit designated by the dispatcher. En route, i.v. access should be obtained, vital signs checked, and fluid therapy initiated. In cases of absent spontaneous respirations, cardiopulmonary resuscitation should be initiated en route. With this theory, speed of transport is critical. Cowley reported a three-fold increase in mortality for every 30 minutes of elapsed time without care [3].

Table 9.1   Basic EMT skills

1. Perform technically sound CPR
2. Maintain an airway (endotracheal intubation?)
3. Obtain IV access and start Ringer lactate therapy
4. Reduction and splintage of fractures
5. Perform primary survey of patient and report findings to destination centre
6. Act in concert with MD in early treatment decisions (radio/telephone contact)

The second philosophy, held by Copass *et al.* [4], is that EMTs can be trained to do procedures which will begin the resuscitation efforts in the field. In cases where spontaneous respiration is absent or where there is profound hypovolaemic hypotension, EMTs can safely intubate the patient and start central lines. Flutter valve needles can be placed intrathoracically to temporarily manage tension pneumothoraces. These procedures are performed under MD supervision via radio contact. Copass' group has shown that significant improvements in morbidity and mortality rates can be expected with this system [4].

Regardless of the philosophy employed, all agree that EMTs should be able to perform certain basic tasks (Table 9.1). There must be frequent open-ended dialogue among the dispatchers, EMTs, and the director of the regional EMT program to improve skills of the EMTs and thus optimize the care of critically injured individuals.

Treatment plan

Wolff *et al.* [5] have identified five phases in the care of the multiply injured patient after arrival at the definitive care centre The five phases are:

1. Resuscitation.
2. Emergency procedures.
3. Stabilization.
4. Delayed operative procedures.
5. Rehabilitation.

Resuscitation

The goal of the resuscitation phase is to establish normal vital signs by dealing with all situations acutely affecting a clear airway, normal ventilatory response, normal blood pressure, pulse, and distal perfusion. In essence, this means establishing an airway by endotracheal intubation or tracheotomy, placing the patient on controlled ventilation, and treating shock. In most instances, this phase of treatment is initiated in the field by the EMTs and is continued upon arrival at the definitive care centre.

In the United States, regional trauma centres have been designed along strict lines. The criteria for a Class I Trauma Centre include thoroughly equipped operating rooms, in-house 24-hour-a-day trauma surgeon presence, surgical subspecialty consultation available within 15 minutes, and the presence of surgical housestaff. Class II criteria are the same, with the exception of the training requirement. In most trauma centres the resuscitation is carried out in the emergency department. These facilities, in general, are equipped for all emergent surgical procedures, standard radiographs, and the institution of ventilatory support. Blood bank support must be quickly accessible for the treatment of shock. The details of the management of shock are completely discussed in Chapter 10.

As long as adequate blood pressure can be maintained in combination with ventilatory support, diagnostic studies can be performed. In many instances, tube thoracostomy, placement of MAST trousers, and/or pericardiocentesis may be required to restore normal blood pressure. If normal blood pressure proves difficult to maintain with appropriate fluid management, abdominal peritoneal tap may be performed to rule out intra-abdominal haemorrhage. If the blood pressure is stable in a moderate range, abdominal CT scanning can be extremely helpful in establishing a diagnosis of a liver or splenic injury, ruptured viscus or renal injury. In the case of a head injury, midface injury, or cervical spine injury, CT scan of the head must be conducted during this phase as well, to rule out intracerebral haemorrhage. Plain radiographs of the entire spine should be obtained at this stage if indicated. These should supplement the initial lateral radiograph of the cervical spine (exposing down to C7), chest, and pelvis radiographs. If the patient's blood pressure is not maintained within a reasonable range at any point, there is no indication for further diagnostic studies and the patient must enter the second phase of treatment.

Immediate surgery

During this phase of treatment the patient is generally moved to the operating theatre. It is during this phase that all maximally invasive life-saving surgical procedures are performed. As noted above, an extremely unstable patient in whom an adequate systolic blood pressure (as indicated by capillary perfusion of the distal extremities and urinary output of 30 ml/h) has not been restored may have to be moved to the operating room before all diagnostic procedures have been performed. In rare circumstances, major surgical procedures may be instituted in the emergency room as typified by a thoracotomy for open cardiac massage. This manoeuvre, however, has generally only been successful for penetrating trauma, and its indications in blunt trauma are subject to debate.

Most patients are brought to the operating room having already been intubated and placed on a volume respirator, with two large bore i.v. access lines (volume replacement ongoing) and a urinary catheter in place. If there has been inadequate opportunity to obtain a clear lateral cervical spine radiograph all the way to C7, the patient must be assumed to have a cervical spine fracture, and a hard cervical collar should be in place. In most instances, trauma victims will have full stomachs and/or have ingested alcohol within 8 hours, and this must be taken into consideration for all victims who arrive in the operating theatre non-intubated. This complicates the situation, and techniques to apply cricothyroid pressure during intubation to minimize the risk of aspiration must be utilized. The trauma anaesthesiologist will generally choose shorter-acting intravenous and inhalation agents along with paralysing drugs for the multiply injured patient.

The majority of life-saving operations in this phase will be performed for ongoing haemorrhage (Table 9.2). This would include laparotomy for splenic, liver, or renal parenchymal injury or thoracotomy for injury to the aorta, vena cava, or pulmonary vessels. Penetrating trauma results in injuries to the same structures, but the types of lesion found will vary according to the type of projectile involved. Neurosurgical procedures for ongoing mass effect of depressed skull fractures or subdural haematoma are also indicated at this stage, and can be performed in

Table 9.2 Indications for immediate surgery

1. Haemorrhage secondary to:
   a. Liver, splenic, renal parenchymal injury –
      laparotomy
   b. Aortic, canal, or pulmonary vessel tears –
      thoracotomy
   c. Depressed skull fracture or acute subdural
      bleed – craniotomy
   d. Pelvic fracture – stabilization

2. Prevention of pulmonary failure:
   a. Femoral shaft fractures
   b. Pelvic fractures

Table 9.3 Evaluation of multiple trauma: patient injury severity score

AIS defined body areas
1. Soft tissue
2. Head and neck
3. Chest
4. Abdomen
5. Extremity and/or pelvis

Severity code
1. Minor
2. Moderate
3. Severe (non-life threatening)
4. Severe (life threatening)
5. Critical (survival uncertain)
6. Fatal (dead on arrival)

$ISS = A^2 + B^2 + C^2$ where A, B, C = individual regional injury severity code

concert with the abdominal or thoracic procedures. Rarely, ongoing haemorrhage due to extremity arterial trauma will require vascular repair in conjunction with stabilization of the fractures by the orthopaedist.

Recent data have indicated that stabilization of femoral and pelvic fractures prevent the pulmonary failure state in blunt trauma [6–8]. Therefore, after haemorrhage due to the above factors has been controlled, femoral shaft fractures and unstable pelvic injuries should be stabilized under the initial anaesthesia. Non-critical orthopaedic injuries to the tibia, foot and ankle, and upper extremities can await the next phase of treatment. If, however, the patient is haemodynamically stable, all open fractures and displaced fractures of the femoral or talar neck should be managed under the initial anaesthesia.

During this phase of treatment, the overall injury severity, age, premorbid nutritional status, and general medical condition of the patient must be taken into consideration. To this end, many systems of trauma scoring have been developed to aid in prognostic decisions in the multiply injured and to assist in research into the problem of polytrauma. These systems include the triage index (TI) [9], trauma score (TS) [10], abbreviated injury scale (AIS) [11], and the injury severity score (ISS) [11,12]. The last-mentioned grew out of the AIS and is the most widely used at this time. In this scale, a severity rating is applied to each injury within each organ system, and the results are squared and summed (Table 9.3). General condition and age cannot be taken into account in this system, but it has been demonstrated that the LD50 for the 15–44 age group is an ISS 40, for 45–64 it is 29, and for 65 and older it is 20. This information must be

considered during the phase of emergent surgery. As an example, a severe crush injury to a tibia associated with an ISS of 40 in a 19-year-old motorcyclist should be managed with debridement and application of an external fixator, while the same injury in a 70-year-old with an ISS of 40 should be managed with an immediate open below-the-knee amputation [13]. This illustrates the importance of communication on the part of the orthopaedist with the team captain general surgeon during this phase of treatment.

Stabilization

The goals for this phase of care of the multiply injured patient and the procedures subsequently performed depend to a large extent on the condition of the patient prior to entry into the phase of immediate surgery. If a stable blood pressure was maintained during the resuscitation and the majority of the major diagnostic work was completed, there will be far less diagnostic work to do during this phase than if the patient was rushed to the operating theatre. Claudi [14] has outlined the goals of this phase of treatment to include:

1. Restoration of stable haemodynamics.
2. Restoration of adequate oxygenation and organ perfusion.
3. Restoration of adequate kidney function.
4. Treatment of bleeding disorders.

This phase of treatment begins after the phase of immediate surgery and after the initial treatment of shock has proven effective. It may last hours to days. During this phase, all open wounds should be optimally managed and all fractures splinted in the position of function. In general, this phase of therapy is conducted in an intensive care unit under the continued direction of the trauma surgeon. In many settings, an intensive care specialist familiar with the evaluation and treatment of the polytrauma victim will take over the stabilization. The goal is to stabilize the patient rapidly to prevent parenchymal damage and to prepare as soon as possible for return to the operating room for other procedures.

In the restoration of stable haemodynamics, the usual monitoring tools are central lines or triple lumen catheters (for measuring pulmonary artery capillary wedge pressures and cardiac output), arterial lines (continuous measurement of arterial blood pressure and access for multiple arterial blood gas samples), and a urinary catheter. Appropriate crystalloid and colloid replacement therapy will be selected based on physiological parameters as well as on frequent packed red blood cell values, arterial blood gas levels, urinary output, cardiac output, wedge pressures, and arterial blood pressure.

For most trauma victims, volume-controlled mechanical ventilation will be selected for this phase. The early use of positive end expiratory pressure (PEEP) is extremely valuable in preventing pulmonary failure [15–17]. Frequent arterial blood gas analyses should direct changes in the mechanical ventilator and PEEP settings. Weaning from mechanical ventilation may be systematically conducted based on the patient's responses to intermittent assisted ventilation and trials of removal from ventilator support once the patient's blood pressure, oxygenation, and ventilation function have stabilized, and if, in the absence of facial or tracheal injury, extubation can safely be performed. Early stabilization of pelvic and femoral fractures to avoid traction is critical in this phase [8].

For the most part, adequate renal function can be maintained by appropriate management of shock. Maintaining adequate blood pressure and urinary output during the two preceding phases is nearly 100% effective in preventing renal failure. Diuretics should be used in a limited fashion in this phase only when sufficient volume has been documented by adequate cardiac output and pulmonary capillary wedge pressure (PCWP) and in general is only indicated in elderly

patients. If hypovolaemic acute renal failure follows high output failure as documented by serum and urinary electrolytes, appropriate use of renal dialysis directed by a nephrologist during this phase is indicated.

Bleeding disorders in the multiply injured patient are nearly always due to haemodilution, i.e. inadequate transfusion of platelets and coagulation factors, and/or shock-related hepatic dysfunction, with the former being far more common. Occasionally, a transfusion reaction may be encountered when O negative or type-specific blood has been used during the resuscitation phase. Wherever possible, cross-matched blood should be used and 6 units of platelets should be given with every 8–10 units of blood transfused. Fresh frozen plasma should be used when prolonged PT and PTT times are evident in patients receiving massive transfusions. Disseminated intravascular coagulation (DIC) is best treated by prevention, as it is very difficult to reverse once the process begins. Adequate initial shock therapy is critical to avoiding these complications.

Delayed operative procedures

As the length of the preceding phase is highly variable, all open wounds must be optimally managed and all fractures splinted in the position of function. This is done in an attempt to minimize the complications of infection, and to offer the pain relief of fracture stability in order to decrease the use of narcotics, which act as CNS depressants as well as respiratory and gastrointestinal function depressants, and should be used as little as possible [13]. In most cases, however, the phase of stabilization is complete within 3–4 hours, and the patient can then be brought to the operating theatre for care of non-life-threatening problems.

As mentioned in the previous section, operative management of femoral fractures and pelvic fractures prevents the pulmonary failure state, and these fractures should be managed whenever possible under the initial anaesthesia. Several other musculoskeletal problems must be treated within the first 6–8 hours for avoidance of complications. Compartmental syndromes, most often associated with fractures of the tibia and forearm in the polytrauma setting, must be managed with fasciotomy early to prevent permanent muscle cell death and/or loss of nerve function. As noted previously, open fractures must also be managed with irrigation and debridement in this time frame to avoid higher rates of infection [18]. Similarly, fractures with associated vascular injury must be reconstructed within 6 hours to avoid loss of muscle and nerve function. When revascularization times are delayed beyond this range, compartmental syndromes distal to the lesion due to prolonged ischemia time must also be considered. There is some evidence to suggest that emergent capsulotomy, open reduction, and internal fixation with compression minimize the risk of late necrosis of the femoral head [19]. These fractures, along with displaced fractures of the talar neck, should be managed in this early acute phase to avoid the devastating complications of bone necrosis in these major weight-bearing joints.

Major fractures of the metaphyseal distal femur, proximal tibia, distal tibia, ankle and foot, and wrist and elbow should be considered in the next line of priority. Especially in the case of severe fractures around the elbow, ankle, and hindfoot, if management is not completed within 8–10 hours of injury, major swelling and fracture blisters ensue, making it wise to delay operative procedures to 8–12 days. Reduction in this time frame will be much more difficult, and therefore early intervention is recommended. Internal fixation of closed tibial fractures should be classed in the next, less-urgent group, especially when associated with an ipsilateral femoral fracture. Conservative treatment in this setting has been shown by Veith *et al.* to be associated with higher rates of nonunion and a greater loss of knee motion [20]. Operative fixation of upper extremity shaft fractures can be grouped here as well.

The management of unstable cervical and thoracolumbar spine fractures varies as to whether the patient is neurologically intact or not. Patients with complete loss of neurological function distal to the fracture who have return of cord level reflexes (i.e. bulbocavernosus reflex) are best managed with early stabilization to enhance the rehabilitation phase. Recumbent, conservative treatment is not indicated in this group. Operative stabilization, which for the most part will be posterior internal fixation and fusion, is best accomplished in the first 5–7 days in this phase to return the patient to the upright position and improve the ventilation–perfusion

efficiency of the pulmonary circulation. These patients, because of their lack of motor function, are at risk for deep venous thrombosis and need to be mobilized early [21]. Patients with cervical, thoracic or lumbar spine fractures and no loss of neurological function should similarly be managed in the same time frame to allow early mobilization and to prevent the complications of prolonged recumbency. Patients with spine fractures and partial loss of neurological function represent a group of different considerations.

Careful attention must be paid to the nutritional status of the patient, as the multiply injured patient has extremely high caloric requirements at this juncture [22]. If the patient, due to head injury, loss of gut or maxillofacial injuries, is unable to take in 2000–3000 calories per day, parenteral nutrition must be initiated. This caloric intake may be accomplished by tube feedings whenever possible, but can be effectively delivered by the total parenteral nutrition (TPN) route. Nutritional consultation and a dietary plan based on calory counts, skin tests, and lymphocyte counts can be extremely useful where the proper nutritional course is in question. Of course, the patient can be weaned from enteral or TPN as head injuries, maxillofacial fractures, and general condition improves.

Recovery/rehabilitation

This is the phase during which musculoskeletal injuries play a critical role. The vast majority of permanent disability following multiple trauma is due to musculoskeletal or CNS trauma. These injuries must be optimally managed in the emergent and delayed operative procedures phases. Closed head injury and complete spinal cord injury are little affected by management, but major improvements can be made by optimum management of musculoskeletal injury. As indicated in prior sections, these injuries are best treated as soon as possible. Fracture reductions are much easier to perform if done before the healing process has begun. Intra-articular fractures are therefore best dealt with operatively in the first 24 hours after injury. Open fractures, fractures with vascular injury, femoral and talar neck fractures, femoral shaft fractures, unstable pelvic fractures and fractures of emergent nature are discussed in preceding sections.

The recovery/rehabilitation phase begins at the

conclusion of the operative phase. In cases of head injury, maxillofacial trauma, or genito-urinary injury, great care must be taken to assure optimal patient nutrition. Therefore, the input of the nutritionist becomes critical at this juncture. Similarly, because of post-trauma depression, the role of the consulting psychologist or psychiatrist becomes important. Physical and occupational therapists play a critical role in optimizing return of function.

In cases of severe multiple musculoskeletal injury, especially those which occur in conjunction with head injuries, transferring the patient to a rehabilitation centre is appropriate at this point. In this setting, a psychiatrist with special-ized training in rehabilitation medicine serves as a critical team leader. This individual organizes the input of the rehabilitation nurse specialists, occupational and physical therapists, and the orthopaedists, urologists, and neurosurgeons. Those patients who do not require speech or occupational therapy, do not have a spinal cord injury, and do not have neurological injuries that would benefit from admission to a rehabilitation unit may be best treated at home. To obtain optimal functional results, the orthopaedist should supervise the physical therapists and visit-ing home nurses. Patients with severe musculo-skeletal injury must be seen by the treating surgeon fairly frequently in the first 6 weeks post-discharge, and at 3- to 4-week intervals thereafter until functional results have been maximized.

Critical musculoskeletal injuries

The patient is too sick!

This is the most common argument against aggressive early management of the multiply injured patient. Frequently, anaesthesiologists and surgeons unfamiliar with the care of this type of patient raise this objection when the ortho-paedist indicates his or her desire to, for example, place intramedullary nails in the femoral and tibial fracture, or to internally fix the intra-articular distal humerus fracture under the initial anaesthesia. Several authors have retrospectively reviewed the efficacy of aggressive early manage-ment in polytrauma, and have concluded that mortality and morbidity are significantly de-creased by early operative intervention in the

management of long bone fractures [5,6,16]. Meek *et al.* reviewed a series of 71 patients with multiple long bone fractures who were assigned to one of two groups according to the treating physician who performed either rigid stabi-lization of long bone fractures within 24 hours or traction/cast treatment [23]. The cases were matched according to ISS scores. Of the 22 patients treated with early stabilization, one expired; and of the 49 treated in traction and casts, 14 expired, which represents a highly signi-ficant difference. Johnson and colleagues reviewed a series of 132 consecutive cases of patients with musculoskeletal injuries (minimum of two long bone fractures) and ISS scores greater than 18 [7]. They compared a group of patients in which all major fractures (long bones, pelvis, and spine) were stabilized in the first 24 hours ($N = 83$) to a group of patients who had their operative stabilization delayed ($N = 49$), basing their analysis of the effect of these treat-ment regimens on adult respiratory distress syn-drome (ARDS). They concluded that there is a significant increase in the incidence of ARDS associated with a delay in operative stabilization of major fractures. This was most dramatic in the group with an ISS of greater than 40. Retro-spective reviews addressing similar issues by Wolff *et al.* [5], Ruedi [24], Riska *et al.* [25], Goris *et al.* [16], Gustillo *et al.* [6] and others have confirmed the fact that early operative stabi-lization of major long bone and pelvic fractures decreases the pulmonary failure state, morbidity, and mortality.

Border's group in Buffalo, New York prospec-tively studied 56 patients with blunt multiple trauma (ISS 22–57) and evaluated the effect of three musculoskeletal injury management schemes on the pulmonary failure septic state [8]. One group had immediate internal fixation of long bone fractures and postoperative ventila-tory support, a second group had 10 days of femur traction and postoperative ventilator sup-port, and the third group was immediately extu-bated after surgery and had 30 days of femur traction. Ten days of femur traction doubled the duration of the pulmonary failure state, in-creased the number of positive blood cultures by a factor of ten, the use of injectable narcotics by a factor of two, and the number of fracture compli-cations by 3.5. Thirty days of femur traction increased the duration of the pulmonary failure state by a factor of three to five (relative to group I), the number of positive blood cultures by a factor of 74, the use of narcotics by a factor of two, and the number of fracture complications by 17.

It is clear from this body of retrospective and prospective work that the concept of the patient being too sick for surgery is incorrect. The sicker the patient (in terms of ISS), the more he or she stands to benefit from immediate stabilization of long bone fractures and the sicker he or she will become if treated conservatively or with traction.

Long bone fracture management

The indications for fixation of long bone fractures are clear and the techniques for this type of management are worthy of discussion. For fractures of the femoral shaft, there is no doubt that closed intramedullary nailing is the procedure of choice. Winquist, in a series of 520 femoral shaft fractures, has demonstrated that the rate of infection is 0.9% and nonunion 0.9% – rates that have not been duplicated with any other method of treatment [26]. Previously, there was concern about increasing the risk of fat embolism in the multiply injured patient by reaming the femoral shaft fracture; however, there has not been any clinical increase in the incidence of ARDS following the nailing of femoral shaft fractures [26]. Bach *et al.* have shown that both in the laboratory and clinically (including 86 open fractures) the reaming of a fractured femur does not produce an increase in fat release [27].

Interlocking nailing has extended the use of the closed nailing technique to include very proximal and distal fractures, as well as highly comminuted fractures. In the vast majority of multiply injured patients, the side-lying position for intramedullary nailing of the femur can be used. After the surgical management of intrathoracic or intra-abdominal haemorrhage, the patient is generally stable once lost blood has been replaced. If the patient's blood pressure has been difficult to maintain, the supine position can be used. The affected limb must be adducted past the midline to allow ease of exposure of the greater trochanter in order to develop the starting point for the intramedullary nail. Another indication for the supine position in nailing the femoral shaft fracture is an associated pelvic fracture. Placing the patient in the side-lying position places stress across the posterior elements of the pelvis and can restart bleeding from fracture surfaces or minor sacral venous plexuses. Many authors prefer the supine position for the nailing of comminuted fractures utilizing interlocking nails, as they feel that the techniques for inserting the distal locking screws are much easier to employ with the patient in this position. In either position, the C-arm must be utilized throughout the procedure for the closed intramedullary nailing technique. Another advantage of the supine nailing position is that surgical conditions of the abdomen, chest, and head can be more easily treated simultaneously by surgical teams working together to expedite the management of the patient.

The closed intramedullary nailing technique has been safely extended to grade I and grade II [26] open fractures in the multiply injured patient with no significant increase in the rate of chronic bone infection. For grade III fractures, however, this technique should generally not be used. To avoid the need for traction following debridement of the wound, external fixation should be employed to allow mobilization of the patient's chest. The fixation should be applied with the patient in the supine position, utilizing the C-arm for pin placement after a thorough debridement of the wound. In general, lateral pin placement is preferred to avoid scarring within the quadriceps muscle mass and subsequent loss of knee motion.

Of all fractures of the long bones, the femur fracture is the most critical. Conservative care of femoral shaft fractures requires the use of traction with the concomitant problems of poor chest position, difficulty with moving the patient for subsequent studies, and the inability to get the patient out of bed. The femoral shaft fracture must receive the orthopaedist's highest priority in the multiply injured and should be stabilized with an intramedullary nail whenever possible.

Occasionally, when a humeral shaft fracture is present, intramedullary nailing is indicated to allow axial weight bearing with crutches early on. This is generally done in the secondary phase of procedures but may be indicated when the patient is stable and tolerating the initial operative session well. Closed tibial fractures may be managed with closed intramedullary or interlocking nailing in the multiply injured patient. Closed fractures can be splinted to partially immobilize the fracture fragments so that stabilization procedures can be delayed to the second visit to the operating room. Reamed or unreamed tibial nailing may be used in this setting. For open fractures, external fixation is currently the procedure of choice. This must be done after the initial debridement during the first anaesthesia to allow for adequate wound care without compromising fracture stability. Half-pin fixation frames have proven to be far superior to the old through-pin Hoffman type of frames. This is because the pins do not impale the muscle–tendon units and allow early motion of the adjacent joints. The half-pin constructs have also proven to have superior biomechanical characteristics. In general, reamed intramedullary nailing has no place in open fractures because of the increased risk of chronic bone infection. Unreamed Enders or Lottes nail fixation may be advantageous, as they allow good care of the soft tissues without the disadvantages of the external fixator. These procedures carry an acceptable risk of chronic infection.

In general, once the femoral shaft fracture has been stabilized and the open long bone fractures debrided and stabilized, the decision to proceed with further intramedullary stabilization of other long bone fractures can be made. The factors to be considered must include expertise of the surgical and nursing staff, availability of implants, condition of the patient, and level of fatigue of the surgical and nursing staff. In most trauma centres, a second surgical or nursing team can be brought in if it is in the patient's best interest to stabilize all the long bone fractures in the first surgical sitting.

Pelvic fracture management

Pelvic fractures are frequently life threatening. Several reported series note mortality rates of 5–20% [28–31]. In reviewing these series, it becomes evident that there is an important difference between simple and complex fractures in terms of morbidity, mortality, and treatment techniques. Simple fractures include simple avulsion fractures of the anterior superior (or inferior) iliac spines, iliac ring fractures and minimally displaced pubic or ischial rami fractures. These are generally low velocity fractures and rarely occur in association with polytrauma.

It is important to classify the complex fractures, as this yields important information with respect to associated injuries, risk of bleeding and mortality.

Classification

Pennal *et al.* [28] have classified pelvic fractures according to the direction of the applied force. Antero-posterior compression fractures, lateral compression fractures, and vertical shear fractures are thereby defined. The anterior half of the pelvis (Table 9.4) includes the pubic and ischial rami, while the posterior portion includes the ilia, the sacroiliac joint, the sacrum and the strong posterior sacroiliac ligaments. In general, injury to the anterior structures is associated with bladder rupture and urethral tears, while injury to the posterior structures is associated with a higher incidence of severe haemorrhage, as well

Table 9.4   Abbreviated injury scale for injuries to the extremity and/or pelvis

Code	Injury
1. Minor	Minor sprains and fractures
	Dislocation of digits
2. Moderate	Compound fracture and digits
	Undisplaced long bone or pelvic fracture
	Major sprains of major joints
3. Serious, non-life-threatening	Displaced simple long bone fracture and/or multiple hand and foot fractures
	Single open long bone fracture
	Pelvic fracture with displacement
	Dislocation of major joints
	Multiple amputation of digits
	Laceration of major nerve or vessels of extremities
4. Severe, life-threatening survival probable	Multiple closed bone fractures
	Amputation of limbs
5. Critical, survival uncertain	Multiple open limb fractures
6. Fatal	Dead on arrival

as injury to the sacral nerve roots. A-P compression fractures include the so-called 'open book' fracture – the widened symphysis pubis, as well as the 'straddle fracture' – displaced fractures of all four anterior rami. A-P compression fractures are generally associated with a higher incidence of bladder and urethral injuries. The lateral compression group of fractures generally consists of an impacted sacral fracture or a fracture through the posterior ilium associated with an ipsilateral or contralateral pubic and ischial rami fracture. These fractures may be associated with injuries to the sacral nerve roots, as well as, less commonly, bladder or urethral injury. Because the critical posterior sacroiliac ligament complex is generally not violated, severe haemorrhage (more than four to six units) is generally not a problem. The vertical shear fracture includes a disruption through the sacroiliac joint, posterior ilium or sacrum associated with a disruption of the symphysis or an ipsilateral fracture of the ischial and pubic rami. The hemipelvis will frequently migrate superiorly and the posterior sacroiliac ligament complex is disrupted. These are the fractures most often associated with major haemorrhage as well as disruption of the sacral plexus.

Based on the initial radiographs, the orthopaedist can focus attention on the associated injuries. With the A-P compression injury, a more careful search for urethral disruption should be conducted if there is blood at the meatus (in the male) or gross blood in the urine. With vertical shear injuries, attention must be given to blood replacement early on [31].

Criteria for emergent fracture care

Patients with severe pelvic fractures may frequently be transported in MAST trousers on backboards. These trousers must be removed after the patient's blood pressure has been stabilized to allow for examination of the pelvis and limbs and for operative procedures to be performed. The use of MAST trousers is not a definitive treatment for pelvic fractures, and the trousers should not be left on the patient indefinitely. Open pelvic fractures carry a 50% mortality rate, as they are frequently the most high energy type of fracture, with the most displacement and

a high risk of deep infection [30]. Generally, the ischial rami produce the open wounds in the perineum. In the female, the pubic rami can produce an open wound into the vagina and a digital pelvic examination is therefore mandatory. In open fractures, a diverting colostomy is indicated, and if the anterior rami fractures are amenable to simple internal fixation with plates and screws and the surgeon has the skills to do so, this should be performed as stability of the fracture fragments will decrease the risk of infection. If the injury is not amenable to this type of management and instability is detectable on examination, an anterior external fixator should be applied.

In the case of continuing haemorrhage, aggressive management of the pelvic fracture is mandatory. If other sources of blood loss have been dealt with and the patient has lost more than four to six units of blood, stabilization of the pelvic fracture is indicated. The simplest way to accomplish this is by applying a bilateral long-leg spica cast with distal femoral pins [13]. This prevents motion of the pelvis when the patient is transported and turned in bed. A large abdominal hole must be cut out for continued observation of the abdomen. The critical point of this treatment is that the legs are stabilized and cannot put loads across the fracture surfaces.

The next simplest way to treat pelvic instability at the first operation is to apply an anterior external fixator. These frames do not offer tremendous support to the posterior disruptions in the case of the vertical shear fractures and cannot hold posterior reductions. They are useful, however, for stabilizing fracture surfaces to markedly decrease their motion and thereby aid in promoting clotting. Ultimately, displaced posterior disruptions should be reduced and internally fixed. The fixation may be accomplished with lag screws across the ilium and into the sacrum placed posteriorly or with small plates placed in screws across the fracture or sacroiliac joint from the anterior side. Although several groups are investigating the role of emergent internal fixation [32], these reconstructions should generally be done as delayed operative procedures, as they often will decompress tamponaded bleeding surfaces and promote further bleeding. As is the case with femoral shaft fractures, traction should play no role in the acute management of pelvic fractures because of the enforced recumbency of the patient and inadequate stabilization of the fracture [8].

Once the pelvis has been adequately stabilized by spica cast, external fixator, or, rarely, internal fixation, haemorrhage will usually cease. For the rare patient who experiences continuing blood loss, pelvic arteriography is indicated. Because only 10–15% of the sources of blood loss are minor arterial in nature, this technique is not indicated as a first-line management of haemorrhage secondary to a pelvic fracture [31]. Eighty-five percent of the sources of bleeding are fracture surfaces or minor pelvic or sacral veins, and the technique cannot address these. After stabilization of the pelvis has been performed, if blood loss continues with loss of six to eight more units over the next 12–24 hours and does not appear to be slowing, the patient should be returned to the radiology suite. Arteriography and embolization with gelfoam or coils can be very effective in experienced hands in controlling blood loss from gluteal or pudendal arteries. Throughout the early course of resuscitation and management, attention must be paid to appropriate replacement of platelets and clotting factors.

Spine fractures

Multiply injured patients with head injuries should be assumed to have a spine fracture until it can be proven otherwise. They should be transported with hard cervical collars and on backboards. The initial screening examination of every multiply injured patient must include a lateral cervical spine film down to C7–T1. In the case of a head injury, during the stabilization phase, complete thoracic and lumbar films must be obtained. Only when the spine films have been cleared should the cervical collar be removed and the patient taken from the backboard.

Patients with spinal cord injuries will have special requirements in regard to fluid replacement during resuscitation. This is due to autonomic dysreflexia and loss of vacular tone. Fluid requirements due to vasodilatation can be massive.

The initial survey in patients with spinal cord injury must include examination for the bulbocavernosus reflex. In the patient with quadriparesis or hemiparesis, the absence of this reflex indicates the presence of spinal shock. The final neurological status of the patient with complete paraplegia or quadriplegia cannot be determined until these cord level reflexes return. Individuals with paraparesis or quadriparesis must be carefully examined for any sign of residual motor or sensory sparing, as this function indicates a partial cord injury and has important prognostic and treatment significance.

Cervical spine fractures

The initial treatment of cervical spine fractures is similar with respect to presence or absence of cord injury. Patients with C1 or C2 fractures are generally neurologically intact on presentation. They should be left in a hard cervical collar until more definitive immobilization can be performed. In general, this means application of a Halo and placement in temporary traction or attachment to a vest or cast. For lower cervical fractures, the patient should remain in a hard cervical collar until a definitive diagnosis of the fracture can be made. Frequently, this will include a CT scan to determine the status of the neural canal. For most lower cervical fractures or single or bilateral dislocated facets, the patient should be placed immediately into a Halo or Gardner–Wells tongs as soon as it has been determined that the patient's other injuries do not require immediate operation.

The three column theory of Denis has been helpful in distinguishing stable from unstable fractures [33]. With an anterior body fracture (the anterior column) with disruption of the posterior wall of the vertebral body (the middle column) and the interspinous ligaments (the posterior column), the fracture is unstable. Disruption of two of the three columns at any single level also indicates instability. Instability implies the potential for further neurological injury. In the face of complete quadriparesis, stabilization of the spine with fusion to the intact levels above and below (generally posterior) is indicated to allow early rehabilitation. In this way, the recumbent position with the concomitant risk of pulmonary problems is avoided. With posterior wiring techniques to supplement bone graft arthrodesis, little more than a cervical collar is necessary for postoperative immobilization. In the instance of partial quadriparesis with distal sparing of function, the general course is a posterior cervical fusion followed by an anterior decompression of the canal (removal of bone fragments). This has been accompanied by an improvement of distal function in many cases.

Thoracolumbar fractures

Once these fractures are properly diagnosed with plain radiographs and CT scans, the patient must be log-rolled, maintaining spinal alignment until the fracture can be definitively treated. Stryker frames or Roto-kinetic beds can be helpful adjuncts, especially when there are associated injuries.

The general principles of treatment for cervical spine fractures apply for fractures of the thoracolumbar spine. If the patient has a complete paraplegia, posterior fusion with rod placement should be carried out to allow mobilization of the patient and a timely rehabilitation. The spine fusion is protected with a plastic thoracic orthosis until the fusion is solid. In the case of a partial injury, a two-staged procedure is preferred, with initial posterior rodding and fusion, followed by an anterior decompression shortly thereafter. Most authors believe that early fusion (within the first 48 hours) is appropriate for patients with partial paraplegia. The indication for an emergent stabilization and decompression is neurological deterioration.

References

1. Baker, S. P. (1987) Injuries: the neglected epidemic: Stone Lecture, 1985 American Trauma Society Meeting. *J. Trauma*, **27**, 343–348.
2. Smith, J. D., Bodai, B. I., Hill, A. S. and Frey, C. F. (1985) Prehospital stabilization of critically injured patients: a failed concept. *J. Trauma*, **25**, 65–70.
3. Cowley, R. A., Hudson, F., Scanlan, E. *et al.* (1973) An economical and proved helicopter program. *J. Trauma*, **13**, 1029–1038.
4. Fortner, G. S., Oreskovich, M. R., Copass, M. K. and Carrico, C. J. (1983) The effects of prehospital trauma care on survival from a 50-meter fall. *J. Trauma*, **23**, 976–981.
5. Wolff, G., Dittman, M., Ruedi, T. *et al.* (1978) Koordination von chirurgie und intensivmedizin zur vermeidung der posttraumatischen respiratorischen insuffizienz. *Unfallheilkunde*, **81**, 425–442.
6. Gustillo, R. B., Corpuz, V. and Sherman, R. E. (1985) Epidemiology, mortality, and morbidity in multiple trauma patients. *Orthopedics*, **8**, 1523–1528.
7. Johnson, K. D., Cadambi, A. and Seibert, G. B. (1985) Incidence of adult respiratory distress syndrome in patients with multiple musculoskeletal injuries: effect of early operative stabilization of fractures. *J. Trauma*, **25**, 375–384.
8. Seibel, R., La Duca, J., Hassett, J. M. *et al.* (1985) Blunt multiple trauma (ISS 36), femur traction, and the pulmonary failure-septic state. *Ann. Surg.*, **202**, 283–295.
9. Champion, H. R., Sacco, W. J., Hannan, D. S. *et al.* (1980) Assessment of injury severity: the triage index. *Crit. Care Med.*, **8**, 201–208.
10. Morris, J. A., Auerbach, P. S., Marshall, G. A. *et al.* (1986) The trauma score as a triage tool in the prehospital setting. *JAMA*, **256**, 1319–1325.
11. Baker, S., O'Neill, B. and Haddlon, W. (1974) The injury severity score: a method for describing patients with multiple injuries and evaluating emergency care. *J. Trauma*, **14**, 187–196.
12. Baker, S. P. and O'Neill, B. (1976) The injury severity score: an update. *J. Trauma*, **16**, 882–885.
13. Hansen, S. (1984) Concomitant fractures in long bones. In *The Multiply Injured Patient with Complex Fractures* (ed. M. Meyers), Lea and Febiger, Philadelphia, pp. 401–411.
14. Claudi, B. F. and Meyers, M. H. (1984) Priority in the treatment of the multiply injured patient with musculoskeletal injuries. In *The Multiply Injured Patient with Complex Fractures* (ed. M. H. Meyers), Lea and Febiger, Philadelphia, pp. 3–8.
15. Blaisdell, F. W. and Lewis, F. R. Jr (1977) Respiratory distress syndrome of shock and trauma. In *Post-Traumatic Failure* (eds F. W. Blaisdell and F. R. Lewis Jr), W. B. Saunders, Philadelphia.
16. Goris, R., Draaisma, J., Van Neikerk, J. *et al.* (1982) Early osteosynthesis and prophylactic mechanical ventilation in the multitrauma patient. *J. Trauma*, **22**, 895–903.
17. Schmidt, G., O'Neill, W., Kotb, K. *et al.* (1976) Continuous positive airway pressure in the prophylaxis of the adult respiratory distress syndrome. *Surg. Gynecol. Obstet.*, **143**, 613–618.
18. Gustillo, R. B. and Anderson, J. T. (1976) Prevention of infection in the treatment of one thousand and twenty-five open fractures of long bones. *J. Bone Joint Surg.*, **58A**, 453–458.
19. Swiontkowski, M. F., Winquist, R. A. and Hansen, S. T. (1984) Fractures of the femoral

neck in patients between the ages of twelve and forty-nine years. *J. Bone Joint Surg.*, **66A**, 837–846.

20. Veith, R. G., Winquist, R. A. and Hansen, S. T. (1984) Ipsilateral fractures of the femur and tibia: a report of fifty-seven consecutive cases. *J. Bone Joint Surg.*, **66A**, 991–1002.

21. Myllynen, P., Kammonen, M., Rokkanen, P. *et al.* (1985) Deep venous thrombosis and pulmonary embolism in patients with acute spinal cord injury: a comparison with nonparalyzed patients immobilized due to spinal fractures. *J. Trauma*, **25**, 541–543.

22. Jensen, J. E., Jensen, T. G., Smith, T. K. *et al.* (1982) Nutrition in orthopaedic surgery. *J. Bone Joint Surg.*, **64A**, 1263–1272.

23. Meek, R., Vivoda, E. and Crichton, A. (1981) A comparison of mortality in patients with multiple injuries according to the method of fracture treatment. *J. Bone Joint Surg.*, **63B**, 456.

24. Ruedi, T. (1985) Priorities in the management of multiple trauma. *Helv. Chir. Acta*, **52**, 331–335.

25. Riska, E., Von Bonsdorff, H. and Hakkinen, S. (1977) Primary operative fixation of long bone fractures in patients with multiple injuries. *J. Trauma*, **17**, 111–121.

26. Winquist, R. A., Hansen, S. T. and Clawson, D. K. (1984) Closed intramedullary nailing of femoral fractures: a report of five hundred and twenty cases. *J. Bone Joint Surg.*, **66A**, 529–539.

27. Manning, J. B., Bach, A. W., Herman, C. M. and Carrico, C. J. (1983) Fat release after femur nailing in the dog. *J. Trauma*, **23**, 322–326.

28. Pennal, G. F., Tile, M., Waddell, J. P. and Garside, H. (1980) Pelvic disruption: assessment and classification. *Clin. Orthop.*, **151**, 12–21.

29. Rothenberger, D. A., Fisher, R. P., Strate, R. and Perry, J. F. Jr (1978) The mortality associated with pelvic fractures. *Surgery*, **84**, 356–361.

30. Rothenberger, D., Velasco, R., Strate, R. *et al.* (1978) Open pelvic fracture: a lethal injury. *J. Trauma*, **18**, 184–187.

31. Slatis, P. and Huittinen, V. M. (1972) Double vertical fractures of the pelvis. *Acta Chir. Scand.*, **138**, 799–807.

32. Goldstein, A., Phillips, T., Sclafani, S. J. *et al.* (1986) Early open reduction and internal fixation of the disrupted pelvic ring. *J. Trauma*, **26**, 325–333.

33. Denis, F. (1983) The three column spine and its significance in the classification of acute thoraco-lumbar spinal injuries. *Spine*, **8(8)**, 817–831.

33. Weigelt, J. Mitchell, R. and Snyder, W. (1979) Early positive end-expiratory pressure in the adult respiratory distress syndrome. *Arch. Surg.*, **114**, 497–501.

10

Traumatic shock and the metabolic responses to injury

R. A. Little and M. Irving

Calls continue for the word 'shock' to be abandoned because it lacks clinical and scientific precision. However, we do not know of any other word which so well conveys the urgency of the clinical problem in the patient suffering from the multifactorial organ/system failure commonly called 'shock' and once graphically defined as a 'momentary pause in the act of dying'. We would, however, agree that the word shock, whilst undoubtedly confirming the seriousness of the clinical problem and indicating the need for urgent treatment, obviously fails to give a scientific dimension or indicate a cause for the problem.

The fundamental defect common to shock of all varieties and aetiologies is a failure of tissue perfusion and oxygen delivery commensurate with the body's needs. This failure of perfusion affects all the body's tissues and organs to a varying degree. The defect has many causes but three broad categories stand out, namely hypovolaemia, pump failure and stagnation. In surgical practice, the most important cause of shock is fluid loss supplemented by nociceptive stimuli from the traumatized tissue. In the case of the traumatized patient or those undergoing surgical operation the lost fluid is usually whole blood. Equally shock may result from loss of serum in the burned patient, water and electrolytes in obstruction of the gastrointestinal tract and third space losses into the retroperitoneum in acute pancreatitis. However, surgical patients are not immune from other causes of shock such as sepsis, myocardial failure, pulmonary embolism, anaphylaxis and neurogenic shock all of which may occur alone or in combination.

In the traumatized patient shock rapidly may supervene if the normal homoeostatic mechanisms that immediately follow injury are overwhelmed. These mechanisms are the starting process of a series of events which lead to restoration of physiological and metabolic normality and the repair of damaged tissues. The interrelationship of these events was described by Cuthbertson in terms of 'ebb and flow' [1]. He divided the responses into an early transient 'ebb' phase, characterized by a reduction in metabolic rate (or oxygen consumption, $\dot{V}o_2$) which was followed, in those going on to recover, by the 'flow' phase with an increase in metabolic rate (Fig. 10.1).

The 'ebb' phase is seen most clearly in experimental animals at ambient temperatures below the thermoneutral zone where it can be attributed to a central impairment of thermoregulation [2]. There is no unequivocal evidence that there is a reduction in metabolic rate shortly after injury in man other than when the injury is so severe that tissue oxygen delivery is compromised. However, there is evidence that both behavioural and autonomic thermoregulation are impaired in man at this time. On the other hand the increase in metabolic rate of the 'flow' phase is best seen in man. It is not a feature of most experimental studies which are of short duration [3,4].

The 'ebb' phase is not to be equated with shock

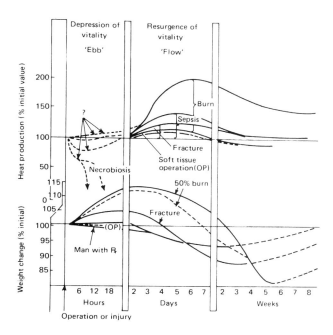

Fig. 10.1 The 'Ebb and Flow' response to injury.

for in this phase oxygen transport to the tissues is often adequate. Shock follows the ebb phase in those who are not resuscitated or who are so seriously traumatized that they will inevitably die. Such a downhill course has been designated necrobiosis (Fig. 10.1) and is characterized by a progressive failure of oxygen transport. In this chapter we will use the ebb and flow concept as a guide to the time course of the responses to injury.

Immediate response to injury

The immediate responses to injury mounted by the body are multifactorial but the most obvious of the responses are those due to activation of the neuro-endocrine system [5]. The principal stimuli of the neuro-endocrine responses are appreciation of danger, fluid loss and afferent nociceptive impulses resulting in, for example, severity related rises in adrenaline and noradrenaline. The former comes from the adrenal medulla and the latter from the sympathetic nerve endings. These hormones cause an im-

mediate response in the cardiovascular system with a tachycardia and a redistribution of the circulating blood volume from non-essential regions such as the skin to essential areas such as the heart, lungs and brain.

The combination of peripheral vasoconstriction and the translocation of interstitial fluid into the intravascular compartment means that arterial blood pressure may remain at near normal levels despite considerable fluid loss. However, when loss from the intravascular compartment exceeds 30% of the normal volume then hypotension supervenes.

Biochemical changes accompany the physiological and are also designed to meet the changed metabolic demands that follow injury. Prominent amongst the changes are measures to mobilize the body's energy stores of glycogen and fat, with the catecholamines, especially adrenaline, again having a major role. There is an injury severity related rise in plasma glucose concentration which is largely the result of a breakdown of liver glycogen and an increase in hepatic gluconeogenesis. This is fuelled by lactate release by skeletal muscle glycogenolysis and by glycerol arising from lipolysis of adipose tissue. Plasma glucose concentration continues to rise over the whole range of injury severity. On the other hand, although there is an increase in plasma nonesterified fatty acid concentrations after minor and moderately severe injuries there is no further rise with increases in severity, a finding which may be related to an increasing impairment of adipose tissue perfusion [6].

Vasopressin is released from the posterior lobe of the pituitary with the result that there is an increase in free water reabsorption from the distal tubules of the kidney. Aldosterone release ensures the retention of sodium and water and the production of ACTH by the anterior lobe of the pituitary leads to release of cortisol from the adrenal cortex. Initially the amount of cortisol in the circulation reflects the severity of the injury suffered by the patient but with increasing severity of injury (injury severity score > 12) the rise flattens off and indeed in the severest injuries the levels tend to fall. As ACTH levels continue to rise with increasing severity of injury it is possible that this failure of the cortisol response is due to a reduction in perfusion of the adrenal cortex.

The purpose of these changes from the teleological point of view is defensive, but when protracted, for example by prolonged inadequate treatment, there is a possibility that aspects of the responses may be harmful.

Clinical picture of shock

The clinical picture of shock is one of a low flow state characterized by skin pallor, sweating, mental confusion, oliguria, tachypnoea and usually, but not always, hypotension and tachycardia. In the early phases of hypovolaemic shock the arterial blood pressure may be raised due to an overvigorous response of the resistance side of the circulation to the evoked sympathetic nervous responses. Although the immediate response to hypovolaemia is a tachycardia this can be followed, as the magnitude of fluid loss increases, by a vagally mediated bradycardia elicited by stimulation of cardiac distortion receptors [7].

Although there may be minor variations in the clinical picture depending upon the cause of the shock state, the basic picture is essentially the same irrespective of the cause. A patient with septic shock may be pyrexial and initially have a warm periphery whilst a patient with cardiogenic shock may have irregularities in the heart rhythm and a raised central venous pressure.

In all types of shock the key to a successful outcome is early reversal of the physiological and biochemical changes by vigorous and adequate treatment.

Pathophysiology of the low flow state

If the changes that occur following injury are not reversed rapidly and thoroughly by treatment then the body enters the downward path to necrobiosis and the patient suffers increased tissue damage.

The deleterious changes possibly have a common pathway through the cardiovascular system. Early in the course of shock changes occur in the characteristics of the blood. Platelets and leucocytes are released into the bloodstream and red cells form rouleaux and begin to sludge. The intrinsic and extrinsic clotting mechanisms and complement are activated with consequent changes in the coagulation/fibrinolytic mechanisms. If normal flow characteristics are not re-

stored by repletion of the fluid volume the changes progress further. There is increased viscosity of the blood and thromboplastins are released from damaged cells and hypoxic endothelium. Thrombin is formed with consequent aggregation of platelets leading to intravascular fibrin deposition. The scene is set for the development of disseminated intravascular coagulation with all the consequences of impaired tissue perfusion.

Although the acute fall in peripheral perfusion triggers many of the changes characteristic of shock, it is important to realize that these are not necessarily reversed by restoration of tissue blood flow. There is increasing recognition that the reflow state is itself associated with adverse changes such as the generation of oxygen free radicals which can exacerbate tissue damage.

One of the principal organs to manifest the changes in tissue perfusion is the lung and indeed in the injured, postoperative or septic patient pulmonary failure is often the cause of death. Innumerable terms have been advanced to describe this heterogenous problem but none is more adequate than the presently accepted ARDS – adult respiratory distress syndrome [8].

Pulmonary responses to injury and shock can be seen immediately after the event. The pulmonary contusion resulting from the direct damage, lung collapse due to air or fluid in the pleural cavity and pulmonary oedema following head injury can all cause respiratory insufficiency.

With the passage of time from the moment of the accident, especially if shock persists or infection supervenes, the full clinical picture of ARDS can arise. The actual pathogenesis of this condition is unclear but the result is an increased vascular permeability in the lung with the accumulation of protein rich fluid in the interstices of the lung which then spills over into the alveoli.

Other organs are similarly affected by the shock state and the effects of DIC and other perfusional changes may be witnessed in the heart, liver, kidneys and brain. Sustained falls in perfusion pressure whilst capable of being tolerated for short intervals will, if sustained, cause permanent cellular damage.

Renal insufficiency in the early stages of shock is a homoeostatic mechanism but if the low flow state is sustained proximal and distal tubular necrosis occurs. In patients with crush injuries myoglobin casts may be present within the tubules. In sustained severe low flow states intestinal mucosal necrosis may be a problem, particularly in the colon. Lesions are also seen in the small intestine; these are thought to be due to hypoxia which can occur, perhaps surprisingly, without a reduction in total blood flow. The hypoxia is a result of the vascular anatomy of the mucosal villi which encourages the exchange of oxygen between the ascending and descending limbs of the mucosal countercurrent exchanger, making the villi very susceptible to a reduction in blood flow velocity [9] A loss of mucosal integrity has been associated with increased translocation of microorganisms and endotoxin into the vascular and lymphatic drainage from the gut, thereby initiating a systemic inflammatory response. Other splanchnic organs can also be adversely affected by hypovolaemia. The pancreas may be especially sensitive releasing, for example, cardiotoxic factors and proteolytic enzymes. The liver can also suffer, despite receiving an increase in the proportion of cardiac output after injury, with an impairment of reticulo-endothelial activity, and whole body energy substrate and metabolite homoeostasis.

The interest in myocardial depressant factors might suggest that the heart is the most susceptible organ in traumatic shock. However, there is little evidence that cardiac performance is impaired in such cases unless there has been direct myocardial injury, although this may not be so in sepsis. Indeed the early response to trauma is often associated with an increase in cardiac contractility. The most important determinants of cardiac function at this time are ventricular preload (end diastolic volume) and afterload (vascular resistance to ejection).

Cerebral blood flow is normally well protected by efficient autoregulatory mechanisms but these too may be impaired by injury. For example, the responsiveness of the cerebral vasculature to carbon dioxide is often lost after head injuries. The impairment of autoregulation may not be limited to direct head injuries. There is experimental evidence that the pattern of change in regional cerebral blood flow produced by haemorrhage can be affected by afferent nociceptive stimuli mimicking injury to peripheral tissues [10]. However, the major threat to cerebral blood flow is a rise in intracranial pressure due to an increase in intracranial mass.

Diagnosis and management of shock

Hypovolaemic shock

Of all the causes of shock, that of most concern to the surgeon is hypovolaemic shock resulting singly or in combination from loss of whole blood, plasma, or water and electrolytes.

The diagnosis of hypovolaemic shock is often, but not always straightforward. The previously mentioned clinical picture is usually apparent and the cause obvious. However, it has to be recognized that the extent of concealed fluid loss can be much more extensive than is clinically appreciated. Thus in traumatized patients a litre of blood can easily surround a fracture of the femur with little obvious swelling and 2 litres of blood can surround a fractured pelvis. Similarly in cases of acute traumatic pancreatitis following blunt abdominal injury large quantities of fluid can be sequestered in the retroperitoneal space – so called third space losses – without any palpable abnormality being apparent.

Today it is almost inevitable that the shocked patient will be subject to intensive clinical monitoring from the moment he presents. However, in most cases of straightforward hypovolaemic shock such measures are unnecessary and all that is usually required is measurement of the pulse rate and arterial blood pressure (perhaps combined to give the Shock Index) together with observation of the state of the superficial veins, skin colour and urine output. However, there is no doubt that in complicated patients, i.e. those with multiple injuries involving the trunk, those with cardiac disease and pulmonary disorders and those who develop complications additional monitoring is required. This will include direct measurement of the arterial blood pressure, right atrial and wedge pressures and estimation of cardiac output. The recording of cardiac output (and hence of oxygen delivery) is important to ensure that $\dot{V}o_2$ is not limited by an inadequate oxygen delivery (Do_2); indeed, improved outcome has been associated with increases in $\dot{V}o_2$ and Do_2 to supra-normal levels.

The interpretation of changes in pulse rate must take into account the biphasic nature of the pulse rate response to haemorrhage (*vide supra*). Also, it should be borne in mind that the persistence of a tachycardia after fluid resuscitation might be due to the inhibition of cardiac vagal activity by trauma and the defence reaction (preparation for fight or flight) rather than to persisting hypovolaemia. A danger here, especially in the elderly, is that attempts to 'titrate' the patient back to a normal pulse rate can lead to fluid overload with all its attendant problems.

Management of hypovolaemic shock

It should not be necessary to emphasize that the priority in hypovolaemic shock is to stop the source of fluid loss. In the case of external bleeding this can be accompanied by pressure and ligation. Bleeding around fracture sites can be lessened by immobilization of the bones. The use of MAST trousers, although superficially logical, has now been shown not to confer any benefit and is not recommended. Internal bleeding usually requires operative intervention but fluid loss from the obstructed gastrointestinal tract may be slowed down by aspiration of the stomach.

Replacement of the lost fluid should proceed at the same time as the loss is being stopped. Fluid should be infused through large cannulae at a rate necessary to reverse the hypovolaemia. Suitable fluids for this are:

1. electrolyte solution – crystalloids;
2. plasma substitutes;
3. blood.

The choice of fluid varies with national opinion. Crystalloids tend to be the preferred choice in the United States whilst colloids are used more frequently in the United Kingdom and Europe [11].

In patients in whom there is continuing loss of blood whole blood should be infused, but the administration of erythrocytes is, perhaps, less important than the maintenance of volume.

Septic shock is treated along similar principles, although in such patients it is necessary to evacuate any abscesses which may be the source of infection and to administer antibiotics. It is now generally accepted that steroids do not have a place in the management of the patient with septic shock or after trauma [12,13] although they may have a role in the acute management of spinal injuries.

Nutritional support for the injured patient

It has long been recognized that following even moderately severe injury patients lose weight, mainly as a result of reduction in the muscle bulk. The loss of weight occurs even in the presence of an apparently normal intake of food. The problem is compounded if, for any reason, the patient cannot eat, for example if he or she is being mechanically ventilated or if the gastrointestinal tract has been injured and requires resting. Yet it is the experience of clinicians dealing with the injured patient that the majority of patients do not require any special nutritional support to recover from their injuries and that the lost weight is soon regained following resumption of normal activity. However, some patients continue to lose weight and progress poorly and in such cases nutritional support has to be considered.

At the present time there is little evidence on which to decide the place of enteral or parenteral nutritional support in the injured patient [14, 15]. However a recent meta-analysis suggests that early enteral feeding reduces postoperative septic complications, when compared with parenteral feeding, in high-risk surgical patients: an effect which was most marked for those patients with trauma [16]. Unlike in general surgery, where there has been considerable interest in the indications for, and value of, nutritional support accidental injury remains a relatively unexplored area despite one or two good publications on the subject (e.g. [15]). On the other hand, enteral nutritional support using defined formula diets is now technically feasible and is administered more readily, especially in the elderly injured patient.

Metabolic consequences of injury

In the early phase of the response to injury there is a mobilization of energy substrates as already described. At this time fat is the main fuel for oxidation and most glucose oxidation can be accounted for by the brain. This preferential oxidation of fat is also seen in other 'stress' states such as sepsis. The early pattern of response is followed by the flow phase characterized by an increase in oxygen consumption which is fuelled by increases in the oxidation of both fat and carbohydrate with only a small contribution from protein [17]. Although glucose is being oxidized in the flow phase there are marked changes in the control of its metabolism, plasma insulin concentrations being much higher than expected from the prevailing glucose levels. The high insulin levels occur at the time of maximum nitrogen excretion. The excreted nitrogen is derived from the breakdown of tissue at the site of injury as well as the generalized wasting of skeletal muscle. Additionally, injury and sepsis appear to be associated with a reduction in protein anabolism.

The hormonal basis of the flow phase and more particularly of insulin resistance is unclear. Attempts at understanding the mechanisms involve using 'triple hormone' infusion of cortisol, adrenaline and glucagon which mimics many of the features of the flow phase [18]. However, the hormone concentrations used in such studies more closely resemble those found in the ebb phase than in the flow phase where the levels of such hormones have almost returned to normal. The monokines interleukin-1 and tumour necrosis factor (cachectin) released from phagocytes may also be involved in the flow phase, although there is no firm evidence for this.

Consequences of malnutrition

It is reasonable to question whether the state resembling malnutrition which follows severe injuries confers any serious disadvantage on the patient. However, there is little doubt that the morbidity and mortality in malnourished patients undergoing major surgery are higher than expected [19]. Malnutrition of moderately severe degree affects virtually every major system in the body [14]. The diminution of muscle bulk, which is due not only to muscle breakdown but also to lack of synthesis, has an adverse effect on respiratory function. Both the vital capacity and the resting minute ventilation are decreased resulting in a greater susceptibility to respiratory infection. Cardiac muscle is also affected, with a reduction in cardiac contractility and therefore reduced arterial pressures. In chronic malnutrition, renal function may also deteriorate as a result of a fall in glomerular filtration rate. The effective surface area of the gastrointestinal tract is decreased and the intestinal transit time increases, resulting in bacterial overgrowth. The effect of both changes is to reduce absorption of nutrients. Malnutrition results in a greater risk of developing infection. Cell-mediated immunity is affected, with a reduction in the numbers of the T cells. Humoral immunity is also affected despite the fact that the B-cell levels are not significantly reduced.

In summary, prolonged malnutrition slows healing and increases morbidity, particularly from infection. Even if the patient should escape these problems, convalescence is likely to be prolonged.

Who needs nutritional support?

Before a decision is made to institute nutritional support, the patient must be resuscitated. The restoration of circulating blood volume to normal is of paramount importance in maintaining perfusion of both the vital organs and the fat depots since free fatty acids released by lipolysis are used as substrates for energy production. The stress caused by pain and fever must if possible be reduced because it results in impairment of mobilization of substrates. In particular, every effort should be made to decrease the size of the injury by, for example, an early decision to amputate a badly damaged limb. Sepsis must be vigorously sought and aggressively treated, for no amount of nutritional support will redress the negative nitrogen balance if infection is allowed to continue unchecked [20].

There are two broad indications for the use of nutritional support in injured patients. First, are those patients in whom malnutrition can be anticipated from the nature and/or the severity of the injury. Second, are patients developing serious complications after initially straightforward injuries. In general terms, the more severe the injury, the more likely will be the need for nutritional support. An objective measurement of the severity can be made using the injury severity score (ISS) [21]. It is recommended that unless the nature of the injury dictates otherwise, nutritional support is likely to be required in patients with an ISS of greater than 14 and is mandatory for those with scores exceeding 20 [22]. Injury of the gastrointestinal tract, and particularly injuries of the pancreas and extensive intestinal injuries, may lead to a prolonged ileus with a diminished appetite and diminished absorption.

The need for mechanical ventilation for any length of time also constitutes an indication for active nutritional support though mechanical ventilation may be beneficial in reducing the patient's energy requirements by taking over the work of breathing.

The patient who develops serious sepsis after an injury, which on its own was not such as to merit nutritional support, must none the less be considered for feeding. The reason for this is that sepsis will lead to further loss of nitrogen with a loss of muscle bulk and a fall in the serum albumin levels.

Indications for parenteral nutrition

It makes sound sense to feed enterally if at all possible. Parenteral feeding is expensive and potentially hazardous, and should be reserved for certain categories of patients. An absolute indication for its use is major gastrointestinal injury from which return of function may be slow. Some patients do not tolerate enteral nutrition despite gradual building up to full-strength solutions and they may have to receive parenteral nutrition. Because of the risk of aspiration, a patient whose level of consciousness is depressed should not be fed enterally unless there is a cuffed endotracheal tube in place.

The advantage of parenteral nutrition over enteral feeding is that it need not be discontinued for surgical procedures or investigations – a distinct benefit for the patient with multiple injuries whose feeding would otherwise be discontinuous because of the many journeys to the operating room for changes or dressings and plasters and other procedures.

It has been shown that the mortality of head injury is reduced by early institution of parenteral nutrition [23]. Rapp and colleagues also showed that parenterally fed patients had a better nitrogen balance and higher albumin levels that enterally fed patients. Considering that the volume of tissue damaged in even a serious head injury is small, such patients have surprisingly high resting metabolic rates. One explanation for this is the spasticity which accompanies serious head injury and another is an increase in metabolism by the central nervous system which, even under normal circumstances, makes up 20% of the total resting metabolic expenditure. Evidence for this comes from Dempsey and associates [24], who showed a considerable reduction in the resting metabolic expenditure by the administration of barbiturates to patients with severe head injury. The case for nutritional support in head injury is further strengthened by the observation that a considerable proportion of such patients ultimately die from infection [25], which, as has been discussed earlier, may be a consequence of malnutrition. Finally, an occasional patient will have such high energy requirements that it is impossible to meet these with conventional enteral feeding formulae.

Which nutrients and how much?

It is possible for a patient to maintain some oral intake, in which case he or she may be able to meet the requirements for electrolytes, otherwise they must be supplied parenterally. The amounts required are calculated from knowledge of normal daily requirements and losses in the urine and any other body fluids. As the patient moves from a catabolic to an anabolic phase, the requirements for potassium, magnesium and phosphorus rise.

Energy requirements are based on resting energy expenditure, which in turn depends on age, sex, size and severity and nature of injury. There are a number of reliable formulae by which the calorie requirements of injured patients can be calculated [26], although it is better, where possible, to measure an individual's energy expenditure by calorimetry. In this way, not only can the optimal level of calories be supplied, but also the form in which they should be taken can be determined. The respiratory quotient will indicate whether fat or carbohydrate is being oxidized [27]. In the past the energy needs of injured patients have been grossly overestimated. In fact, few patients need more than 2000 kcal/day [28]. Even in patients with multiple organ failure the resting energy expenditure rarely exceeds 2500 kcal/day. Only seriously burned patients require more [29]. To give more calories than the patient needs is not only wasteful but may be harmful. Additionally, glucose which is surplus to needs is converted into fat with the generation of 'excess' carbon dioxide, which has to be excreted by the lungs and this requires extra respiratory effort. In a patient with compromised respiratory function this may be enough to precipitate respiratory failure [30].

Calories must be supplied as a mixture of fat and glucose, with about one-third as fat. However, should the patient be septic or have a respiratory disorder, the ratio can, with benefit, be reversed.

Protein requirements are not difficult to assess if facilities are available for measuring urinary nitrogen losses. Generally, the patient requires 2–3g/day more than the daily loss [20]. If urinary nitrogen losses cannot be measured directly, a useful rule of thumb is to give approximately 0.2 g of nitrogen/day per kg of body weight. Standard commercial amino acid preparations are based on the aminogram of egg protein. They contain mixtures of synthetic L-amino acids, approximately 25% of which are the branched-chain amino acids (BCAA) leucine, isoleucine and valine. Recent work suggests that in stress the BCAAs are readily utilized as calorie sources by skeletal muscle. BCAAs are also known to exert an anabolic effect by decreasing protein catabolism and stimulating synthesis. BCAA-enriched amino acid solutions have been shown to have a greater effect on restoring nitrogen balance and immune competence than standard solutions. It must, however, be clearly stated that the role of BCAA-enriched solutions in clinical practice has yet to be clarified, for despite the apparent biochemical advantages described above they have not been shown to provide clinical benefit.

Both fat-soluble and water-soluble vitamins should be supplied. The stores of fat-soluble vitamins are greater and their half-life longer than those of the water-soluble vitamins. However, the water-soluble vitamins should be supplied daily, bearing in mind that injured and septic patients may have increased requirements, especially for the B group of vitamins. Supplements of the trace metals zinc, copper, etc. are unlikely to be required unless prolonged parenteral nutrition is needed, or the patient has abnormally high losses from fistulae, diarrhoea, etc. Certainly, even a modest oral intake in the form of drinks such as tea will supply these elements in sufficient quantities.

Parenteral nutrition: avoiding complications

Figures for catheter-related complications vary widely, depending on the experience of individual units. There is no doubt, however, that complications such as pneumothorax, misplacement of the catheter and sepsis can be kept at very low levels by observing a few simple rules. Feeding catheters should be inserted in the operating theatre, using full aseptic technique and with X-ray screening facilities available. Once inserted, the catheter must not be used for any purpose other than parenteral nutrition. There should be a strict protocol for dressing of the catheter and connecting and disconnecting it from the nutrient solutions. It is now well recognized that it is strict catheter-care protocol and not subcutaneous tunnelling of the catheter which leads to a low catheter sepsis rate.

Initially, feeding should be spread over 24 hours. Over a period of 4–5 days the infusion can be gradually speeded up until, ideally, the patient receives his entire daily requirements during an overnight 12 hour period. This is good for morale, as not only is there one less tube to worry about during the waking hours but also the patient can be more mobile. During the period that the catheter is not in use it is locked with 1000–1500 i.u. of heparin to prevent clotting. The rate of infusion must be slowed down towards the end of the feeding period to prevent reactive hypoglycaemia, which often follows abrupt cessation of the large carbohydrate load. Although the nutrient solution may be given in the form of 500 ml bottles, a 3 litre bag containing all the daily requirements is more convenient. The contents can be infused using a pump, a great advantage for overnight infusion because constant checks on the infusion rate are not necessary.

Monitoring

It is important to make frequent estimations of serum electrolytes, certainly until the patient is well stabilized on a particular feeding regimen. Knowledge of these, together with measurement of losses of body fluids will help in formulating the regimen. Haematological indices should be measured at regular intervals. In particular, the mean corpuscular volume, and prothrombin time will give a clue to deficiencies of folate, vitamin B12 and vitamin K.

Objective evidence of benefit from providing nutritional support is often difficult to obtain.

Body weight is a poor indicator of nutritional status because early changes are often due to water retention. In any case, it is not always possible to weigh patients who are confined to their beds and connected to traction, ventilators, etc. Thickness of the skin fold over the triceps is more useful, as is the trend in the serum albumin levels. Subjectively, however, it is usually rewarding simply to see a patient looking and feeling better.

Nutritional support is continued until the patient is able to meet his or her metabolic needs with a normal diet. It is important to remember that exercise is important for maintaining muscle bulk during feeding.

The decision to feed injured patients parenterally must be taken early and only if enteral feeding is thought to be contraindicated, inappropriate or inadequate. Attention to detail will keep the complication rate low. There is little doubt that the early institution of nutritional support in the severely injured patient reduces morbidity and, in some situations, even mortality.

References

1. Cuthbertson, D. P. (1942) Post shock metabolic response. *Lancet*, **1**, 433–437.
2. Stoner, H. B. (1981) Thermoregulation after trauma. In *Homeostasis in Injury and Shock* (eds Z. Biro *et al.*), Pergamon, New York, pp. 25–33.
3. Little, R. A. (1985) Heat production after injury. *Br. Med. Bull.*, **41**, 226–231.
4. Heath, D. F. (1985) Experimental studies on energy metabolism after injury and during sepsis. In *The Scientific Basis for the Care of the Critically Ill* (eds R. A. Little and K. N. Frayn), Manchester University Press, Manchester, pp. 75–101.
5. Gann, D. S. and Lilly, M. P. (1984) The endocrine response to injury. In *Progress in Critical Care Medicine Vol 1. Multiple Trauma* (ed. R. J. Wilder), Karger, Basel, pp. 15–47.
6. Stoner, H. B., Frayn, K. N., Barton, R. N. *et al.* (1979) The relationship between plasma substrates and hormones and the severity of injury in 277 recently injured patients. *Clin. Sci.*, **56**, 563–573.
7. Thoren, P. (1979) Role of cardiac vagal C. fibres in cardiovascular control. *Rev. Physiol. Biochem. Pharmacol.*, **86**, 1–94.
8. Chamberlin, W. H., Rice, C. L. and Moss, G. (1983) Pulmonary dysfunction in shock. In *Hand-book of Shock and Trauma, Vol 1: Basic Science* (eds B. M. Altura *et al.*) Raven Press, New York, pp. 105–112.
9. Haglund, U. (1973) The small intestine in hypotension and haemorrhage. *Acta Physiol. Scand.*, **Suppl.**, 387.
10. Sandor, P., Demchenko, I. T., Kovach, A. G. B. and Moskalenko, Y. E. (1976) Hypothalamic and thalamic blood flow during somatic efferent stimulation in dogs. *Am. J. Physiol.*, **231**, 270–274.
11. Yates, D. W. and Magill, P. J. (eds) (1978) Plasma volume replacement. *Arch. Emerg. Med.*, **1 (4)** (supplement), 1–58.
12. Dearden, N. M., Gibson, J. S., McDowall, D. G. *et al.* (1986) Effect of high-dose dexamethasone on outcome from severe head injury. *J. Neurosurg.*, **64**, 81–88.
13. Bone, R. C., Fisher, C. J., Clemmer, T. P., Slotman, G. J., Metz, C. A. and Balk, R. A. (1987) A controlled clinical trial of high-dose methylprednisolone in the treatment of severe sepsis and septic shock. *New Engl. J. Med.*, **317**, 653–658.
14. Mughal, M. M. (1987) Parenteral nutrition in injury. *Injury*, **18**, 82–86.
15. Kudsk, K. A., Stone, J. M. and Sheldon, G. F. (1982) Nutrition in trauma and burns. *Surg. Clin. North Am.*, **62**, 183–192.
16. Moore, F. A., Feliciano, D. V., Andrassy, R. J. *et al.* (1992) Early enteral feeding, compared with parenteral, reduces postoperative septic complications. *Ann. Surg.*, **216**, 172–183.
17. Frayn, K. N., Little, R. A., Stoner, H. B. and Galasko, C. S. B. (1984) Metabolic control in non-septic patients with musculoskeletal injuries. *Injury*, **16**, 73–79.
18. Bessey, P. Q., Walters, J. M., Acki, T. T. and Wilmore, D. W. (1984) Combined hormonal infusion simulates the metabolic response to injury. *Ann. Surg.*, **200**, 264–281.
19. Mullen, J. L., Buzby, G. P., Matthews, D. C. *et al.* (1980) Reduction of operative morbidity and mortality by combined preoperative and post-operation nutritional support. *Ann. Surg.*, **192**, 604–613.
20. Alexander-Williams, J. and Irving, M. (1982) *Intestinal Fistulas*. John Wright, Bristol.
21. Baker, S. P., O'Neill, B., Hadden, W. and Long, W. D. (1974) The injury severity score: a method for describing patients with multiple injuries and evaluating emergency care. *J. Trauma*, **14**, 187–196.
22. Stoner, H. B. (1984) The therapeutic implications of some recent research on trauma. *Arch. Emerg. Med.*, **1**, 5–16.

23. Rapp, R. P., Young, B., Twyman, D. *et al.* (1983) The favourable effect of early parenteral feeding on survival in head-injured patients. *J. Neurosurg.*, **58**, 906–912.

24. Dempsey, D. T., Guenter, P., Mullen, J. L. *et al.* (1985) Energy expenditure in acute trauma to the head with and without barbiturate therapy. *Surg. Gynecol. Obstet.*, **10**, 128–134.

25. Becker, D. P., Miller, J. D., Ward, J. D. *et al.* (1977) The outcome from severe head injury with early diagnosis and intensive management. *J. Neurosurg.*, **47**, 491–502.

26. Wilmore, D. W. (1977) *The Metabolic Management of the Critically Ill.* Plenum Press, New York.

27. Frayn, K. N. (1983) Calculation of substrate oxidation rates in vivo from gaseous exchange. *J. Appl. Physiol.*, **55**, 628–634.

28. Macfie, J. (1986) Towards cheaper intravenous nutrition. *Br. Med. J.*, **292**, 107–110.

29. Davies, J. W. L. (1982) *Physiological Responses to Burning Injury.* Academic Press, New York.

30. Askanazi, J., Rosenbaum, S. H., Hyman, A. I. *et al.* (1980) Respiratory changes induced by the large glucose loads of total parenteral nutrition. *JAMA*, **243**, 1444–1447.

11

Reconstructive orthopaedic surgery: skin cover following injury to a limb

P. L. G. Townsend

Acute injury

After debriding any injury, a decision has to be made whether the wound can, or should be closed. It the viability of skin is in doubt, closing a wound under tension is likely to lead to skin necrosis with infection complicating subsequent management.

A possible degloving injury should be looked for, especially in lower limb injuries. The history may be of help, for example if a limb is held against a rigid object such as a kerb, and a wheel passes over the limb, the effect may be to sheer the skin off the underlying structures, and with it its source of blood supply. Where the skin is completely degloved, the injury may be very obvious but where there are only small lacerations, the extent of the injury may not be immediately apparent. The wound should be explored, haematoma evacuated and if the degloving is extensive, circulation to the skin should be carefully assessed. If loss of an extensive area of skin is inevitable, removal of this skin should be carried out and the subcutaneous fat excised, leaving full thickness skin, which can then be stored in a skin bank or fridge at +4°C for secondary application.

Primary skin grafting of wounds is not often carried out except in facial injuries and in this situation it is important to remember the best subsequent cosmetic result is achieved by donor skin grafts taken as close as possible to the recipient site, so that a graft taken from the leg and placed on the face will be yellow in comparison with the adjacent skin.

Skin grafts will only take if there is a suitable vascular bed such as muscle or deep fascia; grafting onto fat is often unsatisfactory and it may be better to remove the fat, the viability of which may very well be in doubt, and graft onto fascia. Grafts will not take where there is no suitable vascular base, for example open joints, tendons without paratenon, bone without periosteum, or cartilage without perichondrium. These situations require some form of cover with its own blood supply and will be dealt with later.

Skin grafts may either be full thickness 'Wolfe' grafts or partial thickness 'Thiersch' grafts. Full thickness grafts require closure of the donor site after removal, which limits the size of the graft, although it is theoretically possible to put a partial thickness graft on the donor site. This is seldom done.

It is more difficult to get a good take of a full thickness graft, therefore their application requires more expertise. Their advantage is that if successful, the grafts do not produce as much fibrosis under them and therefore do not shrink. This is particularly important in, for example, finger contractures or syndactyly, where after release such a graft may be required.

The usual donor site for full thickness grafts is the groin, where quite a large ellipse of skin can be removed and the defect closed. The skin preferably should be taken from the left groin so there is no confusion subsequently about whether the appendix has been removed. An alternative site is the inner aspect of the upper arm, where quite large grafts can be taken and used, for example after release of recurrent Depuytren's contractures.

On the face small grafts can be taken from behind the ear, what is known as a post-auricular 'Wolfe' graft. In older people, similar grafts can be taken from in front of the ear. The defects can then again be closed directly.

Where a large graft is necessary, the supraclavicular fossa can be a suitable donor site. If even larger areas of skin graft are required, initial partial thickness grafts can be applied and after all the swelling has gone down, with shrinking of the graft, this may be excised and the area reconstructed with a better matching full thickness graft.

Partial thickness grafts in the acute situation often do not take well, due to difficulty in determining viability of tissues with wound contamination. As part of the initial management of a large wound at the time of debridement, skin grafts can be taken and stored. The wound site can then be dressed with an antiseptic dressing such as Flamazine or Betadine. After 24–48 hours the skin can be applied often without sedation directly onto the wound surface, the chance of haematoma under the graft is reduced and the prospects of infection diminished. Clinically, the percentage take of graft is enhanced and the wound can often be exposed.

It should not be forgotten that skin can act as a biological dressing reducing fluid loss and preventing infection; as a temporary expedient with exposed bone, it may provide cover until a suitable flap can be carried out as a delayed primary procedure.

In extensive wounds partial thickness grafts can be meshed using a suitable machine; this allows expansion up to three to five times the original size. Epithelium then grows into the gaps between the strands of skin usually within 2 weeks, depending on the amount of meshing and stretching. If the skin is meshed, but not expanded, this helps to allow skin grafts to drape over irregular wounds and at the same time allows blood and serous fluid to drain out through the slits.

Partial thickness grafts, if suitably stored, remain viable for up to 2 weeks; after this viability rapidly falls off. As indicated before, partial thickness grafts do heal with a larger amount of fibrosis underneath and therefore tend to contract.

Flap cover

As indicated, where there is no suitable bed for a graft, skin with its own blood supply must be used to cover exposed bone, cartilage, tendons or joints. To achieve acceptable results, there must be some understanding of the blood supply of the skin. Within skin, there are plexuses at dermal and subdermal levels; within the fat (often less well developed) and on the surface of the fascia, which itself is a relatively avascular structure. There is no longer felt to be an important plexus underneath the fascia. These plexuses all interconnect.

The arterial supply to the skin which vascularizes these plexuses can arise either be direct or indirect vessels. In the 'direct' cutaneous blood supply, there is an anatomically recognizable arteriovenous system, which supplies an area of skin which is the same on equivalent areas of the body. Unlike nerves, the blood supply of any particular area is not so fixed, so if one vessel is divided, alternative adjacent vessels may be able to open up and take over supply and drainage. 'Indirect' vascular supply occurs after blood vessels have supplied bone/muscle or fascia and then provide perforators to the skin.

When raising a flap, understanding the underlying anatomy is therefore vital.

Flaps can be described as:

1. Cutaneous – random;
   – axial;
2. Fascio-cutaneous;
3. Musculo-cutaneous;
4. Osteo-musculo-cutaneous.

Cutaneous random

For many years the concept of random pattern flaps was firmly adhered to, so that if a flap was raised, the breadth would correspond to the length on a one to one basis. Experimentally in pigs, this does seem to apply up to about 3 cm, but after that viability depends more on whether a large vessel is included in the flap.

An example of the use of a random pattern flap

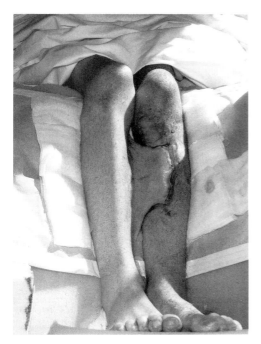

Fig. 11.1 Cross leg flap in position inset to cover exposed bone.

is (Fig. 11.1) the cross leg flap in the lower leg, for example, following skin loss with exposed bone, in the central third of the lower leg. The flap is raised from the inner aspect of the undamaged leg, leaving a graftable bed. The limbs are brought together and the skin of the flap is sutured to the edges of the wound. After about 3 weeks, the flap is divided across its base; by this time there has been extensive re-anastomosis of vessels between the edge and base of the flap and vessels on the damaged limb to maintain the blood supply of the transferred skin.

Axial pattern flaps

One of the great advances in plastic surgery was the discovery that a skin flap containing one of theses anatomically recognized direct cutaneous vessels can be made many times longer than its breadth. The first one described was the groin flap [1] in which skin from the lateral groin extending medially from the area of the anterior iliac spine, can be raised down to its supplying artery, the superficial circumflex iliac artery with accompanying vein.

The groin flap has been used especially on the hand where following injury or removal of malignant tumours; the flap can be raised and then inset onto the hand to cover the exposed tendons or bone. Usually after 3 weeks, often after initial delay by clamping the feeding vessels, the groin flap can be separated, the flap on the surface of the hand, having picked up an alternative supply via re-anastomosis with other vessels on its periphery and base.

Fascio-cutaneous flaps

In the lower limb, simple transposition of skin flaps, even with a ratio of 1:1, containing skin and subcutaneous tissue is fraught with difficulty and often unsuccessful.

Ponten [2], however, described flaps in the lower limb up to 22 cm long, incorporating skin and fascia. This incorporation of the fascia with its vascular plexus on the upper surface obviously increases the integrity and viability of the flap (Fig. 11.2).

Some flaps are difficult to categorize. An example is the valuable radial forearm flap, first described by Yang [3] in China and in the West-

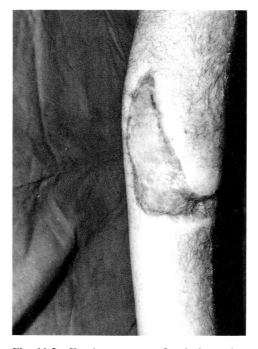

Fig. 11.2 Fascio-cutaneous flap in lower leg rotated to cover defect. Donor site grafted.

ern literature [4]. This flap, supplied by the radial artery, is composed of skin, subcutaneous tissue and fascia and can include segments of radius, or tendons such as palmaris longus or flexor carpi radialis.

The flap is nourished by vessels arising from the radial artery, which pass between the brachioradialis and pronator teres in the upper forearm and flexor carpi radialis and brachioradialis tendon distally. This flap can be based on the central or more distal parts of the radial artery. It has been used as a local flap, or a free flap, the latter to be discussed later. Subject to a satisfactory Allen test, the blood supply of the hand may be maintained via the ulnar artery and palmar arches, thus nourishing the radial artery retrogradely. This flap can be raised after division of the artery proximally and rotated distally. Of considerable interest is the fact that the venous return is then backwards via the vena comitans and the superficial draining veins. This flap can then be rotated to be used in reconstruction of hand injuries, either in the acute situation, where, for example, there has been loss of skin or tendons on the dorsum of the hand; or in later reconstruction, for example after a traumatic amputation where the skin is draped around a segment of radius it can be used in thumb reconstruction (Fig. 11.3).

The advantages of this flap over groin flaps are that only the damaged limb is involved and the patient does not have to be bed bound, the hand can be elevated and mobilization achieved

earlier, with less morbidity. Where the flap has been raised, the defect is skin grafted.

Muscle and musculo-cutaneous flaps

Where there are muscles running under the skin, the blood supply to these muscles often give perforators to the overlying skin. If the muscle is raised with its blood supply, skin overlying the muscle can be taken with it, or alternatively, muscle can be raised as a flap and a skin graft applied on top, as muscle provides an excellent bed for grafting.

The lower leg can be divided into thirds, in the upper third and around the knee, injuries exposing the upper tibia or the knee joint may be covered by use of one or other bellies of the gastrocnemius muscle [5], still attached by its predominant blood supply from the popliteal fossa. Muscle drapes well, can be moulded into cavities and resists infection well. When more complicated reconstruction is likely on the underlying bone or joint, gastrocnemius with overlying skin is preferable (a musculo-cutaneous flap; Fig. 11.4) it can be more easily raised subsequently with skin-to-skin closure.

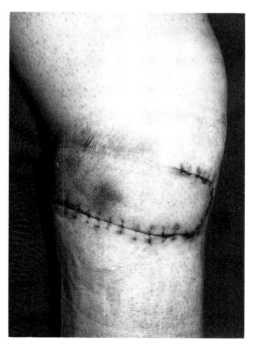

Fig. 11.4 Compound gastrocnemius–skin flap to cover defect below knee. Photo taken after thinning of flap.

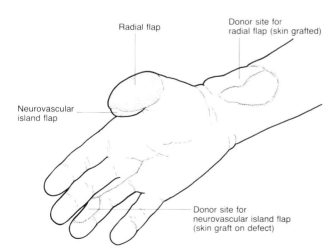

Fig. 11.3 Radial flap used to reconstruct thumb. Note neuro-vascular island flap from ring finger.

In the central tibial area the muscle flap used usually without overlying skin is soleus muscle. This can be separated from the gastrocnemius in a relatively avascular plane, divided off the Achilles tendon and rotated to cover the exposed tibia. Unlike the gastrocnemius, the blood supply is segmental from the posterior tibial vessels and the upper lateral part is also provided by the peroneal artery. In mobilization, some of these segmental vessels will have to be divided.

In the lower third, many muscles become tendons and muscle bulk available is small. If fascio-cutaneous flaps have either failed or are not possible, this is the area where free flaps are often indicated.

Free flaps

Local flap alternatives to covering ungraftable exposed structures should first be considered before use of microvascular 'free flaps'. Other injuries such as a fractured pelvis or injury to the other limb may make a cross-leg flap out of the question, or there may be so much local damage to exclude muscular, or fascio-cutaneous flaps, or else the site in the lower part of the leg may be such that no suitable muscle bellies can be used for cover.

The term 'free flap' is used where the donor flap is detached from its blood supply, transferred to the recipient area and revascularized. The first free flap was carried out by Daniel and Taylor [6] on the groin flap. It was found possible to maintain the viability of the groin flap on the predominant feeding artery, either superficial circumflex iliac artery, or superficial epigastric, together with the draining vein. Lymphatic re-anastomosis was therefore not essential.

Re-vascularization on the damaged leg depends on finding a suitable segment of un-damaged artery and draining vein. The vascular anastomoses are carried out under a microscope. Arterial anastomosis may be either end-to-end, or if possible, end-to-side, so that the peripheral run-off of the recipient vessel is still possible at the same time as nourishing the flap. Vein anastomosis is usually carried out by end-to-end anastomosis. In the situation where suitable recipient vessels are too far from the site for attachment of the flap, vein grafts may be required, reversed in the case of an arterial gap.

Microvascular surgery requires considerable training in the laboratory to achieve an acceptable level of clinical success and for this reason is best carried out in units where such surgery (including a replantation service) is a routine part of surgical practice.

The advantage of a 'free flap' is that it is usually a single stage procedure. While the surgery may take a long time, alternative techniques such as tube pedicles require a longer time in total and much longer in hospital. For this reason the latter technique is now seldom carried out. Another advantage of the free flap is that it brings an increased blood supply to the injured area which enhances healing of adjacent tissue such as an underlying fracture site.

Use of free flaps in an acute injury

Of considerable importance is the timing of the free flap. If bone is exposed and left to dry, it is likely to die off. Emergency free flaps have been carried out after debridement, but this is often an impractical situation. Often the best alternative, especially in a grossly contaminated wound, is initial debridement of the wound; exposed bone and tendons must then be kept moist, either by saturated dressings or using skin as a biological dressing. A delayed primary free flap can then be carried out, preferably within 48 hours, at which time a further debridement, if indicated, is carried out.

At the initial operation if there is an exposed fracture, or in a fractured limb where there are other non-graftable structures involved, some

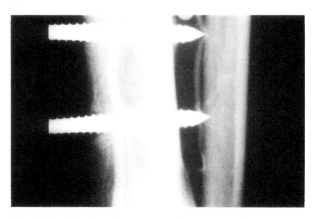

Fig. 11.5   Fixator pins compressing peroneal artery.

form of external fixation may be required. Obviously the pins must not be placed into the exposed bone as this will be the site of cover of the flap. Discussion should be made with the team responsible for the free flap, so the pins do not interfere with exploration or anastomosis of vessels (Fig. 11.5). Also, it should be borne in mind that if pins are passed from the medial side of the tibia, it is possible to damage the peroneal vessels (Fig. 11.5). Again, if pin sites have to be changed later, this undoubtedly reduces the viability of the bone and many produce annular sequestra.

Use of free flaps in chronic injury

Many cases are in this category, although any bone loss will be known from the time of the accident. Traumatized skin may die off under a plaster, a situation which is perhaps more likely to occur where internal fixation is carried out in an area of poor circulation which requires extra soft tissue mobilization to achieve.

Exposed bone and plates provide a difficult situation clinically. Gault and Quaba [7] found that in cases where there was an exposed fracture fixation device, or prosthetic joint, if preoperative wound cultures were negative, or only showed commensals, success rate of cover was high. If pathogenic bacteria were demonstrated preoperatively, then even covering the area with a well vascularized flap, allowing antibiotics to reach the affected area, success rate was low often resulting in chronic infection down to the metal.

In cases showing pathogenic bacteria, removal of the fixation device should be carried out and alternative fixation applied, preferably by external fixation, bearing in mind previous comments. The limb can be held out to length while all obvious dead bone is removed. Radical debridement is essential to prevent long term problems of osteomyelitis. This is preferably done in two stages. After initial debridement, daily antiseptic dressings can be carried out, such as Betadine. After a further week, further debridement can be carried out prior to reconstruction.

The choice of free flap depends on reconstructional requirements: skin, skin and tendons, or skin and bone.

Skin only

The first free flap, as indicated, was a groin flap (Fig. 11.6); its disadvantages are a short vascular pedicle, variability of vascular pattern and small vessels (range 0.8–3 mm). For this reason other

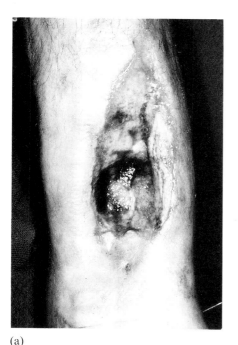

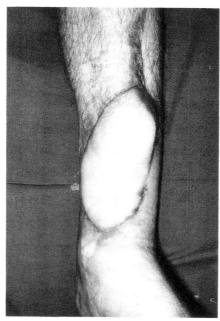

Fig. 11.6 (a) Skin loss and exposed bone lower leg. (b) Free groin flap. Note back cut to expose anterior tibial vessels away from site of trauma.

(a)   (b)

flaps have been developed; however, the groin area remains a good donor site as the wound can often be closed directly.

The radial forearm flap, mentioned earlier, may be used as a free, instead of transposition, flap, usually to resurface the other hand. The advantage of using it as a free flap is that the radial artery on the donor hand can be reconstituted using a vein graft.

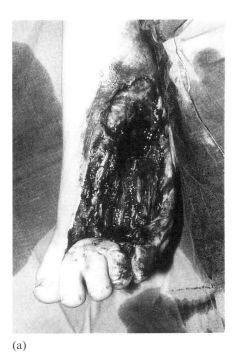

(a)

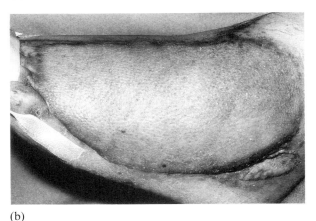

(b)

Fig. 11.7 (a) Degloving injury over foot prior to debridement with skin loss and tendon damage. (b) Free latissimus dorsi flap carried out as delayed primary procedure at 48 hours.

Latissimus dorsi flap

This is a musculo-cutaneous flap that can be used for local transposition or as a free flap (Fig. 11.7a, b). The flap can be used as 'free' muscle alone based on the thoraco-dorsal branch of the subscapular artery, whose origin lies in the axilla. After revascularization, skin grafts can be applied over the muscle. Postoperative management of continuing perfusion may be more difficult than if a cutaneous element is included. Muscle contraction in response to stimulation persists for a number of days after transfer if it remains viable.

The flap taken usually incorporates a skin 'paddle', being nourished by skin perforators coming through the muscle. In this situation, only a lateral strip of muscle need to be dissected with the skin flap, together with the perforating vessels.

The advantages of this flap are its long pedicle, about 10 cm, its versatility, incorporating skin/muscle, or even via its vascular branch to the serratus anterior. Segments of vascularized ribs can be mobilized with the flap. Depending on the size of the flap required the donor site can usually be closed. Disadvantages are a rather bulky flap and the necessity of dividing the nerve to the latissimus dorsi; however, it is sometimes possible to preserve one of the motor branches.

In cases of Volkmann's contracture, it is possible to get motor and therefore good functional recovery after micro-neuro-vascular anastomosis to the transferred latissimus dorsi muscle. The distal end of the thoraco-dorsal vessel can also be used to repair a defect in the radial or ulnar artery if present, producing a flow-through situation, as well as perfusion of the muscle.

Skin and tendon

The combined loss of skin and tendons, for example, over the dorsum of the hand or back of the heel, is a difficult problem, previously requiring firstly flap cover and secondary repair with tendon grafts. This may also require initial use of silastic rods.

Taylor and Townsend [8] showed it was possible to raise segments of tendons with a free flap maintaining their vascularity; for example, with the dorsalis pedis flap it is possible to use seg-

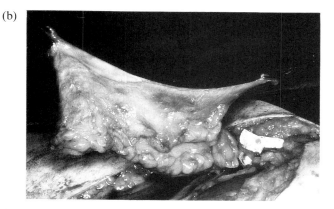

(b)

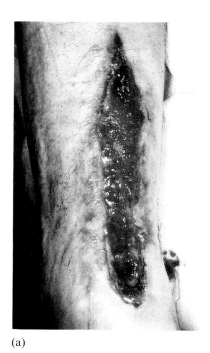

(a)

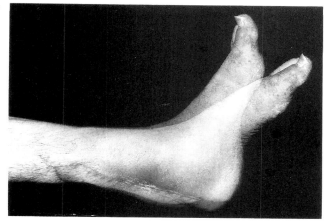

(c)

Fig. 11.8 (a) Skin and tendon loss on back of lower leg. (b) Composite groin flap containing skin, subcutaneous tissue and strip of external oblique aponeurosis. Background material placed behind superficial circumflex artery and vein. (c) Result following reconstruction. Note free flap inset on back of leg.

ments of foot extensor tendons to reconstruct the extensors of the fingers. For longer defects, segments of external oblique aponeurosis can be taken with the groin flap to reconstruct either a similar situation above, or for example the Achilles tendon under free flap cover (Fig. 11.8a–c).

As the tendons or tendon graft (external oblique aponeurosis) are still surrounded by normal vascularized connective tissue, gliding of these structures under the flap still occurs together with more rapid healing from the ends of the vascularized grafts.

More recently, it has been demonstrated that it is possible to take the radial forearm flap with palmaris longus and part of flexor carpi radialis tendons.

Innervated free flap transfer

Reconstruction, especially of a denuded thumb or over the heel, is best achieved if reinnervation is also carried out. Although some form of protective sensation occurs after a long time in the flaps already mentioned, it is possible to improve this by identifying the nerve supply to the skin being used in reconstruction and reanastomosing it to the divided nerves. For example, the terminal branches of the peroneal nerve can be identified while raising a dorsalis pedis flap, and after transfer to the thumb can be reanastomosed to the divided digital or other cutaneous nerves with much improved long term two point discrimination.

Skin and bone loss

The associated loss of skin and bone, especially in the lower leg, is perhaps one of the most difficult reconstruction problems. In the past, often a tube pedicle would be necessary to resurface the area and then subsequently bone grafts placed in position. The success rate was low and morbidity high.

Bone grafts placed as chips or pieces depend on revascularization to provide bony union and any infection diminishes the chance of success. Vascularized bone grafts, as part of a free flap, behave like a double fracture producing callus at both ends and if stressed undergo remodelling, there is therefore a very important fundamental difference between the types of graft. Vascularized bone also has a much greater resistence to infection.

In the hand, where often only a small segment of bone is required the radial forearm flap, either by pedicle or free flap incorporating a segment of radius, can be very useful in reconstruction, for example an amputated thumb [9].

The groin flap (superficial circumflex flap)

It was initially found possible to raise the crest of the ilium together with a groin flap, the bone remaining perfused via its periosteal supply. Although this was a considerable advance, there was a limit to the size of the bone graft which could be taken and would remain vascularized.

Deep circumflex iliac flap (DCIA) [8]

Perfusion studies of the DCIA vessel have shown that not only is skin perfused over the iliac crest, but that via the endosteal and periosteal circulation the whole of the ilium can be nourished by this vessel. For cases of bone loss between 6 and 12 cm this flap should now be considered.

The DCIA (1.5–3 mm in diameter) arises from the external iliac artery. The vena comitans draining the area usually join to form a single vessel draining into the external iliac vein.

The vessels can be identified posterior to the inguinal canal and be traced laterally behind the anterior superior iliac spine, allowing this to be left with the attachment of the inguinal ligament. Near this point, the vessels pierce the fascia transversalis and transversus abdominis and run close to the rim of the ilium between this latter muscle and the internal oblique. In this position, the artery gives off musculo-cutaneous branches. The flap can be raised, cutting a required segment of ilium together with a small cuff of muscles and skin flap according to need (Fig. 11.9).

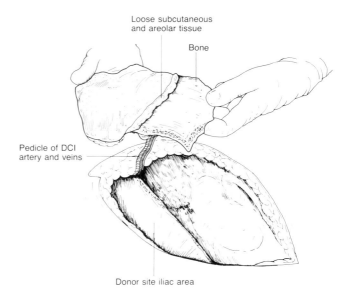

Fig. 11.9 DCIA flap raised, showing skin and bone composite flap still attached by feeding vessels.

The typical case referred to earlier is a lower limb injury where bone loss has occurred either following the accident or subsequently (Fig. 11.10). The limb is held out to length by external fixators (Fig. 11.11) and all dead skin, bone and muscle extensively debrided.

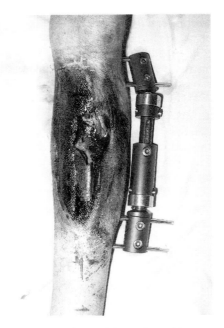

Fig. 11.10 Injury of lower leg with exposed dead bone and skin loss.

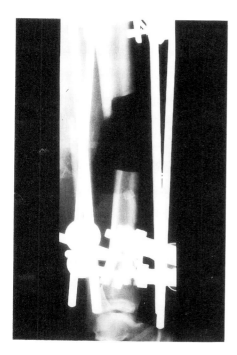

Fig. 11.11 After removal of dead bone, limb being held out to length by external fixators.

The pedicle of the DCIA flap is about 6 cm long, allowing anastomosis some distance away from the area of the bone loss. The bone graft is often stepped to allow locking into the ends of the tibia and then the anastomosis is carried out usually end-to-side to the anterior or posterior tibial artery, and end-to-end of the vena comitans to appropriate vena comitans, or to the long saphenous vein. The latter tends to go into spasm so the former is preferable.

If insufficient bony stability is provided by stepping the graft and tibia, a limited amount of fixation with wire may be required.

If the flap is successful (Fig. 11.12a, b) post-operative infection is usually not a problem unless bone chips or screws have been added.

In certain cases limb injuries are so severe, for example extensive skin loss with multiple fractures, or history of ischaemia within the limb, that anastomosis within the limb may add to the possible complications in view of the extra dissection required. There may be insufficient vascularized skin to cover either the pedicle, or long vein grafts which may be required to provide a blood supply from more proximal undamaged vessels.

In this situation a cross leg DCIA flap can be considered, the vessels being anastomosed to the posterior tibial vessels of the opposite leg. The legs are held together by rigid Hoffman fixation,

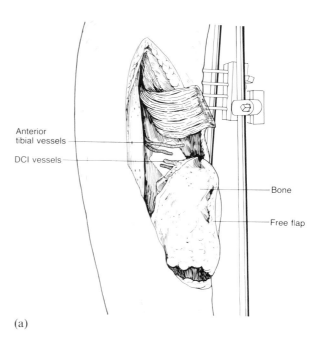

Anterior tibial vessels

DCI vessels

Bone

Free flap

(a)

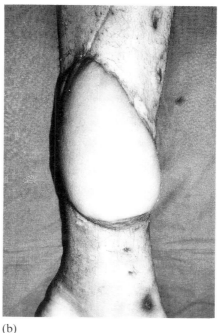

(b)

Fig. 11.12 (a) DCI vessels and flap placed adjacent to anterior tibial vessels prior to anastomosis. (b) Successful free DCIA flap in position over lower leg. Secondary skin thinning may be required later.

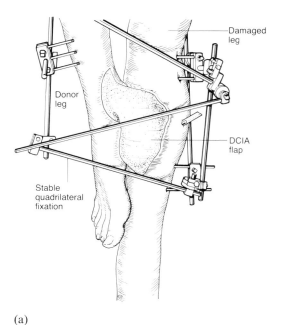

(a)

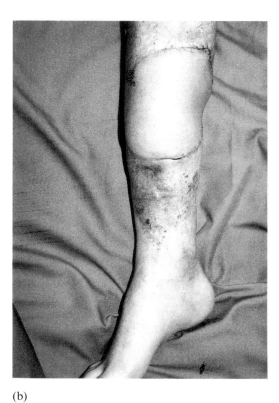

(b)

Fig. 11.13   (a) Cross leg free DCIA flap. Vessels anastomosed normal vessels right leg and flap inset into defect left leg. (b) Flap after division of DCIA vessels at 5 weeks.

thus allowing elevation of the limb and mobilization of ankle, knee and hip joints (Fig. 11.13a, b).

The vessels and flaps are divided later than a traditional cross leg flap at 5 weeks, by which time anastomosis of vessels occurs between the cancellous bone to bone contact and skin to skin contact. Back bleeding from the damaged leg can usually be demonstrated from the DCIA after division.

That the flap and bone remain vascularized is confirmed by comparison between DCIA flaps with anastomosis based on the damaged leg and by the cross leg flap technique [10] of 23 cases, 13 based on the same leg and 10 cross leg cases. Time to clinical union with full weight bearing without external support in both groups was between 6 and 7 months. Following operation, the reconstructive situation is similar to a double fracture and in three of the former and one in the latter group, there was delayed or non-union. Further cancellous chips were added later after

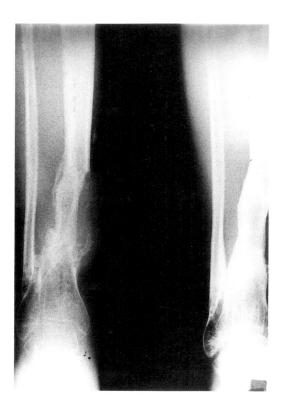

Fig. 11.14   Radiographs to illustrate remodelling of bone with vascularized bone graft. Left side at 6 months, right side at 18 months.

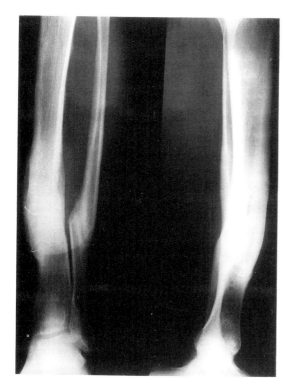

Fig. 11.15 Further case AP and lateral radiographs illustrating late remodelling. Bone graft area between wire loops.

freshening the ends. Extra time for this is taken into account in the overall figures quoted.

The normal postoperative treatment is to remove the Hoffman fixation when skin healing is achieved. The limb is then placed in a plaster of Paris cast and partial weight bearing started as soon as possible (Figs 11.14 and 11.15).

Vascularized fibula

Where there is a bony defect larger than 12 cm, the DCIA flap is unable to be used and in this situation the vascularized fibula based on the peroneal vessels can be considered. Provided about 6 cm are left at either end, the rest of the fibula can be taken as a free graft. To maintain stability in the ankle joint, a distal screw stabilizing the fibula remnant to the tibia is advised.

Even a small segment of fibula can be taken with a cuff of surrounding muscle. The nutrient artery lies in the middle third. In the case of congenital pseudoarthrosis of the tibia, this is probably the operation of choice. Vascularized fibula can, after removing the fibrous tissue between the tibial ends, be passed up and down the tibial medullary cavity ([11]).

Long term follow-up of a vascularized fibula indicates that with stress, the fibula hypertrophy remodels. This process may actually be enhanced if a greenstick or other fracture occurs. After about 2 years it may even be difficult to identify which is tibia and which fibula. Unlike the DCIA flap, the affected limb needs a lot longer external support, often over a year.

The vascularized fibula can be used in reconstruction of the forearm where there is loss of segments of both radius and ulna bones, converting it to a single bone forearm (Fig. 11.16a–d).

Although it is possible to take some skin with the fibula, it is quite small in comparison with a DCIA flap and it may be necessary to resurface the area of skin loss firstly by, for example, a cross leg flap prior to the microvascular procedure.

Replantation

The techniques used in replantation are of relevance to reconstructional problems; the indications are therefore worth briefly considering.

Amputation leading to ischaemia of part of a limb or digits may be partial or complete. In the former if revascularization is not carried out, necrosis of the end will occur.

Amputation may result from a clean cut, crushing, avulsion injury, or a combination of these.

The aim of any replantation should be not only to repair arteries, veins, but also tendons and nerves, as secondary surgery is more difficult to carry out.

The best results from revascularization occur if circulation is restored within 8 hours of injury, cooling the severed part increases this time.

Treatment of severed part

Without using any disinfectant for cleaning, the parts should be kept wrapped in a swab soaked in physiological saline and then placed within a plastic bag. Ice from a domestic refrigerator may

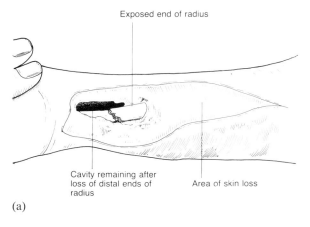

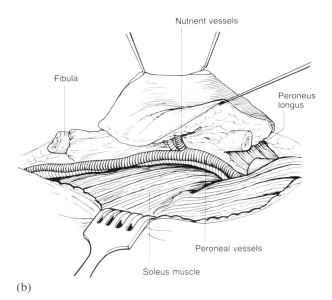

(a)

(b)

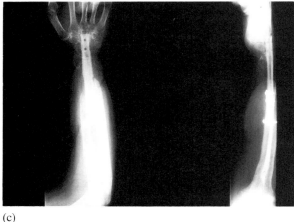

(c)

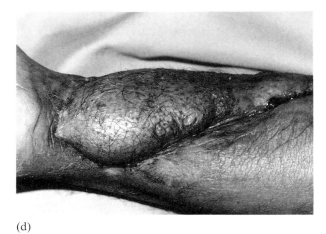

(d)

Fig. 11.16 (a) Compound injury left forearm, with skin loss and exposed dead bone. (b) Vascularized fibula being raised from leg with skin. Note feeding peroneal vessels (arrow). (c) Vascularized fibula in position forming single bone forearm. (d) Skin of flap inset on forearm.

be placed in an outer bag and an equal amount of water added.

On no account should a part be allowed to freeze, and the bag should not be placed in a thermos flask or an insulated container. The two bags can be sealed with one seal and placed in an open container. Cooling is especially important with larger amounts of muscle present in higher amputations, as they are more sensitive to anoxia.

Choice of cases suitable for replantation

Not every amputated digit is worth replanting, clean cut amputations do best. A narrow rim of

crushing can be compensated for by adequate debridement and if necessary vein grafts. Avulsion injuries on the whole do badly.

Replantation of a single digit within no man's land is seldom indicated. Although successful replants should get metacarpo-phalangeal joint movement, there will be interphalangeal joint stiffness and if the other fingers are unaffected the patient will tend to exclude this digit and even demand amputation subsequently.

Indications for replantation are: thumb loss, multiple digit amputations, hand, and distal limb.

Other factors may have to be taken into account: age, sex, dominance of hand and social factors.

The centre which provides a replantation service should be notified, firstly to confirm indications and secondly to mobilize surgical teams and theatre, as time is obviously important. Two teams are preferable. One team debrides and identifies the structures on the amputated part and the other does the same on the stump.

Amputations at wrist level do well, as there are mainly tendons here. The more proximal the amputation, the more ischaemic muscle mass is involved and with it, an increasing risk to the patient's life from toxic breakdown products of anoxia being released into the general circulation after revascularization.

The results of proximal upper limb reimplantation can be unrewarding, mainly due to the poor nerve regeneration at this level. Motor and sensory modalities are more intermixed and accurate reapposition at axonal level is poor.

Incomplete lower limb amputations are usually well worth revascularizing. Replantation of complete amputation may not be so rewarding, as even if sensory return is achieved patients may complain of hyperaesthesia and this possibility has to be compared with the excellent functional results using a prosthesis after below knee amputation.

In multiple amputations where parts are not suitable for replantation, thought should be given to the possibility of providing spare tissue, such as vein or arterial grafts, or even a free flap. For example [12] in an arm and leg amputation where it was not possible to revascularize the arm, a radial forearm flap was raised from the amputated limb and transferred to cover the exposed tibia, allowing him to finish with a below, rather than above, knee amputation (Fig. 11.17a, b).

Reconstructional techniques used in replantation can be used in congenital or traumatic loss of a thumb or digits.

In trauma and in congenital loss due to amniotic bands, the anatomy proximal to the site of amputation is normal. In congenital hypoplasia, or aplasia, for example transverse arrest with loss of all fingers, this does not occur, so alternative tendons or nerves may have to be used, such as wrist flexors and extensors and a cutaneous nerve. The results are therefore very difficult to predict before exploration.

Thumb reconstruction was originally carried out using the big toe, although in many patients this is too large. The wrap-around flap [13] is designed from the big toe, taking, the equivalent size of nail and skin to the remaining normal thumb, together with sensory and vascular supply on one side. The donor site is then skin

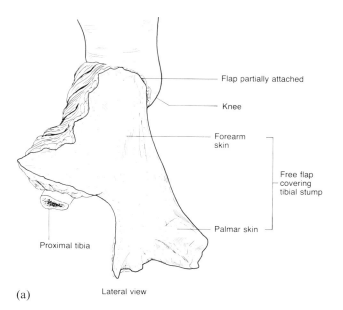

(a)   Lateral view

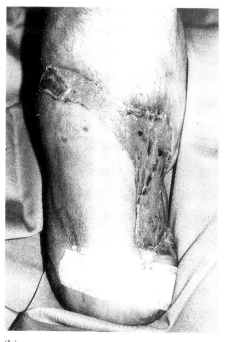

(b)

Fig. 11.17   (a) Free flap of forearm and hand. Skin draped over exposed upper tibia. (b) Amputation stump after healing. Palmar skin placed to cover end of stump.

grafted. The flap is then wrapped around an iliac bone graft and pegged into position into the site of the amputated thumb this flap is then revascularized. This technique provides a better match and reduces the morbidity of the donor big toe. To enhance bone graft take, a segment of distal phalanx is usually taken.

Digital reconstruction is usually from the second toe. This is based on the first dorsal metatarsal artery, a branch of the dorsalis pedis. If this toe is taken out together with the metatarso-phalangeal joint and a segment of the metatarsal, it is then possible to collapse in the donor deficit with a good cosmetic and functional result. Second toe transfer can produce a good sensory mobile digit, although not as powerful as the big toe.

In conclusion, the possibilities available of skin and composite reconstruction have considerably increased in recent years and it is important prior to making a decision on treatment to realize what these possibilities are, especially if local flaps or microvascular surgery are considered as this may affect the mode and placement of fixation. Also, by planning composite reconstruction of the various tissues lost the number of operations may be reduced with earlier rehabilitation of the patient.

References

1. McGregor, I. A. and Jackson, I. T. (1972) The groin flap. *Br. J. Plast. Surg.*, **25**, 3–16.
2. Ponten, B. (1981) The fasciocutaneous flap; its use in soft tissue defects of the lower leg. *Br. J. Plast. Surg.*, **34**, 215–220.
3. Yang, G., Chen, B., Gao, Y. *et al.* (1981) Forearm free skin flap transplantation. *Natl Med. J. China*, **61**, 139–141.
4. Song, R., Gao, Y., Song, Y. *et al.* (1982) The forearm flap. *Clin. Plast. Surg.*, **9(1)**, 21–26.
5. Ger, R. C. (1968) The management of pretibial skin loss. *Surgery*, **63**, 757.
6. Daniel, R. K. and Taylor, G. I. (1973) Distant transfer of an island flap by microvascular anastomosis. *Plast. Reconstr. Surg.*, **52**, 111–117.
7. Gault, D. T. and Quaba, A. (1986) Is free flap cases of exposed metalwork worthwhile? A review of 28 cases. *Br. J. Plast. Surg.*, **39**, 505–509.
8. Taylor, G. I. and Townsend, P. L. G. (1979) Composite free flaps and tendon transfer: an anatomical study and clinical technique. *Br. J. Plast. Surg.*, **32**, 170–183.
9. Biemer, E. and Stock, W. (1983) Total thumb reconstruction: one-stage reconstruction using an osteo-cutaneous forearm flap. *Br. J. Plast. Surg.*, **36**, 52–55.
10. Townsend, P. L. G. (1987) Indications and long term assessment of ten cases of cross leg free DCIA flaps. *Ann. Plast. Surg*, **19**.
11. Zhong-Wei, C., Dong Yue, Y. and Di-Sheng Chang, C. (1982) *Microsurgery*. Shanghai Scientific and Technical Publishers, Springer-Verlag Berlin, Heidelberg, New York, pp. 277–279.
12. Waterhouse, N., Moss, A. L. H and Townsend, P. L. G. (1984) Lower limb salvage using an extended free radial forearm flap. *Br. J. Plast. Surg.*, **38**, 394–397.
13. Morrison, W. A., O'Brien, B. M. and MacLeod, A. M. (1981) Thumb reconstruction with a free neurovascular wrap-around flap from the big toe. *J. Hand Surg.*, **5**, 575.

12

Arthroscopy of the knee

J. L. Pozo

Introduction

The advent of diagnostic arthroscopy and arthroscopic surgery in the last 10–15 years has greatly extended the accuracy of investigation, diagnosis, understanding and treatment of many of the common intra-articular pathologies of the knee.

Historical background

First reports of endoscopic practice date back to Philip Bozzini in Vienna around 1806 [1]. His 'lichtlieiter' or light conductor used candle light reflected down a bifid silver tube to visualize the interior of the nasopharynx, anal canal, vagina, urethra and orthopaedically the sinus of bones affected by osteomyelitis. In order to avoid burns to the surgeons' hands Herteloupe [2] resorted to *Lampyris noctiluca,* the female glow worm (the male only flashing intermittently) as an alternative source of illumination.

More conventional techniques of illumination were developed over the subsequent 50 years: Desormaux [3] used alcohol and turpentine, others experimented with camphor and petrol or burning magnesium filaments in the early cystoscope. The use of electricity to heat the platinum elements to white heat proved a more reliable and controllable source of illumination with David Newman in Glasgow in 1883 first using an incandescent lamp applied to an endoscope.

However, it was the development of the rod lens system by Professor Hopkins at Reading University which dramatically improved the clinical use of the endoscope.

Arthroscopy

In 1918 Professor Tagaki in Tokyo initially examined the inside of a knee in cadavers using a 7.3 mm cystoscope. Two years later he developed an instrument specifically for the examination of the knee: 'the arthroscope'. Although the first instruments did not have a lens system, rapid evolution led to the development of instruments which allowed still photography and cinematography [4] and colour photography by 1939.

In 1921 Bircher [5], working separately in Switzerland, presented the results of his knee examinations using the laparo-thoracoscope and nitrogen or oxygen to distend the joint.

In the USA, Burman, Finkelstein and Mayer [6], at the Hospital for Joint Diseases developed a 4 mm arthroscope which was used not only to examine the knee but also the elbow, ankle and shoulder. In 1934 they went on to describe their arthroscopic observations on 30 knees. There was little further advance in the subject until after the Second World War. Dr Watanabe [7], again in Japan, continued the technological development of the arthroscope, with publication of his water colour atlas of arthroscopy (1957) enhanced in 1969 with photographic material.

The first concrete report of arthroscopic surgery of the knee was the excision of posterior flap of the medial meniscus by Dr. Watanabe in 1962. However, it has been the enthusiastic work and teaching of Dr. R. Jackson on his return from Dr. Watanabe's unit, which led to the great interest and subsequent rapid development of arthroscopic surgery. In 1972 Jackson and Abe [8] reported 200 arthroscopic examinations of knee joints. It seems surprising that it was not until 1978 that the first clinical results of arthroscopic surgery were formally reported by Dandy [9]. By 1981 Johnson [10] was introducing the use of power instrumentation in the knee to trim menisci, excise synovium, shave articular cartilage and abrade articular surfaces.

Work is now being undertaken to investigate and develop the use of lasers in arthroscopic surgery. However, this remains largely restricted to specialist centres and the advantages of these techniques remain undefined.

Advantages and complications of arthroscopic surgery

Advantages

It is now universally agreed that arthroscopic surgery offers many major advantages, particularly when compared to similar procedures undertaken by open arthrotomy.

Diagnostic accuracy

Arthroscopy is reported to have a diagnostic accuracy of 97% in experienced hands [11]. It will often define multiple abnormalities where clinically only one pathology is evident. The findings may differ markedly from the clinical diagnosis, where accuracy ranges only from 60 to 75% [12]. Johnson [10] found that in 229 patients with a clinical diagnosis of a torn medial meniscus, only 21% had this isolated injury. Twenty-three percent had additional pathology and in 56% the diagnosis was completely different.

Access to all compartments and multiple pathologies

Arthroscopic surgery offers the facility to undertake multiple procedures, e.g. partial meni-

scectomy of torn medial and lateral menisci. It allows trimming of the torn posterior quadrant of the meniscus which is inaccessible through an arthrotomy. Drilling of osteochondral lesions can be undertaken with minimal postoperative morbidity. Debridement of joints with early degenerative disease, where more than one compartment may be affected, can produce excellent symptomatic improvement which would be impossible without multiple arthrotomy incisions.

Cost effectiveness

Patients undergoing arthroscopic surgery may be treated as day cases and the older population may require one overnight stay when the procedure is undertaken under general anaesthesia. By contrast after arthrotomy most patients require a minimum of 3–5 days as an inpatient.

Earlier mobilization and rehabilitation

Patients can readily mobilize with crutches or a walking stick and attain independent gait within a few days. Return to work of a sedentary nature is possible soon after, and to more strenuous activities, including driving, in one to two weeks. This contrasts with 10–14 days immobilization to allow sound healing of an arthrotomy incision and the invariable need for physiotherapy to regain full knee mobility over the subsequent 6–8 weeks. However, recent work suggests that incomplete motor control may persist for up to 8 weeks after arthroscopic meniscal surgery [13].

Cosmetic

Scars are minimum, often becoming virtually invisible over a few months. An arthrotomy scar can be unsightly and is not infrequently associated with an area of numbness or reduced sensation adjacent to the incision.

Low morbidity

Postoperative pain is minimal unless the procedure is complicated by a major haemarthrosis. The incidence of complications following arthroscopic procedures remains remarkably low. This allows for second procedures to be undertaken where necessary with little anticipated morbidity.

Complications

The complications of arthroscopic surgery are few and most are regarded as minor. A large study which scrutinized every single problem in a series of 2640 patients reported an overall complication rate of 8.2% [14]. The major complications amounted to 4.8% when cardiovascular episodes, paraesthesias, haemarthroses and effusions were excluded. Some surgeons would regard some of these minor and transient postoperative effusions and haemarthroses as almost inevitable in some procedures. The complication rate following open arthrotomy for meniscal procedures has been reported as 14.6% [15]. The major reduction has been in serious complications such as infection, neurological injury and venous thrombosis and embolism.

a) Any intra-articular structure can be damaged, but usually the anterior horn of the meniscus, the fat pad and the articular cartilage can be lacerated in making the portal incisions. The anterior cruciate ligament is most susceptible to injury during meniscal surgery in the intercondylar notch and during the use of motorized cutters.

b) Haemarthrosis, residual effusions, and fluid leakage from the posterior aspect of the knee represent some of the commoner complications.

c) Excessive or injudicious force in the use of the fine arthroscopic instruments in tight compartments can result in breakage within the knee joint; this is most often encountered in the course of lateral meniscectomies.

d) More serious complications include damage to the popliteal vessels from insertion of instruments via the posteromedial or posterolateral portals, or deep penetration of instruments through the intercondylar notch. The use of power instrumentation has also been associated with damage to the popliteal vessels. The blind passage of the meniscal suture needles has resulted in lacerations of these vessels and the peroneal nerves.

e) In general neurological complications are few. Delee's [16] review of 118 000 procedures revealed 65 neurological injuries, involving pero-

neal, saphenous, femoral, tibial and sciatic nerves. However, in a prospective study of 8791 procedures undertaken by experienced arthroscopists there was only one neurological complication–damage to the saphenous nerve during a medial meniscal suture. Tourniquet paresis seems uncommon, usually mild and undergoes early resolution [17].

f) The incidence of infection remains very low in all reported series, ranging from 0.04 to 0.08%:

Johnson *et al.* [10]: 5 cases in 12 500 arthroscopies;
Mullhollan [18]: 7 cases in 9000 arthroscopies;
Delee [16]: 95 cases in 118 590 arthroscopies.

The possibility that intra-articular steroid injection following arthroscopy may increase the risk of infection has been raised by Montgomery and Campbell [19] following three cases of septic arthritis in their series of 15 500 patients, most of whom had such steroid injections.

g) As with all procedures involving general anaesthesia and tourniquet, there is a small incidence of deep vein thrombosis ranging from 0.1 to 3.2% [20].

Arthroscopic techniques

The low morbidity of arthroscopic examination has made the procedure justifiable as an adjunct to diagnosis, prognosis and treatment. However, these advantages must not allow arthroscopy to become a simple replacement for the clinical skills of a careful history and examination which so often provide an accurate diagnosis and assessment of the need for surgical intervention.

Anaesthesia

Arthroscopy can be undertaken under local, regional or general anaesthesia. The choice of anaesthesia is influenced by many factors including patient co-operation, the surgeon's expertise and the complexity of any surgical procedure.

Local anaesthesia

The use of local anaesthetic within the knee appears safe since blood levels have been shown to remain low during arthroscopic procedures [21]. Although local anaesthesia can be employed for routine diagnostic examination of the knee, the experience of the surgeon, the patient's tolerance and co-operation are of paramount importance. Furthermore, if a treatable lesion is encountered, it may not be possible to proceed, and a second operative procedure under general anaesthesia required at a second admission. In experienced hands, however, straightforward arthroscopic procedures can be undertaken safely and proficiently. It should be stressed that surgery under local anaesthesia requires well drilled, experienced nursing and theatre assistant staff and may nevertheless take longer than the same procedure undertaken under a general anaesthetic. A dose of 20–30 ml of 0.25% or 0.5% bupivacaine with 1:200 000 adrenaline can be used to infiltrate the skin, subcutaneous and capsular tissues and for anaesthetizing the joint [22]. The use of a tourniquet is optional but most patients find it too uncomfortable, and in its absence, intra-articular bleeding can make accurate visualization troublesome. Access for operative procedures can also prove difficult because of the lack of muscle relaxation. Local anaesthetic techniques tend to be time consuming and somewhat variable but eliminate the problems of general anaesthesia, including cardio-pulmonary and thrombotic complications.

Regional anaesthesia

Spinal or regional anaesthesia with femoral nerve block [23] can be employed in patients where there are specific contraindications to general anaesthesia. However, this is rarely used as patients frequently complain of discomfort from the tourniquet despite adequate lower extremity anaesthesia. Femoral blocks fail to anaesthetize the posterior part of the knee and any manipulative procedures in this area can prove very painful. Quadriceps paralysis for 6–8 hours may delay patient discharge or require the use of rather cumbersome splints.

General anaesthesia

With these qualifications and the anticipation of an intra-articular surgical procedure, general anaesthesia is generally more widely employed. Overall, general anaesthesia appears to have a higher patient acceptance and is also more acceptable to the surgeon and the theatre staff as it seems much more efficient [21,23]. It has the further advantage that should the arthroscopic procedure fail, open arthrotomy can be promptly undertaken without the need for the patient to be readmitted for a second procedure.

Surgical techniques

The expertise, instrumentation and techniques necessary for arthroscopic diagnosis and surgery are now familiar and thoroughly covered in an extensive literature and in excellent hands-on courses. In this chapter these are not detailed and only specific points of interest are considered.

Tourniquet

A tourniquet is normally applied to the thigh but need not be inflated if only a diagnostic examination is undertaken. Tourniquet inflation tends to blanch the synovium and may impair the assessment of synovial disorders. If an intra-articular procedure is anticipated, then the use of a tourniquet following exsanguination of the limb is advantageous. In the presence of specific contraindications such as a history of thromboembolic disease it is preferable to proceed without inflating the tourniquet if possible. Impaired visualization due to bleeding can often be overcome by the assistance of low pressure suction through an outlet portal.

Patient position and leg holders

With the patient lying supine, one of three main techniques are employed for examination:

a) Using a leg holder: the patient lies with the legs hanging over the end of the operating table and the leg to be examined firmly held in a special leg holder. This allows the application of stress primarily to open the posteromedial compartment. However, leg holders restrict the range of positions the knee can be manoeuvred into and tend to disadvantage access to the patellofemoral and lateral compartments and interfere with instrumentation through superior portals. These supports incur further expenditure and are not without the potential hazard of damaging ligaments and even fracture to the femur in overforceful manoeuvres to open a tight joint.

b) Lateral post: other surgeons prefer to use a lateral post attached to the operating table, against which the femur can be levered to access the postero medial compartment. The post still allows the knee to be placed in almost any position, including the figure of four configuration to examine the lateral compartment.

c) Surgical assistant: some surgeons prefer to have the patient with the leg hanging over the side of the operating table and the foot supported and controlled on their lap. A varus or valgus stress, when necessary, can be applied by a surgical assistant. The technique tends to suffer from the inconsistent force applied to the knee as fatigue affects the assistant.

All these techniques have their strong proponents and essentially it is a question of trying out each technique before establishing a personal preference which the operator finds comfortable and efficient.

Arthroscopic equipment

Visualization of the intra-articular structures and operative field is now routinely undertaken via a television screen. This requires adequate illumination, with the use of a high intensity or xenon light source. Repeated direct viewing through the arthroscope with a xenon light source has been reputed to result in retinal burns. Video accessories allow the imaging of operations for record and teaching purposes. Efficient routine arthroscopic work requires a considerable financial outlay in specialized equipment, including a light source, camera unit and television monitor, a power unit to drive the motorized instruments and video recorder.

Arthroscopic instruments

The spectrum of manual instruments for intra-articular surgery is now extensive and very reliable. The advent of motorized power driven instruments has extended the arthroscopists'

armamentarium, not only facilitating existing techniques but improving and allowing the development of new procedures. These include, among others, meniscectomy, synovectomy, chondroplasty and abrader blades. It must be emphasized that these instruments are extremely powerful and although excellent in experienced hands they are capable of considerable damage not only to the intra-articular structures, particularly the anterior cruciate ligament, but also to the popliteal vessels, as reported in some studies. It is important to note that the negative pressure from the suction system used with these powered instruments can be sufficient to draw contaminated fluid back into the knee from a bucket at ground level collecting fluid from an accessory drainage tube in the knee.

Disposable cannula systems have also been developed to allow the repeated insertion of instruments through the same portal without repeatedly traumatizing the portal of entry.

Conventional entry portals

The success, safety and efficiency of arthroscopic surgery is highly dependent on the precise placement of the entry portals for adequate visualization and instrument access.

a) The anterolateral portal gives the most comprehensive view of all the compartments.

b) The anteromedial portal allows visualization of the lateral compartment.

c) The central transpatellar tendon portal: the entry point is approximately 1 cm distal to the inferior pole of the patella with the knee at 90° of flexion. The arthroscope is then introduced toward the superomedial quadrant with the knee in 90° of flexion to ensure the arthroscope passes above the fat pad. This central position can free the anteromedial and anterolateral portals for bimanual instrument manipulation. Proponents of this approach argue a better access to the posterior structures through the intercondylar notch, but usually only to best advantage if the 70° arthroscope is used. However, if the fat pad becomes swollen with irrigation fluid, visibility can become rapidly impaired.

d) The superolateral portal: this is the most valuable portal for assessing the patello-femoral articulation. This can also be used to visualize the anterior aspects of the medial compartment and conversely a superomedial portal used to view the anterior aspects of the lateral compartment.

e) The posteromedial portal can be safely accessed if the bony landmarks of the postero-medial edge of the femoral condyle and postero-medial border of the tibia are marked prior to distension, the joint is fully distended and the knee flexed to 90°. This portal allows visualiza-tion of the posterior horn of the medial meniscus and the posterior cruciate ligament.

f) The posterolateral portal: this lies approxi-mately 2 cm above the posterolateral joint line at the posterior edge of the iliotibial band and the anterior margin of the biceps tendon. Entrance is along the posterior edge of the femoral condyle with the trocar directed slightly inferiorly.

Insertion of the arthroscope

Distension of the knee joint with normal saline is undertaken prior to insertion of the sharp tro-car which is directed medially and superiorly through the skin towards the intercondylar notch with the knee in 30° of flexion. As soon as the synovium is penetrated, the sharp trocar is re-placed with the blunt trocar. The knee is allowed to come slowly into full extension and the trocar, with a brisk push through the synovium, is nego-tiated under the patella towards the suprapatellar pouch. Distension of the knee joint can be ad-equately maintained using a 3 litre normal saline bag suspended about 2 metres above floor level. Whether delivered via the arthroscope or through the superolateral portal is a matter of the surgeon's preference.

Postoperative care

Portals may be closed with steristrip or nylon sutures removed 10–14 days after surgery. Except following specific procedures, most patients can fully weight bear immediately after surgery and most are walking freely by 48 hours. However, it is advisable to afford the patient the use of a walking stick or crutches for 1 or 2 days until they have regained their confidence following the general anaesthetic and their initial discomfort has settled.

Diversity of arthroscopic surgery

As expertise and confidence grew in the use of arthroscopy as a diagnostic tool, direct surgical intervention through arthroscopic visualization developed rapidly. This impetus was further pro-moted by the development of instruments and technology particularly adapted to arthroscopic surgery. The result has been an enormous expan-sion in the variety and complexity of surgical procedures which can now be safely undertaken arthroscopically, extending from relatively simple resection of synovial plicae, through re-section and suturing of meniscal tears, to arthro-scopically assisted anterior cruciate ligament reconstructions. The spectrum of arthroscopic operations is considered in further detail in the following sections.

Arthroscopy in the diagnosis of the acute haemarthrosis

It has become fashionable to arthroscope the knee presenting with an acute haemarthrosis [24–26].

Noyes et al. [21] found some damage to the anterior cruciate ligament in 72% of knees. Similarly Jones and Allum [27] found that 54% of their unselected group of patients had acute ACL tears. The incidence of meniscal tears was 22% compared to 62% by Noyes et al. [24] and 66% by Dehaven et al. [26], possibly reflecting the fact that these latter were studies exclusively on sports injured patients. Only 30% required definitive treatment at arthroscopy and no patient over 35 years required an operative procedure.

There are strong proponents of early arthro-scopy since the diagnosis of an acute meniscal tear followed by immediate suture may increase the chances of successful healing. In athletes, early reconstruction of a torn anterior cruciate may be appropriate in order to return the patient to sporting activities with the minimum delay. It would seem preferable to be able to provide a definitive diagnosis and plan for rehabilitation based on arthroscopic examination. However, if primary reconstruction is not entertained at this point there is little to be lost by delay, since there may be resolution in 70% of patients without the necessity of an invasive surgical procedure and general anaesthetic.

Kannus and Jarvinen [28] have reported the outcome of 84 patients with an acute haemarthrosis after injury without instability as defined by clinical examination without anaesthesia. This group, which represented 25% of all knees attending with an acute haemarthrosis, underwent intensive rehabilitation. After an average 8-year follow-up, 86% were asymptomatic, suggesting that the stable knee with a haemarthrosis could sometimes be treated expectantly and was not always associated with an unstable prognosis.

Given the demands on the acute services, and the likelihood of resolution in 70% cases, it would seem appropriate to consider early arthroscopy largely in those patients in whom diagnosis of a major correctable injury would be followed by a definitive procedure at the same operation. It is important to emphasize that arthroscopy of the acutely injured knee is a difficult procedure.

If elective arthroscopy is difficult for the beginner, accurate identification of the sustained damage in the presence of continuous bleeding or when the synovium of the intercondylar notch is grossly swollen and haemorrhagic can present major difficulties of visualization. This type of surgery should only be undertaken by someone experienced in arthroscopic work. This is particularly so if identification of the damage then requires surgical intervention in the acute situation, where visualization can be so much more difficult than in the elective case. When persistent fresh bleeding is a problem, gentle continuous suction through a superolateral portal can clear the field of vision effectively to allow surgical procedures to be undertaken if a good flow of fluid can be achieved to maintain distension of the joint and flush the blood out the joint.

Meniscal surgery

It was as recent as the early 1980s that reports of large series of arthroscopic meniscectomies began to appear in the literature and hence establish the technique as a valuable tool in the orthopaedic armamentarium [29]. The very evident advantages of arthroscopic partial meniscectomy over open arthrotomy established the value of this type of surgery: in particular, the ability for surgery to be undertaken as a day case, the minimal requirement for postoperative analgesia,

and the early return to work and sports [30]. In a large series of 230 patients Simpson *et al.* [31] found that only 25% of patients following open meniscectomy had returned to sports by the 6th postoperative week compared with 86% of the patients who had undergone a similar procedure arthroscopically.

Though the basic techniques of partial meniscectomy will not be considered in this text it is essential to emphasize that accurate definition of the anatomy of the tear is crucial to an understanding and planning of successful arthroscopic meniscal surgery. O'Connor's classification [32] would appear to be eminently simple and valuable in this respect: a) longitudinal tears; b) horizontal tears; c) oblique tears; d) radial tears; e) variations or complex tears; e) degenerative tears. The use of a probe is therefore crucial to define the extent, type and configuration of the tear in the meniscal substance. A more detailed analysis has been presented by Dandy [33] in a report of 1000 symptomatic meniscal lesions. Eighty-one percent of the patients were male. The medial meniscus was involved in 70.5% and the lateral in 29.5%. Of the medial meniscal lesions 75% were vertical, 23% horizontal, the former occurring most frequently in the fourth and the latter in the fifth decade of life. Of the tears in the lateral meniscus, 54% were vertical, 15% oblique, 15% myxoid, 4% inverted and 5% discoid, the most common lesion being a vertical tear involving half the length and half the width of the meniscus. Each different morphological type of tear requires a particular technique to achieve the general objective of removing the unstable fragments whilst being as conservative as possible in retaining a stable rim.

The work of Cargill and Jackson [34], showing that patients with open partial meniscectomy for bucket handle tears did better than those who underwent open total meniscectomy, initiated a trend towards more conservative resection of only the damaged part of the meniscus. This was confirmed by McGinty *et al.* [15] in a study amply demonstrating that after 6 years the partial meniscectomy patients exhibited better functional results and 50% fewer radiological degenerative changes.

Arthroscopy has allowed clarification of the pathology of meniscal tears and has proved to be the ideal technique for further implementing the concept of a more conservative approach to meniscal surgery, allowing removal of only the damaged area of the meniscus. The objective is to remove the torn, mobile fragments and contour the peripheral edge, leaving a residual stable meniscal rim. The rim left after removal of a bucket handle can transmit up to 35% of the load across the joint [35]. Partial meniscectomy may not always be possible if the tear extends to the periphery and a subtotal excision would seem preferable to a total meniscectomy.

Developments in meniscal surgery are now being extended to the use of laser technology. The most commonly used are the Nd-Yag, CO_2 and argon lasers. All have limitations, but the development of a contact probe using a sapphire crystal for the Nd-Yag laser may have considerably advanced the application of the technique. O'Brien and Miller [36] have reported work on canine and rabbit samples which appears to indicate that the laser cuts meniscus tissue more effectively than articular cartilage. In their series of 15 patients there were no complications other than breakage of one contact tip which required retrieval from the joint. The advantages appeared to be mainly in the access to difficult areas of the joint. The system as a whole remains limited largely to research groups and the costs are not inconsiderable.

Meniscal suture

The important role which the meniscus plays in the function of the knee has become increasingly apparent over the last 10 years. It provides stability, transfers loads, lubricates and allows the nutrition of the articular cartilage. Biomechanical studies have demonstrated that in extension 50% of the compressive load of the knee joint is transmitted through the meniscus. In 90° of flexion this increases to approximately 85% of the load [37]. Complete meniscectomy reduces the contact area by 50% significantly increasing the load per unit area. The result is a marked incidence of early degenerative osteoarthritis in the subsequent 15–20 years [38,39]. There has therefore been great interest in the possibility of meniscal salvage by suture to encourage healing. The outer 10–20% of the meniscus is known to have reasonable blood supply provided by the perimeniscal capillary plexus [40].

Open meniscal suture was reported to be associated with a high incidence of healing in chronic peripheral tears and higher rates for acute tears [41]. The development of arthroscopic suture techniques has resulted in renewed interest and enthusiasm for the repair of the torn meniscus.

Reported results are impressive with healing rates of 78–100%. However, these results are not entirely based on second look arthroscopy but include arthrography and the absence of clinical symptoms. Keene and Paterson [42] reported healing in 10 of 11 re-arthroscoped knees out of a cohort of 20 patients with medial meniscal repairs. The most important factors contributing to successful resuture are a) acute tears, b) within 5 mm of the periphery of the meniscus (in the red-red or red-white area) c) in knees which do exhibit instability.

Two suture methods are generally in use: the inside-out technique uses long flexible needles passed into the knee through a curved cannula under arthroscopic vision and across the meniscal tear to emerge through the capsule. In the outside-in technique a needle is placed across the tear from the outside in. A suture is threaded through the needle, picked up in the joint and brought out of an anterior portal. A large knot is made in the end of the suture, which is then drawn back into the joint and against the meniscal surface. This is repeated and the free ends of the sutures tied on the capsular surface.

The potential for serious complications in terms of damage to the peroneal nerve and popliteal artery is considerable. The importance of ensuring that the needles emerge anterior to the semitendinosus tendon for medial repairs and anterior to the biceps tendon for lateral repairs cannot be sufficiently stressed. To ensure these problems are avoided a small incision down to the capsule allows retraction under direct vision of the structures at risk and permits access to emerging needles and suture ligation over the capsular tissues: so-called arthroscopically assisted meniscal repair.

Role of arthroscopy in the treatment of osteoarthritis

Debridement of osteoarthritic knees long precedes the development of arthroscopy. Magnuson [43] reported complete recovery of symptoms in a large number of knee joints following open debridement. Open removal of osteophytes and drilling of exposed subchondral bone became popular as the 'Pridie Procedure' following his reports of good results in 65% of his patients.

However, as far back as 1934, Burman *et al.* [6] noted a marked symptomatic improvement in two patients following diagnostic arthroscopy of their arthritic knees. Jackson and Rouse in 1982 reaffirmed this simple observation that lavage of the joint without any operative procedure resulted in persisting symptomatic benefit. This has now been confirmed by other workers. Attempts to further improve the outcome of simple arthroscopic lavage have led to the inclusion of added procedures to 'tidy up' the knee joint. These have included drilling of exposed bone areas, resection of unstable meniscal segments [44], removal of unstable chondral flaps, debridement of osteophytes and loose fragments of articular cartilage [45] and abrasion arthroplasty to permit capillary bleeding through to the joint surface.

Which of these procedures, or if all, contribute to symptomatic improvement remains largely unknown. However, some pointers are beginning to emerge. Jackson and Rouse [44] reported that excision of unstable, torn meniscal fragments proved beneficial. However, extensive partial meniscectomy of stable fragments appeared to be detrimental [45]. Salisbury *et al.* [46] report that normally aligned knees appear to do better than those with either varus or valgus deformities. Younger patients tended to do better than older patients and those with early degenerative disease again achieved more improvement than those with advanced changes [47]. Bird and Ring [48] confirmed these findings but felt that the procedure was of much less value in rheumatoid and seronegative knees.

In a prospective study of 276 knees with osteoarthritis followed for a mean of 44 months, Patel *et al.* [49] reported good beneficial results in 75% patients. Knees requiring meniscal debridement alone did better than those needing both meniscal and surface debridement and patients under the age of 60 years did better. Bert and Maschka [47] have found that abrasion arthroplasty offers no advantage over other procedures. In their series good results were maintained in 66% of their patients five years after arthroscopic debridement.

The indications for this type of surgery again require clearer definition. However, in certain groups the benefits appear to have been substantial. There seems to be an increasing impression that the older athlete with early degenerative changes can often benefit sufficiently to allow a return to some sporting activities. In some elderly patients conservative methods may fail, but their symptoms are not severe enough to warrant prosthetic replacement. This group may derive major symptomatic benefit from arthroscopic debridement and allow a considerable delay in major surgery.

The mechanism whereby significant symptomatic relief is achieved remains unknown. Whether it is the debridement or the simple act of distension followed by the washing out of debris that is responsible for the observed benefit is difficult to ascertain. However, it seems likely that removal of cartilage debris, crystals and inflammatory factors probably all play a contributary role. Similarly, the likely duration of the symptomatic improvement remains uncertain. Further detailed analyses are necessary before these answers emerge and more accurate indications for this type of treatment can be defined.

Arthroscopic synovectomy

Open synovectomy of the knee in rheumatoid arthritis is known to achieve a reduction in pain and severity of effusions, but only for a period of time due to recurrence of the synovitis [50]. Enthusiasm for this procedure waned because of the prolonged hospitalisation necessary to execute the painful rehabilitation required to regain the range of movement. Sometimes manipulation under anaesthesia became necessary and loss of the range of excursion was well documented [51].

The advent of arthroscopy and the introduction of motorized synovial resectors has led to renewed interest in the procedure particularly in the hope that some lasting benefits could be achieved without the marked drawbacks of open synovectomy.

Early studies were reported by Matsui *et al.* in 1989 [52] where they compared the long term results of arthroscopic (41 knees) versus open (26 knees) synovectomies using large punches. The outcome over ten years was similar in both groups, with 80% of the knees being rated as good at 3 years but deteriorating to 57% good at 8 years. However, the authors found that the radiological changes of deterioration were less marked after arthroscopic synovectomy. Their findings at 2–3 years have been confirmed by Klein and Jensen [53] in a series of 45 patients using a powered synovectomy system. All the patients showed a reduction in pain and swelling and an improvement in the activities of daily living. The majority maintained an increase in the range of movement achieved postoperatively. Where articular damage was established the benefits were less substantial.

Although there are few large studies, and in some series, patients with different inflammatory conditions were included, the general impression appears to be that arthroscopic synovectomy offers many major early advantages.

There was little postoperative pain and both knees could be operated at the same admission. Hospitalization was only over a few days and return to work was rapid. One major advantage was that the majority of patients gained and maintained an improved range of movement. Because of the low morbidity repeat operations were felt to be acceptable in the longer term management. In patients with marked disease and grade IV articular damage, total knee replacement was postponed by more than 2 years.

It must be emphasized that arthroscopic synovectomy is an incomplete synovectomy. It may retard synovial growth. Regrowth is inevitable but then rheumatoid synovium recurs even in complete synovectomy performed by open arthrotomy [54].

Further large detailed studies are necessary in this field before an accurate assessment of the value of this procedure, not only in rheumatoid arthritis but also in other synovial proliferative diseases, can be ascertained.

Synovial plicae

Synovial plicae represent unresolved partition remnants of the three synovial compartments which fuse to form the single knee cavity during embryological development:

a) The infrapatellar plica or ligamentum mucosum is usually a thin band of synovium running from the fat pad to the superior aspect of the intercondylar notch. It can sometimes interfere with the passage of the arthroscope to other compartments. It should not be mistaken for the anterior cruciate ligament, in front of which it lies, initially obscuring the ligament.

b) The suprapatellar plica can divide the suprapatellar pouch into two separate compartments. As with the ligamentum mucosum, it is not thought to be responsible for any symptomatic complaints.

c) The lateral patellar plica is very rare, though described.

d) The medial patellar plica arises superior to the patella and runs down the medial side of the joint over the medial femoral condyle to insert into the fat pad. It is thought that trauma, usually a direct blow, to the overlying part of the knee can result in chronic inflammation and thickening of the plica which can then become symptomatic. The patient complains of pain in the anteromedial aspect of the knee, worse on activity, and sometimes of a clicking sensation and pain on flexion of the knee, often in the arc of 45–60° of the range. This represents the thickened plica flicking across the medial femoral condyle on flexion. Tenderness can be elicited about 1 cm above the medial condyle and the plica can sometimes be palpated or rolled under the finger.

In the absence of other pathology which might account for symptoms in this part of the knee, the presence of a thickened inelastic tough plica on arthroscopic examination, may account for the patient's symptoms.

Initially simple division of the plica was thought to be sufficient treatment. However, in view of the recurrence of symptoms in some patients, probably due to the development of dense fibrous tissue at the site of the previous incision, resection or saucerization of the plica down to the side wall is preferable. This can usually be undertaken with relative ease by introducing the cutting instruments or a powered synovial resector through the superomedial portal or superolateral portal. The patients often report an immediate improvement or resolution of their symptoms.

Loose bodies

The majority of loose bodies are either a) cartilagenous or b) osteochondral in nature. The former usually arise as the result of trauma to the hyaline cartilage of the articular surfaces. The radioopaque osteochondral loose bodies usually arise from osteochondritis dissecans, osteochondral fractures, osteophytic processes, or synovial chondromatosis. 'Rice bodies' represent multiple fibrinous lesions secondary to chronic inflammatory conditions, such as rheumatoid arthritis and sometimes tuberculosis.

The removal of the loose bodies must be allied to identification and treatment of the underlying pathology causing the formation of these fragments. A recent radiograph prior to surgery may be of considerable value in identifying the location and number of radio-opaque loose bodies. A thorough systematic examination of the knee is essential to locate all the fragments. Sometimes difficulty may be encountered when a loose body is obscured behind a large plica or small fragments may come to lie under the meniscus. Once located, the fragment can be pierced with a needle or 'incarcerated' between two needles if it cannot be effectively pierced. A strong grasper is essential to secure a hold on larger loose bodies. On removal, it is best to ensure an adequately sized exit portal than to risk losing the fragment back into the joint.

Small loose bodies in the posterior compartment of the knee may be completely asymptomatic and do not always require removal. Where appropriate, visualization can be undertaken through posteromedial or posterolateral portals. Visualization through the intercondylar notch may then allow instrument access via posteromedial or posterolateral portals. These techniques can however present considerable difficulties.

Multiple loose bodies can be removed without difficulty by repeated washouts and suction of the joint cavity. The removal of small foreign bodies follows the same basic principles. However, when instrument breakage occurs, it is essential to keep the piece on vision until it can be grasped and removed. Small fragments can be held at the tip of a small bore sucker until they can be grasped with an appropriate instrument. Magnetic instruments are now available to immobilize metal foreign bodies until they can be secured and removed.

Lateral release of the patella

Arthroscopic lateral release or perhaps percutaneous arthroscopically assisted lateral release of the patella offers more rapid recovery, less pain, and easier rehabilitation than the equivalent open procedure. The knee is always fully examined before the release is undertaken in order to identify any coincidental pathology, and to assess the congruency of the patello-femoral articulation and the condition of the articular cartilage. The lateral portal can be slightly enlarged and the skin undermined from the margin of the lateral tibial plateau, along the lateral border of the patella tendon and patella to beyond the superior pole border of the patella into the fibres of vastus lateralis, 4 cm above the patella being recommended by Dandy and Griffiths [55]. An incision is made through the capsular retinaculum and into the joint, although some surgeons prefer to maintain the integrity of the synovium. Either using scissors or a special lateral release knife the structures are then split longitudinally from tibial margin to vastus lateralis. It is suggested that unless the patella can be tilted through 90° from the femoral articulation the release is incomplete and further dissection is necessary to ensure the likelihood of an effective procedure. A drain may be left in the line of the release. A compression pad is applied to contain the haemarthrosis when the tourniquet is released. After 48 hours knee flexion and static quadriceps exercises are initiated.

The main difficulties however, have been not so much with the technique of the procedure as to the selection of appropriate cases for this operation. Dandy and Griffiths [55] reporting on their series of 41 knees recommended the procedure as highly successful in patients with recurrent dislocation of the patella in flexion but not for those with subluxation in extension. The procedure again seemed less satisfactory in patients with ligamentous laxity. Although many studies have been reported, difficulties of interpretation arise because few define the type of patellar instability being addressed, and a miscellaneous group of patella subluxation and dislocation often forms the basis of such studies [56]. The problem is further compounded by the fact that the lateral release may have been undertaken specifically for pain in association with instability. Reported success rates vary widely from 44% [57] to 75% [58].

In cases where there is a tight lateral retinaculum with patella tilting or in the lateral facet compression syndrome an isolated lateral release can be considered justifiable when properly supervised conservative treatment has failed to improve symptoms over three to six months.

Arthroscopy in children

The accurate diagnosis of knee problems, particularly acute presentations, in children can be extremely difficult. Arthroscopy provides a minimally invasive technique to reach a diagnosis and afford definitive treatment where appropriate. A clinical diagnostic accuracy ranging from 42% [59] to 55% [60, 61] in the under 13 years-old age-group appears consistent in the literature.

a) Acute injuries: The presentation of a significant haemarthrosis and a very painful knee invariably requires arthroscopic examination. The importance and prevalence of injuries to the anterior cruciate ligament in children is becoming increasingly appreciated. Bergstrom [62] reported damage to the ACL in 43% and Eiskjaer and Larsen [63] in 45% of older children arthroscoped because of an acute haemarthrosis. The injury may be partial or full mid-substance tear and overall represents the single most common diagnosis in these patients with a haemarthrosis. When there is avulsion of the tibial insertion of the ACL with a bone attachment, it may be possible to relocate the fragment accurately either arthroscopically or by open arthrotomy. Tears of the meniscus can be particularly difficult to diagnose. Meniscal injuries, including medial bucket handle tears, occur more frequently than originally expected and are commoner than injuries to the lateral meniscus [60, 63]. Early diagnosis of an osteochondral fracture, usually of the femoral condyle, will allow easier relocation of the fragment for pinning or Herbert screw fixation depending on the size of the lesion.

b) Discoid lateral meniscus: Although initially thought to represent an arrested stage of development of the lateral meniscus, Kaplan [64] did not find any stage at which the meniscus had the discoid configuration. It is rather postulated that as the result of the abnormal posterior ligamentous attachments, the meniscus cannot move back with the femur and with time is pushed into the joint, so that the central concavity becomes obliterated and a discoid shape develops. In the past, the symptomatic discoid meniscus was treated by open resection of the whole meniscus. The advent of arthroscopy has allowed a more accurate diagnosis and a more conservative partial meniscectomy leaving a residual rim in cases of midsubstance tears. Watanabe *et al.* [65] have classified the discoid meniscus as i) complete, ii) incomplete and iii) Wrisberg ligament type. The discoid meniscus, because of its relative immobility, poor vascularization and posterior attachment, is more susceptible to injury. The majority of patients are aged 10–15 years on presentation and complain of pain clicking, snapping, locking and giving way. Lack of extension and a positive McMurray's test may be found in a proportion of these patients. The decision to operate on a suspected discoid meniscus can be difficult, particularly when the history is only of clicking and there is little pain or giving way and with few objective signs. However, Hayashi *et al.* [66] propose that the symptomatic discoid lateral meniscus indicates a tear in the substance of the meniscus or a peripheral detachment. Identification of tears in the midsubstance may be difficult even at arthroscopy. Excision of the meniscus in one piece is the only way to confirm a tear postoperatively. Hayashi *et al.* [66] argue that all discoid menisci have a posterior attachment which then ruptures as part of the mechanism of the posterior tear or peripheral detachment and indicate that in their series of 46 children they did not identify any Wrisberg ligament type of lesions. They recommend complete excision of the meniscus if the lesion is near the periphery, or if the fascicle in the popliteal area is torn, i.e. the Wrisberg ligament type. For a midsubstance tear, about 4 mm–6 mm rim can be left in situ. Surgery can be technically difficult and sometimes a combination of arthroscopic and open techniques becomes necessary to remove the discoid fragment effectively. Long-term data is lacking on whether meniscectomy, partial or total, in these children results in early osteoarthritis of the lateral compartment.

c) Chondromalacia patella: The diagnosis of chondromalacia patella is based on clinical examination and findings, and the absence of any radiological abnormalities. The role and value of arthroscopy in the management of adolescent knee pain remains a matter of vigorous contention. However, there seems to be little to be gained by submitting patients, particularly those with a classical history, clinical findings, the absence of an effusion and normal radiograph, to an intrusive and invasive procedure when the chance of discovering any abnormal findings remains small, the significance of these uncertain and the likelihood of symptomatic improvement little if any. Furthermore the natural history of the condition suggests that spontaneous improvement would occur without surgical interference in at least 50% of the cases and there is no evidence that arthroscopy has improved on this natural outcome [68].

d) Osteochondritis dissecans: The diagnosis of osteochondritis dissecans is generally straightforward and based on radiological examination. Its management is considered in a separate section.

e) Septic arthritis: Arthroscopic techniques of drainage and lavage have been found to be very successful in the treatment of septic arthritis of the knee in children [60, 68, 69]. It allows for thorough débridement and lavage, and may be repeated if necessary. Treatment must include the appropriate antibiotics in adequate doses. The use of passive continuous motion techniques may be used as an adjunct to help maintain the range of movement during the recovery phase of treatment.

Osteochondritis dissecans

The exact aetiology of osteochondritis dissecans remains unknown. The generally accepted view is that a localized area of subchondral bone undergoes infarction, probably against a background of a traumatic event, allowing separation of the overlying articular cartilage.

Arthroscopy has allowed ready access and visualization of the osteochondritis dissecans fragment and an understanding of the natural history of the disease. The locations of the lesions are described as classical (69%), extended classical (6%) and inferocentral (10%) on the medial condyle and inferocentral (13%) and anterior (2%) the lateral condyle [70].

Undisplaced lesions in young children may heal if further trauma is avoided particularly if located in the non-weightbearing area. No treatment is usually necessary other than careful follow-up until the lesion is noted to be incorporated radiologically. In the older age groups, where surgical treatment is indicated, arthro-

scopy is becoming the commonest approach to surgical intervention.

Guhl [71] recommends arthroscopic examination and treatment of children over the age of 12 with lesions larger than 1 cm in diameter.

a) In patients with no overt loosening of the fragment, careful probing is necessary to define its location as there is often no obvious break in the continuity of the articular surface. The preferred treatment is multiple drilling with a small diameter K wire through the fragment into the underlying subchondral bone to stimulate vascularity and healing [72].

b) If the fragment is not completely loose but still attached by a tissue hinge, it can be turned back to expose the base which is then curetted. The fragment is secured with two slightly divergent K wires which are drilled through the fragment and condyle to emerge through the condyle in the area of the femoral epicondyle. Once the wires appear under the skin they can be withdrawn retrogradely whilst the intra-articular end is viewed directly via the arthroscope until it is just below the articular surface. The K wires are cut off under the skin to allow for easy removal 6–8 weeks later. The patient can be maintained in a partial or non-weightbearing status for 6–8 weeks.

Care should be taken not to damage the epiphysis by drilling the K wire through epiphyseal plates which are still open.

c) In the older patient with a well established hinged fragment, the latter may be excised and the underlying crater curetted or drilled as above to stimulate the development of fibrous or fibrocartilaginous growth. If the fragment is free as a loose body, it should be removed and the crater treated as above. If the lesion is fragmented, multiple fixation is unlikely to achieve healing and the fragments are best removed and the crater treated appropriately.

Osteochondral fractures

In the adult, articular cartilage shears at the junction between the calcified and uncalcified zones. The adolescent cartilage does not have a calcified zone and the shear forces are transmitted directly to the subchondral bone resulting in an osteochondral fracture [73]. In these cases, diagnosis is usually early because of the acute presentation following the injury. The patient invariably has a significant haemarthrosis and the knee may be locked. The fresh detached fragment can usually be reattached into the crater with stability, and secured by the pinning technique described above.

Arthroscopically assisted anterior cruciate reconstruction

Numerous methods are available for augmentation or reconstruction of the torn anterior cruciate ligament, using prosthetics, allografts or autografts. The development of interference screw fixation allowing early mobilization, together with the early success of the bone–patella tendon–bone graft technique, accurate drill guides and reproducible isometry techniques, has resulted in an enormous interest and work in ACL reconstruction. The results of open arthrotomy techniques appear to be reproducible and reliable with Clancy et al. [74] and O'Brien et al. [75] reporting 90% good results in the short to medium term. However, many of these cases were protected with an extra-articular reinforcement.

One of the technical problems in reconstruction has been the placement of the graft material at the exact anatomic location of the anterior cruciate ligament on the distal femur. The advances in arthroscopic techniques and technological equipment, has encouraged arthroscopic or arthroscopically assisted ACL reconstruction to try and overcome some of the problems presented by conventional arthrotomy.

Arthroscopically assisted reconstruction is said to offer superior visualization of the anatomic cruciate attachments and site for graft placement. The notchplasty can be undertaken with greater ease. There is improved cosmesis for the patient because of the smaller scars. There are no major incisions through the extensor retinaculum or joint capsule which theoretically should result in less quadriceps inhibition and easier rehabilitation [76].

In a comparison of arthroscopically assisted reconstruction versus a miniarthrotomy using dacron grafts, Gilquist and Oldesten [77] reported the operation time was significantly longer in the former but the Lysholm scores and activity levels were the same in both groups. No benefit was defined in terms of rehabilitation and they found the access for the notchplasty was easier through a miniarthrotomy. In the series reported by Buss et al. [78] the average operating time for arthroscopic reconstruction was 173 minutes (range 109–254 minutes). Short term reviews of miniarthrotomy or arthroscopic reconstruction using bone-patellar tendon–bone autografts have shown no statistically significant differences [79]. The short term success rate of 87% for the arthroscopic assisted procedure [78] appears no different from that achieved by open techniques. In a study with a 4-year average follow-up, Aglietti and co-workers [80] reported an 81% satisfactory outcome, but 23% of the group had undergone a lateral tenodesis. The need for an extra-articular reinforcement, particularly when arthroscopic techniques are used remains undefined. No long-term prospective study of the arthroscopic and open techniques is available as yet and therefore the final verdict remains to be established.

Role of magnetic resonance imaging

In experienced hands arthroscopy can reach a diagnostic accuracy of 98%, with correspondingly high levels of specificity and sensitivity [81]. Magnetic resonance imaging now provides a non-invasive method of assessing injury particularly to the soft tissues of the knee. This may significantly reduce the number of patients undergoing arthroscopy with normal findings and without the need for definitive surgical treatment.

Recent MRI studies followed by arthroscopic examinations have confirmed the high diagnostic accuracy of MRI. An accuracy of 78 to 97% for lesions of the anterior cruciate ligament and 99% for the posterior cruciate tears have been reported by Fischer et al. [82] from their multicentre study of 1014 patients. Diagnostic accuracy for medial meniscal tears at 89–91% – sensitivity 96% and specificity of 91% – is lower than for lateral meniscal injuries where the diagnostic accuracy is rated at 88–97% – sensitivity 96% and specificity 98% [82,83]. The main contentious area remains the over-diagnosis of tears in the posterior horn of the medial meniscus.

Some of these may be inferior incomplete tears not identified at arthroscopy or simple degenerative myxoid change within this area of the meniscus not extending to the surface. The false positive group is of considerable concern and emphasizes the need to match clinical to MRI findings.

With increasing experience and rapidly advancing technology producing higher quality imaging, the diagnostic reliability of the technique will undoubtedly improve. As yet, it remains a very expensive and time-consuming diagnostic modality. The indications for its use must as always be considered as an aid to diagnosis and not simply supplant the clinical skills and management of the physician. Boden *et al.* [84] showed that in 74 asymptomatic volunteers who underwent MRI, 13% under, and 36% over, the age of 45 years were diagnosed as having meniscal tears.

The commonsense and pragmatic approach as defined by Richard Senghas [85] cannot be more simply and succinctly expressed: 'If an arthroscopy is indicated by the severity or duration of the patient's symptoms, what is the point in doing an MRI. If a negative result would mean the continuation of non-operative treatment, whilst a positive result would mean arthroscopy is indicated, then an MRI might save the patient an invasive procedure under anaesthesia.' Nevertheless, MRI will undoubtedly contribute enormously to the pre-operative management of difficult cases and help clarify the need for arthroscopy where the significance of clinical history and findings are uncertain.

References

1. Bozzini, P. (1806) Lichtleiter, eine Erfindung zur Anschauung innerer Thiele und Krakenheiten nebst der Abbildung. In *Journal der practishen Arzneykunde und Wundarzneykunst Berlin* (ed. C. W. Hufenland), **24**, 107–124.
2. Herteloupe, C. L. S. (1827) *La Lithotritie*. Academie des Sciences, Paris.
3. Desormaux, A. J. (1853) De L'Endoscope. *Bull. Acad. Med. Academie des Sciences.*
4. Tagaki, K. (1933) Practical experience using Tagaki's arthroscope. *J. Jpn Orthop. Assoc.*, **8**, 132.
5. Bircher, E. (1921) Die arthroendoskopie. *Zentralbl. Chir.*, **48**, 1460.
6. Burman, M. S., Finkelstein, H. and Mayer, L. (1934) Arthroscopy of the knee joint. *J. Bone Joint Surg.*, **16**, 225–268.
7. Watanabe, M., Takeda, S. and Ikeuchi, H. (1957) *Atlas of Arthroscopy*. Igaku Shoin, Tokyo.
8. Jackson, R. and Abe, I. (1972) The role of arthroscopy in the management of the knee: an analysis of two hundred cases. *J. Bone Joint Surg.*, **54-B**, 310.
9. Dandy, D. J. (1978) Early results of closed partial meniscectomy. *Br. Med. J.*, **1**, 1099–1100.
10. Johnson, L. L. (1981) *Diagnostic Surgical Arthroscopy: the Knee and Other Joints*. Mosby, New York.
11. Dandy, D. J. and Jackson, R. W. (1975) The impact of arthroscopy in the management of disorders of the knee. *J. Bone Joint Surg.*, **57B**, 346.
12. Curran, W. P. and Woodward, E. P. (1980) Arthroscopy: its role in diagnosis and treatment of athletic knee injuries. *Am. J. Sports Med.*, **8**, 415.
13. Durand, A., Richards, C. L., Moulin, F. and Bravo, G. (1993) Motor recovery after arthroscopic partial meniscectomy. *J. Bone Joint Surg.*, **75A**, 202–213.
14. Sherman, O. H., Fox, J. M., Synder, S. J. *et al.* (1986) Arthroscopy – 'no problem surgery'. *J. Bone Joint Surg.*, **68A**, 256–265.
15. McGinty, J. B., Guess, L. F. and Marvin, R. A. (1977) Partial or total meniscectomy. A comparative analysis. *J. Bone Joint Surg.*, **59A**, 763–766.
16. Delee, J. C. (1983) Complications of arthroscopy and arthroscopic surgery. Results of a national survey. *J. Arthroscopic Rel. Res.*, **1**, 214–220.
17. Small, N. C. (1988) Complications in arthroscopic surgery performed by experienced arthroscopists. *Arthroscopy*, **2**, 253–252.
18. Mulhollan, J. S. (1982) Swedish arthroscopic system. *Orthop. Clin. North Am.*, **13**, 349.
19. Montgomery, S. C. and Campbell, J. (1989) Septic arthritis following arthroscopy and intra-articular steroids. *J. Bone Joint Surg.*, **71B**, 540.
20. Walker, R. H. and Illingham, M. (1983) Thrombophlebitis following arthroscopic surgery. *Contemp. Orthop.*, **6**, 29–33.
21. Eriksson, E., Haggmark, T., Saartok, T. *et al.* (1986) Knee arthroscopy with local anesthesia in ambulatory patients. *Orthopaedics*, **8**, 186–188.
22. Fairclough, J. A., Graham, G. P. and Pemberton, D. (1990) Local or general anaesthesia in day case arthroscopy. *Ann. R. Coll. Surg. Eng.*, **72**, 104–107.
23. Fairclough, J. A., Graham, G. P. and Pemberton, D. (1990) Local or general anaesthesia in day case arthroscopy. *Ann. R. Coll. Surg. Eng.*, **72**, 104–107.
24. Noyes, F. R., Bassett, R. W., Grood, E. S. and

Butler, D. L. (1980) Arthroscopy in acute traumatic haemarthosis of the knee. *J. Bone Joint Surg.*, **62A**, 687–697.

25. Gilquist, J., Hagberg, G. and Oretorp, N. (1977) Arthroscopy in acute injuries of the knee joint. *Acta Orthop. Scand.*, **48**, 190–196.

26. Dehaven, K. E. (1983) Arthroscopy in the diagnosis and management of the anterior cruciate ligament deficient knee. *Clin. Orthop.*, **172**, 52–56.

27. Jones, J. and Allum, R. (1977) Acute traumatic Haemarthrosis of the knee, expectant treatment or arthroscopy. *Ann. R. Coll. Surg. Eng.*, **48**, 190–196.

28. Kannus, P. and Jarvinen, M. (1987) Long term prognosis of nonoperatively treated acute knee distortions having primary haemarthrosis without clinical instability. *Am. J. Sports Med.*, **15**, 138–143.

29. Hamburg, P., Gilquist, J. and Lysholm, J. (1983) Suture of new and old peripheral meniscus tear. *J. Bone Joint Surg.*, **65A**, 193–197.

30. Firer, P. (1985) Arthroscopic meniscectomy. South African experience. *J. Bone Joint Surg.*, **67B**, 507.

31. Simpson, D. A., Thomas, N. P. and Aichcroth, P. M. (1986) Open and closed meniscectomy, a comparative study. *J. Bone Joint Surg.*, **68B**, 301–304.

32. O'Connor, R. L. (1977) Arthroscopy of the knee. *Surg. Ann.*, **9**, 265.

33. Dandy, D. J. (1990) The arthroscopic anatomy of symptomatic meniscal lesions. *J. Bone Joint Surg.*, **72B**, 628–633.

34. Cargill, A. O. and Jackson, J. O. (1976) Bucket handle tear of the medial meniscus. *J. Bone Joint Surg.*, **58A**, 248.

35. Hargreaves, D. J. and Seedhom, B. B. (1979) On the 'bucket handle tear': Partial or total meniscectomy? a quantitative study. *J. Bone Joint Surg.*, **61B**, 381.

36. O'Brien, S. J. and Miller, D. V. (1990) The contact Nd-yttrium-aluminium garnet laser – a new approach to arthroscopic laser surgery. *Clin. Orthop. Rel. Res.*, **252**, 95–100.

37. Seedhom, B. B., Dowson, D. and Wright, V. (1974) Functions of the menisci – a preliminary report. *J. Bone Joint Surg.*, **56B**, 381.

38. Fairbank, T. J. (1948) Knee joint changes after meniscectomy. *J. Bone Joint Surg.*, **30**, 664.

39. Jackson, J. P. (1968) Degenerative changes in the knee after meniscectomy. *Br. Med. J.*, **2**, 525–527.

40. Arnoczky, S. P. and Warren, R. F. (1982) Microvasculature of the human meniscus. *Am. J. Sports Med.*, **10**, 90–95.

41. Hamburg, P., Gilquist, J. and Lysholm, J. (1983) Suture of new and old peripheral meniscus tear. *J. Bone Joint Surg.*, **65A**, 193–197.

42. Keene, G. C. R. and Paterson, R. S. (1987) Arthroscopic meniscal suture. *J. Bone Joint Surg.*, **69B**, 162.

43. Magnuson, P. B. (1941) Joint debridement: a surgical treatment of degenerative arthritis. *Surg. Gynecol. Obstet.*, **73**, 1–9.

44. Jackson, R. W. and Rouse, D. W. (1982) The results of partial arthroscopic meniscectomy in patients over 40 years of age. *J. Bone Joint Surg.*, **64B**, 481–485.

45. Salisbury, R. B., Nottage, W. M. and Gardner, V. (1985) The effect of alignment on results in arthroscopic debridement of the degenerative knee. *Clin. Orthop.*, **198**, 268–272.

46. Jones, R. E., Smith, E. C. and Reisch, J. S. (1978) The effects of medial meiscectomy in patients older than 40 years. *J. Bone Joint Surg.*, **60A**, 783–786.

47. Bert, J. M. and Maschka, K. (1989) The arthroscopic treatment of unicompartmental gonarthrosis: a five year follow-up study of abrasion arthroplasty plus arthroscopic debridement and arthroscopic debridement alone. *Arthroscopy*, **5**, 25–32.

48. Bird, H. A. and Ring, E. F. (1978) Therapeutic value of arthroscopy. *Ann. Rheum. Dis.*, **37**, 78–79.

49. Patel, D. V., Aichroth, P. M. and Mayes, S. T. (1990) Arthroplastic debridement for degenerative arthritis of the knee. *J. Bone Joint Surg.*, **72B**, 1091.

50. Taylor, A. R. (1973) Synovectomy of the knee: long term results. *J. Bone Joint Surg.*, **61B**, 121.

51. Laurin, C. A., Desmarchais, J., Daziano, L. et al. (1974) Long term results of synovectomy of the knee in rheumatoid patients. *J. Bone Joint Surg.*, **56A**, 521–531.

52. Matsui, M., Taneda, Y., Ohta., S., Itoh, T. and Tsuboguchi, S. (1989) Arthroscopic versus open synovectomy in the rheumatoid knee. *Int. Orthop.*, **13**, 17–20.

53. Klein, W. and Jensen, K. U. (1988) Arthroscopic synovectomy of the knee joint: indication, technique and follow-up results. *J. Arthrosc. Rel. Surg.*, **4**, 63–71.

54. Gschwend, N. (1981) Synovectomy. In *Textbook of Rheumatology*. Saunders, Philadelphia, p. 1874.

55. Dandy, D. and Griffiths, D. (1989) Lateral release for recurrent dislocation of the patella. *J. Bone Joint Surg.*, **71B**, 121–125.

56. Aglietti, P., Pisaneschi, A., Buzzi, R. et al. (1989) Arthroscopic lateral release for pateller pain or instability. *Arthroscopy*, **5**, 176–183.

57. Ogilvie-Harris, D. J. and Jackson, R. W. (1984) The arthroscopic treatment of chondromalacia patellae. *J. Bone Joint Surg.*, **66B**, 660–665.

58. Sherman, O. H., Fox, J. M., Sperling, H. et al.

(1987) Patellar instability treatment by arthroscopic electrosurgical lateral release. *Arthroscopy*, **3**, 152–160.

59. Suman, R., Stother, I. G. and Illingworth, G. (1985) Diagnostic arthroscopy of the knee in children. *J. Bone Joint Surg.*, **67B**, 675.

60. Angel, K. A. and Hall, D. J. (1989) The role of arthroscopy in children and adolescents. *J. Arthr. Rel. Surg.*, **5**, 192–196.

61. Harvell, J. C., Fu, F. H. and Stanistsk, C. L. (1989) Diagnostic arthroscopy of the knee in children and adolescents. *Orthopaedics*, **12**, 1555–1560.

62. Bergstrom, R., Gilquist, J., Lysholm, J. and Hamburg, P. (1984) Arthroscopy of the knee in Children. *J. Paed. Orthop.*, **4**, 542–545.

63. Eiskjar, S. and Larsen, S. T. (1987) Arthroscopy of the knee in children. *Acta Orthop. Scand.*, **58**, 273–276.

64. Kaplan, E. B. (1957) Discoid lateral meniscus of the knee joint: nature, mechanism and operative treatment. *J. Bone Joint Surg.*, **39A**, 77.

65. Watanabe, M., Takeda, S. and Ikeuchi, H. (1978) *Atlas of Arthroscopy*. 3rd edn, Igaku-Shoin, Tokyo, p. 88.

66. Hayashi, L. K., Yamaga, H., Ida, K. and Miura, T. (1988) Arthroscopic meniscectomy for discoid lateral meniscus in children. *J. Bone Joint Surg.*, **70A**, 1495–1500.

67. Goodfellow, J. W. and Sandow, M. J. (1985) The natural history of anterior knee pain in adolescents. *J. Bone Joint Surg.*, **67B**, 36–38.

68. Nade, S. (1983) Acute septic arthritis in infancy and childhood. *J. Bone Joint Surg.*, **65B**, 234–241.

69. Smith, M. J. (1986) Arthoscopic treatment of the septic knee. *Arthroscopy*, **2**, 30–34.

70. Aichroth, P. M. (1971) Osteochondritis dissecans of the knee. *J. Bone Joint Surg.*, **53B**, 440–447.

71. Guhl, J. F. (1982) Arthroscopic treatment of osteochondritis dissecans. *Clin. Orthop.*, **65**, 167.

72. Bradley, J. and Dandy, D. J. (1989) Results of drilling osteochondritis dissecans before skeletal maturity. *J. Bone Joint Surg.*, **71B**, 642–644.

73. Rosenberg, N. J. (1964) Osteochondral fractures of the lateral femoral condyle. *J. Bone Joint Surg.*, **62A**, 2.

74. Clancy, W. G., Nelson, D. S., Reider, B. and Narchania, R. G. (1982) Anterior cruciate ligament reconstruction using one-third patellar ligament, augmented by extra-articular tendon transfers. *J. Bone Joint Surg.*, **64A**, 353–359.

75. O'Brien, S. J., Warren, R. E., Pavlov, H., Panariello, R. and Wickiewicz, T. L. (1991) Reconstruction of the chronically insufficient anterior cruciate ligament with the central third of the patellar ligament. *J. Bone Joint Surg.*, **73A**, 278–286.

76. Rosenberg, T. D., Paulos, L. E., Victoroff, B. N. and Abbott, P. J. (1988) Arthroscopic cruciate repair and reconstruction. In *The Crucial Ligaments* (ed. J. A. Feagin), Churchill Livingstone, New York, Edinburgh.

77. Gilquist, J. and Odensten, M. (1988) Arthroscopic reconstruction of the anterior cruciate ligament. *Arthroscopy*, **4**, 5–9.

78. Buss, D. D., Warren, R. F., Wickiewicz, T. L., Galinat, B. J. and Panariello, R. (1993) Arthroscopically assisted reconstruction of the anterior cruciate ligament with use of autogenous Patella-Ligament grafts. Results after twenty-four to forty-two months. *J. Bone Joint Surg.*, **75-A**, 1346–1355.

79. Shelbourne, K. D., Rettig, A. C., Hardin, G. and Williams, R. I. (1993) Miniarthrotomy versus arthroscopic assisted ACL reconstruction with autogenous patellar tendon graft. *Arthroscopy*, **9**, 72–75.

80. Aglietti, P., Buzzi, R. and D'Andria, S. (1991) Arthoscopic anterior cruciate ligament reconstruction with patella tendon. *Arthroscopy*, **8**, 5–10.

81. Jackson, R. W. and Dehaven, K. E. (1975) Arthroscopy of the knee. *Clin. Orthop.*, **107**, 87–92.

82. Fischer, S. P., Fox, J. M., Del Pizzo, W. *et al.* (1991) Accuracy of diagnosis from magnetic resonance imaging of the knee. *J. Bone Joint Surg.*, **73A**, 2–10.

83. Boree, N. R., Watkinson, A. F., Ackroyd, C. E. and Johnson, C. (1991) Magnetic resonance imaging of meniscal and cruciate injuries of the knee. *J. Bone Joint Surg.*, **73B**, 452–457.

84. Boden, A. D., Davis, D. O., Dina, T. S. *et al.* (1992) A prospective and blinded investigation of magnetic resonance imaging of the knee. Abnormal findings in asymptomatic patients. *Clin. Orth.*, **282**, 177–185.

85. Senghas, R. E. (1991) Indications for magnetic resonance imaging. *J. Bone Joint Surg.*, **73A**, 1.

13

Flexor tendon surgery

C. Semple

Flexor tendon surgery continues to present considerable problems to the surgeon, despite numerous advances in scientific knowledge, and applied surgical techniques over the past two decades. Most population centres now have two or three surgeons who specialize in hand surgery and are capable of carrying out effective primary tendon repair and this has now supplanted the previous enthusiasm for tendon grafting, carried out at a later stage once the original wound had healed.

Applied anatomy and physiology

The basic topographical anatomy of the flexor tendons has been understood for many years, but recently the precise anatomy of the tendon sheaths, their vincula, associated blood supply and synovial fluid nourishment of the tendon has been explained in considerable detail. Bunnell coined the phrase 'no man's land' for the area of the flexor tendon sheath between the distal palmar crease and up to the proximal interphalangeal joint including both tendons; and he felt that repair of tendons in this region was extremely complex and advocated delayed repair rather than attempting surgery in such a difficult area. Doyle has described the fibrous flexor sheath of the flexor tendon in a way which has now become standard (Fig. 13.1), and this should be understood by all surgeons carrying out operations on flexor tendons. From the point of view of damaged flexor tendons and their repair

the A2 and A4 annular pulleys are the most important, and significant problems will occur postoperatively, with bow-stringing of tendons and other difficulties if the A2 pulley is com-

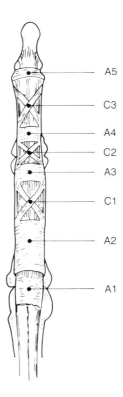

Fig. 13.1 Fibrous flexor sheath. A2 and A4 are the most important. Bow stringing will occur if A2 is removed; A3 and C pulleys can be removed if absolutely necessary to gain access.

pletely removed or divided. The A3 pulley is a very short one and does not contribute significantly to the overall integrity of the sheath, and the cruciate, or C pulleys can also be divided if necessary to obtain access to tendons.

Inside the fibrous flexor sheaths the synovial sheath maintains a valuable fluid environment, and there is good evidence that this fluid environment provides at least as much nourishment to the tendon as the intratendinous vascular network. Indeed in some it may even supply the majority of such nutrition. Removal of portions of the synovial sheaths at the end of a surgical repair, as advocated by some surgeons, is bound to affect the synovial fluid environment of the tendon and disturb the healing process.

The vascular network of flexor tendons is now well understood, although some debate still exists regarding the exact movement of nutrients in and out of the tendon in the natural human situation. The majority of the blood supply to the tendon comes from the vincular vessels. Some of it comes from the proximal portion of the musculotendonous junction, and probably very little comes from the distal portion of the tendon at its osseous insertion. The vincula to the tendons vary considerably in their position and length, particularly in the ring and little finger. Armenta and Lehrman have described these vincula as arising from four levels of the volar aspect of the phalanges and define them as V1, V2, V3 and V4; these small vascular reflexions have some relevance, particularly in the region of the superficialis decussation, as fairly short strong vincula may prevent tendons from retracting, and on the other hand a long thin vinculum may be torn resulting in bleeding in the sheath and some damage to a tendon, particularly the profundus tendon.

For many years it was considered that flexor tendons were incapable of healing from their own intrinsic cellular tissues and that adhesions of one type or another were necessary in order to bring fibrocytes in from external areas to unite the two tendon ends. It now appears clear, however, that given appropriate circumstances flexor tendons are capable of healing satisfactorily from their own tissues, and this is particularly so when they lie in a natural synovial fluid environment. Lundborg's careful studies have shown that isolated small portions of tendon can commence healing when totally isolated in the knee joint of a rabbit,

devoid of any blood supply or external cellular factors. In practice, many factors are involved, including damage to the tendon sheath, and vascular elements of the vincula.

The overall message appears clear; tendon repair must be carried out as carefully as possible, preserving all potential blood supply to the tendon and respecting the synovial sheath at all levels.

Surgical repair of flexor tendons

The diagnosis of a divided flexor tendon might appear straight forward to someone experienced in hand surgery, but a disturbing number of damaged flexor tendons remain undiagnosed until the patient turns up some weeks later with a healed wound and an inability to flex a finger. At this stage the treatment options are restricted, as the flexor tendon may well have shortened into the palm, the fibrous sheath may have collapsed particularly at the level of the proximal phalanx, and considerable skill will be required to obtain a satisfactory result.

Assuming, however, that the divided flexor tendon is diagnosed shortly after the injury it is now standard practice to recommend *primary repair* of that tendon or tendons, providing an experienced hand surgeon and appropriate surgical facilities are available. It is also vitally important to have good quality follow-up facilities, including physiotherapy and occupational therapy. Given good quality facilities, and a co-operative patient, it should be possible to obtain 70% good or excellent results following primary flexor tendon repair, and these are the sort of results which have been published over the last decade, generally coming from good quality hand surgery units. A number of technical aspects of flexor tendon surgery are common to all surgical units, while in other fields there is some difference in approach or technique. All surgeons carry out such surgery under an exsanguinating tourniquet, a bloodless field, and there is an increasing use of brachial block anaesthesia, rather than general anaesthesia for such surgery. Brachial block anaesthesia has a number of advantages, particularly that one can instruct the patient on how to take care of his hand in the immediate postoperative period and obtain his immediate cooperation. With an increased knowledge of anatomy, and good quality surgical instruments it is possible to make a neat approach to the damaged tendon and its sheath without harming the neighbouring structures such as vessels or nerves, generally making use of the original wound which is usually transverse in the finger.The great majority of flexor tendon injuries occur in young males, between the ages of 10 and 30, and the vast majority of wounds are caused by glass or knife and occasionally by sharp machinery. The type of tendon suture used very much dictates the type of exposure of the finger and tendon sheath. If a long Bunnell type zig zag suture is to be used then a considerable amount of tendon will have to be exposed in order to place the suture, whereas a shorter H-shaped suture (such as a Kessler or its variants) enables a much smaller exposure of the tendon to be used. The general trend now is to use a short core suture to hold the two ends of the tendon together and supplement this by some fine circumferential sutures to tidy up and closely approximate the epitenon, or synovial surface of the tendon to reduce any rough areas which might cause adhesions. Most core sutures which have been described recently are variations on the Kessler/Mason/Allan suture (Fig. 13.2), although other methods such as Tsuge (Fig. 13.3) and Becker (Fig. 13.4) have been described.

Some surgeons prefer to release the tourniquet and achieve haemostasis before suturing the skin, whereas others are prepared to suture the skin and completely close the wound before releasing the tourniquet. There is general agreement that some form of protected motion is necessary after flexor tendon surgery, and the method popularized by Kleinert is widely used. This involves

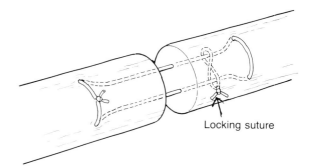

Fig. 13.3   Tsuge suture.

attaching an elastic band to the relevant finger or fingers and thereby preventing the patient from producing an active pull on their repaired tendon, yet allowing active extension of the finger and passive flexion so that the flexor tendon can move passively in its sheath without undue tension being applied to it. Various refinements of this type of controlled motion have been described; most surgeons and therapists allow a

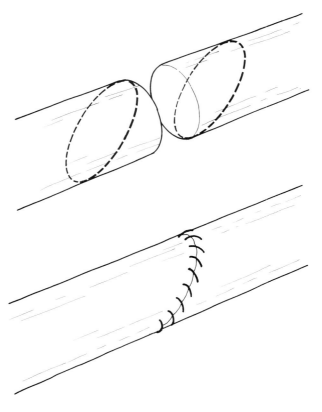

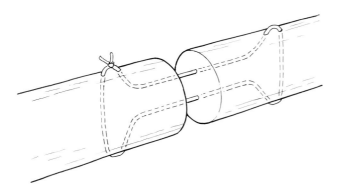

Fig. 13.2   Kessler/Mason Allen suture.

Fig. 13.4   Becker suture.

graduated release from this type of controlled movement over a period of 4–6 weeks. Careful control of such movements is necessary by the hand therapist, together with a considerable degree of patient cooperation.

After repair of the tendon, debate continues about the need for formal repair of the tendon sheath over the tendon repair. It appears clear from physiological evidence that the synovial lining of the sheath is extremely important in providing an appropriate nutritional milieu for the healing tendon, but it is often difficult or impossible to formally close the sheath. In some situations where a considerable amount of damage has occurred to the finger, the tendon sheath may be deficient over a significant length and reconstruction of tendon sheaths/annular pulleys may be necessary. This is always difficult and a number of substitutes have been suggested such as palmaris longus, as a weave between the remnants of the original tendon sheath, or a piece of fascia lata or palmaris longus taken right round the proximal phalanx of the finger to reconstruct an A2 pulley. Lister has described a neat method using a portion of the extensor retinaculum, which has the advantage of including a portion of synovial lining which can be used to cover the tendon at the A2 level.

Author's preferred technique

The fact that a tendon division has occurred does not automatically mean that a tendon requires repair, and certainly when the patient presents late, after the original wound has healed, the actual deficit of function following loss of one tendon only in the finger is often remarkably small. The matter should be carefully discussed with the patient before proceeding to tendon repair. A number of papers have been published which recommend repair of both superficial and profundus tendons in no mans land, that is at the level of the distal palm/proximal phalanx, and have shown that statistically these are likely to produce better results than repair of one tendon only and excision of the other tendons. The reasons for this are not entirely clear, but are almost certainly related to the better preservation of the vascular circulation and the pulley system when both tendons are carefully repaired at that level.

Primary tendon repair is carried out in a bloodless field under a pneumatic tourniquet, and brachial block anaesthesia. If the wound in the finger is a transverse one then it is open via a bayonet extension, or alternatively a Bruner type of incision may be used, particularly in the central two fingers. Exposure of the tendon is by careful trap door extension of the original wound in the tendon sheath, and the two tendon ends are delivered into the wound by flexing the finger at the relevant joints, although occasionally the proximal end of the profundus tendon may require to be retrieved by means of a separate incision in the distal palm. The tendon surfaces are not handled at all with any forceps or instruments, although once the tendon has been retrieved it can be held in the wound by means of fine hypodermic needles passed through the tendon sheath. A core suture of the Kessler type is placed using 4/0 braided polyester suture (Ethibond), with the knot generally placed in the gap between the tendon ends. If the tendon ends lie easily together with no irregularities then no further sutures are placed, but generally a few further sutures, and sometimes a complete circumferential suture of fine 8/0 nylon is required to tidy up the tendon ends and encourage them to lie easily flush with each other. Both flexor tendons are repaired at all levels unless there is significant tearing or crushing of the tendon ends which make the prospect of a successful outcome remote, in which case one tendon only will be repaired and the other one removed. If the trap door in the sheath can be easily repaired this is done, but this may produce excessive tightness over the repaired tendon and the trap door may simply be laid across the tendon with one or two very slack sutures. Care is taken to ensure that the A2 pulley system is at least 50% intact. Digital nerves are repaired at this stage if they were also damaged in the original wound. A suture of 4/0 nylon or prolene is inserted into the finger nail, avoiding the nailbed so that elastic traction can be applied to the finger postoperatively. If the finger nail is badly bitten or otherwise damaged, traction on the finger can be achieved by a button hook glued onto the nail postoperatively. The wound is closed and a complete hand dressing applied with careful compression, using a crepe bandage and small dressings to each individual finger and plaster support applied on volar and dorsal aspects before the tourniquet is released. All hand surgeons have their own particular way of applying bandages and dressings, and it is important to gain experience and confidence in a particular style of applying a bandage so that the circulation to the hand is not impeded but also that effective support of the soft tissues and prevention of haematoma formation occurs.

On the day following surgery the patient is seen by the hand therapist, who carefully instructs the patient in the degree of movement that he/she may use, involving elastic band traction to encourage gentle movement of the repaired tendon in its sheath, yet avoid excessive tension at the repair. Plaster protection of the wrist and hand is used, with the wrist moderately flexed, about 30°, and with a dorsal hood to prevent full extension of the finger yet allowing an almost full range of flexion. Considerable care has to be taken over this type of postoperative splintage and elastic traction, and the therapist has to carefully control the patient so that the proper joints, particularly the proximal interphalangeal joint, are flexing adequately; it is all too easy for the metacarpophalangeal joint to do all the movement and leave the interphalangeal joints stiff. Routine antibiotics are not used and the patient is followed up in the dressings clinic until the wound has healed and sutures have been removed. Regular hand therapy sessions continue initially two or three times a week, decreasing as the patient gains more confidence and use in the finger. The patient is generally fit for discharge from follow-up at the 2- or 3-month stage.

The above comments relate essentially to damage to the flexor tendons at the level of the proximal phalanx, but similar techniques are used at all levels, although one generally expects a better result in patients with divisions of the flexor tendons in the distal forearm or wrist: divisions of the flexor profundus tendon only, in the distal portion of the finger, may be more easily dealt with by simple advancement of the flexor tendon by 1.5 cm, which can generally be managed without difficulty. As implied above, a number of authors have described good or excellent results in 75% of patients undergoing primary tendon repair, but we have found this level of success difficult to achieve. We feel that at least part of this difficulty may lie in the unselected nature of patients dealt with in an NHS hospital in the UK and the varied level of patient co-operation and drive which exists.

Delayed repair

Primary tendon repair, as described above is generally taken to mean repair within 24 hours of the original injury, but the patient may not present for a day or two, and other factors may make such prompt repair impossible. Delayed primary repair up to a week is perfectly possible, although much depends on the state of the wound and if there is any suggestion of infection then the wound must be cleaned and left to heal naturally before contemplating any tendon surgery. When the wound has healed tendon repair may still be possible, although much will depend on the position of the proximal end of the tendon: if this has contracted back to the palm, and the superficialis decussation has closed, or the fibrous flexor sheath has collapsed, particularly at the level of the A2 pulley, then the prospect of achieving a good result is diminished. When discussing flexor tendon surgery with the patient it is extremely important to explain the potential risks and disadvantages of such surgery. While some series describe success rates of 75%, it must be stressed that these are generally private clinics in the United States run by very experienced hand surgeons and the general results of flexor tendon surgery in public hospitals in the United States, and the NHS in the UK are generally much poorer. It must be remembered that patients are likely to strongly resent a lot of time, surgery and rehabilitation spent on a finger which ends up stiff and useless, and indeed they occasionally take this resentment to Court. For the patient with a healed wound and a divided tendon or tendons it is important to clearly define the advantages and disadvantages of prospective flexor tendon surgery, and the patient may well be better off with his hand as it is, rather than embarking on a long and complex period of surgery and rehabilitation, with only a possibility of improving matters.

Tendon grafting

When direct tendon repair is impossible, either due to the long delay which has occurred since the original injury, or to the degree of damage to the tendon, its sheath or the finger as a whole, then some form of tendon replacement may be appropriate. Free tendon grafting, as described by Pulvertaft, requires considerable care with regard to surgical technique and postoperative rehabilitation, and furthermore the finger should have a good or excellent range of passive movement preoperatively. It must be stressed that no form of tendon grafting can ever improve on the preoperative passive range of movement. All too often flexor tendon reconstructive surgery fails because the patient does not start off with a good passive range of movements. The essential techniques of free tendon grafting have not changed since Pulvertaft's original descriptions, and the reader is referred to his article for a description of that surgery. The concept of a staged tendon reconstruction, using a silicone spacer rod to form a pseudosheath has gained popularity since Hunter's original description and this is the method of choice in situations where the tendon sheath is badly damaged by scarring, previous burns, etc. It must be stressed, however, that this technique which is time-consuming and difficult to carry out, is no substitute for standard free tendon grafting which is still the appropriate method if the tissues of the finger are satisfactory. With the staged tendon reconstruction technique the initial surgery involves removing all scarred and unsatisfactory tissue from the region of the tendon and its sheath, repairing or reconstructing tendon pulleys, particularly the A2 pulley, and inserting a silicon rod to run from the distal phalanx to the palm or wrist. The proximal portion of the rod is left free, and it simply moves in and out in a pistoning fashion with passive movements of the finger and thereby forms a sheath around itself. It is important to appreciate that the sheath which is formed is not a true synovial sheath, as Lundborg has shown, but is simply a sheath lined by granulation tissue and this is one of the factors which can complicate the second stage of the procedure when the formal tendon graft is inserted. Significant scarring and adhesions may form between the granulation tissue and the new tendon. The time between the first and second stages is generally 3 or 4 months, as long as the skin and subcutaneous tissues of the finger have healed satisfactorily and the finger has regained a full passive range of movements at all joints. The second stage operation should be a

very much less traumatic one than the first stage, with simple retrieval of both ends of the tendon and insertion of a free tendon graft, generally palmaris longus or plantaris. An appropriate suture will secure the graft firmly into the distal phalanx and an 'in and out weave' and/or 'fish mouth suture' is made proximally in the palm or wrist. Controlled gentle active movement is commenced once the wounds have healed, generally at the 10 day stage and remains under the care of the hand therapist for at least 3 months. In all types of tendon surgery, but particularly following tendon grafting, some adhesions are always likely to form and they are most likely to resolve following repeated small active movements of the tendon rather than by any attempts at passive manipulation. La Salle and Strickland found that in their series of 43 patients with two stage tendon grafting, different types of rod designs made no particular difference to the results, nor did placement of the proximal end of the rod in the palm or wrist, or the degree of immobilization/mobilization used postoperatively. They also found that it made no significant difference whether the profundus or superficialis was used as the motor for the tendon graft, although most surgeons consider that the most appropriate motor muscle is that which has the easiest excursion at the time of the grafting procedure.

Further reading

Armenta, E. and Lehrman, A. (1980) The vincula to the flexor tendons of the hand. *J. Hand Surg.*, **5**, 127–134.

Doyle, J. R. and Blyth, W. (1975) The finger flexor sheath. *AAOS, Symposium on Tendon Surgery in the Hand*, pp. 81–87.

Hunter, J. M. and Schneider, L. H. (1977) *Staged Flexor Tendon Reconstruction*, AAOS Instructional Course Lecture, 26, Mosby, St Louis.

La Salle, W. B. and Strickland, J. W. (1983) An evaluation of digital performance following two-stage flexor tendon reconstruction. *J. Hand Surg.*, **8**, 263–267.

Lister, G. D. (1979) Reconstruction of pulleys employing extensor retinaculum. *J. Hand Surg.*, **4**, 461.

Lundborg, G. and Rank, F. (1978) Experimental healing of flexor tendons based on synovial fluid nutrition. *J. Hand Surg.*, **3**, 21–31.

Lundborg, G. *et al.* (1980) Superficial repair of

severed flexor tendons in synovial environment. *J. Hand Surg.*, **5**, 451–461.

Manske, P. R. and Lesker, P. A. (1982) Nutrient pathways of flexor tendons in primates. *J. Hand Surg.*, **7**, 436-444.

Neilsen, A. B. and Jensen, P. O. (1985) Methods of evaluation of flexor tendon results. *J. Hand Surg.*, **10B**, 60–61.

Pulvertaft, R. G. (1959) Experience in flexor tendon grafting. *J. Bone Joint Surg.*, **41B**, 629.

14

Musculoskeletal trauma: nerve

D. Marsh and N. J. Barton

Division of a peripheral nerve is a unique injury. In laceration of any other tissue, one group of cells is separated from another group of cells. Even when a hollow tube is cut, such as a blood vessel or ureter, the two ends consist of independent masses of viable cells, with the potential for the divided structure to *repair* itself by formation of scar tissue. A peripheral nerve injury is different; the nerve cells themselves are cut into two pieces. The distal portion of the neuron, amputated from the cell body, must die. Repair, in the sense of a join between tissues, is therefore impossible. The only hope for restoration of communication lies in a totally different process – *regeneration*.

Surgeons must therefore understand something of the unique and fascinating nature of nerve cells and their response to injury. They must approach the divided nerve in the full knowledge that they cannot truly repair it; they can only give it the best environment in which to regenerate.

Structure and function of normal nerve

Each peripheral nerve (Fig. 14.1) consists of thousands of axons, whose cell bodies lie either in the dorsal root ganglion (for sensory fibres) or in the anterior horn of the spinal cord (for motor fibres), held together by connective tissue elements. The latter are of fundamental impor-

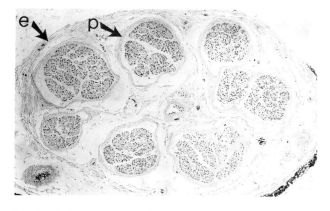

Fig. 14.1 Transverse section of sural nerve, showing epineurium (e) and perineurium (p). Haematoxylin and eosin × 50.

tance in the processes of recovery from peripheral nerve injury and in our attempts to help.

Axons may be a metre or more in length, but even the thicker myelinated fibres are only 20 microns wide; this is equivalent to a 5/0 nylon suture 5 m long. Such a formidable arrangement is sustained by virtue of a highly efficient axoplasmic transport system, capable of moving chemicals and cellular organelles in both directions at rates up to 400 mm/day. The Nissl granules in the cell body (Fig. 14.2) are the enzyme manufacturing endoplasmic reticulum; their profusion is evidence of the Herculean metabolic task of sustaining a total volume of axoplasm which may be 200 times that of the cell body.

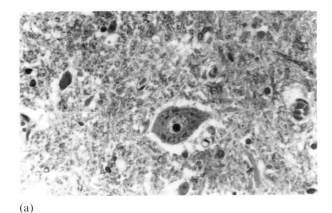

(a)

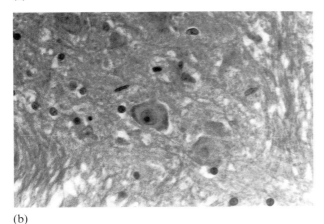

(b)

Fig. 14.2   (a) Anterior horn neuron with Nissl substance in clumps in the cytoplasm (haematoxylin and eosin × 650). (b) Anterior horn cell showing chromatolysis (× 800).

Every nerve fibre has associated Schwann cells; in a minority, these produce a myelin sheath. This allows up to a 100-fold increase in conduction velocity for a relatively small increase in diameter. Equally important, it allows many more action potentials to be transmitted per second. The Schwann cells are also gifted in other ways and their versatility is given full play after injury, as we shall see. They sit on a basement membrane, which forms the inner lining of the endoneurial tube, whose great significance is that it forms a conduit, specific to each fibre, leading directly to the correct target organ.

Nerve fibres are grouped together in fascicles which are ensheathed in perineurium. This membrane is mainly responsible for the biochemical environment in which the nerve fibres lie and has been described as the blood–nerve barrier due to its highly selective permeability. Fascicular grouping varies greatly from nerve to nerve, ranging from a few large to many small fascicles. The pattern of fascicles also varies along the length of a given nerve, as Sunderland [1] showed, although towards the periphery it is more constant [2].

The membrane surrounding the whole nerve trunk is the epineurium, whose chief characteristic is its physical strength. It normally lies in some longitudinal tension, so that the two ends of a divided nerve spring apart. Considerable longitudinal traction on the nerve can be sustained by the epineurium without the nerve fibres suffering rupture. However, this is *not* true at the points of emergence of the nerves from the spinal cord, where the epineurium is relatively deficient and small tensile forces can cause enormous damage.

Degeneration and regeneration

Damage to axons, severe enough to lead to their death distal to the lesion, may be due to stretch, crush, or a cut. The outcome of these different types of injury is vastly different, but all produce one constant feature: an apparently preprogrammed response to injury by the parent cell body proximally and the Schwann cells below the lesion. This response can be divided into degenerative and regenerative phases, though these overlap in time and are both highly constructive in what they achieve.

Degenerative phase

This consists of changes in the cell body and Wallerian degeneration in the distal axons. The former is called chromatolysis, because of the observed dissolution of the deeply staining Nissl granules, signalling a change in the synthetic machinery of the cell, like a factory re-tooling. Ribosomes which were designed for production of transmitter substances are replaced by new ones, dedicated to the production of cellular building material. Energy production, previously geared to transmission of action potentials, is switched to the pentose phosphate pathway, more suited to the work of chemical synthesis. Glial cells proliferate over the surface of the injured cell and prise loose the synaptic endings from other CNS cells, as if taking the cell out of service to concentrate on the business of regeneration. These changes begin within hours of injury and the signal initiating them is presumably brought from the site of injury in the axoplasmic transport system.

Wallerian degeneration is the work primarily of the Schwann cells. It does not necessarily start at once; transmission of action potentials below a complete transection has been observed for up to a week. Myelin surrounding the axons is rapidly broken down followed by the axons themselves, the Schwann cells acting as phagocytes. The basement membrane remains intact and the Schwann cells, increased in number, form solid columns (the bands of Büngner) within the endoneurial tubes. These extend from both cut ends of the nerve toward each other and unite, forming an attractive surface down which the regenerating axon sprouts can grow. Evidence is accumulating that the Schwann cells also create gradients of neurotropic substances which draw axon sprouts in their direction.

Augustus Waller (1816–1870) was a busy general practitioner at St Mary Abbott's Terrace in Kensington, London where he carried out the research on degeneration of nerves in frogs with which his name is associated and for which he was elected a Fellow of the Royal Society at the age of 35. This shows that one need not be prevented from doing research by shortage of time or facilities; the real impediment is the lack of will to do it. Waller was also interested in the ability of white blood corpuscles to escape from capillaries and such was his dedication that he courageously attempted to study the microcirculation in his own prepuce, though after a few attempts he changed to the frog's tongue and was able to demonstrate that pus contained extravasated leucocytes. In the same period he also published papers on the physiology of vision, the microscopy of hailstones, and the formation of coloured films by the action of halogens on metals. After 10 years in practice, he moved first to Bonn and then to Paris to obtain more favourable opportunities for carrying out his scientific work, and returned to England in 1858 as Professor of Physiology in Queens College, Birmingham (which has since become the University) and Consultant Physician to the Queen's Hospital in Bath Row (whose buildings now house the Birmingham Accident Hospital).

Regenerative phase

The 'degenerative' process creates the conditions under which regeneration proper can proceed. The first stage is a sprouting of new axons at the level of the lesion; several fine filaments of axoplasm reach out from each axon. This is not a passive process, like toothpaste being squeezed from a tube; the tip of the advancing axon sprout has a specialized structure, known as the growth cone and containing actin and myosin, which burrows actively through the tissues and drags the axon after it. If the endoneurial tubes are intact (as in axonotmesis due to crush) the axon sprouts have an easy job and can progress to their correct target organs at a rate of about 1 mm per day.

However, in the case of a cut, the sprouts must first find their way through granulation tissue into the endoneurial tubes of the distal stump and this is a powerful factor working against the reestablishment of useful connections. Some sprouts will never find the distal stump and will only contribute to a tender neuroma at the suture site. Whatever chemotactic signals are being produced by the ever-resourceful Schwann cells, the chances of any axon finding its old, correct, conduit are remote. Even if a sensory axon finds a sensory tube, it is likely to lead to the wrong species of touch receptor, located in the wrong area of skin. An enormous degree of topographic disorganization is inevitable.

The new axons must then undergo a process of maturation, including remyelination. Finally, the quality of sensibility regained will depend crucially on the re-establishment of useful connections with the specialized sensory receptors [3].

Much effort is being directed towards unravelling the mechanisms by which these processes are initiated and controlled. There is certainly room for improvement: experimental studies involving ideal sutures in primates have shown that about half of the axons fail to regenerate. A few adjuvant treatments, apparently effective in laboratory animals, have been shown to enhance the vigour of the regenerative response after suture. However, at the time of writing, no safe and reliable method for enhancing regeneration in the clinical context exists.

The above gloomy facts underly the poor results obtained after peripheral nerve repair, at least on the sensory side. They suggest two cardinal principles which should guide the surgical approach:

- Do nothing to interfere with the process of axonal regeneration. In particular, *minimize fibrosis.*
- Minimize the spatial disorganization by trying to appose fascicles correctly to one another.

Different surgeons apply these two principles with different emphasis. To some it is a transgression of the first to suture individual fascicles; to others it is necessary to do precisely that in order to satisfy the second. There is no reliable evidence which indicates that either point of view has more to commend it.

Factors influencing results

The most powerful factors determining the outcome of peripheral nerve injuries are not under the control of the surgeon. These are the age of the patient and the level and nature of the lesion. Young patients with lesions in continuity or clean cuts, sustained at a distal level, do well.

We all hope that in future years we will be able to do more to determine the quality of the outcome, whether by improved surgery or adjuvant chemical therapy, but at present, the single most effective step in improving results overall would be the elimination of delay in diagnosis and treatment.

Avoidable delay in diagnosis

From the moment of injury, patients begin to learn how to cope without the function that they have lost. Skills for which the injured hand may previously have been preferred begin to be transferred. Evidence is accumulating that structural changes occur in the CNS due to the loss of afferent input from the denervated part. These processes will continue until reinnervation takes place and the longer that is, the less complete will be the eventual recovery of function. The end organs, whether motor or sensory, also deteriorate; therefore suture of a divided nerve should be carried out with minimal delay. The most

frequent cause of delay is missed diagnosis at the time of injury.

There are six reasons why it may not be realized that a nerve has been cut:

1. The relevant nerve is not examined. Sometimes the patient does not consult a doctor, but if he does then *failure to examine* the function of any nerves which may be divided is *negligence* and will be so judged in the Courts. The diagnosis is made by testing the motor and sensory function of the nerve distal to the cut, not by looking at or poking around in the wound. This includes all nerves which could conceivably be cut, remembering that a long thin blade or sliver of glass may pass deeply and obliquely into the tissues and divide structures far from the cut in the skin: we have seen an injury with an entry wound on the lateral side of the upper arm which divided the *ulnar* nerve only, just falling short of coming out again through the skin on the medial side of the arm.

2. Sensory testing may be inadequate. Remember that a patient may take some time to realize that part of the body has become anaesthetic. It is totally inadequate to test sensibility by touching the part and asking 'can you feel that?'; an affirmative reply cannot be trusted even from the scrupulously honest. Also dangerous is 'tell me when I touch you'; a falsely reassuring picture may be obtained due to tiny movements or vibrations caused by the touch which are picked up by highly sensitive receptors in adjacent nerve territories.

Better is to ask the patient 'does this feel different from normal?' (or 'different from this?' – comparing it with an area of skin supplied by a different nerve). If it does feel different, you must assume that the nerve is divided until proved otherwise. Best is to set some sort of discrimination task ('am I touching you with the sharp end or the blunt end?' – Fig. 14.3). In applying such a test, take care to eliminate vision and *repeat* the test a few times in random sequence; with only one application, the patient with a divided nerve will get it right 50% of the time.

These sorts of tests are hard to perform in young children. Here it is best to follow Dellon's [4] advice and use the innocuous tuning fork (the pronged end), the feeling is one of tickling and they laugh; with sharp pins they cry. Again, do not be misled by the ability to *detect* the buzz;

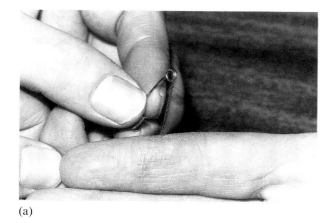

(a)

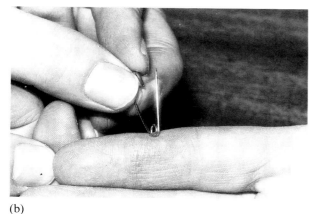

(b)

Fig. 14.3 Testing the ability to distinguish (a) sharp from (b) blunt.

vibrations travel far across the skin. Ask for a difference in quality of sensation between two sides or two nerve territories. Another innocuous test suitable for children is to immerse the digits in warm water for 30 minutes and check for wrinkling of the pulp skin [5].

3. Important clues, provided by the consequences of autonomic denervation, are ignored. Affected digits are warm, due to vasodilatation, and dry, due to cessation of sweat production. The skin dries within a few minutes of division of sudomotor fibres and a simple means of assessing this is to feel the frictional drag in moving a plastic pen across the skin – dry skin shows low friction. A more precise (and documentable) measure is obtainable with a cheap skin resistance meter [6]. In either case it is obviously necessary to avoid confusion by blood or cleansing agents on the skin.

4. A partial division may lead to error: there may be a cut in the median nerve but the patient may have normal sensibility in, say, the thumb. There are ten digital nerves and with any cut on the front of the palm, wrist or arm the territories of all ten must be examined.

5. There may be unexpected anatomical variation. For example, every fifth patient with complete division of the median nerve can still oppose the thumb because the opponens pollicis is ulnar-innervated. It is important to record this, because after repair of the nerve, a functioning opponens may be wrongly interpreted as evidence of recovery. Similarly, one patient in five has a sensory frontier between the median and ulnar nerves which does *not* run down the centre of the ring finger.

6. Even after the most rigorous testing, suspicion must be maintained whenever a penetrating injury *could* have damaged a nerve. At the time of writing two authors have provided evidence that divided nerves, lying in contact, can transmit action potentials across the gap in the first few hours after injury, albeit unphysiologically evoked synchronized action potentials [7,8]. This ceases, of course, after Wallerian degeneration begins.

There is only one sensible response to all these pitfalls: have a low threshold for exploring the wound, or at the very least arrange an immediate review by an experienced surgeon.

Timing of repair

Seddon and his co-workers [9] favoured secondary repair of nerve lacerations. However, their main experience was with nerves injured in war, where both the nature of the wounds and the circumstances of early surgery are very different from those usually occurring in civilian practice. It should be possible in the 1990s to get the patient to a surgeon experienced in this type of work with a fully equipped operating theatre and plenty of time, within a short time after the injury.

If, as is generally the case, the wound is a clean-cut and tidy one, and direct apposition of the cut ends is possible, then current opinion is that the best chance for regeneration is given by primary repair [10]. Primary repair is now preferred, because the cut fascicles can be directly matched (not possible after a scarred section has been resected), the nerve can be repaired under no more tension than it normally has, and regeneration can start straight away.

Suture should be done immediately whenever possible, within the limits of common sense. A patient not available for surgery until late at night will probably gain more than he or she loses if the surgeon sleeps and then performs the operation the following morning, *provided* the limb is elevated in the meantime to minimize oedema. A wait of up to 24 hours does no harm (unless arterial repair is also necessary, in which case there must be no delay at all).

The desire for primary repair must be tempered by basic surgical principles and there are three main reasons why delayed repair may be indicated. The first is that the wound is too contaminated (including an initially clean wound in which diagnosis has been delayed beyond 24 hours). The second is that the nerve injury involves an element of crush or traction and it is not possible to judge how much of the proximal stump needs to be resected to find viable axons. The third is that there is a skeletal injury which for some reason cannot be stabilized immediately, so that a nerve repair is at risk of subsequent disruption.

If delay is appropriate, then a preliminary operation must be performed, during which the wound is cleaned and the cut ends of the nerve are *apposed*, not just marked. This is to prevent retraction of the nerve ends, which would necessitate a graft rather than direct suture subsequently.

Principles of wound care

Remember that a cardinal aim of treatment is avoidance of fibrosis:

- prevent oedema formation. Insist on elevation of the injured hand above the level of the patient's head at all times both while waiting for surgery and for several days afterwards. A sling is not enough;
- prevent ischaemia. The main blood supply to a peripheral nerve is via longitudinal internal plexuses and these are compromised by stretch; therefore tension is a very bad

thing. This argues for generous mobilization of nerve to avoid tension, but this must be tempered by awareness of the risk of damaging feeder vessels, particularly in the distal stump; dissect outside the adventitia. In the case of the ulnar nerve, divided at the wrist, use the ulnar artery. If it is also divided, repair it (or at least suture together the tied-off ends); this takes most of the tension off the nerve as well as improving arterial supply;

- prevent haematoma. Expose the nerve under tourniquet; insist on having a fine bipolar diathermy and use it, after removal of the tourniquet but before suture of the nerve, to prevent intraneural haematoma. This is particularly important when dealing with the median nerve, which may have a large artery within it;
- prevent drying out of the tissues. Keep the nerve moist with saline at all times;
- avoid unnecessary interfascicular dissection and suture. If you suture fascicles, then use a monofilament synthetic suture of 10/0 grade or finer. Do not excise epineurium.

Use of microsurgical technique

Twenty-five years ago the argument was about *when* the nerve should be sutured; since then the area of debate has shifted and the main question now is how the nerve should be repaired. Many experts believe that results are better when the

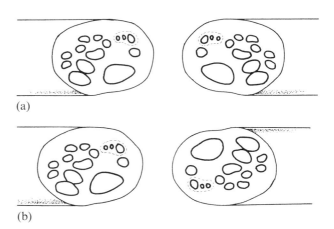

(a)

(b)

Fig. 14.4   (a) Correct and (b) incorrect alignment of fascicles.

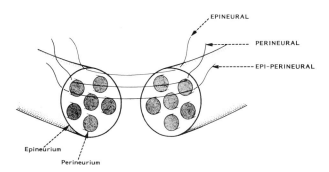

Fig. 14.5 Epineural, perineural and epi-perineural sutures.

operating microscope, microsurgical instruments and microsurgical techniques are used for nerve repair [11].

Microsurgical repair does not necessarily mean fascicular suture; with the microscope it is possible to orient the nerve ends better (Fig. 14.4) and insert the sutures more accurately, whether they are epineural, perineural or epi-perineural (Fig. 14.5). However, although the naked eye can discern the fascicles as well as the epineurium, it is only with the microscope that one can see and therefore suture the perineurium. Advocates of immediate fascicular suture argue that the formal coaptation of matching fasciculi must reduce misdirection of regenerating axons.

Although one would expect this gentler and more precise surgery to produce a better result, the place of microsurgery is not so firmly established for nerves as it is for small blood vessels. It is important to remember that it is not axons, but large groups of axons which are being coapted; the evidence for significant benefit from improved topographic accuracy is inconsistent:

Animal experiments have the advantage that at a later date the repaired nerve can be removed and studied in various ways; in particular they allow histological assessment of axon regeneration. Dog peroneal, cat sciatic and, rarely, primate median nerve have been used as models. Approximately half of the published studies report improved histological appearances and electrophysiological function after perineural repair performed under the microscope. However, the other half (by and large the more recent studies) reported that epineural repair, sometimes performed with the aid of the microscope, sometimes not, was just as good.

Clinical studies have the advantage that humans can cooperate with much more sophisticated tests of function of the sutured nerves, particularly sensory function. This ought to allow measurement of the ability to transmit information accurately, and thus demonstrate the advantage of better fascicular orientation and coaptation, if there is any.

However, this is not as easy as it sounds and there has been a remarkable dearth of comparative clinical trials of different suture techniques. Series reported by Salvi [12] and Donoso *et al.* [13] suggested there might be some advantage to microscopic perineural repair. Neither Young *et al.* [14] nor Marsh and Barton [15] could demonstrate any benefit.

What, therefore, should you do?

If you work in a hospital which possesses a suitable operating microscope (one with pedals controlling focus and magnification and binocular eyepieces for an assistant) together with microsurgical instruments and sutures, and you have learned how to use all these, we would recommend that you do so. However, be careful that you do not in the process contaminate your field or prolong tourniquet time beyond acceptable limits. Consider also that, if there is a choice between an early operation with magnifying spectacles versus a late one with the microscope, the former is preferable. You may say this choice should never have to be made, but under pressure of many cases waiting for theatre time, it can happen. It is more likely to happen if you get a reputation among nurses and anaesthetists for making a prolonged circus out of nerve repair, so if you use the microscope be quiet and efficient about it.

Make sure in advance that *you* know how to set it up and operate all its features. Adjust it for the intended field before you scrub, then roll it back and expose the nerve under tourniquet using ordinary instruments. Then release the tourniquet, use the diathermy (bipolar near the nerve) and pack the wound with swabs while you bring the microscope in again. It is a good idea for your assistant to let the scrub nurse have a look every now and then to relieve boredom.

Fascicular suture is not something you should embark upon without expert instruction. You are likely to do more harm (by production of intraneural fibrosis) than good (by accurate co-

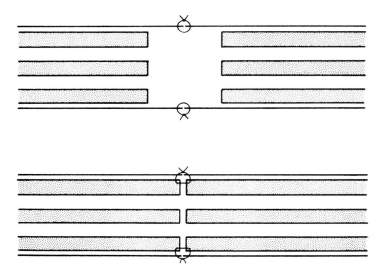

Fig. 14.6   Improved fascicular coaptation with epi-perineural sutures.

aptation). If you need to read this before operating on a nerve, then do an epineural repair – with or without the microscope – but as carefully and accurately as you can, and with the finest possible non-absorbable and non-reactive suture material.

Our own preference is for an epi-perineural suture because an epineural suture may drag the epineurium forwards (Fig. 14.6), like a sleeve pulled down over the end of the fingers, leaving the cut fascicles separated. The suture must pass through connective tissue (epineurium or perineurium), not nerve tissue.

Rehabilitation

After the nerve has regenerated, the information passing along it to and from the patient's brain will be scrambled. No electronic device could function after such an insult, but people can, due to the plasticity which is a feature of the CNS. Almquist *et al.* [16] suggest that it is because childrens' brains are more adaptable that they do better following nerve repair, not because the nerve actually regenerates better.

In order to make the most of their potential, patients need help in two respects. First, they need to know the time-course of regeneration. If they know what to expect they will not become dismayed or demoralized by the prolonged and imperfect recovery and will make the best of what they have. Warn them that:

• the affected part will remain numb for some months after the operation; they must be very careful not to burn themselves during this time;
• the first sensation to return will be 'protopathic': unpleasant and abnormal, but usefully protective;
• discriminatory touch sensibility will come more slowly and may continue to improve for 4 or 5 years;
• sensibility will never return to normal (in adults);
• they will experience many and varied paraesthesiae during regeneration.

Second, they need hand therapy. For the first few weeks, the nerve repair must be protected from tension by suitable splintage. Following this, they need to be helped to regain full mobility. In addition, they may be helped at a later stage by formal sensory re-education: graded sensory exercises under supervision. This depends on there being an enthusiast in your physiotherapy or occupational therapy departments. For many patients, their normal work constitutes much the best form of re-education.

Surgical methods

If it is possible to appose the two cut ends without undue tension, then direct suture is the method of choice.

Early direct suture

Having made a prompt diagnosis of nerve division, cover the wound with a betadine-soaked swab and start antibiotics. Admit the patient and organize theatre and the most experienced surgeon available. We have already discussed the use of magnification and the principles of wound care.

Expose the cut ends and study the pattern of the fascicles, with the aim of matching them accurately. Even without the microscope, one can get some idea by matching up the small blood vessels on the surface of the nerve, and if the cut is oblique then there is no difficulty in getting the rotation correct.

In our opinion, it is unwise to try to trim the ends of the nerve. If it was a clean sharp cut, you will probably only make it worse, as it is very difficult to hold the nerve still while you cut it whereas, when the patient cut it, it was held steady by surrounding tissues. Moreover, if you resect the bulging endoneurium, it only forms another bulge quite quickly. If the cut was not a clean sharp one, you should not be doing primary repair.

The essential point in technique is that the nerve ends must not be dragged together under tension. That is one reason for using fine suture material (not larger than 6/0); if there is tension, the suture breaks. However, the elasticity in the nerve does make the ends retract from each other, and to help yourself get in the first two stitches you may flex the adjacent joint through about half its range. You should not stick needles across the nerve as this may cause further injury, but we find it helpful to use a strong sub-epineural stay suture to take the tension while the finer sutures are put in.

The initial stay suture is the one which determines the rotation and the nerve ends must be carefully aligned before it is inserted. The main sutures are then inserted and, as we have said, a fine accurately placed epineural stitch is perfectly acceptable. A few epi-perineural sutures are preferable, after which the gaps are filled in by simple epineural sutures, and the stay suture is removed.

After completion of the repair, it should be possible to relax the adjacent joint into an almost neutral position, though it is wise to splint it in slight flexion for 2 weeks and in a neutral position for another 2 weeks.

Late direct suture

If it was not possible or desirable to repair the nerve within 24, or at most 48 hours, it is better to wait for about 8 weeks and then do a secondary procedure. The argument for this used to be that the epineurium thickened up and made it easier to suture, but with modern techniques we do not need this extra assistance. What is more important is to ensure that the initial phase of healing and deposition of scar has taken place.

In a secondary procedure it is necessary, even if the nerve ends have been apposed, to resect both ends back to healthy unscarred nerve tissue. This can be the most difficult part of the operation. You need a very sharp straight cutting edge: half of a razor blade (cut longitudinally) held in a strong needle holder is best. You also need something to hold the nerve still; special instruments are made, but if you have not got them you can sterilize one of the plastic bracelets used to identify patients, wrap it around the nerve, and then cut through bracelet and nerve together on to a wooden or metal spatula. It is better to press than to saw.

Then inspect the cut surface and see whether you have got back to healthy white bundles or can still see homogeneous grey scar tissue, in which case further resection is necessary. For this, the microscope is very helpful. In practice, any visible neuroma swelling is full of scar so you must cut back to where the nerve is of normal diameter.

Now is the time of decision. Can the cut ends be brought together easily or not? You are allowed some, but not full, flexion of adjacent joints, but mobilization of the nerve for several inches on either side is discouraged because of damage to its blood supply. A gap of 1 cm can usually be closed using the same technique as for primary repair; with a gap of more than 2 cm, this will produce unacceptable tension.

Grafting

The alternative is a nerve graft. Although this means two suture lines instead of one and an intervening segment of initially avascular connective tissue elements, it is better than suture under tension [17]. The absence of need for prolonged splintage with flexed joints also allows earlier hand therapy and use of the hand.

The usual donor site is the sural nerve and it is possible to obtain 35 cm from each leg. Three or four strands are used and the epineurium of the graft is sutured to the epineurium or perineurium of the main nerve. It is wise to use two stitches at each end to prevent rotation and thus loss of apposition of the cut ends at the junction. The most extensive use of nerve grafts is in reconstruction of the brachial plexus and, to save time, various sorts of nerve 'glue' have been used. These are not new, and nerve grafting used to be done by gluing together several parallel strands of sural nerve and then suturing them, as one, into the defect; this was called a cable graft. Nowadays it is preferred to spread the strands of graft apart so that each can acquire a blood supply as soon as possible.

Better still, the blood supply can be brought with the nerve, a vascularized nerve graft, with microvascular suture of the vessels from which the blood supply of the nerve is derived. The problem is in finding a suitable donor and at present the method is largely confined to brachial plexus injuries in which the prognosis for recovery of the ulnar nerve is considered hopeless; this nerve is then used as a vascularized graft to the trunks and cords which lead to the median and radial nerves. The long-term results are not yet known.

The future: adjunctive therapy

Many surgeons now believe that there is a limit, a low limit, to the quality of reinnervation following nerve transection which can be achieved by prompt diagnosis and optimal surgical technique. This is set by the regenerative power of the nerves themselves and by the problem of topographic disorganization (regenerating axons failing to find their correct end-organs). It would seem that any further improvement in results, and any progress in treatment of more central lesions which show no, or hardly any, regeneration, requires a leap in understanding of the process at the level of neurobiology.

We may speculate that new knowledge may enable us to intervene biochemically, as an adjunct to physical coaptation of the divided nerve. We may one day be able to switch back on the growth potential of the embryonic neurones, perhaps even utilize mechanisms by which axons find their correct target organs in the first place.

At present, we have only a few animal studies to encourage us, showing some enhancement of regeneration by a variety of agents, none of which is yet ready for clinical application. Physical agents showing some effect include pulsed electromagnetic fields and low-dose lasers. Biochemical agents include gangliosides, leupeptin, laminin and triamcinolone.

Assessment of results

There are two completely separate reasons for assessing the results of nerve repair. The first is clinical: to check, in the individual case, that regeneration is proceeding at a reasonable pace and that re-suture or grafting is not required. The second is in a research context, to compare two different methods of treatment. These two objectives require different methods.

Checking regeneration

Here there is little point in trying to express quantitatively the regeneration which has taken place. One is interested primarily in the *rate* at which things are happening; simple, qualitative tests suffice, but must be carried out regularly. As far as motor fibres are concerned, the matter is simple, pick a muscle which is recorded as having been completely paralysed at the time of the nerve injury, and whose function can be unambiguously detected without confusion from trick movements.

The return of function in sensory fibres can be detected by application of stimuli either to the nerve trunk or to the skin innervated by it. The former includes Tinel's sign – an 'electric' sensation in the territory of the nerve produced by percussion over the nerve trunk. The most distal point at which this is elicited is the level the regenerating axon tips have reached and should progress at about 1 mm per day. It is important to start distally and work proximally, or you flood the hand with paraesthesiae and cannot continue the examination. Another approach is to keep the site of stimulation constant and vary the power of the (electrical) stimulus. This is the idea of sensory threshold measurement [8].

In applying stimuli to the skin in the territory of the nerve, one is seeking answers to two questions. When does protective sensibility recover? When does the sense of light touch recover (if at all)? Protective sensibility can be tested by asking the patient to discriminate between the sharp and blunt ends of a pin. Touch sense implies tactile gnosis: the ability to discriminate different textures, shapes of coins or other objects and so on. For those who like to describe events in terms of grades and numbers, the return of skin sensibility is more easily recorded by use of the Medical Research Council sensory scale of S0 to S4 [18]. However, the numbers should not obscure the fact that this is a qualitative, descriptive grading only.

The decision to re-suture because of failure of regeneration is very difficult. The cost (in lost time) of starting again from scratch is high and there is no guarantee of better luck next time. Much would depend on what the patient's wishes are and the level of experience of the surgeon who did the first operation. Rarely is such a decision taken because of dissatisfaction with the quality of tactile gnosis, when protective sensibility and some motor function have returned.

Comparing different treatments

Injuries to neural tissue throughout the body remain the source of massive morbidity. As already stated, much basic neurobiological work is in progress, aimed at finding ways to reawaken or enhance the ability of nerve cells to regenerate. Transections of peripheral nerves in the upper limb are the most likely human test bed for such new treatments because they are common and do show at least some regenerative ability. Comparative trials between different treatments could be very helpful.

Qualitative measures, such as the MRC S 0–4 scale, are of little use in this context. For these purposes, a quantitative expression of the end result is exactly what is needed.

This has proved very elusive, so much so that it is impossible to compare the results of one author with those of another. Again the problem is

mainly on the sensory side; unlike muscle function, which an outside observer can measure, sensation is known only to the subject. Although psychologists have many elaborate methods for investigating mechanisms underlying sensation, few have addressed themselves to the problems of applying them to people whose sensations are abnormal, as they are after peripheral nerve suture. Their methods are apt to be misleading, since patients do not recover a certain proportion of normal sensation, rather a new kind of sensation.

For example, a test such as two-point discrimination is very difficult to apply reliably in people with disordered sensation. False positives are common unless a rigorous testing technique is employed and most values obtained in outpatient clinics or occupational therapy departments are probably worthless [19]. Particularly misleading is the habit of using two-point discrimination as a summary measure of sensibility; there is no evidence that performance of any one sensory task adequately sums up sensory function in the normal hand, let alone the highly abnormal.

Overall function is probably best assessed by tests which involve the performance of integrated tasks with a high sensory component, such, as picking up small objects (Fig. 14.7), discriminating shapes or textures and so on [20]. These can be so arranged to give a quantitative result by scoring speed and accuracy. The score must be expressed as a ratio to performance by the patient's normal hand, not by reference to population norms: variation between people is far

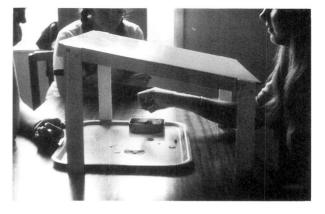

Fig. 14.7 The picking-up test, performed against the clock, developed from Moberg [20].

higher than variation between dominant and non-dominant hands.

More detailed assessment of sensory function is a specialist topic; ideally one would like to estimate both the numbers of the various populations of touch receptors reinnervated and the degree of topographic disorganization, but that is beyond the scope of this chapter.

Summary

The present situation is that results of nerve suture in adults are at best poor, because of the limited regenerative power of nerve cells and the topographic disorganization caused by transection of the endoneurial tubes. This will not change until huge strides have been made in understanding the neurobiology of regeneration.

In practice, even worse results often occur because of delay in diagnosis; this is avoidable by application of known principles. Immediate careful direct suture is the best treatment for the clean cut nerve. One should strive to

- appose the fascicles accurately;
- avoid intraneural fibrosis by gentle tissue handling.

References

1. Sunderland, S. (1945) The intraneural topography of the radial, median and ulnar nerves. *Brain*, **68**, 243–298.
2. Jabaley, M. E., Wallace, W. H. and Heckler, F. R. (1980) Internal topography of major nerves of the forearm and hand: a current view. *J. Hand Surg.*, **5**, 1–18
3. Mackel, R. (1985) Human cutaneous mechanoreceptors during regeneration: physiology and interpretation. *Ann. Neurol.*, **18**, 165–172.
4. Dellon, A. L. (1981) *Evaluation of Sensibility and Re-education of Sensation in the Hand.* Williams & Wilkins, Baltimore.
5. O'Riain, S. (1973) New and simple test of nerve function in the hand. *Br. Med. J.*, **3**, 615–616.
6. Wilson, G. R. (1985) A simple device for the objective evaluation of peripheral nerve injuries. *J. Hand Surg.*, **10B**, 324–330.
7. Lynch, G. and Quinlan, D. (1986). Jump function following nerve division. *Br. J. Plast. Surg.*, **39**, 364–366.
8. Smith, P. J. and Mott, G. (1986) Sensory threshold and conductance testing in nerve injuries. *J. Hand Surg.*, **11B**, 157–162.
9. Seddon, H. (1975) *Surgical Disorders of the Peripheral Nerves*, Churchill Livingstone, London, p. 275.
10. Birch, R. (1986) Lesions of peripheral nerves: the present position. *J. Bone Joint Surg.*, **68B**, 2–8.
11. Narakas, A. (1986) Editorial. *Peripheral Nerve. Repair and Regeneration*, **1**, 3–4.
12. Salvi, V. (1973) Problems connected with the repair of nerve sections. *Hand*, **5**, 25–32.
13. Donoso, R. S., Ballantyne, J. P. and Hansen, S. (1979) Regeneration of sutured human peripheral nerves: an electrophysiological study. *J. Neurol. Neurosurg. Psychiatry*, **42**, 97–106.
14. Young, L., Wray, C. and Weeks, P. M. (1981) A randomised prospective comparison of fascicular and epineural digital nerve repairs. *Plast. Reconstr. Surg.*, **68**, 89–93.
15. Marsh, D. and Barton, N. (1987) Does the use of the operating microscope improve the results of peripheral nerve suture? *J. Bone Joint Surg.*, **69B**, 625–630.
16. Almquist, E. E., Smith, O. A. and Fry, L. (1983) Nerve conduction velocity, microscopic, and electron microscopy studies comparing repaired adult and baby monkey median nerves. *J. Hand Surg.*, **8**, 406–410.
17. Millesi, H., Meissl, G. and Berger, A. (1972) The interfascicular grafting of the median and ulnar nerves. *J. Bone Joint Surg.*, **54A**, 727–750.
18. Medical Research Council (1954) Special Report Series no. 282. *Peripheral Nerve Injuries.* HMSO, London.
19. Moberg, E. (1987) Personal Communication.
20. Moberg, E. (1958) Objective methods for determining the functional value of sensibility in the hand. *J. Bone Joint Surg.*, **40B**, 454–476.

15

External skeletal fixation for the treatment of fractures

J. Kenwright

Introduction

External skeletal fixation was used in the last century and developed extensively by Hoffmann in 1938, who employed fixation for various types of fracture including fractures of the facial bones. Enthusiasm for the treatment method has waxed and waned, but since 1980 there has been a surge of increased use for many different types of fracture and it is interesting to define why this has occurred.

There have been major advances in plastic surgical techniques for replacing lost or severely damaged soft tissue, and these treatments rely on effective skeletal stabilization. Modern external skeletal fixation systems can always supply this need. Similarly, operations are available for reconstruction of large segmental bone defects, and an increased use of such methods has led to a greater need for external skeletal fixation. Infected fractures still present some of the most difficult problems in orthopaedic surgery and lead to prolonged morbidity. Although improved wound care has decreased the incidence of such disasters, the widespread use of internal fixation and the salvage of many limbs which might previously have been amputated has resulted in many infected pseudarthroses. External skeletal fixation is one of the mainstays of treatment for such problems. There have also been major advances in frame technology, so that complex fractures can be effectively stabilized.

These include fractures of the pelvis and juxta-articular regions as well as those of short bones.

More confident management of screw tracks has led to reduced fear of complications associated with infected tracks. Finally, the transfer of experiences through international communication has led to a widened use of external skeletal fixation in many countries over the last 10 years.

In the following sections the main indications for the use of external skeletal fixation in the treatment of the injured will be discussed. External fixator frame technology and application, the principles of treatment and the problems created will also be presented.

Indications

Fractures associated with severe soft tissue injury

External skeletal fixation has become the method of choice for stabilization of fractures associated with severe open or closed soft tissue injury (Fig. 15.1). Dramatic results have now been described from many sources, demonstrating that early stabilization of severe injuries can lead regularly to sound healing with a painless and functioning limb. Most of the studies are retrospective analyses of large numbers of patients but they do show clearly that effective stabilization by whatever means leads to lower rates of infection than seen for injuries of equivalent severity treated in casts. Hicks [1] first demonstrated this influence of stability using internal fixation; primary and secondary amputation rates were decreased for

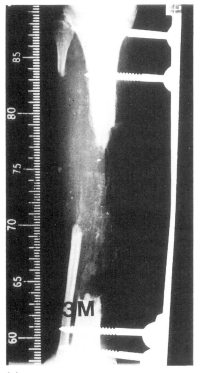

(a)

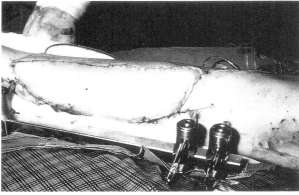

(b)

Fig. 15.1   Frames may need to meet considerable mechanical demands as seen here in (a) where there has been major bone loss. The patient could mobilize freely (b) following free vascularized grafting with skin, muscle and bone.

open tibial diaphyseal fractures if early stabilization with plates was used. In general, external skeletal fixation is now used for stabilizing such fractures, though internal fixation should still be considered first in the forearm and in femoral fractures. Internal fixation usually means increas-

ing local soft tissue damage in order to apply the implant, and such dissection is unnecessary with external skeletal fixation. Many of these injuries can now be treated by reamed or unreamed intramedullary nailing. For most open diaphyseal fractures there is little difference seen in the results from either nailing or treatment by external fixture.

With the use of effective stabilization, fracture infection rates for tibial diaphyseal fractures can be reduced to approximately 2% for grade I and II open fractures [2]. Infection rates of between 20% and 40% are still recorded for grade III open wounds even when employing modern methods of stabilization. In order to maintain these low rates of infection for lesser wounds and to try and reduce the infection rates for major wounds, it would seem important to stabilize fractures effectively very early after injury. The importance of obtaining vascularized soft tissue closure within 72 hours of injury has now also been demonstrated. There is little place for the use of skeletal traction or fracture stabilization with casts in the primary treatment of grade II or III open fractures, as neither offers sufficient stability for wound healing.

Less severe soft tissue injuries with skin of doubtful viability

Apparent simple skin contusion is often unmasked as necrosis several days from injury. This necrosis will then need excision, and fracture stabilization with external skeletal fixation will be required if the bone is subcutaneous. Such contusion with suspect skin is often treated best by stabilization of the fracture using external skeletal fixation as the primary treatment on the first day. This allows stable healing conditions for the damaged skin and may limit the extent of the subsequent necrosis. The serious and often unrecognized nature of many closed soft tissue injuries has been stressed by Tscherne and incorporated in his most useful system of classification of fractures in which closed fractures are classified into four types according to the scale CO–CIII [3].

Neurovascular injuries

If surgical repair of a major vascular or neurological structure is to be made, stabilization of the skeleton is needed. External skeletal fixation as a preliminary to vessel repair is usually the method of choice in such circumstances.

Compartment syndrome

If this crisis arises in the leg or forearm, the wide decompression needed invariably destabilizes the fracture completely and external skeletal fixation should be applied.

Multiple injuries

It has been shown recently that stabilization of multiple fractures within the first 24 hours of injury reduces the incidence and severity of adult respiratory distress syndrome (ARDS) [4]. External skeletal fixation can usually be applied to one or more fractures and be built into the operative programme so that several fractures are stabilized simultaneously. Such a plan of combined surgery is needed for multiple fractures to reduce the time of the initial emergency surgical programme.

Early application of external skeletal frames may even be needed in the receiving area of the Accident Department in order to reduce haemorrhage associated with severe pelvic fractures. The application of anterior frames under such circumstances may reduce pelvic volume and add just sufficient stability to reduce blood loss even if there is incomplete stabilization of the posterior elements of a fracture dislocation; this can be a life saving procedure.

The use of early external skeletal fixation of the tibia combined with closed nailing of a femoral fracture sustained in the same leg is especially indicated in order to facilitate early rehabilitation of the knee joint, and of muscle function in the leg.

Acute bone loss

Such loss is usually associated with severe soft tissue wounds and external skeletal fixation is the method usually chosen for fracture stabilization (Fig. 15.1). The defect can be treated by grafting, or acute shortening and remote distraction osteogenesis.

Fracture instability

External skeletal fixation is indicated frequently for treatment of unstable juxta-articular fractures of the radius and for fractures of the pelvis, where the main objective is to control fracture position, and where the degree of comminution or displacement may make internal fixation difficult. The use of external skeletal fixation for treatment of unstable closed fractures of the tibia or femur is advocated by some surgeons [5,6]; though fracture control is very effective the method is not universally popular, however, due to the significant incidence of screw track infections, and the prolonged healing times often seen with this method of treatment. Closed intramedullary nailing with locking screws is now the most effective treatment for such unstable fractures. The combination of external fixation and limited internal fixation is very safe and useful for pilon fractures.

Fracture infection

External skeletal fixation has revolutionized the treatment of fracture infection. The main principle of such treatment is the uncompromising excision of dead bone and creation of a healthy wound. Once this is accomplished, one of the following procedures for reconstruction of soft tissue or bony defect is selected.

i. Pappineau method with massive cancellous graft.
ii. Fibular transposition for tibial fractures.
iii. Free vascularized transfer of bone and soft tissue.
iv. Bone transport by the Ilizarov technique.

Each of these methods depends upon stabilization of the bony fragments in the presence of bone loss, this stabilization to be maintained for 6–12 months in many instances. This is a demanding situation for fixation which can now be treated effectively by external skeletal fixation.

Non-union

Stabilization is usually needed for the treatment of any atrophic, hypertrophic or infected non-union and external skeletal fixation should be considered for each problem. External fixation allows wound care, stabilization of fragments and mobilization of adjacent joints, and this often in patients in whom there are stiff joints due to previous prolonged conservative treatment. Bone graft can be applied through incisions remote from damaged skin.

External skeletal fixation may also be indicated for the treatment of many short bone fractures in the hand or wrist, for dislocations, for the correction of post-fracture deformity, or for arthrodesis performed early after devastating joint injuries.

Frames, screws and the bone screw interface

The ideal system

Many different external fixation frames are available, each designed to try to meet the specifications for an ideal fixation system. These are that frames should be (i) simple to apply by relatively inexperienced operators; (ii) convenient for the patient allowing overall mobility as well as muscle and joint rehabilitation; (iii) adjustable so that fracture position can be corrected after application and so that the mechanical conditions at the fracture site can be adjusted i.e., dynamization should be possible; (iv) versatile so that fractures in long and short bones as well as in the pelvis can be treated; (v) inexpensive and re-usable; and (vi) have standardized instruments designed for their application. Each available system has attempted to embrace many of the features that would make it 'ideal' but each has limitations because several of these specifications for the perfect frame are mutually exclusive.

In clinical practice it is probably necessary to have two types of frame available in an accident unit, including a simple unilateral system for diaphyseal fractures which represent the vast majority of fractures requiring treatment; a versatile complex system for pelvic, short bone, and complicated fractures is also essential. Circular frames are rarely needed for acute treatment of injuries.

Frame stability

Knowledge of frame stability has accumulated from clinical experience and from investigations made on material testing machines. The scientific literature and the manuals accompanying the frames describe the geometrical configurations which will give adequate stability and prevent loss of fracture position during rehabilitation for most fracture patterns [7,8].

The weakest link in all systems is the screw clamp junction, and loss of fracture position is usually due to failure at this point. When stiffness of the frame/fracture system is considered as opposed to failure strength all unilateral frames are considerably less stiff in antero-posterior bending than in other axes [7] Stiffness of the frame system depends on the material properties of the frame and on the geometry of the frame and screws as applied. Simple measures which give predictable increases in stability include decreasing the offset of the frame from the bone, increasing the number of screws, increasing the distance between screws and changing the angle of the screws so that they are not all in one plane. In the lower leg the bending moments are principally sagittal: if mechanical conditions alone were the most important ones then one set of screws should be inserted in the antero-posterior plane so as to resist effectively this

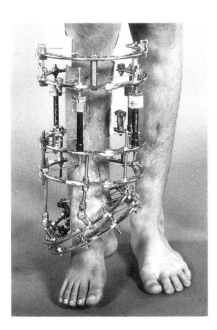

Fig. 15.2 Circular frames with tensioned thin wires give high degrees of bending stiffness but allow axial flexibility on weight bearing. Their main use is for correcting fracture deformity and for bone transport.

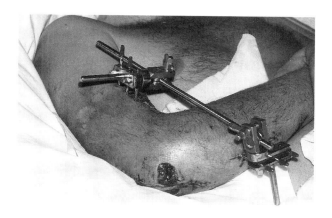

Fig. 15.3 Frames bridging joints should be removed as soon as possible; the wrist and inferior radio-ulnar joints will tolerate frames for approximately 4 weeks. The elbow joint is less tolerant.

bending moment. For very unstable fractures major modifications may be needed such as triangulation of the frame, the use of a dual frame configuration or change to a circular frame (Fig. 15.2).

A lot of emphasis has been placed upon the results obtained from tests upon simulated fractures fixed by frames and loaded in material testing machines. The conditions within these tests are often ideal with perfectly applied bone screws, a situation which is not always possible to achieve in clinical practice. In patients there may be very unstable or comminuted fractures, and the bone itself may be osteoporotic. Hence in clinical practice allowance needs to be made for these factors when planning application of a frame and when planning postoperative weight-bearing.

There is a considerable body of opinion now which advocates decreasing the stability of frames in one or more axis during the early or later stages of fracture healing to improve the mechanical environment for the healing fracture. Progressive dismantling of frames can be performed [9] or frames selected with features which allow dynamization [5,10]. It should, however, be noted that decreasing rigidity (and hence stiffness) in one axis may lead to a decrease in stiffness in another axis. For example, torsional stiffness may be reduced unevenly by such manoeuvres and this may lead to an inappropriate shear at the fracture on loading [8].

Choice of frame

In general unilateral frames are satisfactory for most diaphyseal fractures. Juxta-articular fractures may cause special problems as will any need to create fixation across a joint (Fig. 15.3), and for such circumstances a more complex frame will be needed. If progressive correction of deformity is required or bone transport is planned, circular frames are the most appropriate.

Bone pins and screws

The geometry of an external fixator results in large bending loads being carried by the screw in addition to some tensile and compressive loads. In experimental cadaveric studies, the application of a moderate value of cyclically applied load has been shown to result in an increased incidence of screw loosening over unloaded or statically loaded screws [11].

The likely mechanism causing this loosening would appear to be related to the amount of relative movement which occurs between the screw and the bone [12,13]. Hence, if the movement between the screw and the bone can be reduced, for example by using a larger stiffer screw, then the incidence of screw loosening may be expected to reduce. Large diameter screws also greatly enhance the stiffness of the fixator system.

Various types of screw threads have been tested, although there is insufficient evidence that one particular type is more effective than another. Most external fixators offer a specific screw for use with the fixator and some offer specific screws for both cancellous and cortical bone.

The concept of inserting crossed thin wires under tension with circular frames is an interesting alternative to the use of conventional screws. With these wires there can be considerable rigidity of a fracture and bone fragments in bending, yet flexibility in axial loading. This mechanical combination is claimed to give the most appropriate environment for fracture healing.

Fatigue failure of screws and pins is uncommon and is not considered to be a practical problem.

On fixator removal, the refracture rate through either small or large diameter screw holes is low. Remodelling occurs rapidly around screw holes which enhances local bone strength unless there is gross and continuing infection.

Application of frames

Planning

Preoperative planning is needed, making allowance for the nature of both the bone and soft tissue injury, as well as the mechanical demands that will be placed upon the fixation system. An overall plan for the type of frame to be used and its configuration should be made before entering the operating theatre so that necessary equipment can be available.

Detailed planning is needed for siting of the screws. Draping should show the whole contour of both limbs so that accurate alignment can be achieved. For many injuries, including fractures of the pelvis and in the distal forearm, certain standard positions for screw insertion have been well tested and are nearly always selected. For tibial and femoral fractures screw positions have to be chosen carefully for individual situations. Screws should be inserted at least 2 cm from the fracture itself, but this rule may have to be broken if there is severe comminution or if there are longitudinal splits through the bone. Under these circumstances fracture fragments may be penetrated and despite occasional infection of such screw tracks infection of fractures does not occur. Sites for screw insertion are chosen, other factors being equal, where there is thin soft tissue coverage between the skin surface and the bone, and where skin moves little during joint function. For tibial fractures the medial surface of the tibia is the most appropriate from this point of view and should be chosen, though the anterior crest is the most sound mechanically when using a unilateral frame. Other factors may predominate when choosing screw sites. These include planning for future plastic or other soft tissue surgery when adequate access to wounds may be a critical factor.

The normal anatomical siting of neurovascular structures will influence the placement of screws and this is a particularly important factor when inserting screws through the femur, tibia or humerus especially with the use of circular frames. The exact site of neurovascular structures should be checked in an atlas preoperatively: safe corridors for insertion for each bone have been defined by both Green [14] and Behrens [9].

Finally, when planning, the mechanical demands on the fixator should be considered carefully. The fracture may be very unstable and a plan must be made to use the appropriate frame and an adequate number of screws, these placed with optimum geometry. Postoperative demands on the fixator are affected by the patient's weight, the weight-bearing programme to be prescribed, and the overall activity related to the personality of the patient will also require consideration.

If there is a strong possibility that subsequent internal fixation may be needed, and exchange nailing is now frequently needed, the screw holes should be placed allowing for future skin incisions.

Insertion of screws

Having planned the sites of insertion for screws, an incision is made approximately 1 cm long so that tenting of the skin is not seen around the screw when joints function: this avoids skin necrosis which is accompanied by inevitable infection. Screw holes should be pre-drilled using a sharp drill bit to reduce thermal necrosis, and the surrounding skin needs protection during drilling. It is very easy to over-penetrate the distal cortex and injure nerves or vessels, this being a particular risk in the central half of the tibia. Screws can be placed accurately using image intensification and should be inserted through the centre of the bone for maximum mechanical effect. The screws should be inserted in a meticulous manner applying similar mechanical principles to those used with internal fixation.

Fracture reduction

Before tightening the clamps upon the screws major efforts should be made to reduce the fracture using any open wound for accurate reduction.

After care

At the end of the procedure, and whilst still within the operating theatre, the screw holes should be assessed in different positions of function to make sure there is no tenting of the skin. The frame should be offset from the limb sufficiently to allow for the considerable oedema which frequently follows serious injury. Reduction is checked on radiographs.

Postoperatively screw-hole management can be performed effectively by many means. Screw holes should be dressed each day and can be left wet with dressings or dry. If there are scabs, these should be removed to allow drainage.

Problem areas and complications

Major complications are rare as a direct result of the use of external skeletal fixation, but there are many minor problems and it is these which sway the surgeon away from the universal use of external skeletal fixation for the treatment of all unstable fractures.

Screw track problems (Fig. 15.4)

Screw track complications rarely cause permanent disability but their high incidence is one of the major objections to the use of external skeletal fixation. Well placed screw tracks, maintained in a meticulous manner can remain trouble free for approximately one month after insertion. There then follows an increasing in-

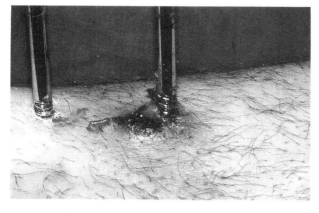

Fig. 15.4 Screw track problems are very common. The screw has to be replaced in infections like this. Skin tenting always leads to necrosis and secondary infection. Despite large residual screw holes in the bone late fracture through these is rare.

cidence of infection with or without loosening associated with increased patient activity. Reddening around the screw hole is seen frequently during excess use and responds well to immobilization for 24 hours, which both reduces the loading of the bone screw interface and the fretting of the screw on the soft tissues. Positive signs of infection require antibiotic therapy as well as rest. If infection continues with discharge, and lysis is seen on radiographs the screw needs replacing at a site at least 1.5 cm from the initial placement. Despite many problems seen with screw tracks, it is unusual to have to abandon the treatment method prematurely because of these complications. When treating complex conditions such as infected non-unions, frames can be maintained for over 1 year.

After removal of screws infection nearly always resolves. Ugly pitted scars may remain but are amenable to minor surgical procedures. Osteomyelitis may persist following screw removal and radiographs including tomograms may show a small ring sequestrum. In this situation the track needs full curettage under general anaesthetic when the condition nearly always resolves. Refracture through screw holes is very unusual even when using 6.0 mm screws.

Loss of fracture position

This complication should be guarded against and usually follows incorrect insertion of screws or gross overloading of the system.

Joint function

Loss of function can be associated with any fracture but is encountered commonly in both the ankle joint after tibial fractures and in the knee joint after stabilization of femoral fractures. When treating tibial fractures equinus deformity develops very readily due mainly to postoperative discomfort with inhibited muscle action: the equinus remains and is often impossible to correct at a later stage; however, this problem is avoidable. An intensive physiotherapy programme is needed with this type of injury, starting immediately after frame application, and it is advisable to apply a plastic or plaster of Paris splint with the foot in the plantargrade position

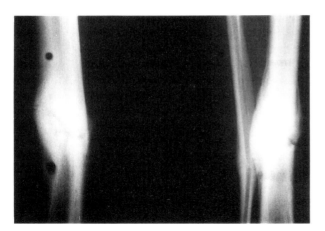

Fig. 15.5 Healing with external callus formation is 'ideal'. There is often a gap at the fracture site, and also rapid healing is needed so that frames can be removed as early as possible.

at the time of initial frame application. If the frame has to be applied on the lateral side of the leg because of soft tissue damage the screws passing through the anterior compartment will increase the risk of equinus deformity and vigorous steps need to be taken to prevent permanent deformity.

When stabilizing femoral fractures through the lower third of the femur the screws pass through the fascia lata: it is crucial that longitudinal division of this fascia is made at the time of frame application and that the knee is put through its normal range of movement in the operating theatre. If this is not done, extensive knee stiffness will follow. Patients need to be encouraged firmly to use the knee during the early days after femoral fixation and adequate sedation and supervision of movement is needed in the first week.

If a joint has to be bridged by a frame the joint will nearly always have permanent substandard function, although bridging the wrist joint during the treatment of lower radial fractures does not appear to lead to major stiffness so long as the frames are removed within 4 weeks.

Problems with fracture healing

Fixation systems and the fracture healing process

Experimental and clinical experiences have shown that the fracture healing process is acutely

sensitive to the mechanical environment at the fracture site. It is also claimed that external skeletal fixation inhibits healing of diaphyseal fractures, and that most frames offer too much rigidity. This latter point is difficult to prove, as external skeletal fixation is used in general for the most severe types of fracture which have very long and varied healing times whatever treatment method is employed.

The pattern of healing when using external skeletal fixation for diaphyseal fractures is that of secondary fracture healing, or healing by external callus formation (Fig. 15.5). Even with meticulous reduction of such fractures at the time of frame application, there is always a significant gap or incongruity at the fracture site so that primary bone healing or 'gap healing' cannot occur. It is now known that under such fracture healing conditions functional stimulation is required, and this at an early stage during the treatment. With serious long bone fractures treated by external skeletal fixation using rigid frames such stimulation is unlikely to occur. This has been confirmed in patients being treated by unilateral external skeletal fixation by measuring the amount of movement that does occur at the fracture site during weightbearing in the early weeks after fracture. It was shown that very little movement occurs at the fracture site in the first 6 weeks after injury [15]. Burny [6] has shown that many fractures of the tibia heal rapidly if treated with external skeletal fixation using 'minimum fixation' with a non-rigid unilateral Hoffmann frame configuration.

Similarly De Bastiani [5] and Behrens [9] have proposed that fractures of the tibia should be dynamized after an interval of 6 weeks, either by adjusting the frame to allow dynamic loading during weightbearing or by progressive dismantling of the frame.

There is also evidence that strain should be applied to fractures within the early weeks after injury, though the timing must vary with the severity of soft tissue injury [10,16].

With the types of programme described in these studies frames were applied as early as possible after injury and maintained at least until clinical union had been reached. There is a school of thought which proposes that frames be removed as soon as the initial soft tissue injury has healed; subsequent treatment would be by a cast. In this way the advantages of external skeletal fixation and functional cast treatment can be embraced so that the most appropriate mechanical environment exists throughout treatment. In our experience removing frames at early stages has nearly always led to unsatisfactory bone healing and if this method is to be used it is suggested that bone grafting is applied at the time of frame removal.

Combinations of internal and external fixation can be employed and accurate reduction be maintained by minimal internal fixation (Fig. 15.6), the external skeletal fixation system supplying the majority of stability. The mechanical environment associated with this type of combined fixation inhibits external callus formation. Healing of the fracture will occur eventually after many months but if the frame is removed before such healing has occurred very careful protection of the fracture will be needed and it is recommended that bone graft should also be applied, with the frame *in situ*.

Failure of healing

Delayed or non-union is common in diaphyseal fractures treated by external skeletal fixation. External fixation is used for the most severe types of injury and long healing times of over 20 weeks are common for tibial fractures. With these types of injury there must be a strong case for adding bone graft if there is any bone loss, or significant comminution. The graft is applied at the initial operation or within the first 6 weeks of injury.

Despite a low threshold for the use of bone graft, non-union may still develop. This can then be treated by further bone grafting of the fracture whilst maintaining the frame *in situ*, but other methods should be considered in this situation. If the soft tissues have healed soundly it may be appropriate to change to internal fixation, preferably with the use of a locked intra-medullary nail for diaphyseal fractures. If this change in treatment method is to be used the limb should be

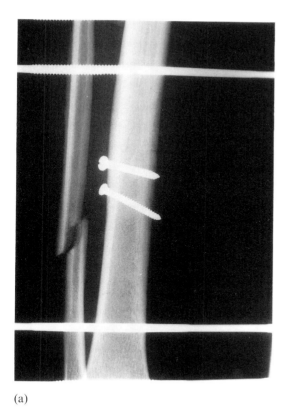

(a)

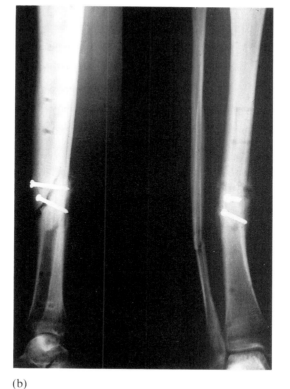

(b)

Fig. 15.6 Combinations of internal and external fixation enable accurate reductions to be maintained as seen in radiograph (a). Such stabilization inhibits external callus formation and predisposes to mechanical failure when the frame is removed (b).

immobilized in a cast for at least 1 month after frame removal before embarking on the internal fixation. This interval allows local screw tracks to heal soundly and reduces the risk of fracture through the screw holes. If internal fixation is planned the screw tracks should be curetted formally at the time of frame removal.

The treatment of infected non-union is a complex subject which cannot be covered within the scope of this chapter. All the principles of external skeletal fixation apply to these difficult problems.

Patient tolerance

Frames are well tolerated by patients despite intermittent screw-track infections and the need for multiple hospital attendances. A few patients have an unfavourable psychological response to external skeletal fixation and develop a strong rejection response to the presence of the appliance on the limb; if this occurs the frame must be removed.

Conclusions

The recent developments in external skeletal fixation have changed the management of many types of fracture and particularly severe open fractures, fractures with bone loss and fracture infection; the method offers safe, atraumatic, and effective stabilization of complex fractures.

Planning is required even in the emergency situation; it is important for subsequent care for the frames to be applied with meticulous attention to mechanical details in the same way as employed with internal fixation. Planning should also take into account the mechanical demands that will be placed upon the leg and the subsequent surgery that might be needed both to bone and soft tissue.

This type of stabilization when used for open fractures is associated with very low rates of fracture infection if there has also been correct wound care. It is, however, becoming clear that certain types of devastating fracture below the knee might still best be treated by primary amputation [17]. Careful review of the long-term results of type III C tibial fractures, with asso-

ciated vascular damage and soft tissue loss, shows that most patients in this group still require a secondary amputation; this end result is seen despite technically satisfactory primary fixation and rescue of a viable limb. If this group is excluded it is probable that external skeletal fixation is the method of choice for stabilization of most diaphyseal fractures with grade 2 or 3 open wounds.

The future for external skeletal fixation for fracture control for severe injuries is clear, but the place of the treatment method for treatment of simple fracture instability is still in doubt.

There is still room for development of frame technology perhaps incorporating new materials, and for further studies of the influence of adjustment of flexibility to enable the most appropriate mechanical environment to be applied at the different stages of fracture healing for an individual fracture.

References

1. Hicks, J. H. (1964) Amputation in fractures of the tibia. *J. Bone Joint Surg.*, **46B**, 388–392.
2. Gustilo, R. B. and Anderson, J. T. (1976) Prevention of infection in the treatment of one thousand and twenty-five open fractures of long bones. *J. Bone Joint Surg.*, **58A**, 453–458.
3. Tscherne, H. and Oestern, H. J. (1982) Quoted in Szyszkowitz, R. (1988) *Curr. Orthop.*, **2**, 14–17.
4. Johnson, K. D., Cadambi, A. and Burton, S. (1985) Incidence of adult respiratory distress syndrome in patients with multiple skeletal injuries. Effects of early operative stabilisation of fractures. *J. Trauma*, **25**, 375–384.
5. De Bastiani, G., Aldegheri, R. and Brivio, L. R. (1984) The treatment of fractures with a dynamic axial fixator. *J. Bone Joint Surg.*, **66B**, 538–545.
6. Burny, F. (1979) Elastic external fixation of tibial fractures: study of 1421 cases. In: *External Fixation: the Current State of the Art* (eds H. F. Brooker and C. C. Edwards), Williams & Wilkins, Baltimore.
7. McCoy, M. T., Kasman, R. A. and Chao, E. Y. (1983) Comparison of mechanical performance in four types of external fixators. *Clin. Orthop. Rel. Res.*, **180**, 23–33.
8. Finlay, J. B., Moroz, T. K., Rorabeck, C. H., Davey, J. R. and Bourne, R. B. (1985) Stability of ten configurations of the Hoffman external fixation frame. *J. Bone Joint Surg.*, **67B**, 734–744.

9. Behrens, F. and Searls, K. (1986) External fixation of the tibia. Basic concepts and prospective evaluation. *J. Bone Joint Surg.*, **68B**, 246–254.
10. Kenwright, J., Goodship, A. E., Kelly, D. J., Newman, J. H., Harris, J. D., Richardson, J. B., Evans, M., Spriggins, A. J., Burrough, S. J. and Rowley, D. I. (1986) Effect of controlled axial micromovement on healing of tibial fractures. *Lancet*, **ii**, 1185–1187.
11. Pettine, K. A., Kelly, P. J., Chao, E. Y. S. and Huiskes, R. (1986) Histologic and biomechanical analysis of external fixator pin-bone interface. *Orthop. Transac.*, **10**, 337.
12. Scatzker, J., Horne, J. G. and Sumner-Smith, G. (1975) The effect of movement on the holding power of screws in bone. *Clin. Orthop. Rel. Res.*, **111**, 257–262.
13. Uthoff, H. K. (1973) Mechanical factors influencing the holding power of screws in compact bone. *J. Bone Joint Surg.*, **55B**, 633–639.
14. Green, S. A. (1981) *Complications of External Skeletal Fixation: Causes, Prevention, Treatment.* C. Thomas, Springfield, Illinois.
15. Cunningham, J. L., Evans, M. and Kenwright, J. (1989) The measurement of fracture movement in patients treated with unilateral external skeletal fixation. *J. Biom. Eng.*, **11(2)**, 118–122.
16. Goodship, A. E. and Kenwright, J. (1985) The influence of induced micromovement upon the healing of experimental tibial fractures. *J. Bone Joint Surg.*, **66B**, 650–655.
17. Hansen, S. T. (1987) Editorial. The type III C tibial fracture, salvage or amputation. *J. Bone Joint Surg.*, **69A**, 799–780.

16

Brachial plexus injuries

A. O. Narakas†, P. M. Yeoman and C. B. Wynn Parry

Part 1 Surgical Reconstruction

A. O. Narakas

Introduction

During the last 22 years the author has been confronted with over 1200 various plexopathies (Tables 16.1 and 16.2), 864 patients being victims of accidents in their postnatal life. It is this latter group which will be presented.

At first sight these 864 patients with traumatic brachial plexus injury (BPI) are numerous enough to yield valuable statistics. In reality, this is hardly the case because we do not see all cases of BPI, but only the severe ones, and many come from neighbouring countries. In the first 500 patients seen only 360 were living in Switzerland, in the last 300 seen only 246. Therefore it is difficult to establish the frequency of BPI in Switzerland. A survey of patients admitted to the University Hospital of Lausanne after trauma

Table 16.1 Aetiology of brachial plexus injuries caused by kinetic displacement (patients seen by the author between 1.1.1965 and 15.5.1988)

		%	Conservative treatment or orthopaedic reconstruction	Operated on their plexus	Operated by other surgeons
Road traffic accidents 669 = 77.4%					
Using motorcycles (125 cc and more)	394	45.6	115	292	7
Using motorcycles (< 125 cc)	76	8.8	33	42	1
Using bicycles	37	4.3	10	27	
Using cars and other vehicles	105	12.2	50	54	1
Pedestrians hit by vehicles	57	6.6	33	24	
Various accidents 195 = 22.6%					
In factories, building sites, forestry, agriculture	59	6.8	41	18	
Sport (mostly skiing)	47	5.4	38	9	
Benign falls (from own height)	78	9.0	77	1	
Severe falls	11	1.3	4	7	
Totals	864	100	401	455	9

† Deceased

Table 16.2 Various plexopathies (referred for diagnosis and treatment between 1.1.1965 and 15.5.1988)

		Conservative treatment or orthopaedic surgery	Operated on their plexus	Operated by other surgeons on the plexus
Obstetrical palsy	162	141*	19	2
Post-radiation	72	34**	36	2
Iatrogenic (sections, ligatures, crush, drills, etc.)	32	13	18	1
Gunshot wounds	19	10	9	
Various tumours	19	4	15	
Pancoast tumour	8	1	7	
Secondary compressions after trauma (callus, fibrous bands, scar)	12	0	12	
Severe paralytic thoracic outlet syndromes	19	0	17	2
Parsonage–Turner syndromes	19	17	2	
Rucksack palsy or analogous	3	3	0	
Cervical disk hernias	3	0	0	3***
Various radicular syndromes	21	2	2	17***
Various myelopathies and encephalopathies	12	3	0	9***
Probable psychogenic (hysterical palsy)	3	2	1	
Post-vaccination	3	1	0	2***
Idiopathic	5	0	0	5***
Totals	412	231	138	43

* Nine patients are on the waiting list for reconstructive orthopaedic surgery.
** One patient on the waiting list for neurolysis and omentoplasty.
*** Referred elsewhere or no treatment prescribed.

has shown a yearly variation (over 7 years) between 3 and 7.5 per 10 000 cases. A survey of patients admitted to hospital after motorcycle accidents or related vehicles has shown a variation of 2% maximum to 0.7% minimum. This does not include patients coming to polyclinics in the departments of neurology, orthopaedics or plastic and reconstructive surgery; the latter is incorporated in our hospital which is primarily involved with hand surgery.

Diagnosis has evolved over the years because of refinements such as CT scan combined with myelography with hydrosoluble dye, magnetic resonance imaging, evoked sensory and nerve action potentials which have become available. The operative treatment has also involved combining nerve reconstructive measures with old and new orthopaedic operative procedures. The requirements of today's patients with BPI have also changed. Young people with persisting complete palsy do not accept amputations and even refuse orthotic devices because it 'stamps' them as invalids. Therefore these 864 cases of BPI are far from homogenous. However, they provided

the author with ever increasing experience in this field, and in this chapter attempts will be made to convey it to the reader.

Classification of brachial plexus injuries

Traditionally BPIs are divided into supraclavicular and infraclavicular palsies, the former being complete or incomplete, the latter sparing usually the suprascapular nerve and the clavicular portion of pectoralis major. However, experience has shown that this classification does not necessarily correspond to levels of injury. A classification into five levels has been proposed by the author [1]. Level I corresponds to roots, level II to the anterior ramus of the spinal nerve, level III to trunks, level IV to cords and level V to the origins of individual peripheral branches of the BP. This classification has to be applied for each anatomical structure originating from the five roots of the BP. For instance, a common type of injury is a rupture of the upper trunk C5–C6 (level III), a rupture of the anterior branch of C7 (level II) and a root avulsion C8 and T1 (level I). However, the same clinical picture will be produced by a rupture of the suprascapular nerve at the scapular notch (level V), rupture of the divisions leaving the upper and middle trunks (level III–IV) to form the cords and a lower root avulsion C8–T1 (level I). Retro- and infraclavicular lesions often show a distal lesion of the suprascapular nerve, of the whole posterior cord or only of the axillary and possibly radial nerves of the lateral cord or only the musculocutaneous nerve. Occasionally the origin of the median and ulnar nerves is also affected. In fact, any classification is condemned to have numerous exceptions or subgroups due to the complex anatomical features of the BP. Total loss of function can be explained by five degrees of severity of injury as proposed by Sunderland [2] each having a totally different prognosis and requiring different types of treatment [3].

For example: degree 1 (Seddon's neurapraxia [4] requires rest only, degrees 2 and 3 (axo-

Table 16.3 **Radicular avulsions as seen at operation in patients with traction injuries of the brachial plexus (*n* = 422, supraclavicular *n* = 219, more distal *n* = 203)**

| Roots avulsed | n *pat.* | n *roots* | *Distribution and* n *of individual roots* | | | | | Remarks |
			C5	C6	C7	C8	T1	
C5 isolated	1 (PRF)	1	1	0	0	0	0	C5 in a prefixed plexus corresponds actually to C6
C6 isolated	14	14	0	14	0	0	0	
C7 isolated	17 (2 POF)	17	0	0	17	0	0	C7 in a post fixed plexus corresponds to C6
C8 isolated	5 (1 POF)	5	0	0	0	5	0	C8 in a POF corresponds to C7 actually
T1 isolated	2	2	0	0	0	0	2	
C5–C6	6	12	6	6	0	0	0	
C6–C7	9 (2 POF)	18	0	9	9	0	0	C6–C7 in POF correspond actually to C5–C6
C7–C8	4 (1 POF)	8	0	0	4	4	0	C7–C8 correspond to C6–C7
C8–T1	32	64	0	0	0	32	32	
C5–through C7	7	21	7	7	7	0	0	In one case C4 was also avulsed
C6–C8–T1	5 (1 POF)	15	0	5	0	5	5	The POF case corresponds to a C5–C7–C8 avulsion
C7–C8–T1	44	132	0	0	44	44	44	
C6–C7–T1	2	6	0	2	2	0	2	
C5 through C8	3	4	3	3	3	3	0	
C5–C6, C8–T1	2	8	2	2	0	2	2	
C5, C7–C8–T1	2	8	2	0	2	2	2	
C6 through T1	39	156	0	39	39	39	39	
C5 through T1	25	125	25	25	25	25	25	In one case C3 and C4 were also avulsed
Totals	219	624	46	112	152	161	153	
%	52		7.4	17.9	24.4	25.8	24.5	

N.B. In 13 additional cases with root avulsions: two of C6, three of C8, two of T1, three of C6–C7, two of C5–C6–C7 and one of C7–C8–T1 have not been recognized at operation (intraforaminal avulsion or in the spinal canal) and diagnosed much later. This increases to 232 (55%) patients with root avulsions and to 646 the roots avulsed, percentages changing to 18, 4 for C6, the others being hardly affected.

notmesis) requires rest followed by physio-therapy, degrees 4 and 5 (neurotmesis), possible surgery. Five roots, five anterior branches of spinal nerves C5–T1, three trunks, three cords, eleven terminal branches and in 5% of cases the accessory spinal and phrenic nerves, can present with any of these five degrees of severity of injury, including avulsion of roots in various combinations. Moreover, traction lesions may extend over a length of the entire plexus which produces a great variety of pathological changes and further confuses a set classification. However, instrumental and surgical explorations of BPI provide us with some information about the frequency of some lesions. Table 16.3 shows the distribution of root avulsions. C5 is the least vulnerable, but C6 and in some cases C7 are tethered by fibrous tissue investing their epineurium to the rims of the foramen, while C8 and T1 have such an anchorage rendering them more vulnerable to avulsion [5]. Table 16.4 shows the frequency of lesional patterns encountered at surgical exploration.

Lesions associated with BPI

Whenever the surgeon is confronted with a traction BPI in the days or weeks after injury presenting with a partial or total palsy, he has to decide which degrees of injury he is dealing with. Treatment will depend on this initial assessment of pathology. Some clues are helpful, such as the evaluation of kinetic deceleration energies caused by the accident. Only violent trauma will rupture or avulse the BP. Such violence will frequently produce regional injuries [6].

Fractures

When associated with BPI, fractures have a sinister significance, e.g. fractures of the transverse processes of the lower cervical vertebrae, and fractures or dislocation of the neck of the first and second ribs are consistent with lower root avulsions.

A rupture of the subclavian or axillary artery in young patients is practically always accompanied by ruptures of nerve trunks, cords, terminal branches or root avulsions. In 57 consecutive cases of injury to these vessels, there has been only one case in a young patient in whom portions of the plexus were not ruptured but only elongated (degrees 2 and 3 of severity of injury), therefore not requiring nerve repair. Conversely, two patients aged over 60 years presented with an axillary artery lesion, one after a fall from her own height dislocating the shoulder, the other after receiving a blow to the upper

Table 16.4(a) Pathology found at operation in 100 consecutive patients with a total BP palsy persisting 2 months or more after the accident

Macroscopical pathology	*N*	*Missed pre- or peroperative diagnosis*
Avulsion of C5 through T1	14	2 partial Brown–Séquard syndromes
Rupture of C5 through T1	4	2 avulsions C8–T1 and one C7–T1
Rupture of C5, avulsion C6 through T1	23	
Elongation of C5, avulsion C6 through T1	3	
Rupture of C5–C6, avulsion C7–C8–T1	22	one C6 avulsion
Rupture of C5–C6, various injuries to C7–C8–T1	3	
Avulsion of C5–C6, elongation C7–C8–T1	1	one avulsion of C7
Elongation of C5–C6–C7, avulsion C8–T1	11	one avulsion of C7
Rupture C5–C6–C7, elongation C8–T1	3	
Rupture C5, avulsion C6, rupture C7–C8–T1	2	
Rupture C5, avulsion C6, rupture C7, elongation C8–T1	1	
Rupture C5–C6, elongation C7, avulsion C8–T1	1	
Avulsion C5, rupture C6, avulsion C7–T1	2	
Elongation of all primary trunks	1	
Elongation of cords and terminal branches	2	one avulsion of C7
Rupture of cords and/or terminal branches	6	

In 76 patients there were root avulsions at operation; in 6 they were missed, giving a total of 82 patients with root avulsions.

Table 16.4(b)   Pathology found at operation in 50 consecutive patients with apparently partial supraclavicular BPI persisting 2–12 months after injury

	N	Remarks
Clinical palsy (C4) C5–C6		
Elongation C5–C6 ± suprascapular nerve	4	
Elongation C5–C6, musculocutaneous and axillary nerves	3	2 partial C5–C6 avulsions not recognized
Elongation C5, avulsion C6	1	
Rupture C5, elongation C6 ± suprascapular nerve	2	
Rupture C5–C6	6	
Rupture C5, avulsion C6	2	
Avulsion C5–C6	4	one partial Brown–Séquard syndrome not recognized
Clinical palsy (C4) C5, C6, C7		
Elongation C5–C6–C7	3	one axillary nerve rupture found and repaired
Rupture C5, avulsion C6, elongation C7	1	one axillary and musculo-cutaneous nerve found and repaired
Rupture C5–C6, elongation C7	2	
Rupture C5–C6–C7	5	
Rupture C5, avulsion C6–C7	3	
Avulsion C5–C6, elongation C7	1	
Avulsion C5–C6–C7	4	one partial Brown–Séquard syndrome not recognized
Clinical palsy C7–C8–T1 or C8–T1		
C5–C6 normal, C7 elongation C8–T1 avulsion	1	
C5–C6 normal, avulsion C7–C8–T1	4	one rupture of musculocutaneous nerve found and one of axillary nerve
C5–C6–C7 normal, elongation C8–T1	2	
C5 to C7 normal, avulsion C8–T1	1	
C5–C6 normal, avulsion C7 ⎫ C8–T1 ruptured ⎬	1	

N.B. In 44% of patients with incomplete supra-clavicular lesions there are root avulsions and in 8% two level injury is present.

chest. The vascular lesion of the brittle artery was similar to a fracture and less like a rupture caused by elongation. Both patients had 2–3 degrees nerve injuries, i.e. without interruption; therefore they did not require nerve repair and the function of their limbs recovered fairly well in 1½ years. The author has seen also three cases of acute thrombosis, one of the axillary and two of the subclavian artery, followed by a complete BP infraclavicular palsy, i.e. without any mechanical trauma. Pathogenesis of BP palsy with 'fractures' of atheromatous arteries after minor trauma could be analogous to the ones seen in thrombosis. Similarly, ulnar artery thrombosis in the Guyon's canal also produces a complete distal ulnar nerve palsy.

Other associated and relatively minor injuries

Table 16.5 give useful information with regards to regional associated lesions seen in BPI. We have studied the frequency of BP in trauma to the cervical spine [7], of the shoulder girdle and arm using the files of Lausanne's University Hospital, and from several main trauma centres in Switzerland. An error varying from 2 to 3% has to be admitted, e.g. shoulder dislocations may present with a suprascapular, an axillary musculo-cutaneous nerve palsy or a mild BP involvement which are not diagnosed during ambulatory treatment or a short stay in hospital. Diagnosis will be made later and will not necessarily appear in the hospital files. In this region with a popu-

Table 16.5   Associated lesions in 300 consecutive patients with traction BPI

Regional trauma	Complete supraclavicular palsies C5 – T1 n = 168		Incomplete supraclavicular palsies				Extended or limited infraclavicular palsies n = 47	
			C5–C6 (C7) n = 79		(C7)C8–T1 n = 6			
	n	%	n	%	n	%	n	%
Lateral fractures of cervical spine	9	5.3	2	2.5	1	16.7	0	0
Fractures and dislocations of first rib, and first and second ribs	10	5.9	0	0	2	33.3	0	0
Fractures of the scapula	43	25.6	8	10.1	0	0	4	8.5
Acromio-clavic ⎱ joint or sterno-clavic ⎰ disloc.	10	5.9	3	3.8	1	16.7	2	4.3
Fractures of clavicle	17	10.1	4	5.1	0	0	2	4.3
Proximal humerus fract.	17	10.1	2	2.5	1	16.7	4	8.5
Fract. of scapula and clavicle and/or of proximal humerus	11	6.5	1	1.3	0	0	2	4.3
Ruptures of the rotator cuff	4	2.4	3	3.8	0	0	5	10.6
Disloc. of the shoulder	3	1.8	6	7.6	1	16.7	6	12.8
Multitrauma to upper limb	12	7.1	0	0	0	0	4	8.5
Partial Brown–Séquard syn.	5	3	1	1.3	0	0	0	0
Rupture of subclavian or axillary artery	32	19	3	3.8	1	16.7	6	12.8
Rupture of artery and vein	4	2.4	0	0	0	0	2	4.3
Rupture of the vein alone	1	0.6	0	0	0	0	1	2.1

lation of half a million, the author sees practically all the cases of BPI and the error rate of our hospital statistics could be ascertained. Initially it is very difficult to diagnose a partial BPI or an isolated nerve palsy in a patient with multiple trauma who is possibly unconscious. Even in shoulder dislocation producing acute distress it requires much experience to establish a supra-scapular or an axillary nerve palsy. We have proceeded to routine EMG in traumatic humero-scapular dislocations in 34 consecutive cases before that study was stopped for ethical reasons. In over 70% of cases (25 patients) there were significant alterations in the deltoid (fibrillations, etc.), showing that a partial lesion of the axillary nerve was present. Only five patients in this group presented with a clinical palsy; three required exploration and the nerve was ruptured in two, continuous in one. The latter did not recover satisfactorily after neurolysis, whereas the other two did well after grafting. We should have resected the rosary type lesion in continuity and grafted the defect. This shows that not only the diagnosis is difficult clinically but even the sever-

ity of lesions can be misinterpreted at operation by an experienced surgeon such as the author who has operated on 103 axillary nerves.

Analysis of 994 cases of trauma to the shoulder girdle (Table 16.6) admitted to three hospitals shows clearly that there is a considerable difference regarding nerve injury between cases with lesions to isolated structures of the shoulder girdle and those who have multiple regional or general injuries from a violent accident. One patient out of three with severe cervical shoulder girdle and general trauma will present a BPI or related nerve injury. Fifty-eight percent of these patients were motorcycle riders or passengers. About 1.3% of patients admitted to hospital with significant multiple injuries to the upper limbs (fractures, dislocations, etc.) after a motorcycle accident present a BP or a related nerve injury, while this incidence is 15 times less in occupants of cars. In 115 consecutive cases with fractures of the cervical spine and no spinal cord injury, three patients (2.6%) presented a BPI all associated with fractures of segments C4 to C7 (51 cases); none with fractures of segments C1 to C3 (64

Table 16.6   Incidence of BP and related nerve injuries in shoulder girdle trauma
n* = 994 patients admitted to 3 hospitals

Diagnosis		n *patients*	n *with diagnosed nerve injuries*	%
A.	Severe blunt trauma including contused wounds but no dislocations nor fractures	48	2	4.2
	One bone or one joint injured	537	7	1.3
	Several shoulder girdle structures injured	349	31	8.9
	Extended shoulder girdle and general trauma	60	19	31.7
		994	59	5.9
B.	1. any shoulder dislocation	219	24	11
	2. proximal humerus fract.	254	8	3.1
	3. fract. clavicle	234	7	3
	4. AC jt dislocation	105	1	0.97
	5. fract. scapula	90	8	8.9
	6. fract. scapula and clavicle	18	4	22.2
	7. AC dislocation, fract. of proximal humerus	5		
	8. shoulder dislocation and fract. prox. humerus	13	2	15.4
	9. scapula and shoulder dislocation	8	2	25
	10. fract. scapula, shoulder and AC joint dislocation	2	1	50
		946	57	

* I am indebted to Dr. R. Blatter from the General Hospital, Bellinzona, to Professors J. J. Livio and S. Krupp from the University Hospital, Lausanne, and to Professor W. Taillard from the University Hospital Geneva, for making their statistics available.

cases). Conversely in 600 consecutive BPI 53 patients (8.8%) presented with fractures of the cervical spine. There were four at the level of C1 to C3 and 49 (92.5%) at the level from C4 to T1 including the first rib. In particular, fractures of transverse processes are frequent in these cases (32 patients of 49, i.e. 65%) while vertebral bodies were fractured in only 16 patients (32.7%) and articular processes in nine patients (18.4%).

Spontaneous recovery

Bonney [8], Yeoman [9], Wynn Parry [10,11], Sedel [12], Ransford and Hughes [13], and the author have followed a certain number of patients with complete palsies of the upper limb after BPI under conservative treatment observing spontaneous recovery. Though these authors have not always used the same criteria for evaluation, a comparison between these studies has been attempted in Table 16.7. This table shows essentially that after excluding those with neuropraxia approximately 45% of patients with a total palsy persisting a few months will stay that way for ever. A detailed study of our series of 50 patients who were not operated on for various reasons (infection, late referral, operations refused, etc.) though they would have been if it had been possible, shows that there are seven patterns of recovery:

Group 1: 2 patients
All recovered well except those with involvement of C7.
Group 2: 8 patients
C5/6 lesions recovered well; C7 poor recovery and C8/T1 no recovery at all.
Group 3: 4 patients
C5 recovered well; C6 and C7 poor recovery and C8/T1 no recovery at all (myelography carried out in only 2 and avulsion of C8 and T1 nerve roots confirmed).
Group 4: 13 patients
Minimal recovery in C5 and C6 but none elsewhere. All had Horner's syndrome. Myelography was carried out in eight patients and all revealed multiple root avulsions.
Group 5: 3 patients
All had Horner's syndrome. One myelograph performed which showed avulsion of C8 and T1 nerve roots. All three patients showed some recovery in C7 but none elsewhere.
Group 6: 14 patients

Table 16.7 Spontaneous recovery in complete traumatic brachial plexus injuries

Authors	n *patients*	n *with recovery*	%	Shoulder %		Elbow %		Wrist %		Fingers %	
				Add	*Abd*	*Fl*	*Ex*	*Fl*	*Ex*	*Fl*	*Ex*
Bonney (4)	19	12	63	63	16	32	32	26	0	21	0
Yeoman (18)	99	53	53	45?	3	50	30	23	7	9	7
Wynn Parry (16)	23*	3	13	13	0	13	0	13	0	13	0
Sedel (12)	65	44	68	?	18	35	25	27	0	23	11
Wynn Parry (17)	several hundred		approx. 67	70	10	50	30	20	?	20	?
Narakas	50	30	60	58	18	30	18	28	4	18	4
	Average percentage of recovery		54	50	11	35	23	23	2	17	4

N.B. External rotation in the shoulder was studied only by Bonney and Narakas, noting recovery respectively in 10.5% and 14%, i.e. an average of 12% of patients.
* 14 amputees in Wynn–Parry series.

All had Horner's syndrome. Myelography carried out in 9; avulsions of lower 3 roots in 4 patients and all roots C6–T1 in the other 5.
Group 7: 6 patients
Some recovery in C8/T1 but none elsewhere. One had Horner's syndrome.

Twenty-three patients in this series which were similar to those reported by Yeoman had marked or severe pain. Thirty-four were involved in a motor cycle accident. The follow-up ranged from 3 to 27 years; mean 5.6 years.

Motor recovery in 50 patients in the non-operative series. Muscle power to M3 [MRC grading (6) = contraction against gravity] or better:

Protective skin sensibility

Eleven patients in groups 1, 2, 3 and 7 recovered protective skin sensibility in the median; and 7 in groups 1, 5 and 7 in the ulnar distribution.

Conclusion

The varied pattern of recovery in this relatively small series of patients who did not undergo operative treatment serves to show the wide area of damage that can be inflicted by traction on the plexus (Table 16.4).

Group 1: C7 involvement

In group 1 there was 1 normal myelogram but a lesion in continuity of the upper and lower trunks and either a rupture of the middle trunk or possible avulsion of C7 nerve root. Isolated rupture of C7 is rare.

The author has seen one case of isolated C7 avulsion without any marked injury to the remaining plexus caused by sudden traction on the arm: a nurse when running down steps was passing her finger along the vertical bars of the rail when her hand got caught. She presented an immediate isolated motor and partially sensory loss of C7 function, with temporary urine retention and transient paraesthesiae in her homolateral lower extremity. Lumbar puncture showed blood in her CSF fluid and twice the normal albumin content. A myelography was refused by the patient whose upper limb recovered almost completely in 2 years. However, she still presents an atrophy of the middle portion of her pectoralis major, upper portion of latissimus dorsi and some weakness of wrist flexion. Power of her grip is diminished by 25% compared to the dominant other hand.

Group 2

Group 2 patients must have had an elongation of the upper trunk, partial rupture of C7 and probably an avulsion of C8–T1 in six patients who had Horner's syndrome (two positive myelographies); a crush injury to the lower trunk in two patients (one normal myelography) with no Horner's syndrome. After 2–3 years their residual palsy was very similar to that of a Klumpke's paralysis.

Group 3

Group 3 patients had an elongation in continuity (degrees 2–3 of Sunderland) of C5, and severe disruptions and/or avulsions of the other roots are even worse.

Group 4

They must have had a degree 3–4 injury to the upper trunk.

Group 5

Group 5 patients probably had a lower root avulsion (all presented with a Horner's syndrome) a rupture of the upper trunk and a degree 3–4 to C7.

Group 6

Group 6 patients had complete either C5–T1 avulsions or rupture of C5, and C6–T1 avulsions.

Group 7

Group 7 had upper root avulsions and/or ruptures, with degrees 2, 3, 4 injury to C8–T1.

Direct operative treatment

Brachial plexus surgery has evolved over the years and there is little sense in detailing what has been done in the past. The indication for operation remains the same: young patients who present with a total palsy after a violent deceleration accident. The operation is then performed as early as the condition of the patient permits,

particularly when a vascular injury is present and the limb is well perfused. Vascular and nerve repair are then carried out simultaneously. In cases when vascular repair is urgent the plexus surgeon or any surgeon belonging to his team are called to evaluate the lesions and the arterial reconstruction is performed when possible outside the plexus. Nerve repair is done later when it is not possible as an emergency. Emergency nerve repair is very rarely carried out in traction injuries. It is, however, performed in low velocity missile wounds or lacerations to produce gratifying results even when lesions are close to the foramen or intraforaminal. This confirms that contrary to traction these type of injuries (as iatrogenic sections) do not produce any important retrograde degeneration. In patients with partial palsy (e.g. Erb's type) repeated clinical examinations are carried out including the study of evoked potentials and when possible in the first few days before distal nerve degeneration occurs. Except for C5, which is difficult to test, the level of lesions of C6 and C7 may be determined. When the surgeon is convinced that ruptures and/or root avulsions are present there is no sense in procrastinating with a persisting palsy, and exploration is carried out as early as possible before scarred tissue occurs. Dissection is thereby facilitated. The extent of injury is often devastating; in half of the cases it was worse than expected. Only in two occasions out of more than 400 operations, was no macroscopical lesion found, one in a case of possible hysteria after a deep wound opening the humero-scapular joint, the other presenting with motor loss inconsistent with the sensory loss. Both patients made a complete recovery within a month from surgery when nothing had been done other than to inspect the supra and infraclavicular plexus by a wide exposure and perform peroperative stimulation.

Delayed operation

Patients were observed and operation was delayed when the degree of trauma overall was insufficient to avulse or rupture the brachial plexus; or in the absence of vascular injury, neighbouring fractures and in particular when the sensory loss was less extensive than the motor. When there is incomplete loss of sensation the patient is always treated conservatively and examined at regular intervals; weekly in the first month; then monthly. EMG and conduction tests are performed from the 18th post-trauma day. CT scan, myelography and MRI are confined to those who are candidates for surgery.

Only four patients with incomplete sensory loss corresponding to their involved motor territory had to come to operation because they failed to recover within their expected time, i.e. 6–9 months after injury. They had either partial trunk or cord lesions requiring grafting in three and neurolysis in one.

Correlation between sensory and motor loss

This is a reliable method of evaluating degrees of injury more severe than degree 1 (neurapraxia), bearing in mind that variations of sensory innervation are less precise than motor distribution.

Degree of damage

The importance of distinguishing between neurapraxia, axonotmesis and neurotmesis has to be stressed because at present only neurotmesis requires early repair (degrees 4 and 5, plus root avulsion). We have never seen neurapraxia affecting the entire plexus, although electrocution will produce a clinical state approaching this widespread neurapraxia. In our experience there was apparent total paralysis but further testing revealed M1 function in most muscle groups and incomplete sensory loss. By contrast, numerous cases have been observed of pure neurapraxia of some structures of the BP while others were normal or totally paralysed. Invariably some degree of sensation could be elicited when palsy seemed to be total, but sometimes involuntary defence movements were possible. Without implying psychogenic attitudes, it seems to the author that sensory and motor functions offer basically different mechanisms. Sensation is a passive function imposed to a large extent on an individual by the environment. Motor function, excluding reflexes, requires volition, i.e. active participation. The former is less likely to be suppressed than the latter. So far the author has seen only three cases of so-called hysterical BP palsy, one ending with a subcapital amputation of the upper limb after 5 years of unsuccessful psychi-

atric treatment. The patient, who because of her palsy, had become a total invalid moving about in a wheelchair, resumed walking 1 week after amputation, regained normal behaviour, returned to a successful professional life, became an international swimming champion, married, had children, etc. She cannot explain today why a simple carpal tunnel operation under plexus block caused a total persisting BP palsy. I did explore her plexus 1 year after the surgery, finding no lesions and all muscles responding to peroperative stimulation. Five years later I amputated her arm which was still functional according to electrophysiological investigations. The reader may imagine how difficult it was after exploring the plexus for a second time and finding no lesions to decide to amputate after receiving advice by several psychiatrists who had treated or seen the patient.

Surgical reconstruction

Goals of repair

The restoration and planning of function of a paralysed upper limb depends on the extent of the paralysis weighed against the known results of available reconstructive operations or prosthetic and orthotic devices [14].

There are contradicting patterns in use depending on the parts affected. A patient with a paralytic hand and a normal shoulder and elbow will use his dominant or non-dominant extremity mainly for coarse activities. Conversely, a patient with a paralytic shoulder, a good elbow and a normal hand will restrict the use of his limb to refined activities provided this extremity is dominant. When it is not, the hand will be only a 'helping hand'; it is rare for that hand to be used to initiate an activity followed by the other. The shoulder, which has the highest mobility of all our joints, serves to position the hand, but there are other important functions concerning balance of the body, protecting it, etc. At present the author considers that the shoulder and elbow function have to be favoured when basic requirements of a non-dominant upper limb have to be satisfied, bearing in mind that good hand function cannot be reconstructed in total BP palsies. Basic hand functions (key-pinch, grasp and protective sensation) have a subsidiary role in recon-

Table 16.8(a)   Graphical representation of function gained by direct surgical treatment (sutures, grafts, neurotizations) in total BP palsies with complete interruptions (lesions in continuity excluded): Root avulsions: ●; Ruptures of nerves: //. The criteria of evaluation are given in Table 16.9. The height of each line represents the result achieved in each individual case. Results improve when more than one proximal stump is available to be connected to the periphery

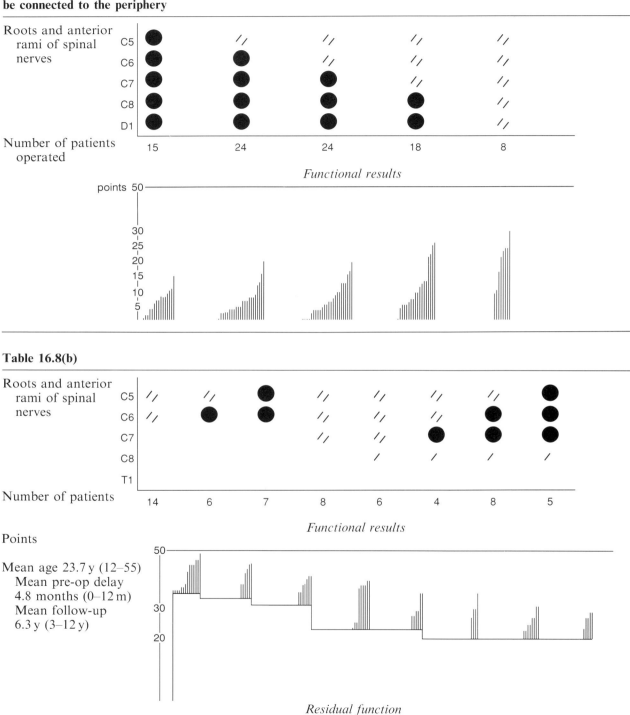

Table 16.8(b)

Residual function

Table 16.8(c)

Posterior cord ruptures

Pattern of ruptures:	Isolated	+ SS	+ MC	+ SS MC	+ MC MED	+ All term branches
Number of patients operated	6	5	5	4	4	4

Mean age 21.7 y (13–34)
  Mean pre-op delay
  4.2 mo (15–7)
  Mean follow-up
  4.8 y (3–10)

Residual function

---

struction. Therefore, the basic requirements in restoring some function to a totally paralysed upper extremity are as follows :

1. Thoraco-humeral grasp, i.e. adduction of the humerus against the chest, and if possible the opening of the pinching element, i.e. abduction of the humerus with a stable humero-scapular joint and sensation on the thorax and opposite inner aspect of the arm.
2. Elbow flexion and internal rotation of the humerus; when possible, some external rotation to allow opening and closing of the antebrachio-thoracic grasp.
3. and 4. Flexion and extension of the wrist. Active flexion allows opening of the fingers provided they are not totally clawed. Extension, particularly when powerful, allows the reconstruction of grasp or pinch with a paralytic hand. Primitive sensation in the radial fingers is also a prerequisite.
5. Active thumb adduction, possibly abduction, to allow a key pinch and a fair sensation in order to use it.
6. Active finger PIP flexion combined to MP flexion produced by a tenodesis effect.
7. Active MP and PIP extension or obtained by any ancillary function (flexion of the wrist) by a tenodesis effect.

8. The last and ultimate is pollici-digital pulp to pulp pinch with a good sensation, and fourth and fifth finger flexion to obtain a locking effect on objects held in the hand.

Techniques of repair according to pathology

In complete root avulsion C5–T1 the goal is to reconstruct thoraco-brachial grasp, stabilize the shoulder, restore elbow flexion and internal and external rotation of the humerus; to restore sensation to the inner aspect of arm (usually preserved by the injury), outer aspect of forearm and even thumb and index (C5–C6 dermatomes). First of all we need scapulo-thoracic and scapulo-humeral function. The serratus anterior is all important to provide abduction of the arm and flexion (anterior projection) when a scapulo-humeral arthrodesis has been performed. The lower digitations of the serratus anterior are more efficient and they are innervated through C7, partially through C6. But these roots are avulsed. This means that either we reinnervate these digitations using intercostal nerves or we give them up for a modest opening and closing of

Table 16.9   Evolution of basic functions of the upper limb points

Shoulder (max. 13 points)	0	1	2	3	4	5
Abduction and/or forward flexion (any of both better prevailing) (max. 5 points)	0° Flail joint, no active function, humero-scapular dislocation >1 cm	0–30° Stable, humero-scapular dislocation <1 cm	30–60°	60–90° With extended extremity	90–120° (at 60° with 1 kg at least at wrist level on extended limb)	>120° or at 90° with 3 kg at wrist with extended arm
External rotation (max. 4 points)	0° Forearm in passive or active flexion of elbow cannot be brought away from chest	Forearm can be brought by 5–10° away from chest	Forearm (elbow flexed) can be brought by 10–30° away from chest	Forearm (elbow flexed) can be brought by 30–60° (60° means that the forearm is in sagittal plane) from chest	Forearm (elbow flexed) can be more than 60° away from chest (outside sagittal plane) or to sagittal plane against resistance	
Thoraco-brachial grasp, i.e. abduction and/or internal rotation when elbow can be actively flexed (max. 2 points)	Cannot hold anything between arm/forearm and chest wall	Can hold a patient's file under arm	Can hold a bag of 1 kg and more between chest and arm			
Posterior projection (max. 2 points)	None	Wrist with elbow in extension can be brought to lateral aspect of gluteus (slit of pocket)	Wrist can be brought behind plane of glutei or better or patient can push something behind him (e.g. shifting gears of a car)			

External rotation arm in abduction is not evaluated. This basic function would deserve at least 2 points. However this additional score would emphasize external rotation as being a very important basic function deserving 6 points, i.e. 4 points for external rotation in the transverse plane (arm in adduction against the chest) and 2 points in the sagittal plane (arm in abduction). There is no doubt that compared to the points awarded for other functions, this way to evaluate would give an undeserved importance to external rotation.

Table 16.9 (continued)

Elbow (max. 9 points)	*0*	*1*	*2*	*3*	*4*	*5*
Flexion (5 points)	Not possible or insignificant	Hand to pocket or belt	To 90° against gravity	To 90° with 1 kg in hand or 1.5 kg at wrist	To 90° and more with 3 kg in hand or 4.5 kg at wrist	Flexes 90° and more with 5 kg or 7.5 kg at wrist
Extension (4 points)	Not possible	Extends arm in passive abduction and full internal rotation to full passive ROM against gravity	Extends with 1 kg in hand or 1.5 kg at wrist	Extends with 3 kg in hand or 4.5 kg at wrist	Better than 3 kg in hand or 4.5 kg at wrist	
Forearm prono-supination (max. 3 points)	None	Only incomplete pronation or supination	Both functions present totalling 50°	Both functions totalling 100°		
Wrist (max. 8 points)		Against gravity (forearm in supination)	With 1 kg in hand	With 3 kg	Better than 3 kg	
Flexion (4 points)	None					
Extension (4 points)	None	Incomplete against gravity	Complete against gravity	With 1 kg in hand or against strong grasp (5–10 kg/cm²)	More than 1 kg or grasp of over 10 kg/cm²	

The position of weights along the limb plays a definite role because of the lever momentum.
Flexion of elbow at 90° with 3 kg suspended on the upper third of the forearm has not the same meaning as the same flexion with the same weight suspended at the wrist level or held in the hand.

the thoraco-brachial pinch being effected by the trapezius, levator scapulae and rhomboids. A very valuable solution is to reinnervate the supra-scapular nerve with a transfer of the distal portion of the accessory nerve; a solution which produces good function of the upper trapezius, sometimes fair function of the middle trapezius because of satellite innervation and an active abduction between scapula and humerus of at least 50°. This will bring the arm almost to 90° away from the thorax provided the scapula can be stabilized against the thorax or rotated outwards due to reinnervation of the lower digitations of the serratus anterior. Internal rotation of the humerus can be obtained by reinnervating the sternal portion of pectoralis major with one intercostal nerve, and flexion of the elbow is obtained using two or three intercostal nerves

Table 16.9 (continued)

Hand (max. 17 points)	0	1	2	3	4	5
Long fingers motor (max. 5 points)	Total palsy (no flexion, no extension). Hand is a passive, flail weight	Passive hook (fingers are flexed in a position either by contracture or active muscle function, an active closure of fist not possible. Patient can hook on something he uses the hand as a kind of shovel or spoon	Active hook by active finger flexion (primitive grasp) from a half open position the long fingers can be brought down to touch the palm. Patient can hold something	Opening and closing of fist. Grasp power less 3 kg/cm² (Jamar dynamometer)	Good function of long fingers for flexion and extension. Grasp power 3–8 kg/cm² (Jamar dynamometer)	Fair independence of fingers. Grasp 8 kg (Jamar dynamometer)
				One point is subtracted if finger extension (opening) is not possible		
		Adduction or flexion present (key pinch) no opening	Closure and opening of key pinch	Pulp to pulp pinch		
Thumb motor (max. 3 points)	Total palsy		Power up to 1 kg/cm²	Key pinch over 1 kg/cm²		
				One point is subtracted if extension of thumb (opening) is not possible.		

It has been admitted, however disputable, that the most primitive function of the hand is to be a 'paper weight' or a kind of spoon or shovel (e.g. arthrogrypotic, sclerodermic and other patients with analogous type of deformity). A totally paralytic hand or unstable as in advanced rheumatoid arthritis has not even that function. The next functional step seems to be a hook enabling the patient to carry a bag whether it is produced by stiffness of the joints or active long finger flexor function. This function in daily life seems to be equivalent to a key pinch. Correlation of motor function of the hand seems to be thumb to pulp pinch and independence of finger motion. In brachial plexus injury sophisticated hand function is beyond the possibilities of nerve repair. Therefore it is only grossly evaluated.

transferred onto the lateral cord. Some sensory rami originating from C4 may also be transferred to the lateral cord to provide protective sensation which is initially referred to the shoulder then, after 2–3 years, referred to the antero-lateral aspect of arm, thumb and index; possibly the middle finger. Transfers of intercostal nerves to the lateral cord may sometimes produce an M2+

Table 16.9 (continued)

	0	*1*	*2*	*3*	*4*	*5*
5th finger motor 1 point	No strong flexion 0	Strong flexion (locking position when a knife or the handle of a tool is held in the hand)	—	—	—	—
Sensory (8 points) median n. area 5 points (pulp of thumb, index and long fingers)	No sensation	Temperature and pain felt, paraesthesias disturbing or not	Touch felt (without disturbing paraesthesias) no dysaesthesia	Light touch felt without paraesthesias gross localisation	Some tactile gnosis Weber above 15 mm	Fair tactile gnosis Weber below 15 mm
Ulnar nerve area 3 points (pulps of 4th and 5th fingers)	No sensation	Temperature and pain felt, paraesthesias disturbing or not	Touch felt (without disturbing paraesthesias) no dysaesthesia	One point is subtracted if dysaesthesia is present, two if hyperpathia is present		

The final result consists of the residual function, the function gained by operation and the function obtained by spontaneous regeneration. In complete paralysis the residual function is nil. When all spinal nerves are interrupted the final result corresponds to the gain obtained by operation. When some nerves are not functional but are not interrupted anatomically (degrees 1 to 3 of Sunderland) recovery by spontaneous regeneration has to be evaluated and subtracted from the final result in order to obtain the gain yielded by surgical nerve reconstruction.
In incomplete paralysis the maximal loss caused by nerve interruption has to be evaluated against the loss caused by degrees 1 to 3 of Sunderland in order to assess the gain obtained by nerve repair of degrees 4 and 5 and root avulsion.

to M3 flexion of the wrist but unfortunately not strong enough to reconstruct a useful key-pinch. The patients ask for it once they have a stable shoulder and M4 elbow flexion.

In C5 rupture and C6 through T1 root avulsion, we use presently the distal spinal accessory nerve to neurotize the suprascapular nerve. Part of C5 is connected to the lateral fascicles of the posterior cord (axillary nerve fibres); the anterior fascicular groups of C5 are connected to fascicles in the lateral cord going to the anterior thoracic nerves for the pectoralis major; the remaining to fascicles innervating the musculo-cutaneous nerve, while one or two intercostal nerves re-innervate the lower digitations of the serratus anterior. Intercostal nerves can be used to rein-nervate the anterior and inferior thoracic nerves as an alternative to C5 which will reinnervate the serratus. There is no doubt at present that healthy nerves such as the spinal accessory, deep motor branches from the cervical plexus and intercostals have a potential for reinnervation superior to that of ruptured C5 when C6 through T1 are avulsed. Histological examination of the last slice cut when trimming the proximal stump of C5 has shown that in more than half of the cases 80% of the fibres were damaged, thus demonstrating the ascending character of traction lesions. In C5–C6 ruptures and lower root avulsions a maximum effort of repair is devoted to the shoulder and elbow, but also attempting to obtain some wrist extensor reinnervation; a goal, alas, we fail to reach in many cases. It is easier to reconstruct a grasp with the hand when powerful wrist extensors are available. C5 can, in conjunction with the spinal accessory nerve or on its own, be connected to nerves commanding the shoulder; while C6 is used for elbow and wrist flexion, elbow extension and/or wrist extension. Combined contractions are frequent and can be used for transfer to an antagonist. Intercostals are used on fascicles originating from C7, either its posterior or anterior division. The former choice gives better results than the latter.

In C5–C6–C7 ruptures with lower root avulsion the BP is reconstructed as anatomically as possible using the XIth nerve for the suprascapular and connecting at least the motor fascicles of C8 to the proximal stump of C7 (plexoplexal neurotization). Intercostals have been used to innervate the median or ulnar nerves with poor results.

In total ruptures of the primary trunks repair is carried out in order to reproduce the normal anatomy. It seems worthwhile to reconstruct the lower trunk C8–T1 when one is certain that the corresponding roots have not been avulsed, provided that the defect is not wider than 4 cm. Some function of the flexor carpi ulnaris and deep flexors of the third, fourth and fifth fingers can be expected. In partial BP palsies reconstruction is also performed according to the pathological findings. When C5 is ruptured and C6 avulsed, reconstruction is carried out by uniting the XIth nerve to the suprascapular nerve while grafts connect C5 to posterior and lateral cords. A marked or partial trumpet sign is always obtained, i.e. the patient compulsively flexes the elbow when he abducts the shoulder. He may, however, flex the elbow without abducting the shoulder using his pectoralis major to counterbalance the abductors. He may flex his arm with-

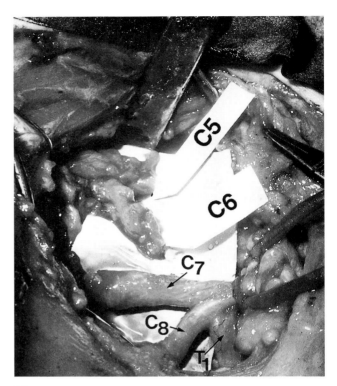

(a)

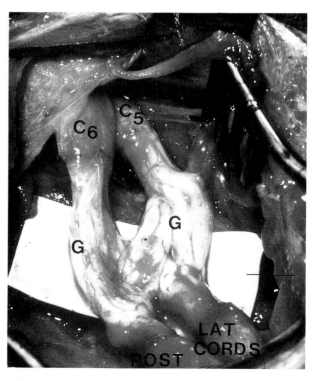

(c)

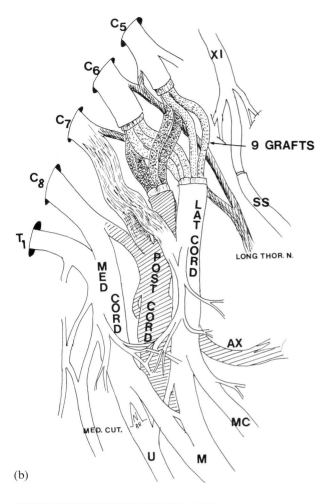

(b)

Fig. 16.1 (a) Lesions seen in a typical Erb's palsy: rupture of C5 and C6, elongation in continuity of C7 while C8 and T1 are normal (left plexus). (b) Drawing showing the repair performed: four grafts cover the proximal stump of C5, five grafts that of C6 while the spinal accessory nerve is used to neurotize the supra-scapular nerve. (c) Repair was performed using fibrin glue and a few stay stitches. The grafts will be spread on their bed (medial scalenus) for better revascularization. (d) Neurotization of the supra-scapular nerve (SS) with the distal branch of the spinal accessory nerve (XI). The preserved ramus for the upper portion of the trapezius can be seen disappearing under the labels.

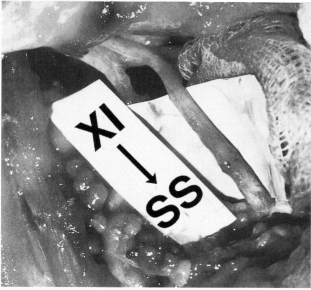

(d)

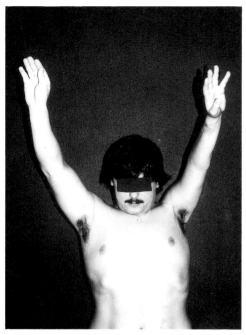

(a)

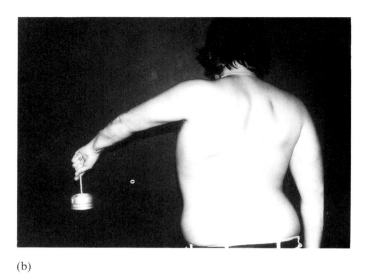

(b)

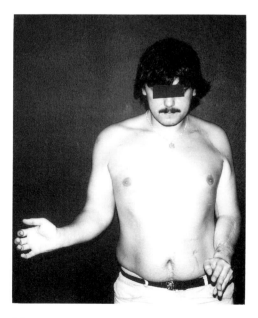

(c)

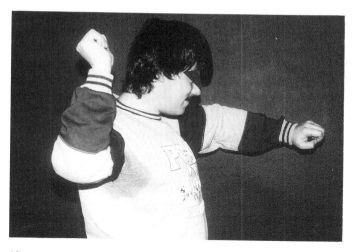

(d)

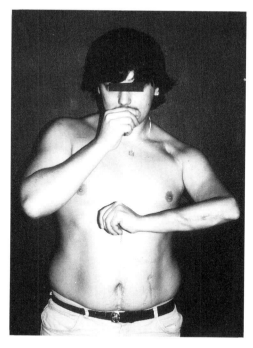

(e)

Fig. 16.2 Result 4 years after the repair illustrated in Fig. 16.1 (b–d). Forward elevation and abduction in the shoulder are good (a). The extremity, however, is in internal rotation (arm and forearm) and the power of abduction not impressive (b) as the patient reaches only 60° of global abduction carrying 2 kg in the hand. Note the paralysis of the lower portion of the trapezius and latissimus dorsi. The forearm is pronated. The lack of external rotation in the transverse and sagittal plane are well demonstrated (c and d). The patient was a victim of a motorcycle accident with multiple lesions. Visible scars relate to a laparotomy for splenic rupture and compound fractures of the forearm with a compartment syndrome (rupture of the subclavian artery). Because of inactivity after the accident he gained 20 kg in weight. The attempt to reach the mouth (e) shows the lack of external rotation of the humerus. Because the patient did not recover digit extension the flexor carpi ulnaris was transferred onto the common extensor of the fingers and onto the long extensor of the thumb with a satisfactory result (a) for the fingers and a poor result for the thumb (a and c). The tendon of the FCU passing over the dorsal aspect of the forearm is clearly visible (e) as well as the hyperactivity of the ulnar nerve (c) which tends to produce a flexion of the MP joints and hyperextension of the DIP joints. Three months later the humeral tendon of teres major was transferred onto the teres minor and infraspinatus tendons with a gain of 20° in external rotation. Note the maintained function of the upper trapezius. The patient can flex the elbow with 5 kg in his hand (not shown on photographs).

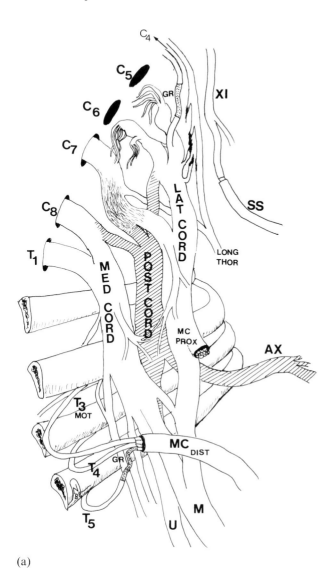

(a)

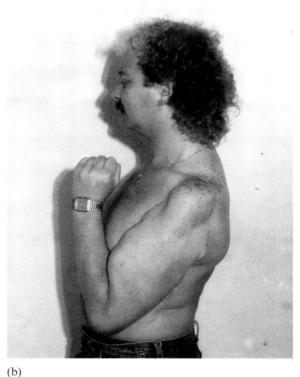

(b)

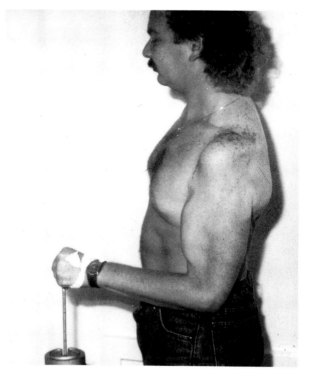

(c)

Fig. 16.3   By contrast, a patient with root avulsion C5–C6. The repair performed is shown in (a). Recovery of shoulder function is almost as good as in Fig. 16.2, but elbow flexion was incomplete and weak (M2+). A latissimus dorsi transfer was performed onto the biceps. Flexion is good (b) but the patient cannot lift more than 1.5 kg (c) held in the hand in spite of the impressive bulk of the muscle transferred. Note the partial winging of the scapula caused by a subtotal denervation of serratus anterior; also note the bulk of recovered deltoid.

out flexing the elbow; however external rotation when obtained is always linked with some abduction of the arm.

In C5–C6 ruptures reconstruction tries to reproduce the normal fascicular distribution, but the author favours the use of the XIth nerve to neurotize the supra-scapular nerve because the abduction between scapula and humerus is essential for acceptable shoulder function. Grafting the suprascapular nerve from C5 rarely gives satisfactory results because the cranial portion of C5 (12 o'clock) is particularly damaged in traction lesions and because simultaneous contractions between the spinati, teres major, subscapularis and pectoralis major are very common.

Reconstruction of cords and individual nerves

The lateral cord is rarely damaged. When it happens care must be taken to reconstruct the anterior thoracic nerves when there is a lower root palsy. Absence of pectoralis major function, usually in conjunction with subscapularis, latissimus dorsi and teres major function is very disturbing; the patient cannot adduct his arm unless he has very powerful biceps and coracobrachialis. He then has the feeling of a flail shoulder.

Lateral cord repair yields good results. The posterior cord is invariably injured in infraclavicular BPI because of its anchorage; isolated injuries to the posterior cord also occur. Reconstruction yields good results except for MP joint extension. The medial cord is rarely injured. Either C8 or T1 is avulsed; rarely, the lower primary trunk is ruptured; or the median, ulnar and medial cutaneous nerves are ruptured close to their origins. It is always worthwhile reconstructing them even if it takes years before recovery is seen in the forearm and hand.

Results of BP repair

In BPI supraclavicular lesions presenting with degrees 4, 5 and root avulsions, normal function of the limb has never been restored even when

lesions were limited to C5 and C6. Useful function has often been obtained but when it is not we question our pre- and peroperative diagnosis. Root avulsions have been misdiagnosed several times – occasionally our choices of repair was incorrect. For instance, the role of serratus anterior in shoulder function has only been recognized in the last 3 years, while the importance of the suprascapular nerve has been known for 2 decades. However, a possible rotator cuff rupture present in 3% of supraclavicular BPI has been identified only during the last 7 years. Brown–Sequard's partial syndromes have been missed initially in more than half of the cases; and the use of intercostal nerves in them has led to a partial or total failure. Avulsion of nerves from muscles (suprascapular from spinati, axillary from deltoid, median and radial from muscles in the forearm, musculo-cutaneous from biceps) have been recognized slowly over the years as well as fibrosis of muscles caused by ischaemia in late revascularizations of the limb. Pitfalls in BPI are more often encountered than thought of and the author has to admit many failures in the past caused by his incapacity to observe and identify pathological conditions which are now evident.

Infraclavicular BPI can yield excellent results provided the median and ulnar and to some extent radial nerve fibres have not been severely damaged. A distinction has to be made between mono- or bifunctional nerves such as the long thoracic, suprascapular, axillary and musculo-cutaneous nerves and the multifunctional nerves such as the radial, particularly ulnar and median nerves which convey impulses to numerous antagonist–agonist muscles and subtle sensory messages. Their normal function cannot be reconstructed satisfactorily whatever the refinement and minuteness of technique. When good or excellent results in their repair are obtained, either there is an anomalous innervation or the result is obtained by chance.

Reporting results of BPI is almost impossible [15–20] due to the complexity of functions in the upper limb. We have attempted together with P. Raimondi and A. Morelli from Legnano, Italy, to create an evaluation which takes into account only the basic functional requirements of the upper extremity (Table 16.8). The results obtained are represented in Table 16.9 and illustrated by Figs 16.1–16.6.

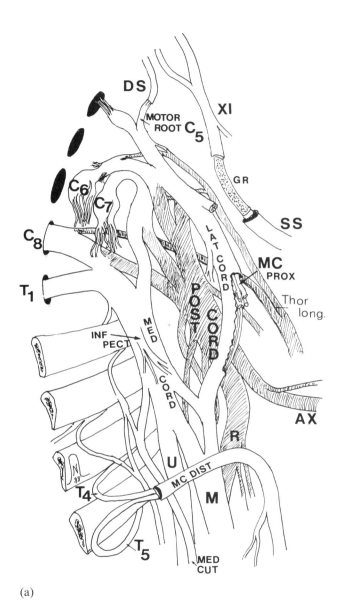

(a)

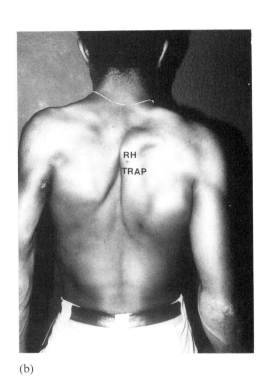

(b)

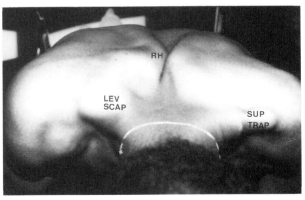

(c)

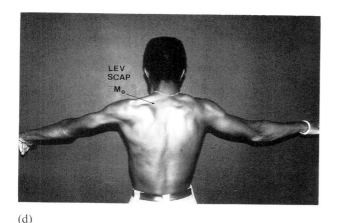

(d)

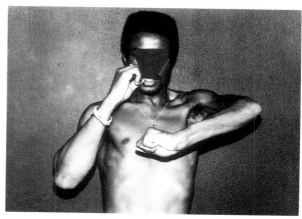

(f)

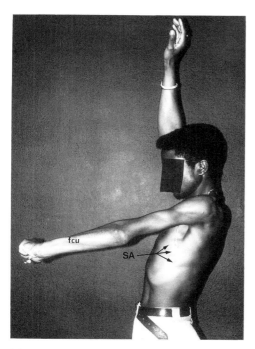

(e)

Fig. 16.4 Patient with root avulsion C5, C6 and C7 and minor stretch injury to C8 after a motorcycle accident operated 3 weeks post-trauma (see (a)). Photographs show the result 3 years and 9 months after operation. (b) demonstrates the palsy of middle and lower trapezius and of levator scapulae confirmed by the axial view (c) which demonstrates that the upper trapezius has recovered half of its bulk; (d) and (e) show the abduction and flexion in the shoulder; the recovery of deltoid and serratus anterior (lower digitations) is well demonstrated, also the transferred FCU onto EDC and EPL, while pronator teres was transferred onto ECRB, causing some radial deviation on extension of the wrist. The patient has full extension of the fingers (not shown here). (f) shows an attempt to bring the hand to the mouth; the lack of external rotation of the humerus is quite evident (e). This could be partially corrected by transferring the teres major (which has recovered to M4) tendon onto the external rotators. The biceps is only at M2+. The latissimus dorsi whose superior portion is at M2 and inferior at M4 could be transferred onto the biceps. The patient is, however, well adapted to his handicap and does not wish any further surgery.

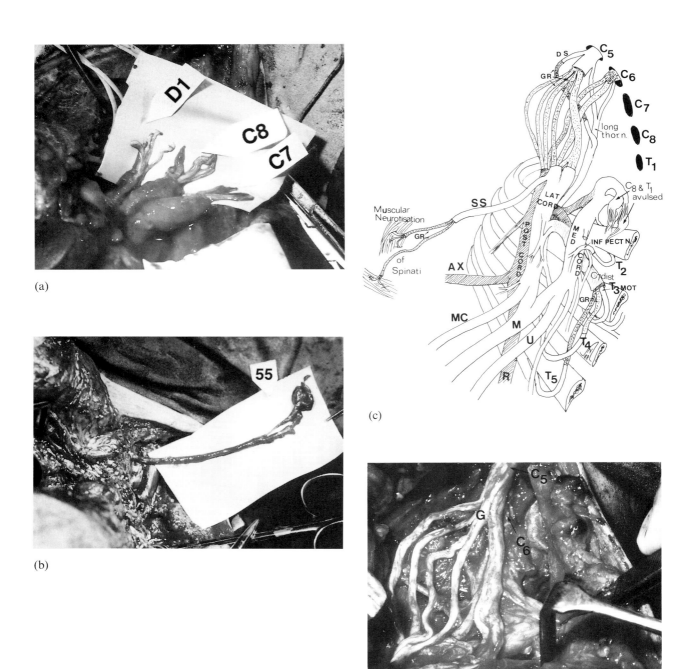

(a)

(b)

(c)

(d)

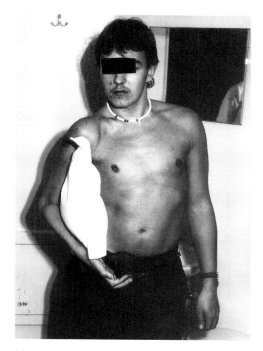

(e)

Fig. 16.5 Rupture of C5 and C6, root avulsion C7, C8 and T1 (a). The suprascapular nerve was avulsed from the spinati (b) and the proximal stump of C6 was poor. The repair was carried out according to drawing (c) and photograph (d). (e) shows the brachio-thoracic grasp (biceps at M3+ and triceps lateral portion at M2 synchronous to biceps, FCR at M2). (f) despite a deltoid at M3 the function of the shoulder is poor (spinati at M2); therefore the humero-scapular angle does not increase on attempted abduction and the scapula is lateralized by a strong serratus anterior (finger of examiner on tip of scapula). This shows the importance of good function of the suprascapular nerve, contrasting with Fig. 16.4.

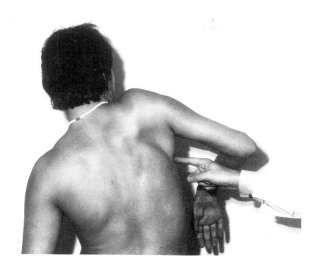

(f)

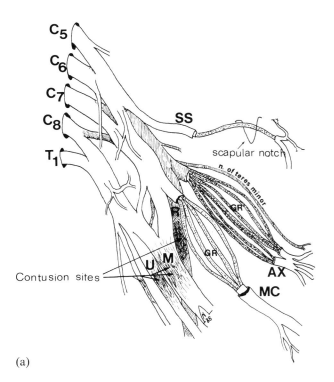

(a)

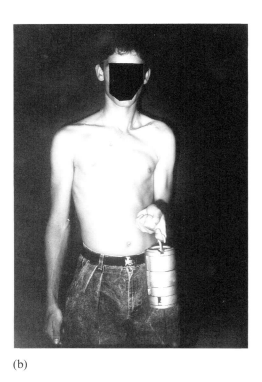

(b)

Fig. 16.6   This patient presented an axillary artery rupture and an extended brachial plexus palsy sparing the pectoralis major, teres major and minor and latissimus dorsi. At operation a suprascapular, axillary and musculo-cutaneous nerve ruptures were found; whereas the radial, median and ulnar nerves were contused but in continuity. Twelve grafts 7 cm long (both sural nerves were harvested) were used for the repair. His shoulder function, not shown here, is complete and powerful except for weak external rotation; the infra-spinatus did not recover for some unknown reason. His biceps is at M4+: he lifts 7 kg easily to 90° with one finger! This result demonstrates the striking contrast between supra-clavicular and more distal lesions with sparing of severe injuries to the ulnar, median and radial nerves.

References

1. Narakas, A. (1977) Indications et résultats du traitement chirurgical direct dans les lésions par élongation du plexus brachial. *Rev. Chir. Orthop. (Paris)*, **63**, 88–106.
2. Sunderland, S. (1951) A classification of peripheral nerve injuries producing loss of function. *Brain*, **74**, 491–516.
3. Medical Research Council (1954) *Peripheral Nerve Injuries*. HMSO, London, p. 4.
4. Seddon, H. J. (1943) Three types of nerve injury. *Brain*, **66**, 17–293.
5. Herzberg, G., Narakas, A., Comtet, J. J. *et al.* (1985) Microsurgical relations of the roots of the brachial plexus. Practical applications (in French and in English). *Ann. Chir. Main.*, **4**, 120–133.
6. Narakas, A. (1977) Les lésions dans les élongations du plexus brachail: différentes possibilités et associations lésionnelles. *Rev. Chir. Orthop. (Paris)*, **63**, 44–54.
7. Narakas, A. (1985) The treatment of brachial plexus injuries. *Int. Orthop. (SICOT)*, **9**, 29–36.
8. Bonney, G. (1959) Prognosis in traction lesions of the brachial plexus. *J. Bone Joint Surg.*, **41B**, 4–35.
9. Yeoman, P. M. (1975) *Traction Injuries of the Brachial Plexus*. Thesis for doctorate of Medicine, Cambridge (unpublished). Data in Seddon, H. J. (1975) *Surgical Disorders of the Peripheral Nerves*, 2nd edn. Churchill Livingstone, Edinburgh, p. 194.
10. Wynn Parry, C. B. (1974) The management of injuries to the brachial plexus. *Proc. R. Soc. Med. (London)*, **67**, 488–490.
11. Wynn Parry, C. B. (1978) Management of peripheral nerve injuries and traction lesions of the brachial plexus. *Int. Rehabil. Med.*, **1**, 9–20.

12. Sedel, L. (1977) Traitement palliatif d'une série de 103 paralysies par élongation du plexus brachial. Evolution spontanée et résultats. *Rev. Chir. Orthop. (Paris)*, **63**, 651–663.

13. Ransford, A. O. and Hughes, S. P. F. (1977) Complete brachial plexus lesions. *J. Bone Joint Surg.*, **59B**, 417–420.

14. Allieu, Y. Triki, F. and de Godebout, J. (1987) Complete brachial plexus paralysis. The value of preservation of the limb and restoration of active elbow flexion (in French). *Rev. Chir. Orthop. (Paris)*, **73**, 665–673.

15. Allieu, Y. Privat, J. M. and Bonel, F. (1984) Paralysis in root avulsion of the brachial plexus. Neurotization by the spinal accessory nerve. *Clin. Plast. Surg.*, **11**, 133–135.

16. Alnot, J. Y., Jolly, A. and Frot, B. (1981) Traitement direct des lésions nerveuses dans les paralysies traumatiques du plexus brachial chez l'adulte. *Int. Orthop. (SICOT)*, **5**, 151–168.

17. Millesi, H. (1987) Brachial plexus injuries: management and results. In: *Microreconstruction of Nerve Injuries* (ed. J. K. Terzis, W. B. Saunders, Philadelphia, pp. 347–360.

18. Narakas, A. (1987) Plexus brachialis und na-heliegende periphere Nervenverkletzungen bei Wirbelfrakturen und anderen Traumen der Halswirbersale. *Orthopäde*, **16**, 81–86.

19. Narakas, A. (1984) Thoughts on neurotization or nerve transfers in irreparable nerve lesions. *Clin. Plast. Surg.*, **11**, 153–159.

20. Sedel, L. (1987) The management of supraclavicular lesions clinical examination, surgical procedures, results. In *Microreconstruction of Nerve Injuries* (ed. J. K. Terzis), W. B. Saunders, Philadelphia, pp. 385–392.

List of abbreviations

AX:	axillary nerve
DS:	dorso-scapular nerve for rhomboids and levator scapulae
GR:	graft
inf pect:	anterior thoracic rami for the sternal portion of pectoralis major
Long. thor.:	thoracicus longus nerve
M:	median
ME:	musculo-cutaneous nerve
MC prox.:	proximal stump of transected musculo-cutaneous nerve
MC distal:	distal stump of the same nerve on which the nerve transfer with intercostal nerves is performed
Med cut:	medial cutaneous nerve of forearm
R:	radial nerve
SS:	suprascapular nerve
sup pect:	rami to the clavicular portion of the pectoralis major
T3 MOT:	motor ramus of third intercostal nerve
XX:	spinal accessory nerve

Part 2 Associated Injuries and Complications

P. M. Yeoman

Vascular lesions associated with injuries of the brachial plexus have already been discussed by Narakas in his experience with 57 cases of injury either to the subclavian or axillary arteries. In my own experience vascular injuries were more commonly associated with infraclavicular lesions of the brachial plexus where the prognosis for the plexus lesion is considered to be more favourable [1] and possibly due to less severe violence. As it happened, the outcome was a disaster in some of my patients who were referred to me for assessment and further care. They had already developed a Volkmann's ischaemic contracture of

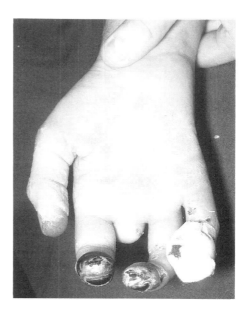

Fig. 16.7 Gangrene of the fingers in a lesion of the brachial artery and an infraclavicular traction injury of the brachial plexus. Appropriate treatment would have prevented the loss of the fingers in a patient whose nerve lesion recovered.

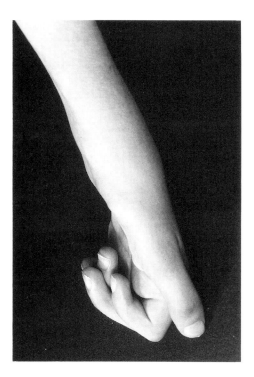

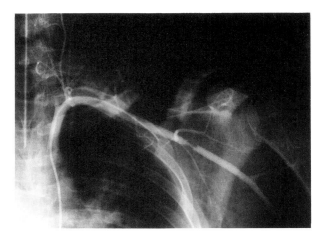

Fig. 16.9 Arteriogram (femoral) revealing a block of the brachial artery in continuity due to avulsion of the intima; associated haemothorax, open fracture of clavicle and complete rupture of infraclavicular brachial plexus. Recovery excellent after arterial and nerve grafts, nerve repairs and internal fixation of clavicle.

Fig. 16.8 Volkmann's ischaemic contracture of the flexor and intrinsic muscles in a patient whose plexus injury recovered.

the flexor muscles of the forearm and the intrinsic muscles of the hand (Fig. 16.8).

Volkmann's ischaemic contracture

It is an agreed fact that ischaemia of muscle is painful, and we teach that, passively to stretch a potentially ischaemic muscle will increase the pain. Hence the important test of stretching the flexor muscles of the forearm or the extensor and/or flexor muscles of the foot and toes when a 'compartment syndrome' is suspected. If a traction lesion of the plexus is superimposed then painful stimuli will be abolished and the ischaemic pattern will persist unrecognized. Twenty-two patients who were referred to me for further care out of a total of 532 were examples of Volkmann's ischaemic contracture superimposed on their brachial plexus traction injuries. I estimate that half of them (11 patients) could have made an excellent recovery if the vascular lesion had been recognized and dealt with. As a result of the author's previous experience at the Institute

of Orthopaedics in London when engaged in assessing patients at a later stage of their plexus injuries [2], it was clear that a surgeon should be advised to exclude a vascular lesion within 4 hours from the time of injury. Delay could be disastrous for the limb.

Arteriography (Fig. 16.9) must be available and indeed used if there is the slightest suggestion of an associated vascular lesion. This may inevitably involve early exploration of the lesion, even if it means calling up a team of experienced surgeons at any time of day or night. Exploration

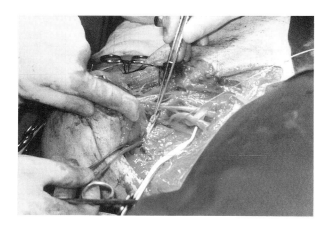

Fig. 16.10 Resection of brachial artery at damaged segment before graft.

is surprisingly easy at the acute stage compared with the lengthy and potentially meddlesome dissections through a minefield of fibrous tissue a few months later. Arteries and veins are restored by direct suture or graft (Fig. 16.10); then the nerves can be traced and the extent of their damage assessed before repair or graft. Fibrin glue is a quick and a well tried alternative [3] to meticulous but lengthy microscopic fascicular suture. The author has first hand experience of 17 such problems in the acute stage and ten went on to worthwhile recovery in that they achieved not only a useful and fairly strong hand grip (power 4: MRC grading) but protective skin sensibility. Sadly the other ten patients failed to recover any satisfactory function because there was either a long drawn out traction injury extending proximally from the site of vascular repair or associated avulsion of nerve roots.

Nerve pedicle graft

The survival of nerve graft has concerned us for years and there is a critical diameter but not necessarily length of free graft that will survive [4]. A vascular bed is an obvious requirement but not always easy to achieve amidst a thick sheet of fibrous tissue. The nerve pedicle graft [5] was designed to by-pass impenetrable and potentially hostile avascular territory for free nerve tissue. The blood supply was carried intact with the projected nerve and because the first stage involved ligature of one end of the loop it was possible to achieve a pre-degenerate length of nerve and thereby satisfy the metabolic requirements as a result of Wallerian degeneration. The final diameter of the graft tube would not be further reduced by fibrous tissue. This led to further research on the relative merits of pre-degenerate nerve grafts; some were impressed [6], others were not [7]. An example of the successful use of a two stage nerve graft is illustrated in a patient aged 24 who was sitting in the front passenger seat of a car when the car skidded off the road and careered through a fence and into a field. A fencing post pierced the front of the car and transfixed him to the seat (Fig. 16.11). The post entered his axilla and chest. In addition to the major wound he sustained a severe haemothorax, lung damage, a fractured shaft of humerus and a complete brachial plexus injury.

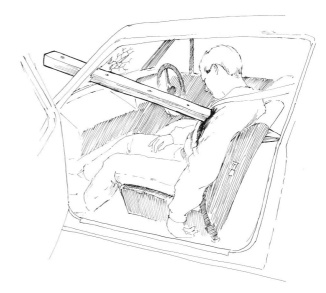

Fig. 16.11 Fencing post transfixed this patient, penetrating the chest, axilla and causing considerable vascular and nerve damage, as well as a fractured humerus.

After the wounds had healed and 3 months after the accident he was referred to me with an un-united fracture of the humerus and a flail arm lacking in shin sensibility. An arteriogram (Fig. 16.12); revealed that the axillary artery was not filling but there was a fairly adequate collateral circulation, and indeed the radial pulse was palpable. The outlook was not favourable; but a myelogram failed to reveal any traumatic meningocoeles or distorsion of the cervical nerve

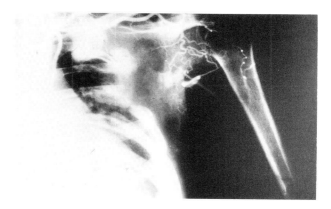

Fig. 16.12 Radiograph and arteriogram revealed an inadequate filling of the brachial artery but a reasonable secondary collateral flow to the distal part of the limb.

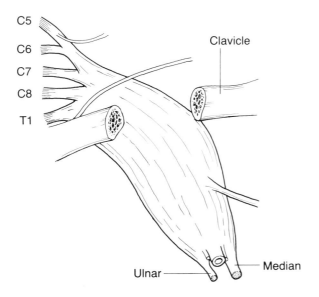

Fig. 16.13 Extensive scar tissue around the clavicle area with intact nerve roots and distal peripheral nerves.

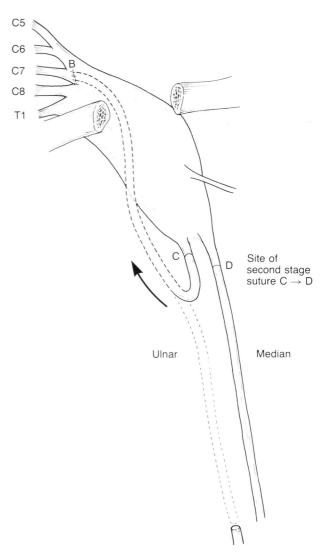

Fig. 16.14 First stage pedicle nerve graft; ulnar nerve mobilized and distal end doubled back to be sutured to C7 nerve root.

roots. A lengthy exploration was made of the supraclavicular part of the brachial plexus and the nerve roots and main nerve trunks were found to be intact (Fig. 16.13). I decided that any dissection around the clavicle and beyond in the axilla might damage the vital collateral vessels and thereby compromise the viability of the upper limb. A second exploration was made below the axilla and the ulnar nerve was mobilized down to the wrist together with its vessels. It was divided just proximal to the wrist and looped up through a tunnel made by a blunt nosed instrument in the scarred axillary area to emerge in the root of the neck where I sutured it to the proximal divided end of the root of C7 (Fig. 16.14). The fracture of the shaft of the humerus was secured with a plate and cancellous bone graft packed round. The second stage was achieved 3 months later and involved a relatively easy dissection to identify the loop of ulnar nerve, divide it and suture it to the distal end of the divided median nerve (Fig. 16.15). At 1 year there was a definite contraction in the flexors of the wrist and at 18 months it was possible to restore reasonable function in the hand by an arthrodesis and tendon transplants to the fingers. At 2 years there was not only recovery in skin sensibility in the median but strangely in the ulnar distribution as well. He must have been one of those fortunate

enough to have cross connections between the ulnar and median nerves in the wrist and hand.

This rather lengthy account must not detract from the later successful free vascularized ulnar nerve grafts including microscopic restoration of the vessels [8]. It serves to focus attention on the sacrifice of the ulnar nerve and its remarkable use in grafting the brachial plexus. The term 'sacrifice' may be misleading but it is written in the context relating to the negligible chances of recovery in the ulnar distribution in the hand after a degenerative lesion of the ulnar nerve in the

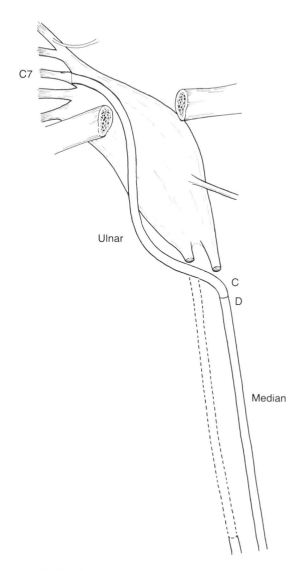

Fig. 16.15 Second stage pedicle nerve graft; ulnar nerve sutured to divided median nerve below level of scar tissue (mid-humerus).

Nerve root avulsion

The nearer the nerve injury is to the spinal cord the worse the prognosis.

It is necessary to determine nerve root avulsion because there is no way at present to successfully re-implant it. Isolated nerve root avulsion is barely possible without some other damage to the plexus in the type of traction injuries which are currently familiar. A myelograph [9] may well reveal a single traumatic meningocoele (Fig. 16.16) but it does not necessarily indicate that all the nerve root is avulsed; a CT or MRI scan would give a more accurate definition. Recovery in that nerve root might be very misleading and would throw doubt on the validity of the abnormal radiographic finding. A pre- or post-fixed plexus would explain the anomaly and there are many deviations from the accepted anatomical patterns [10]. Multiple meningocoeles (Fig.

axilla. The quality of recovery in the intrinsic muscles is very poor indeed because of the long distance between the axilla and hand and the time taken for any recovering nerve fibrils to reach an intrinsic muscle; which in the long interval degeneration has taken place not only in the motor end-plate but in the muscle fibres.

We can afford to lose the ulnar nerve in those circumstances because it has an important part to play in restoration of function in the proximal part of the totally paralysed upper limb.

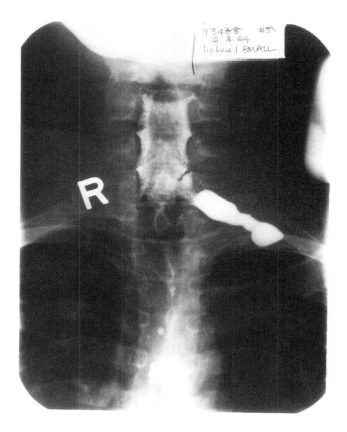

Fig. 16.16 A single traumatic meningocoele.

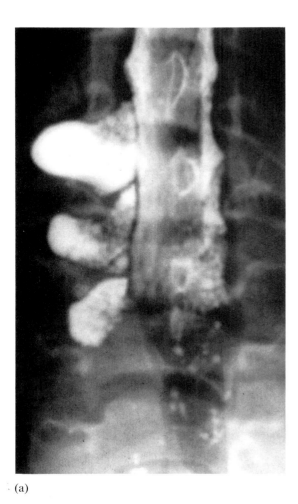

(a)

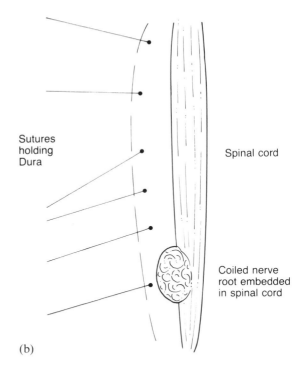

Sutures holding Dura

Spinal cord

Coiled nerve root embedded in spinal cord

(b)

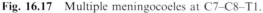

Fig. 16.17   Multiple meningocoeles at C7–C8–T1.

16.17) are much more serious and when combined with the clinical picture of a painful flail arm, lacking sensibility, produced by an accident of high velocity and with an associated Horner's syndrome (Fig. 16.18) the outlook is very gloomy.

Haemorrhage into the subarachnoid space has been mentioned by Narakas and the author has confirmed this on three occasions when a lumbar puncture was performed on three patients who had been struck on the shoulder by a heavy object on a building site; there was no associated head injury. It is not surprising that bleeding occurs when a nerve root is torn because it is enveloped by small nutrient vessels both within and on the surface of the meningeal sleeve; it is, however, surprising to find relatively few reports of spinal cord damage. Exploration of the spinal

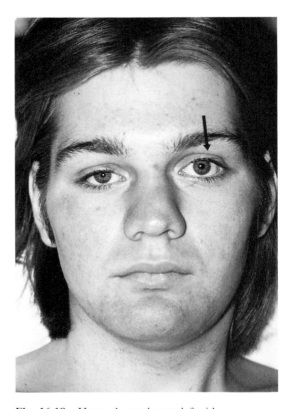

Fig. 16.18   Horner's syndrome left side.

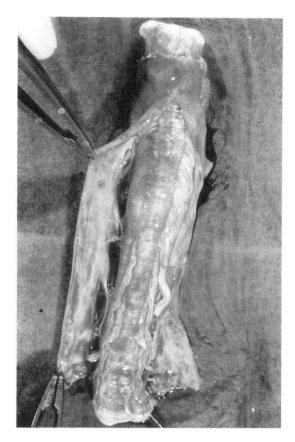

Fig. 16.19   Nerve roots totally avulsed from the spinal cord (autopsy specimen).

cord frequently reveals that the nerve rootlets have been avulsed, leaving a clean surface on the side of the spinal cord (Fig. 16.19). It is likely that pain is one of the unfortunate consequences of local spinal cord trauma.

Long term complications of nerve root avulsion

The author has seen two patients with long tract signs leading to spasticity and later more widespread signs of multiple sclerosis arising 15 and 18 years after a complete traction injury of the brachial plexus. The immediate diagnosis was not evident and it was hoped that the abnormal late onset spasticity was due to fibrous adhesions withdrawing the spinal cord into the mouth of a traumatic meningocoele [11], but sadly other

signs were found which discounted the mechanical cause. Another patient sustained a severe traction injury to the plexus at the age of 10 when tobogganing and 20 years later he was referred owing to difficulty in walking over a period of 2 years. There was no doubt that he had a spastic gait with all the signs of an upper motor neurone lesion. A myelograph revealed a filling defect compressing the lower cervical spinal cord. At operation the author found a coiled up piece of nerve root which was adherent to the cord (Fig. 16.20). The compression was relieved by removal of the coiled stump of nerve root and there was worthwhile but not full improvement in his gait over the next 3 years.

In conclusion, there has undoubtedly been an advance in both the diagnosis and management of brachial plexus injuries during the last decade. It is likely that further advances will be made, particularly with nerve grafts [12], fibrin glue for nerve repair and more detailed knowledge of the pharmacological activity at nerve endings. The more severe injuries could be reduced immediately by banning motor cycles.

References

1. Leffert, R. D. (1985) *Brachial Plexus Injuries*, Churchill Livingstone, New York, pp. 3–57.
2. Yeoman, P. M. and Seddon, H. J. (1961) Brachial plexus injuries: treatment of the flail arm. *J. Bone Joint Surg.*, **43B**, 493.
3. Seddon, H. J. and Medawar, P. B. (1942) Fibrin suture of human nerves. *Lancet*, **2**, 87.
4. Seddon, H. J. (1972) *Surgical Disorders of the Peripheral Nerves*. Churchill Livingstone, London, pp. 16–286.
5. Strange, F. G., St. C. (1950) Case report on pedicled nerve graft. *Br. J. Surg.*, **37**, 331.
6. Ballance, C. and Duel, A. B. (1932) Operative treatment of facial palsy by the introduction of nerve grafts into the fallopian canal and by other intratemporal methods. *Archs Otolaryngol.*, **15**, 1.
7. Bunnell, S. and Boyes, J. H. (1939) Nerve grafts. *Am. J. Surg.*, **44**, 64.
8. Bonney, G., Birch, R., Jamieson, A. J. and Eames, R. A. (1984) Experience with vascularized nerve grafts. *Clin. Plast. Surg.*, **2,1**, 137.
9. Yeoman, P. M. (1968) Cervical myelography in traction injuries of the brachial plexus. *J. Bone Joint Surg.*, **50B**, 253.
10. Kaplan, E. B. and Spinner, M. (1980) Normal and anomalous innervation patterns in the upper ex-

tremity. In *Management of Peripheral Nerve Problems* (ed. G. E. Omer and M. Spinner), Saunders, Philadelphia, pp. 77–89.

11. Penfield, W. (1972) Late spinal paralysis after avulsion of the brachial plexus. *J. Bone Joint Surg.*, **31B**, 40.

12. Glasby, M. A., Gilmour, J. A., Gschmeissner, S. E. *et al.* (1990) The repair of large peripheral nerves using skeletal muscle autografts: a comparison with cable grafts in the sheep femoral nerve. *Br. J. Plast. Surg.*, **43**, 169.

Part 3   Rehabilitation

C. B. Wynn Parry

Lesions of the brachial plexus are ideally explored immediately after injury or within the first 2 or 3 weeks. The operation is much less difficult than at a later stage. However this is often not possible, either because of the co-existence of head injuries or chest injuries or the lack of availability of a specialist unit. Thus many patients with brachial plexus lesions are seen months after injury. Elevation and the wearing of an appropriate sling will prevent formation and organization of oedema, and trophic lesions can be avoided by careful education of the patient to avoid damage to the insensitive hand. Should these basic principles have been neglected, patients may present for consideration of surgery some months after injury with a very stiff shoulder and an oedematous brawny arm and very stiff hand. The shoulder is particularly likely to stiffen as are the metacarpophalangeal joints and the thumb web. It is essential to have a good range of external rotation to allow adequate exposure of the plexus at operation and it may therefore be necessary to insist on a preoperative spell of intensive rehabilitation to prepare the patient for surgery. This is best done as an inpatient with an intensive programme of physiotherapy and occupational therapy, but at the very least, several hours a day as an outpatient should be required with progressive passive stretching of stiff joints, hydrotherapy and intensive re-education of spared muscles. If any oedema has organized then a spell of elevation may be necessary. It is surprising how rapidly even chronic oedema can subside if continuous elevation in

bed is insisted upon. At this stage it is necessary to establish whether the patient has a pre- or post-ganglionic lesion. If the lesion is preganglionic then there is no hope of repairing the plexus although some form of reconstruction such as neurotization may be considered. If the lesion is postganglionic it may be either in continuity or there may be ruptures of one or more roots.

Electromyography can be most valuable to assess the situation. Routine electromyography in our unit comprises sampling of at least two muscles supplied by each root to determine if there are any surviving motor units indicating that the lesion is not total.

Secondly, sensory conduction studies stimulating the index, middle and little fingers and recording over the median and ulnar nerves at the wrist; stimulating the radial nerve in the midforearm, and recording over the first dorsal interosseous space; stimulating the ulnar nerve at the wrist and recording over the ulnar nerve above the elbow. In the presence of total anaesthesia the presence of an action potential will indicate a preganglionic lesion. The absence of sensory action potentials in an anaesthetic digit unfortunately does not mean that the lesion is certainly postganglionic, for it is possible to have pre- and post-ganglionic elements and the post-ganglionic element will show on electrical investigation. Sensory evoked potentials can be very helpful. Median and ulnar nerves are stimulated at the wrist and recordings made over the brachial plexus, over the cervical spine at the level of C2 and over the contralateral parietal cortex. The detection of a potential over the plexus at the root of the neck in the presence of anaesthesia in the distribution stimulated, will indicate a preganglionic lesion and the degree of attenuation between that and C2 will indicate the relative degree of post- and pre-ganglionic involvement. We have shown that the most valuable results are obtained by a combination of the two techniques [1].

Myelography has been disappointing in the past for it is possible to have a meningocele and yet an intact root, and conversely it is possible to have a normal myelogram but an intra-dural root avulsion. However the combination of a CT scan and myelography appears to be giving very promising results.

The more information that can be gathered

before operation, the more certainly the diagnosis of the exact type and level of the lesion can be made.

Whether there has been rupture of nerve roots which are repaired at operation or whether spontaneous recovery is going to occur after a degenerative lesion in continuity, it is going to be months or years before the patient regains function; and in the case of a total avulsion lesion proved at surgery, it is clear that recovery will never occur.

For suitable patients with a permanent paralysis of the plexus and for the months or years before recovery occurs in those with reparable or recoverable lesions, functional splinting has been adopted in our unit. For the patient with a total paralysis, the full flail arm splint is provided. This is, in effect, an artificial arm over the patient's own limb. It consists of a shoulder support, elbow locking device, forearm support and a platform on the wrist piece into which a variety of tools may be fitted. The tools can be operated by a harness from movement of the contralateral shoulder, just as in a standard artificial arm, so that the patient has his good hand free to operate tools. The splint is ready-made and modular and comes in three sizes. The orthotist makes adjustments to suit the individual patient and the occupational therapist supervises a detailed training programme in which the patient learns to use the splint for a variety of activities of daily living, hobbies, recreations and appropriate work. The occupational therapist and the workshop technician will make every effort to simulate the patient's normal work and try out the splint in this realistic situation. Ten days is allowed for intensive training by which time the majority of patients will be fully conversant with its use (Fig. 16.20). The value of these splints is that they allow the patient to retain the arm in his body image during the stage of paralysis. It relieves the strain on the shoulder and it allows a variety of functional uses. It is in effect a mobile vice and is most valuable for steadying tools while the other hand directs the operation. A wide range of trades and professions have been made possible using this splint including draughtsmanship, spray painting, spot welding, engineering, car maintenance, gardening and a whole variety of recreations and hobbies. We have three patients who are able to go deep sea fishing with totally paralysed arms using the flail arm splint and we

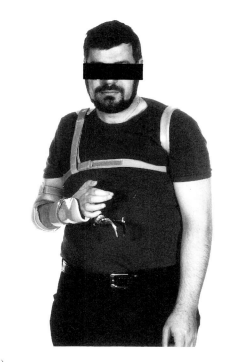

(a)

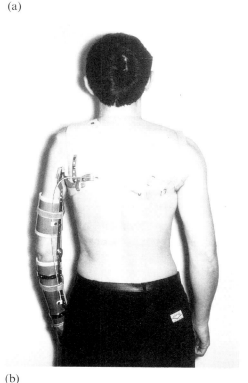

(b)

Fig. 16.20 Front (a) and rear (b) views of the flail arm splint. On rear view note shoulder support, shoulder joint and elbow ratchet.

have patients who can play golf, cricket and carry out all activities around the house, including painting and decorating [2].

Clearly patients must be motivated towards use of the splint and somebody who rejects it as clumsy and has no wish to try it should not be coerced into so doing. With experience the occupational therapist and the workshop technician can assess within a day or two whether a patient is likely to be a splint user. At a recent 2-year follow-up, 70% of patients were using the splint for hobbies, recreation or work. Patients may use the splint for a few months and then discard it, either when recovery occurs or when they become used to working. If it can be demonstrated to an employer that the patient has useful function with his paralysed arm, he may be much more ready to accept him for employment.

There are a variety of modifications of this splint for less severe paralysis. For example a patient with a C5/6 palsy who has no elbow flexion, a simple elbow lock splint is provided which weighs virtually nothing and allows the patient to position his arm in one of five positions. We have many patients who have been able to return to full work immediately on provision of this splint. For a patient with a C5/6/7 palsy with added paralysis of wrist and finger extension, a dropped wrist and finger appliance can be added. In a patient who has either recovered or has spared proximal muscle function and there is paralysis below the elbow, the forearm trough alone is all that is required and the shoulder piece can be discarded. A number of patients in the Armed Forces with total paralysis following brachial plexus lesions have been fitted with this splint and as a result of proving that they have excellent function they have been retained for full service careers. It is particularly important to help these patients get back to employment. In many cases they may well not be able to return to their former employment, e.g. labourers, brick layers, and the like. Many, however, by simple adjustments at work may be able to return to work and it is here that the services of a Resettlement Officer are invaluable. In our unit we have a full-time Resettlement Officer who is experienced in industry and in the niceties of trade union law. His role is to make immediate contact with the employer and indicate to him the extent of the injury and the likely time the patient will be off

work. Throughout the course of rehabilitation, he will contact the employer and keep him informed of progress. The vast majority of employers are perfectly happy to keep the job open for a patient and to modify it accordingly if only they are kept informed. So often the employer hears nothing for many months or years and naturally gives up hope and employs someone else in his place. In many instances the Resettlement Officer will visit the place of work and discuss with the personnel officer and the foreman what modifications could be made to allow the patient to return to work. It is very helpful if a trial period of work for a day or two can be arranged at an early stage of the rehabilitation so that the patient does not lose hope.

Seventy-four patients with total paralysis of the arm were referred to our Resettlement Officer and 81% were able to be returned to work.

Some 30 years ago, the standard treatment for a person with a total avulsion lesion of the brachial plexus was early amputation, arthrodesis of the shoulder and fitting of a prosthesis. It was shown that few patients actually use their artificial limb. The situation is even more radical now because well over half our patients have total avulsion lesions which involve avulsion of all five roots of the spinal cord. In such a situation there is total loss of proximal control and even with amputation and arthrodesis, such patients will never be able to operate a prosthesis because they have paralysis of the thoracoscapular muscles. Twelve of our patients had been advised elsewhere to have immediate amputation and 11 of them regained significant shoulder and elbow function some years later. Very few patients wish to have amputation. Young men do not want to be seen on the beach and in the swimming pool with a stump but most people are unobservant enough not to notice a withered arm. Only one out of our series of over a thousand patients with total paralysis of the arm developed trophic lesions severe enough to require amputation. The main indication for amputation is in an athletic person in whom the limb gets in the way when running or in a rugger scrum. Amputation of course has no effect whatsoever on the severe pain that so many of these patients suffer. It is deeply distressing for the patient to wake up after an amputation to find that his pain has not improved.

Reconstructive surgery

There are various procedures to restore elbow flexion, such as the Steindler operation, pectoralis major transfer, triceps to biceps transfer and the latissimus dorsi transfer. For a patient with a C7 paralysis, the standard radial nerve tendon transfers are appropriate to restore wrist and finger extension. However, re-education after tendon transfers for the brachial plexus lesions present greater problems than after peripheral nerve injuries. Joints are often stiff and there may well be contractures, there is often cross innervation causing co-contraction which makes re-education difficult and muscles may not be as strong for transfer as in the standard peripheral nerve lesion. In brachial plexus lesions objectives are more limited and it is common practice to transfer a muscle that is less strong than one would like, e.g. a 3 plus muscle. Although only limited power may develop it may make all the difference to the patient's function [3].

Pain

One of the most devastating effects of these tragic lesions is the severe pain that so many patients with avulsion lesions of the plexus suffer. Wynn Parry [4] showed that some 90% of patients with avulsion lesions of the plexus suffer severe pain at some stage. The pain is characteristically crushing or burning and felt in the anaesthetic and paralysed hand. The pain may feel as if the hand is being tightened in a vice or is having boiling water poured all over it. This pain is usually constant and unremitting, In addition, there may be severe shooting pains of the paroxysmal type lasting a few seconds and being particularly violent, causing the patient to cry out or turn away and double up in pain. These paroxysms are often quite unpredictable and may occur many times an hour throughout the day. It is these paroxysmal attacks of pain that are the most devastating and to which the patient finds most difficulty in adjusting. When the spinal cord is deafferented by avulsion of nerve roots, the nerve cells in the dorsal horn that have lost their input begin to discharge with high frequency impulses, increasing in frequency and intensity as

times goes on. This is the cause of the severe pain. Anderson *et al.* [5] showed in an experimental model in the cat that within 8 days of deafferentation of the spinal cord, nerve cells start firing spontaneously and more cells discharge with an increasing frequency so that by a month there was massive discharge throughout the whole of the dorsal horn. This pain may come immediately after the accident but we have patients in whom the onset has been delayed by 3 or 4 months. This pain is notoriously resistant to standard analgesics and indeed does not respond to the narcotics such as morphine or heroin. The single most helpful way of coping with this pain is by mental distraction. This allows the patient to bring in his own central inhibitory pathways, for it is known that there is an inhibitory pathway for pain running from the hypothalamus through the para-ventricular grey through the raphe nucleus in the medulla down to laminae 1 and 5 in the dorsal horn where all the nociceptive traffic is arriving. Involvement in absorbing work or hobbies can often either completely or materially reduce this pain. Often the patients find that when they relax in the evening, the pain comes back with a vengeance and many patients have taken a second job in order to try and cope with the pain [4].

By far the most valuable modality in our hands has been transcutaneous electrical stimulation. Electrodes are applied just proximal to the site of lesion. In a total lesion, for example, the electrodes will be placed on the neck and on the front of the chest over the C3/4 dermatomes and over the inner side of the upper arm over the T2 dermatome. The aim is to stimulate the afferent input above and below the lesion in order to produce maximum release of endorphins at that site to try and damp down the transmission of the spontaneous firing. We insist that all our patients are admitted to our intensive rehabilitation unit where our physiotherapists, who are particularly skilled in this technique, will try various positions of the electrodes and various settings of the parameters, stimulating for many hours a day for 2 weeks before the treatment is abandoned as unhelpful. Far too often we have found that patients have been given stimulators at pain clinics without proper instruction in their use and advised to try it for half an hour at a time. This is quite useless. The stimulation has a cumulative effect as is well shown by Melzak [6]. The patients must be encouraged to use the stimulator for many hours a day, if necessary all day and sometimes all night for long periods before giving up [7].

Sixty percent of the patients we have treated with severe pain from avulsion lesions have had substantial or complete relief. Most patients can give up the treatment within 6 months but some have continued to use it for up to a year and keep the stimulator by them if there is an exacerbation of pain with an intercurrent infection or a particularly stressful period in their lives.

We cannot emphasize enough the importance of the correct use of this invaluable technique. Fortunately the vast majority of patients either lose their pain within an average time of 3 years or come to terms with it to the extent that it no longer impinges on their life. Many patients respond to transcutaneous stimulation but a few – some 1% of all our patients with severe pain – find themselves in a desperate state with unremitting pain which gradually increases with time and totally destroys their life. Such patients are quite unable to work and the whole family suffers. It is for these patients that the dorsal root entry zone lesion is suitable. Nashold [8] described an operation to destroy the nerve cells in laminae 1 and 5 and although it is a destructive lesion it is aimed at the seat of the problem rather than tracts carrying nociceptive information. It is well recognized by neurosurgeons that destruction of tracts such as cordotomies, rhizotomies and mesencephalic tractotomies is no longer indicated in 'benign' pain. Sooner or later pain will certainly recur and usually at a considerably greater intensity than before. Thomas at the National Hospital for Nervous Diseases in London has carried out operations on 27 of our patients with severe unremitting intractable plexus pain. These are patients in whom the whole family has been affected by the pain and in which it is quite clear that desperate measures are required. Patients must of course be subjected to the full rehabilitation programme already described with a trial of return to work, functional splinting, transcutaneous stimulation and anti-paroxysmal drugs such as Tegretol and Tripatfen. In both Nashold's [9] and Thomas's [10,11] series, between 60 and 70% of patients can be expected to achieve substantial and complete relief of pain. There are, however, serious drawbacks to the operation for there is a significant incidence of complications. In Thomas's series, 10% of patients had significant neurological defects such as weakness of the ipsilateral leg, unpleasant dysaesthesiae of the trunk, weakness of the neck muscles and affection of balance. One of our patients was rendered impotent and two were impotent for 6 months. It is therefore vital to make sure the patient understands the serious risk that he may be running, the least of which may be a lack of relief of pain and at the worst a neurological disability in addition. Provided the patient is psychologically robust and has been carefully assessed by the clinical psychologist, and provided the rehabilitation team is satisfied that every possible measure has been tried exhaustively and that the patient is in a really desperate state, then he is referred for this procedure.

Conclusions

Surgery is only one episode, albeit an all important one, in an ongoing saga in patients with brachial plexus lesions. The best results cannot be expected without the backup of a comprehensive and intensive rehabilitation regime. The rehabilitation team will provide the best conditions for surgery by restoring as full a range of passive movement to joints as possible and reducing oedema and regaining maximum function in spared muscles. They will provide skilled re-education after surgery, whether reparative or reconstructive. They will make determined attempts to help the pain and explain to the patient the nature of the pain and how he can best cope with it. They will provide appropriate functional splinting and help the patient return to work.

References

1. Jones, S. J., Wynn Parry, C. B. and Landi, A. (1980) Diagnosis of brachial plexus traction lesions by sensory nerve action potentials and somatosensory evoked potentials. *Injury*, **12**, 376–382.
2. Wynn Parry, C. B. (1980) Management of traction lesion of the brachial plexus and peripheral

nerve injuries in the upper limb. The Ruscoe Clark Memorial Lecture for 1979. *Injury*, **11**, 265–285.

3. Frampton, V. M. (1986) Problems involved in the management of reconstructive surgery in brachial plexus lesions contrasted with peripheral nerve injuries. *J. Hand Surg.*, **11**, 3–9.

4. Wynn Parry, C. B. (1980) Pain in avulsion lesions of the brachial plexus. *Pain*, **9**, 41–53.

5. Anderson, L. S., Black, R. G., Abraham, J. *et al.* (1971) Neuronal hyperactivity in experimental trigeminal deafferentation. *J. Neurosurg.*, **35**, 444.

6. Melzack, R. (1975) Prolonged relief of pain by brief intense transcutaneous stimulation. *Pain*, **1**, 357–374.

7. Frampton, V. (1982) Pain control with the aid of the transcutaneous stimulator. *Physiotherapy*, **68**, 77–71.

8. Nashold, B. S., Urban, B. and Zorab, D. S. (1976) Phantom pain relief by focal destruction of the substantia gelatinosa of Rolando. In: *Advances in Pain and Research Therapy* (eds J. J. Bonica and D. Albe Fessard) Vol. 1. Raven Press, New York, pp. 959–963.

9. Nashold, B. S. and Ostdahl, R. H. (1979) Dorsal root entry zone lesions for pain relief. *J. Neurosurg.*, **57**, 9–69.

10. Thomas, D. G. T. and Sheehy, J. R. R. (1983) Dorsal root entry zone lesions (Nashold's procedure for pain relief following brachial plexus avulsion. *J. Neurol. Neurosurg. Psychiat.*, **46**, 924–928.

11. Thomas, D. G. T. and Jones, S. J. (1984) Dorsal root entry zone lesions (Nashold's procedure) in brachial plexus avulsion. *Neurosurgery*, **15**, 966–967.

17

Rotator cuff injury

M. F. Swiontkowski

The rotator cuff is the term given to the confluence of the supraspinatus, infraspinatus, teres minor, and subscapularis. Its structure and function are essential to the stability and motion of the glenohumeral joint. The unconstrained articulation of the large radius convexity of the humeral head and the very shallow concavity of the glenoid surface must be enhanced by this confluence of tendons. Degeneration of this essential structure leads to pain, weakness, and sometimes stiffness of the glenohumeral joint. When degeneration progresses to a complete tear, superior instability of the glenohumeral joint can result. This phenomenon, with its resultant weakness of abduction and external rotation as well as pain, can lead to permanent, irreversible worsening of shoulder function.

Smith [1] credited by Codman [2] as the first investigator to report tears in the region of the insertion of the supraspinatus tendon. Smith was also the first to note the association of ruptures of the long head of the biceps with these tears. Additionally, he observed that 'the undersurface of the acromion process was found hardened by the friction of the head of the humerus and covered by a peculiar enamel-like secretion'. This was, of course, a description of an associated osteophyte of the undersurface of the acromion process. In the majority of the younger-aged cadavers Smith examined, he suspected acute trauma was the cause of the tendon avulsions. In two older cadavers he reported bilateral findings with communication of larger tears with the subacromial bursae, and noted synovial hyper-

trophy. One hundred years later Smith's findings were confirmed by Codman [2], Skinner [3], and Cotton [4], who reported a high incidence of these findings in older patients and frequent bilaterality. Codman was the first to recommend prompt recognition and repair to avoid 'much pain and disability as well as great economic loss' [2]. Functional improvement following repair was later confirmed by McLaughlin [5].

Presentation

Patients with tears of the rotator cuff are frequently older than 40 years of age and present with pain and weakness. Most patients have a prolonged history of intermittent aching in the shoulder associated with forward elevation and internal rotation of the arm. Older patients will often have no history of trauma, while those in the 40–55 year age group, particularly males, generally report a fall or forced abduction–external rotation of the arm [6].

Unless an element of adhesive capsulitis is associated with a longstanding rotator cuff tear, the patient will have a full passive range of glenohumeral motion. Initiation of abduction is typically severely limited, as is active internal rotation and forward elevation. These findings contrast with the partial tear stage or earlier 'impingement lesions', in that weakness and loss of active motion are present. The pain reported in both conditions is frequently aggravated by use of the arm in internal rotation and forward elevation. Patients report a dull, moderate to severe ache in the shoulder region. A frequent complaint is the inability to sleep on the affected side. The pain frequently radiates to the deltoid insertion and occasionally to the lateral elbow region. Deltoid motor function and axillary nerve sensation should be normal.

Diagnostic methods

Because of variability in history, degree of weakness of external rotation, initiation of abduction, and degree of pain, it is often impossible to make a definitive diagnosis of a rotator cuff tear. For this reason, ancillary diagnostic methods are of critical importance. Arthrography remains the cornerstone of diagnostic technique; however, the importance of plain radiography is frequently underestimated. In patients with large cuff tears, the classic radiographic findings are a decreased space between the superior humerus and undersurface of the acromion (less than 7 mm), cyst formation at the insertion of the supraspinatus, sclerosis of the undersurface of the acromion, irregularity of the greater tuberosity, and deepening of the groove between the articular surface and cuff attachment. A high quality AP of the scapula (allowing the clear visualization of the glenohumeral articular surface) and an axillary view must be obtained in every patient where the diagnosis of a rotator cuff tear is considered.

Standard arthrography has correlated with surgical findings in 90–100% of cases in multiple series of rotator cuff tears [7,8]. Pneumoarthrotomography is thought by several authors to improve the accuracy of diagnosis, but this is generally restricted to partial tears of the inferior surface of the cuff. The size of the tear is difficult to estimate from the arthrogram, and the differentiation of a small to medium size tear from a massive tear is best made on the basis of clinical examination and plain radiographs.

Recently, the use of ultrasonography has been shown to be an excellent alternative to the use of arthrography. A newer design probe head is required, as well as an interested and experienced ultrasonographer. Using these criteria, Mack *et al.* have demonstrated a 91% sensitivity and a 100% specificity compared to surgical findings [9]. This diagnostic tool is especially useful in patients with contrast allergies. Shoulder arthroscopy, although useful in treating labral tears and

lesions of the biceps tendon, is of little help in the management of rotator cuff tear [10].

Rotator cuff anatomy and physiology

The confluence of the tendons of the subscapularis anteriorly with the teres minor, infraspinatus, and supraspinatus tendons posteriorly to superiorly is illustrated in Fig. 17.1. As shown by Smith [1] and Codman [2], the supraspinatus is involved with the vast majority of rotator cuff tears. This is due to its function in initiating abduction as well as to its position in relation to the inferior acromion and coracoacromial ligament.

Rotator cuff vascular anatomy may play a critical role in the degeneration of the rotator cuff [11]. Using injection studies, Laing investigated the arterial supply of the humerus in detail [12]. He noted the perforation of vessels of the anterior humeral circumflex into the humeral head and rotator cuff in the region of attachment of the supraspinatus tendon. Lindblom and Palmer were the first to demonstrate hypovascular areas in the region of the rotator cuff [13]. They noted a low perfusion area near the insertion of the supraspinatus tendon into the tuberosity, and a second region within the long head of the biceps near its origin at the superior glenoid. Based on clinical experience, Codman [2] had pointed to a 'critical portion' of the supraspinatus tendon which was renamed the 'critical zone' by Neer [14]. This region was shown in the injection studies of Rothman and Parke to have relatively low perfusion [15]. Rathburn and MacNab's study confirmed this finding and hypothesized that the resting position of the arm in adduction and vertical rotation causes the humeral head to place pressure on this region, which further decreases perfusion and predisposes this region to degeneration [16]. In the author's experience, preliminary studies utilizing laser Doppler flowmetry have shown this region to be hypervascular in terms of real-time measurement of capillary level blood flow [17]. It may be that repeated trauma to the tendon due to impingement on the undersurface of the acromion (see below) produces hyperaemia, which weakens the substance of the tendon and predisposes this region to rupture. This may correspond to Neer's phase I (haemorrhage and oedema) at the periphery of a cuff disruption [18].

The spectrum of rotator cuff disease

Neer has carefully and clearly delineated the spectrum of rotator cuff disease, based on experience in the anatomy laboratory and in surgery [18]. Stage I is oedema and haemorrhage within the 'critical zone' due to repeated trauma of the humeral head riding superiorly and crushing the tendon against the anterior surface of the acromion. Statistically, this is more common in the under 30 age group and is associated with overhead sports (i.e. tennis), but can occur in any patient with a new onset of activity above the horizontal plane. A common scenario is the 50-year-old weekend house painter or tree trimmer. With this history and mechanism of injury, conservative treatment is successful in all but the rarest cases. Treatment includes the use of an anti-inflammatory drug and resistive internal and external rotator strengthening exercises. Isometric exercises using surgical tubing for mechanical resistance have proven very effective, but must be performed at least three times a day for several weeks and then continued on an intermittent basis for several months. This treatment should be employed when there is no element of adhesive capsulitis restricting the active and passive range of shoulder motion. When adhesive capsulitis is present, assisted ROM exercises and/or manipulation should be included in the treatment plan. In the athlete, shoulder subluxation may play a role in the development of these symptoms. Shoulder instability and apprehension with the arm in abduction and external rotation must be examined for and treated appropriately. In all three stages of the disease, Radiographs must be carefully studied for osteophytes and narrowing of the acromioclavicular (AC) joint, reflecting AC arthritis which can mimic the symptoms of rotator cuff disease. A careful examination will often reveal direct tenderness over the AC joint, and the symptoms in this case can be relieved by a 2–3 ml injection of lidocaine into this joint. The cross body adduction test, which produces pain both in subacromial impingement stage I and AC arthritis, can thereby be eliminated.

The second stage of rotator cuff disease is that of fibrosis and tendinitis. With prolonged, repeated impingement of the rotator cuff on the undersurface of the acromion and coracoacromial (CA) ligament, the single cell layer, thin, overlying subacromial bursae becomes hypertrophied, and fibrotic. Because of the chronicity of the condition, this population of patients is generally 10–15 years older than the first stage patient. The history is that of refractory shoulder pain exacerbated by forward flexion and internal rotation. Frequently, patients presenting with this history of symptoms of intermittent severity for several years will have had multiple subacromial injections of steroids. This provides excellent temporary relief of the condition due to the patent anti-inflammatory properties of these compounds. Unfortunately, these compounds also result in weakening of the tensile strength of tendons and predispose to rupture of the rotator cuff – the next stage in the natural history of the disease. The use of these compounds on a chronic basis of this disease process must therefore be condemned.

As with the patient presenting in stage I, an element of adhesive capsulitis may be present in the stage II patient. This patient would present with limitations of active *and* passive ROM, evident primarily in loss of forward elevation and internal rotation. As the age of presentation moves into the 40–50 year age group, calcific tendinitis must enter the differential diagnosis. On the initial screening X-rays, calcific deposits in the insertion of the supraspinatus will be evident. The history is most often quite different from that of impingement syndrome with the rapid onset of severe shoulder pain unprovoked by activity. Calcific tendinitis is effectively managed by heat and anti-inflammatory drugs or with aspiration of the calcific deposit followed by administration of a single dose of long-acting steroid into the area of calcific degeneration.

In the second stage of impingement, correct conservative treatment as outlined for stage I should be employed for at least 12 months. In refractory cases, surgical management is recommended. This consists of resection of the thickened bursae, removal of the CA ligament, inspection of the tendon for a tear, and an anterior acromioplasty of the type advocated by Neer [14,18]. Removal of the lateral acromion is to be condemned, as it does not address the problem of the zone of impingement and weakens the deltoid origin [18]. The anterior–inferior one-third of the acromion should be inspected for overhang or osteophytes and if either of these is present, this segment of the acromion should be removed with a thin beveled osteotome or high-speed burr. The approach to the region should be an oblique incision one finger breadth lateral to the acomion in Langer's lines to optimize cosmesis. The interval between the anterior and middle one-third of the deltoid should be split $1\frac{1}{2}$–$2\frac{1}{2}$ cm distal from the tip of the acromion within the tendinous portion. Minimal deltoid (1 cm or less) from the lateral portion of the acromion as well as the anterior portion should be taken down. Care must be taken to leave enough deltoid fascia on the superior acromion to allow repair and, when this is not possible, repair should be performed with non-absorbable sutures through drill holes.

The final phase of the disease spectrum is that of acromial bone spurs and tendon ruptures. As this represents the endpoint on a continuum of chronic disease, patients in this phase are generally 45 or more years old. Almost invariably, the symptoms are of many years' duration. As noted earlier, patients presenting with tendon ruptures have frequently had multiple steroid injections, which play a role in pathogenesis. Because of the older age range of these patients, the differential diagnosis of chronic shoulder pain must include cervical radiculopathy, superior sulcus (Pancoast) tumors, and coronary artery disease. The biceps tendon is involved in the zone of impingement, and irritation of the biceps tendon is often present with tenderness in the bicepital groove. Neer has stated that the biceps tendon ruptures infrequently in this stage, and that the ratio of rupture of the supraspinatus to rupture of the long head of the biceps is seven to one [18]. Anatomical variability within the bicipital groove (shallowness, sharp lateral margin) may predispose some patients to early rupture of the long head of the biceps.

With further impingement on a fibrotic cuff, two phenomena develop. The anterior–inferior edge of the acromion becomes hypertrophic, and osteophytes and bone cysts develop in response to the pressure phenomenon. The second development is thinning and atrophy of the rotator cuff. The cuff tendon in the zone of impingement has become hypervascular from irritation [17] and eventually becomes weakened in terms of tensile strength. At this point, minor trauma leads to a rupture of the tendon. Routine radiographs may reveal the acromial changes and in cases of moderate to large size tears the distance

between the humeral head and the acromion may be narrowed. Other than these radiographic signs present in large tears, there are no plain radiographic findings diagnostic for a cuff tear. The utility of arthrography and ultrasound has been referred to previously.

It is unlikely that partial or full thickness rotator cuff ruptures will heal if they remain untreated. This is due to the pathophysiology which produced the tensile weakness and the continued stress on the tendon in the region of the tear. In the setting of chronic shoulder pain where the indications for anterior acromioplasty are present (positive impingement test with symptoms refractory to conservative care for 12 months) in association with a proven cuff rupture, the acromioplasty should be performed as outlined by Neer and the rotator cuff concomitantly repaired directly using non-absorbable inverted sutures or brought into a groove in the greater tuberosity and sutured into bone through drill holes. Every effort must be made to mobilize the edges of the retracted cuff in the case of large (greater than 4 cm) tears and repair the tendon to bone. Where this is not possible, interposed synthetic materials or freeze dried dura or fascia lata have not proven effective and a simple debridement of the tendon combined with resection of the CA ligament, bursal resection, and inferior acromioplasty should be performed. Advancement of the supraspinatus posteriorly as described by Debeyre may be an effective alternative [19]. Great care must be taken to evaluate the acromioclavicular joint preoperatively as noted above. A resection of the lateral 1.5 cm of the calvicle should be performed when the AC joint is arthritic and pain is relieved by preoperative local anaesthetic injection or when an inferior osteophyte is impinging on the rotator cuff.

If a full thickness rotator cuff tear remains untreated, the disease may progress further. This progression takes the form of further superior migration of the humeral head until it eventually articulates with the acromion and loss of glenohumeral joint space results, with cyst formation and erosion of the atrophic humeral head and glenoid. The later articular changes occur because of the pathomechanical joint forces which introduce extreme shear forces across the glenohumeral joint and result in cartilage degradation and subchondral bone atrophy. Neer has termed this process 'cuff tear arthropathy' [20]. The recommended treatment is total shoulder arthroplasty with repair of the cuff whenever (although this occurs rarely) possible. Following this procedure, a special rehabilitation program must be designed to offset the loss of the constraining function of the rotator cuff and, in fact, special glenoid components may be necessary to prevent excess shear force across the glenoid surface with subsequent increased risk of loosening. It is not suggested that all rotator cuff tears result in this severe joint destruction, but this must be taken into consideration when recommending treatment of a full thickness rotator cuff rupture.

In the continuum of rotator cuff impingement disease, the impingement sign is helpful in differentiating symptoms referable to the rotator cuff from those due to calcium deposit tendinitis, AC arthritis, instability, and other non-glenohumeral aetiologies. As the test for the sign is described by Neer [18], the examiner stands to the rear of the seated patient and stabilizes the scapula with one hand and raises the arm with the other into forward elevation. Prevention of scapular rotation forces impingement of haemorrhagic, fibrotic, or torn supraspinatus region onto the anterior–inferior edge of the acromion, which reproduces the patient's complaint. This manoeuvre will also produce pain with glenohumeral arthritis, mild adhesive capsulitis, subluxation, and calcium deposition disease. The final confirmation of the diagnosis of impingement related rotator cuff disease can be made with the 'impingement test', also described by Neer [18]. The subacromial space is injected with 10 ml of 1.0% xylocaine and the above-described manoeuvre repeated. This is best accomplished with the patient seated, the shoulder sterilely prepared, using a long $1\frac{1}{2}$ inch 25 gauge needle, and with an assistant pulling the arm distally. This injection will not relieve symptoms due to the other problems listed above.

Results of operative repair

When ruptures of the rotator cuff are repaired primarily after debriding the frayed edges or suturing them into bone troughs in the greater tuberosity, excellent results in terms of pain relief can be expected in 84–95% of patients [7,8].

Patients with smaller tears tend to have better results, although the size of the tear is not the critical indicator. Duration of symptoms is inversely proportional to the percentage of excellent results, which mandates an early investigation into the possibility of rotator cuff rupture. Duration of symptoms is directly related to the size of the tear and to the distance between the humeral head and acromion, both of which directly influence the results. Loss of passive ROM and strength of abduction and external rotation preoperatively negatively affect the results of surgical treatment and suggest that an element of adhesive capsulitis negatively influences final motion and function in terms of pain [4]. Loss of strength, however, is not directly related to the size of the cuff defect. Despite the fact that many of the cuff repairs are not 'water tight' when reexamined arthrographically postoperatively, pain relief and improvement in function are achieved in approximately 98% of patients [8]. Because the majority of patients with irreparable cuff tears improve after debridement and acromioplasty, the author believes that the key to relieving pain and improving function is the acromioplasty. The implication is that removing the compressive forces on a thickened, hyperaemic tendon, torn or not, produces pain relief.

The future

The educational efforts of Neer, Hawkins, Rockwood *et al.* will continue to have the effect of improving both the knowledge base and the experience of the general orthopaedist, which will most likely result in earlier diagnosis and treatment of the impingement syndrome. The best approach to the treatment of massive rotator cuff tears and cuff-tear arthropathy is to prevent them from developing. New information on the response of the rotator cuff to injury and repair will be forthcoming, due in part to the development of new techniques for studying soft tissue blood flow and repair [17]. Improved techniques for arthroscopy may play an important role in the clinical study of the rotator cuff, as well as investigations into less traumatic techniques for its repair [10]. Improved substitutional materials may one day make the repair of massive cuff tears with interpositional material a reality, which should yield improved functional results. Much investigative work is being conducted into the clinical problems of rotator cuff function degeneration and repair.

References

1. Smith, J. G. (1834) Pathological appearances of seven cases of injury of the shoulder joints with remarks. *London Med. Gaz.*, **14**, 280.
2. Codman, E. A. (1937) Rupture of the supraspinatus – 1834 to 1934. *J. Bone Joint Surg.*, **19**, 643–652.
3. Skinner, H. A. (1937) Anatomical considerations relative to rupture of the supraspinatus tendon. *J. Bone Joint Surg.*, **19**, 137.
4. Cotton, R. E. and Rideout, D. F. (1964) Tears of the humeral rotator cuff – a radiological and pathological necropsy survey. *J. Bone Joint Surg.*, **46B**, 314–328.
5. McLaughlin, H. L. (1944) Lesions of the musculotendinous cuff of the shoulder – the exposure and treatment of tears with retraction. *J. Bone Joint Surg.*, **26**, 31–51.
6. Post, M., Silver, R. and Singh, M. (1983) Rotator cuff tear, diagnosis and treatment. *Clin. Orthop.*, **173**, 78–91.
7. Ellman, H., Hanker, G. and Bayer, M. (1986) Repair of the rotator cuff – end result study of factors influencing reconstruction. *J. Bone Joint Surg.*, **68A**, 1136–1144.
8. Hawkins, R. J., Misamore, G. W. and Hobeika, P. A. (1985) Surgery for full thickness rotator cuff tears. *J. Bone Joint Surg.*, **67A**, 1349–1355.
9. Mack, L. A., Matsen, F. A. III, Kilcoyne, R. F., Davies, P. K. and Sickler, M. E. (1985) US evaluation of the rotator cuff. *Radiology*, **157**, 205–209.
10. Ogilvie-Harris, D. J. and Wiley, A. M. (1986) Arthroscopic surgery of the shoulder – a general appraisal. *J. Bone Joint Surg.*, **68B**, 201–207.
11. Moseley, H. F. and Goldie, I. (1963) The arterial pattern of the rotator cuff of the shoulder. *J. Bone Joint Surg.*, **45B**, 780–789.
12. Laing, P. G. (1956) The arterial supply of the adult humerus. *J. Bone Joint Surg.*, **38A**, 1105–1116.
13. Lindblom, K. and Palmer, I. (1939) Ruptures of the tendon aponeurosis of the shoulder joint – the so-called supraspinatus rupture. *Acta Chir. Scand.*, **82**, 133–142.
14. Neer, C. S. (1972) Anterior acromioplasty for the chronic impingement syndrome in the shoulder – a preliminary report. *J. Bone Joint Surg.*, **54A**, 41–50.
15. Rothman, R. H. and Parke, W. W. (1965) The vascular anatomy of the rotator cuff. *Clin. Orthop.*, **41**, 176–186.
16. Rathburn, J. B. and MacNab, I. (1970) The microvascular pattern of the rotator cuff. *J. Bone Joint Surg.*, **52B**, 540–553.
17. Swiontkowski, M. F. Unpublished data.
18. Neer, C. S. (1983) Impingement lesions. *Clin. Orthop.*, **173**, 70–77.
19. Debeyre, J., Patte, D. and Elmelik, E. Repair of ruptures of the rotator cuff of the shoulder – with a note on advancement of the supraspinatus muscle. *J. Bone Joint Surg.*, **47B**, 36–42.
20. Neer, C. S., Craig, E. V. and Fukuda, H. (1983) Cuff tear arthroplasty. *J. Bone Joint Surg.*, **65A**, 1232–1244.

Osteoarthritis of the hip

C. H. Wynn Jones

Incidence

Population surveys show the incidence of osteoarthritis of the hip increases with age. In females almost all have pain with marked radiological changes but in males only just over half those with moderate radiographic changes admitted to pain.

The overall incidence in female and male adults of all ages was 1%.

Aetiology and pathogenesis

Primary, idiopathic

This group is diminishing as identifiable causes or related factors are discovered.

Secondary, congenital

Skeletal dysplasia generalized.
Congenital hip dysplasia [1].
Strong inherited tendency yet no actual identified lesion.

Secondary, acquired

Acute injury and late effects.
Overload or repetitive minor injury.

Infection.
Suppuration/T.B.
Nutrition, rickets, metabolic and endocrine disorders, gout, acromegaly, slipped upper femoral epiphysis.
Inflammatory.
Immune deficiency disorder, rheumatoid arthritis.
Lysozome or storage diseases.
Following avascular necrosis:
Perthes' disease;
Idiopathic;
Associated with alcohol;
Other storage diseases, Gaucher's etc.;
Steroids.

Histological, biochemical and mechanical changes in cartilage and bone in osteoarthritis

Histology

The earlier changes can be seen as a natural process of aging and may not be associated with osteoarthritis either clinically or radiologically.

The earliest findings are zones of granularity especially of the anterior head.

Cartilage fibrillation may vary from minor to full thickness crevices down to bone. There may be cartilage loss, subchondral sclerosis and trabecular thickening.

Synovial inflammation is evident with increased vascularity, mononuclear cell infiltrate, fibrin deposits and villous hypertrophy.

Crystals are frequently associated with a high degree of inflammation in the synovium and may be of monosodium urate, as seen in gout or calcium pyrophosphate in chondrocalcinosis.

Biochemical changes

Proteoglycan molecules become smaller, synthesized at an increased rate and they appear to aggregate less well. There is overall less proteoglycan and there is an increased chondroitin component compared to the keratin sulphate component within the cartilage. The water content in arthritic cartilage is increased and the collagen bundle arrangement is altered; the meshwork structure becomes deficient.

Mechanical changes

Failure of lubrication cannot be implicated at present. There are glycoproteins in the synovium fluid that have particular lubricating qualities. Pseudonym 'Lubricin'.

Cartilage mechanical strength

The creep test under load of cartilage shows that the cartilage is softer and there is an increased rate of creep with an overall reduction in the compressive stiffness. The cartilage is thinned down overall. Freeman found that the cartilage at the zenith of the femoral head was much thicker and had different compression qualities from the cartilage at the antero inferior aspect of the head.

Vascular changes in osteoarthritis

These may be secondary to the initial development of osteoarthritis. There is certainly increased flow in the subchondral area in the cancellous bone beneath arthritic joints as demonstrated by isotope investigations There is also an increased venous intraosseus pressure.

Classification

Radiographic morphology of hip osteoarthrosis

There is no generally agreed radiological classification of osteoarthritis of the hip. Wroblewski and Charnley [2] describe such a classification but do not relate it to the outcome in total hip replacement. Such a classification becomes more important if osteotomies of various types are considered because it is now generally agreed that certain types of osteotomy may be better for specific radiological varieties of osteoarthritis.

Bombelli, in his classic monograph on osteoarthritis [3] of the hip treated by osteotomy, describes such a classification. The author commends the following (differs little from Charnley's).

Superolateral (Fig. 18.1)

Type a

Spherical head polar osteoarthritis, i.e. superior narrowing of the joint space with sclerosis or cyst formation. The medial cartilage joint space may be normal and there are minimal osteophytes.

Type b

Ellipsoid head. The acetabulum is more oblique and the head in the corresponding plane is flattened. There are major medial osteophytes on the femoral head with a capital drop. The head is beginning to glide antero-cranially out of the acetabulum.

Type c

Subluxated. There is extreme obliquity of the articular acetabular surface with uncovering of the femoral head. Shenton's line is severely interrupted and there are often marked floor osteophytes.

Type d

Lateralized.

(i) Early stage.
(ii) Middle stage.
(iii) Later stage.

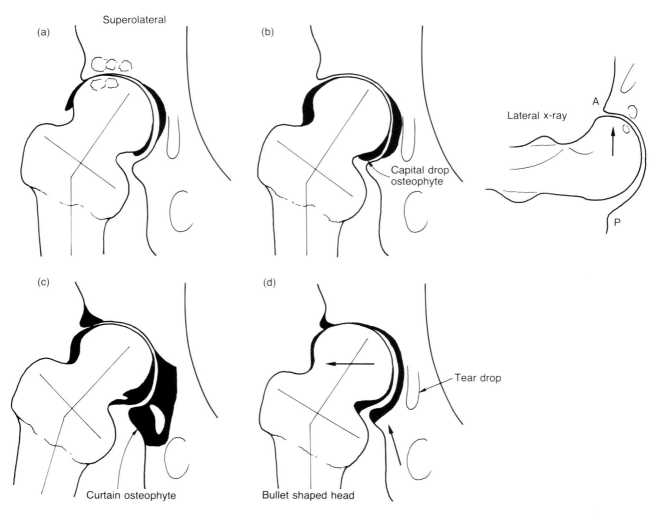

Fig. 18.1   (a) Loss of joint space superiorly and anteriorly polar OA. Neck slightly valgus (normal CCD < 126° 3). Weight bearing surface horizontal. (b) As (a) but head gliding more anterosuperior – WBS oblique. Valgus neck (CCD > 126°). (c) Congenital abnormal acetabulum with severe obliquity. Valgus anteverted femoral neck (new acetabulum formed). (d) Floor curtain osteophytes, extruding head, i.e., floor very deep. Often normal neck shaft angle.

The femoral head tends to migrate laterally. The head is usually fairly round, the weight bearing surface is horizontal and according to the grade the capital drop, i.e. the medial head osteophyte and the curtain osteophyte, i.e. the inferior floor osteophyte, become well developed. There may be a small roof osteophyte. (dii may be confused with type a.)

The superolateral group a,b,c belong to those arthritides that result from hip dysplasia and Perthes' disease. (The lateral radiograph demonstrates anterior osteoarthritis between femoral head and acetabulum and there may be a great deal of anteversion of the femoral neck in the congenital varieties.) There may be a strong preceding history of injury or heavy sport in superolateral type d.

Concentric (Fig. 18.2)

The head is spherical and well centred even on a lateral radiograph and there is even cartilage wear on acetabulum and femoral head. Osteophytes are scarce. The bone may be eburnated and sclerotic. There may not be widespread cyst formation because of even stress on the femoral head and acetabulum.

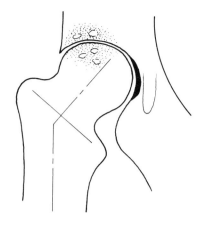

Fig. 18.2 Concentric round head, even wear acetabular cartilage and femoral head.

Medial (Fig. 18.3)

Type a (equatorial)

The femoral head points to the deeper aspect of the acetabulum. There is loss of joint space medially. Good superolateral cartilage joint space can be seen to be preserved. There may be a lateral acetabular osteophyte and a modest varus disposition on the femoral neck.

Type b (coxa profunda)

In such a case there is often a very varus disposition of the femoral neck, perhaps CCD angle 110. Superolateral cartilage joint space may be well preserved. In the main there is inferomedial

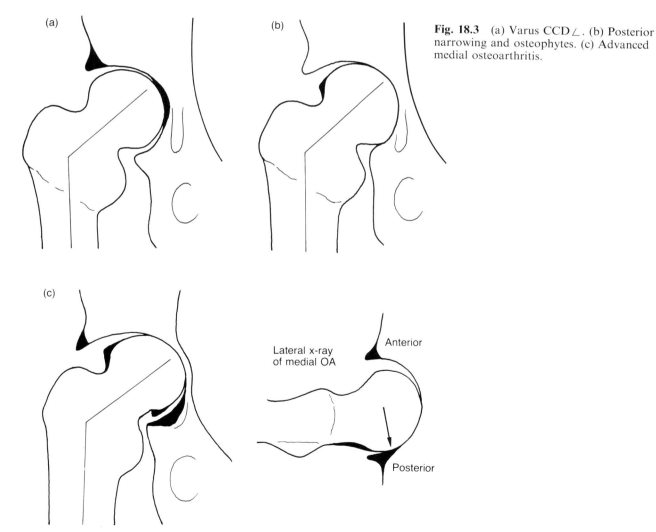

Fig. 18.3 (a) Varus CCD∠. (b) Posterior narrowing and osteophytes. (c) Advanced medial osteoarthritis.

narrowing of the joint space. The head is well sunk into the acetabulum, the medial wall of which may be very thin.

Type c (protrusio acetabuli)

The floor of the acetabulum is often interrupted and the head deeply penetrates into the acetabulum with medial osteoarthritis. The femoral head often loses its normal shape. On the lateral radiograph there is often good anterior joint space but posteriorly it may be lost and the head may be directed posteriorly, i.e. retroverted.

Other features that can be radiologically interpreted are the biological reaction of the bone to the arthritic process. The reaction may be atrophic, normotrophic or hypertrophic. In the former there is often collapse of the femoral head with very little attempt at osteophyte formation. It could be considered a metabolic problem and in such cases there are often marked inflammatory synovial changes, oedema and a high degree of vascularity. The latter hypertrophic osteoarthrosis is where the hip has a completely distorted shape and there is marked over growth of osteophytes. There are often protruding roof osteophytes and the capital drop is often high and with a large medial osteophyte in the acetabular floor; a so-called curtain osteophyte. It could be interpreted that in such cases the bone is still very reactive. Frequently there is a good cortical thickness in the femoral shaft. Such cases often respond well to osteotomy because the bone is reactive. A concomitant of this radiological feature is often marked stiffness which may be a contraindication to osteotomy.

Such a classification is helpful in choosing which sort of osteotomy to undertake. In terms of success rate after conventional cemented arthroplasty there are the obvious problems that may be predicted. For example, a gross protrusio with loss of the medial floor may mean that special measures will have to be undertaken to lateralize the cup into its anatomical position perhaps with bone grafting or the use of a noncement cup with perimeter bearing. Similarly, a superolateral type b or in particular c with a marked degree of subluxation, an arthritic high false acetabulum is formed which has a very deficient roof. Special techniques are required to obtain the correct relationship of the prosthesis

and true acetabulum; bone grafting or a small acetabular component may be required.

In osteotomy the implications for classification are much more profound as the success in any particular sort of osteotomy depends upon the type of arthritis.

Although not widely practised now, resurfacing arthroplasty is generally unwise for patients with radiological features more of metabolic inactivity than mechanically reactive osteoarthritis. The incidence of femoral neck failure is high in such patients. The bone density can be quantified with CT scans and should not be under 200 CT units.

Biomechanics of the hip

1. Normal.
2. The hip after osteotomy.
3. Biomechanical aspects of T.H.R. and design.

Normal hip joint

To assess the forces across the hip joint one has to simplify the hip down to a simple system of levers. A static analysis in one plane only is the simplest.

Uniplanar static analysis

The magnitude and direction of the forces acting on the joint are represented in Figs 18.4 and 18.5.

Figure 18.6 represents the analysis of the hip joint force with the subject standing on one leg,

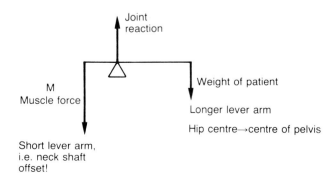

Fig. 18.4 Torque equilibrium in one-legged stance.

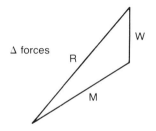

Fig. 18.5   Where length is proportionate to amount. direction is direction of force.

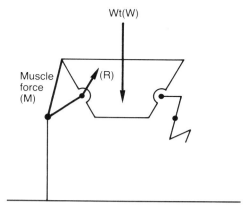

Fig. 18.6   One leg weight-bearing stance: W = weight of patient; M = muscle force of abductors; R = joint reaction force.

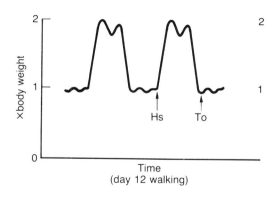

Fig. 18.7   Load trace from instrumented femoral component during walking.

when the subject is in equilibrium and Newton's first law is fulfilled. Newton's third law states that in equilibrium for each force there is an equal and opposite force. A simple balance principle, as in the diagram above, shows this.

Due to its small lever arm about the hip joint the abductor force must be large to achieve equilibrium. The sum of the abductor force and the body weight must equal the force on the hip joint to achieve force equilibrium. The force across the hip joint is large, for example four times the body weight.

The femoral neck must therefore withstand a large bending moment.

Dynamic stress analysis

The more sophisticated analyses consider the body in locomotion. Skin markers and light emitting diodes are placed over bony prominences in relation to the axial points of the joints of the lower limb. The patient is filmed in two planes at right angles during walking. Simultaneously, ground to foot forces readings in various directions are measured by a force-plate recessed in the floor, and thus the components of total joint force can be obtained by computer analysis. The phasic actions of muscles can be recorded by EMG synchronous recordings and relayed by trailing leads or telemetry. From these studies Paul suggested a figure of four times the body weight as a peak during walking. Walking up an incline or going upstairs increases this to about five times body weight [4].

It is estimated that certain sporting activities may increase the hip joint load to 15 times body weight, but these figures are difficult to analyse.

In vivo prosthetic joint force recordings have been undertaken English [5] implanted prostheses from which direct readings of force transmitted during ambulation were recorded. The load cycle achieved with walking by English is shown in Fig. 18.7.

Figure 18.8a shows that the resultant force across the hip joint varies according to the gait phase. When seen after total hip replacement the angle varies less. The inclination of R as viewed laterally is shown in Fig. 18.8b. This implies a twisting force which is applied to the proximal femur (Fig. 18.8c).

These findings in general suggest that load variability induced by walking and physical activity has a greater effect upon the magnitude and direction of R; thus the stress across the hip joint has a bearing on implant design and/or surgical technique.

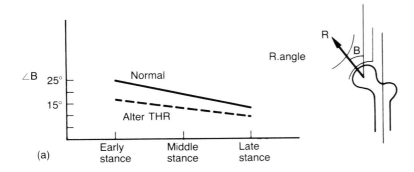

(a)

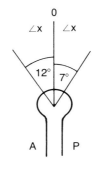

Fig. 18.8 Load angle and direction during walking. (a) ∠ of **R** in coronal plane. (b) Load ∠ change during walking: sagittal plane. (c) Torsional moment on femoral component induced by alternating ∠ **R** with respect to coronal plane.

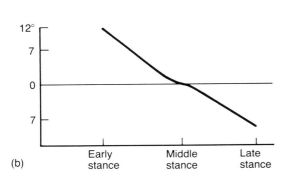

(b)

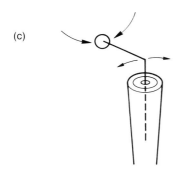

(c)

Biomechanics of the hip joint and osteotomy

Osteotomy and the soft tissue release can affect the forces across the hip joint in three ways:

(1) Alteration of the neck shaft angle alters the lever arm. The effect of this can be considered in the coronal and sagittal planes. A more varus disposition of the neck shaft angle reduces the joint force and medializes R, because it effectively increases the load taken by the abductor muscles. Valgus osteotomy on the other hand increases R and makes it more steeply inclined (Fig. 18.9a). As viewed in the horizontal plane the extension component to an osteotomy must tend to put R posterior to the vertical line of the hip joint (Fig. 18.9b).

(2) Osteotomy can influence the load distribution within the joint, an osteotomy (Fig. 18.9c) can improve congruency increasing the load bearing area. A valgus osteotomy brings osteophytes that were previously not load bearing into load contact with the acetabulum and must reduce joint stress (Fig. 18.9d). Muscle or tendon release (Voss procedure) can also reduce hip joint force.

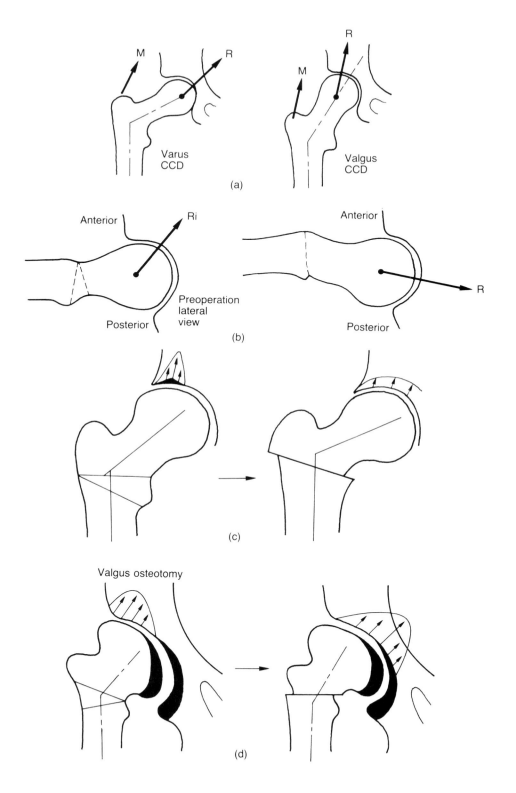

Fig. 18.9   (a–d) Alterations of Resultant force R with osteotomy. Improving congruency 'evens up' bad distribution.

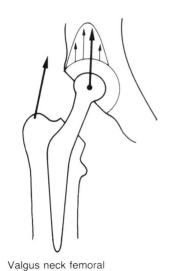

Valgus neck femoral
component

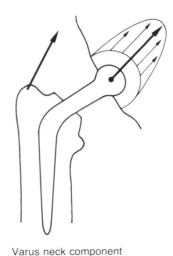

Varus neck component

Fig. 18.10   (a) Valgus neck femoral component. (b) Varus neck component.

Biomechanical alterations after hip joint replacement

Femoral component

Wroblewski's analysis of fractured femoral stems demonstrates that the initiation point for a fatigue failure is the anterolateral corner of the prosthesis. This supports the biomechanical analysis demonstrating a torsional force on the proximal femur. An increased offset prosthesis would increase the anterolateral load on the prosthesis. Anteversion of the prosthetic component tends to reduce the torsional moment. Similarly, a very valgus disposition of the neck shaft angle would decrease the torsional moment. A valgus neck shaft angle can minimize the lateral skin stress in the prosthesis but a side effect of the use of such a prosthesis would be to localize force R more superolaterally within the acetabular component with the potential for uneven load distribution at the cement bone interface (Fig. 18.10).

Implant design

An intramedullary femoral prosthesis alters the load distribution within the femur. Abnormal bending, shear and hoop stresses are induced. The design of the prosthesis and fixation must be such as to minimize each of these.

Axial

Calcar contact theoretically facilitates proximal load transmission but clinical studies when cemented arthroplasty is used suggest that calcar contact is quickly lost and there is remodelling of the calcar with rounding and loss of the axial loading. However, theoretical and experimental analysis supports the use of a collar. With an uncemented component, however, with a collar, definite axial loading can be determined as evidenced by sclerosis.

Radial and hoop stress

A wedge type of prosthesis, either cemented or uncemented, can induce these. The induction of hoop stresses in the more proximal femur may be beneficial. With cemented arthroplasty loss of bone density proximally suggests that weight is taken more distally through the prosthesis and this may enhance implant fatigue. Hoop stresses may be uniformally induced in the femur if the prosthesis is evenly tapered. Certainly any proximal muscle attachment forces will compliment the implant-induced hoop stresses.

Choices of treatment in hip osteoarthritis including historical perspectives

Conservative management

The obvious straight forward lines of management should not be forgotten, weight reduction is paramount but not always easily achieved. A whole range of non-steroidals are available but none obvious best in osteoarthritis.

Physiotherapy is usually tried but the results are disappointing. There are two specific areas where physiotherapy in the author's opinion is definitely beneficial:

(a) The occasional patient has minimal radiological changes and yet a marked degree of stiffness. If associated with a great deal of pain, an intra-articular injection of steroid and Marcain combined with intensive physiotherapy can produce a long lasting improvement.

(b) There are patients who without gross radiological changes appear to have developed quite a severe fixed flexion deformity. This can be aided greatly by preoperative advice from a physiotherapist and hydrotherapy. Hydrotherapy is an important line of treatment in the slightly stiff younger male patient where the symptoms are not quite bad enough for total hip replacement and the surgeon may be undecided about the benefits of osteotomy. Hydrotherapy can be used as a waiting manoeuvre before total hip replacement and the increased range of movement produced may be very beneficial, though pain may not be much reduced.

Operative treatment

The choice in general terms is between osteotomy or total hip replacement and the latter may be cemented or non-cemented. The choice is fairly straight forward in a patient over about 60 years. Cemented arthroplasty of a conventional design gives very satisfactory results in more than 90% of patients.

In active, very young patients the results of conventional cemented total hip replacement are worse than osteotomy. If there are the ideal indications for osteotomy, i.e. a moderate fixed flexion deformity and one of the more classic

indications for osteotomy (see later under subsection osteotomy), then this treatment should be preferred. Osteotomy does not preclude a satisfactory total hip replacement, because modern osteotomy does not involve much displacement of femoral shaft.

Between the ages of 45 and 60 many surgeons would use conventional and time tested cemented total hip replacement and it is the author's view that it is much better to use a well cemented total hip replacement performed by a surgeon familiar with a good technique than the occasional non-cemented total hip replacement.

A non-cemented prosthesis can be used if there is excellent quality of bone stock and the geometry of the bone can be matched by an appropriate well fitted non-cemented prosthesis. There are patients, however, particularly those who have had osteotomy previously, where the accurate reaming required for non-cement prosthesis would be extremely difficult. In this small group of patients with advanced changes with abnormal bone geometry resurfacing may still have a place. The bone density of the femoral head and neck must be above 200 units as measured by CT scan.

Arthrodesis in the younger patient should be considered. A young male patient of short stature probably does best with this operation. The other hip and ipsilateral knee must be entirely normal. The technique of arthrodesis is not described as it is outside the scope of this chapter, but a method should be adopted probably using internal fixation and bone grafting, that does not derange the geometry of the proximal femur and acetabulum. The arthrodesis can then be converted to a total hip replacement if required years later.

Historical perspectives

The reader is referred to the original papers to obtain detail of osteotomies used historically and for the techniques and results of the early workers in total hip replacement. McMurray popularized the high offset osteotomy which was not internally fixed; later Wainwright described internal fixation methods leading up to Pauwell's work published in 1976. This latter is the forerunner of the modern osteotomy technique.

In hip arthroplasty the very earliest varieties were those of Rehn: 'Interposition arthroplasty'

1930 [6], although Girdlestone's operation is in a sense an excision arthroplasty. Wiles in London in 1938 was probably the first to use replacement of both the acetabular and femoral surfaces. Thompson (1954) and Moore (1952) popularized the hemiarthroplasty (femoral) for arthritis.

Indications, techniques and follow-up of osteotomy of the hip

General indications for osteotomy

Generally patients less than 50 years of age.
No obesity.
A good range of movement; preferably 90° of flexion.
A clerical rather than a manual worker.
Good congruence in a functional radiograph.
The radiographs should show signs of mechanical overload with secondary arthritis rather than atrophic or inflammatory arthritis.
Patients must be motivated to comply with the rehabiliation process with partial weight bearing and intensive exercises.
Morphological radiographic classification is vital to determine which osteotomy is likely to give the best result.
The key to the choice of osteotomy is the size, shape and direction of the weight bearing surface; 'sourcil' of Pauwells and Bombelli.

Options

Femoral osteotomy:

Varus, plus or minus extension and derotation component.
Valgus, plus an extension or flexion component.
Trochanteric lateralization procedure (Maquet).

Pelvic osteotomy:

Chiari operation.

Pelvic rotation operation including cover:

Salter
Triple (Berne or Steele).
Wagner osteotomy.

Often included particularly with the valgus

femoral osteotomy is the Voss procedure with a widespread soft tissue release further decreasing the stress on the hip. A femoral osteotomy is best utilized when there is adequate cover of the femoral head. If the head is uncovered in early disease in the younger patient a rotational osteotomy of the acetabulum would be preferred but the acetabulum must be congruous with the femoral head. In an older person with more major secondary arthritic changes and loss of cover an operation such as a Chiari may be more suitable. The neck shaft angle, i.e. CCD angle, is a guide to which osteotomy might be used. Coxa valga tending to give an extrusive arthritis might suggest that the varus femoral osteotomy is preferred to render the neck shaft angle more normal, and vice versa for a congenital coxa vara tending to produce a protrusive arthritis when a valgus osteotomy is often indicated.

Choice of osteotomy according to classification of osteoarthritis
(See previous subsection)

Superolateral

(a) Varus osteotomy.
(b) Early stage pelvic rotational osteotomy later valgus osteotomy alone or with pelvic osteotomy.
(c) Early stage pelvic osteotomy or shelf later valgus osteotomy.
(d) (i) Varus extension osteotomy
    (ii) Valgus extension osteotomy.
    (iii) Total hip replacement.

In dealing with (b) (c) and (d)ii, potential adduction of at least 15° range of movement should be available. Patients with a flattened head do well with a valgus osteotomy.

Medial osteoarthritis

(a) and (b) valgus extension osteotomy
(c) total hip replacement.

Principles of osteotomy

Anteroposterior radiographs centred on the hip and lateral radiographs are required. A weight bearing 60° oblique (Berne View) shows the loss of cover of the anterior head. The two methods available to plan the angular correction by osteotomy are:

(a) Tracings are made of the femur and acetabulum from the neutral position as in the original radiograph. Where a valgus osteotomy is considered an ideal may be perfect congruence with placement of the femur in adduction. It is advisable to plan extra superolateral clearance. The capital drop should approximate to the curtain osteophyte.

(b) The patient can be examined under image intensifier with films taken in adduction and abduction. Similarly, the extension component can be assessed by examining the abduction and adduction with the hip in flexion. If there appears to be increased joint space and superolateral opening out of the joint space the actual position of the leg in relationship to the image intensifier table determines the correct position for osteotomy. An ordinary lateral radiograph may give some idea of the anteversion of the neck. The extension component overcomes this. If there is clinically a fixed flexion deformity, enough extension must be put into the osteotomy to align the leg normally. With the joint capsule open the hip can be flexed until the anterior uncovered head is covered. Modern imaging with 3D CT reconstruction allows accurate planning. Some centres are using computer assisted techniques derived from the CT information to plan 3 dimensional corrections possible with a pelvic rotational operation.

Other points to assess in planning:

1. *Leg lengthening.* Leg length is increased with valgus osteotomy and vice versa with varus – with a valgus of 30° and extension component of 10° in a patient with a CCD of 130° there will be approximately 5 mm lengthening.
2. *Trochanteric osteotomy.* This can be added (a) to a valgus osteotomy. A bone graft can be wedged underneath to effectively lateralize the greater trochanter to maintain abductor power. (b) In a varus osteotomy of more than 20° the greater trochanter can be brought back to a more anatomical level to produce correct tension on the abductors and reduce the tendency to a postoperative limp.
3. Correction of a rotational element, i.e. severe external rotation deformity.

4. Reduction of the stress on the hip by muscle release (a). The abductors are in small part released in such a valgus osteotomy by lateralizing the greater trochanter and allowing the trochanter to ride up slightly but maintaining some soft tissue connection to stabilize the bone graft. (b) Adductor and psoas release is performed in a valgus osteotomy as the valgus would otherwise increase tension (Voss procedure).
5. Maintenance of load line in relationship to the knee. If a valgus osteotomy is undertaken the shaft should be lateralized to keep the load line satisfactory and to prevent a tendency to valgus deformity of the knee. *Vice versa* with a varus osteotomy.
6. Any major obstructing osteophyte should be identified, such as a so-called elephant trunk osteophyte on the head or a hypertrophic acetabular floor osteophyte.
7. If the valgus has been planned by plain radiographs the valgus component achieved may be under estimated, i.e. if a planned valgus of 20° is required and this is to be associated with an extension component of 15° or so, the surgeon will actually need to perform a 25° valgus angulation at operation in order to achieve the planned valgus as on the preoperative radiographs. The reverse is true in varus osteotomy. For more details the reader is referred to Bombelli's classic text [3].

Technique of valgus osteotomy

The patient should be supine on the operating table. An incision along the line of the shaft of the femur going from the tip of the greater trochanter to the anterior superior iliac spine is used. The femur is reached by deepening along the line of the skin incision through the fascia. Vastus lateralis is lifted forward. The capsule is exposed and opened and it is suggested that an AO angle blade plate of 130° is utilized. Figure 18.11 illustrates the calculation for the insertion angle for the seating chisel.

The line of the seating chisel is easy to find after direct inspection of the femoral neck. Operative radiographs are not required in general but an inexperienced surgeon might find them useful. Attention must be paid to the plane of insertion of the seating chisel, the coronal plane for the valgus component, the sagittal plane for the

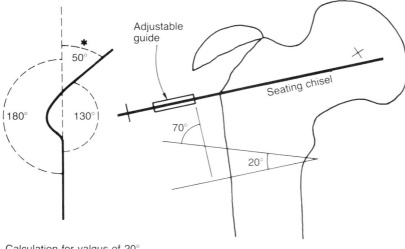

Fig. 18.11   Planning calculations for a 20° valgus osteotomy using a 130° blade plate.

Calculation for valgus of 20°

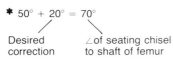

∗ 50° + 20° = 70°

Desired   ∠ of seating chisel
correction   to shaft of femur

extension component and the horizontal plane for the rotational component.

It is recommended that a long cancellous or cortical screw be inserted into the proximal osteotomy fragment to prevent the blade pulling out of the head and neck when compression is undertaken.

N.B. When the bone is sectioned the ilio-psoas muscle can be transected. The adductor release should be through a separate incision and due allowance must be made for this when draping.

Postoperative rehabilitation

(a) No passive movements; hydrotherapy.
(b) Six months elbow crutches if possible with partial weight bearing and graduated increments of weight bearing over this period.

Varus osteotomy

In general this osteotomy is beneficial in a rather earlier stage of osteoarthritis with minimal osteophytes, a valgoid femoral neck and a round femoral head. A particular indication may be in coxa vara subluxans when the weight bearing surface is horizontal and osteoarthritis is at its most early stage. It is in this sort of case that progressive arthritis can be predicted with certainty and a prophylactic operation may be justified. A varus osteotomy is not indicated when the head is flattened or osteophytes are too bulky.

The approach is much as in a valgus osteotomy. There is no need for adductor release or a psoas release. If more than 20° of varus is planned it is necessary to osteotomize the greater trochanter and more distally fix it. If 25° of varus is planned from a radiograph and there is an extension component also planned, it is necessary to under form the osteotomy at the actual operation. If in the coronal plane a 25° angle of varus from radiograph template is planned it would be necessary to put in only 20° of varus at the operation. A 90° AO blade plate is suggested with an offset and this automatically tends to maintain the knee alignment. To minimize shortening bone should not be resected; the calcar area of the proximal femur can be impacted into the shaft of the femur and securely held with a blade plate.

Assessment of angle of insertion of seating chisel

Using a 90° blade plate, if a varus of 20° is planned it is obvious that a 70° angle of the seating chisel is required in relationship to the long axis of the shaft of the femur.

Postoperative management as in valgus.

Follow-up after proximal femoral osteotomy

Bombelli [3] reports in a 6–8 year follow-up of valgus extension osteotomy that the results of pain relief are very good, i.e. 308 patients out of 471 had no pain. With medial osteoarthritis grade a and b Maquet [7] reports on the results of a valgus extension osteotomy that in an 8-year follow-up of 150 cases 83% were painfree. Bombelli on the follow-up of varus osteotomy over a similar period of time reports that 198 patients out of 212 had no pain. A fifth of patients had a slight limp after varus osteotomy. Morscher [8] reports from a multicentric continental trial that 80% had a good relief of pain and an improvement in 60% walking ability.

Cemented total hip arthroplasty. General principles and techniques including approaches to the hip joint

General principles

The general success rate after primary hip cemented arthroplasty is more than 90%. Some 350 000 are performed each year worldwide and it competes with heart and renal transplant surgery in reducing disability. The results of primary surgery are so much better than revisional surgery and there is no doubt the principle of 'get it right first time' applies.

A cemented total hip replacement will always have a finite life span. It is only with improvements in materials and techniques that survivorship will continue to improve. Major design changes are unlikely. The success rate in terms of prosthetic survival are higher in low demand users, i.e. the older patient and in patients with multiple joint problems. The clinical test bed for any hip replacement implant is a younger more active patient.

Whilst cemented total hip replacement may not be denied to patients who are in higher risk groups there are factors that have been identified that can be modified to improve implant survival.

High body weight has been related to early failure in many studies. High activity levels after surgery have been correlated with increased failure rates. Importantly positively restricting activity levels after surgery in younger patients can enhance implant survival. In this study the failures frequently did not use walking aids in the early postoperative period. More controlled trials are needed in such patients.

Careful planning and choice of implant is critical to the early success of insertion and a trouble free perioperative period. Clinical assessment demonstrates any severe degree of fixed flexion, external rotation or adduction deformity. Mild deformities need no special attention, but, for example, failure to correct a severe external rotation deformity by radical release of the posterior capsule and piriformis may spoil the result and the author considers that if this is not done at the time of operation, no amount of physiotherapy postoperatively will correct such a rotational deformity.

A fixed flexion deformity in a unilateral hip will correct spontaneously after pain relieving surgery. If the deformity is present in a younger patient with bilateral disease both hips should be replaced followed by hydrotherapy.

Preoperative counselling of the patient should be undertaken well before surgery. The choice of type of operation and implant suggested must be spelled out and the potential complications of note.

A full and frank discussion of these including overlengthening – nerve palsy and infection may save later medico-legal difficulties – the notes must include the details of the counselling.

Bilateral hip replacement

In patients with bilateral hip arthritis an extremely careful evaluation of the overall medical status of the patient is required. The author's experience is that patients under 60 who are slim and have no other medical problems can safely undertake this procedure particularly if anti-embolic measures are undertaken. In patients over 70 it is only the exception that bilateral simultaneous hip arthroplasty can be safely undertaken.

There is no authoritative agreement on the optimum interval between two hip operations.

The author's experience is that in the older patient where the primary indication is relief of pain a planned second admission is acceptable; between 6 months and a year after the first. For a younger patient the best results after bilateral operations are obtained within a smaller time interval.

Leg length inequality needs to be assessed. Often this is apparent due to an adduction contracture and is relieved in the painful stiff hip by arthroplasty. Occasionally, a severe contracture merits an adductor release which is performed percutaneously at the end of the hip operation. True leg length inequality of 1–1.5 cm can be corrected during ordinary arthroplasty and capsulotomy, but for greater length of inequality special measures need to be undertaken.

Planning for this needs to be undertaken prior to operation. Again a balance should be struck. In an elderly patient often the quickest operation consistent with a good straightforward technique may not equalize the leg length but is acceptable; the patient needs to be warned before the operation. A younger patient will seek perfection and the leg length can be achieved by a longer operation involving greater blood loss because of the wide capsular and muscular release; instability in the early stages is a likely hazard.

Accurate measurement of leg length discrepancy is required before operation and any fixed deformity is taken into account. At operation fixed reference points are determined either by:

(a) The most accurate; parallel pins are driven into the pelvis and femur prior to dislocation.
(b) The radiological tear drop, often obscured by floor osteophyte or ossification of the transverse ligament is identified and a point on the femur best made by burning a deep diathermy mark.

The desired length can be achieved by measurement after transecting in this order (a) capsule, (b) psoas, (c) piriformis and lastly (d) gluteus maximus tendinous insertion at the linea aspera.

Surgical Approach

Osborne [9] has described the history of surgical access for hip replacement. There are occasion-ally specific indications for particular approaches to the hip and these need to be assessed pre-operatively. The author's view is that a severe fixed flexion deformity is better approached by an anterolateral or trochanteric osteotomy approach following a radical anterior release. A very severe fixed external rotation deformity is more easily corrected by a posterior approach. If the patient has a spastic element which is due to coincidental disease an anterior approach is preferable as the spasm tends to produce a flexion contracture and instability is likely with a posterior approach.

In all these approaches it is vital that soft tissue tension be determined from trial insertion and reduction of the femoral component. Gross pistoning of the femoral prosthetic head out of the acetabulum must not occur. In the posterior or anterior approaches trial reduction is critical, as no easy adjustment of the soft tissue tension can be undertaken once the prosthesis is inserted with cement.

In the trochanteric osteotomy approach the trochanter can be attached a little more distally to tighten up the soft tissues but the leg may be short. With the modified McFarland approach there is only a minimal capacity to tighten up soft tissues. In this approach the hip is usually perfectly stable in full internal rotation but if put in rather slackly in external rotation it may dislocate. It is vital that the hip is inserted with neutrality of both components with a 22 mm head prosthesis. If, for example, slight anteversion of the femoral component is combined with slight anteversion of the acetabular component then dislocation at trial reduction can be very apparent. The only safeguard against this is very accurate repair of the anterior fibres of medius. It is better to rely in the greater part on the stability from the prosthetic component position than the repair of anterior fibres of gluteus medius.

It is vital that the nursing staff understand the principles of the approaches used for the hip joint. In any one unit varying approaches may be used and various protocols of postoperative management may be instituted. This frequently leaves the nursing staff confused unless the principles of possible instability with the different approaches are explained. With any of the approaches described, if there is adequate soft tissue tension and correct component positioning, no special safeguards in postoperative re-habilitation are required.

Bone cement surgical technique

Improvement in mechanical properties of polymerized methacrylate

Inclusions of blood, air, radio-opaque agents and antibiotics should be minimized. Ling, Lee *et al.* [10], describe an elegant study of these factors. To avoid admixture of too much air the cement should be mixed rather than beaten like egg white. The dough should be used early so re-ducing laminations. Any technique that mini-mizes the amount of blood in the acetabulum or the femur and preventing lamination of blood in the cement should be utilized. The mechanical properties of the cement are enhanced if after delivery the cement is highly contained and preferably polymerized under pressure. There is clearly an overlap between the factors improving mechanical properties of cement and improving cement penetration into bony irregularities.

The recently advocated method of limiting air admixture into the cement is for the cement to be mixed in a vacuum and the cement to be centri-fuged. It does alter the cement handling charac-teristics and laboratory rehearsal is advised. This may produce more cement shrinkage and is not widely adopted.

Under this context the overall mechanical be-haviour of the cement mantle can be considered. There is no doubt that an even cement mantle is required. There may be sites that for particular mechanical reasons concerned with cement properties the cement should be thicker, e.g. in the superomedial femoral area. The techniques to achieve the above principles are described later.

Improved fixation of cement to the bone

First generation techniques did not involve brushing or lavage. The so-called second gener-ation techniques have produced the greatest advances.

Halawa [11], working in Ling's unit describes the benefits of washing the trabecular bone with a pulsatile lavage system. The debris is thereby removed and there is enchanced cement penetra-tion into the trabecular bone. Subcortical strong trabecular bone should be pressurized for fixa-tion. The penetration of cement into trabecular bone can be enhanced by pressurizing the cement. On the femoral side this can be under-taken by inserting the cement from distal to proximal using either a gun or a vent tube and digitally inserting the cement. The cement can be pressurized if a less viscous cement is used and a dam is applied to the proximal femur or the mouth of the acetabulum; it is easier where the cement is fully contained.

If in doubt the inexperienced surgeon should not use very non-viscous cement because it is difficult to handle and a deficient technique may provide a worse result than a sensibly used ordi-nary dough. It must be remembered that Charnley in his earlier work did not use these sophisticated methods and he inserted the cement dough with digital thrusts into the medullary cavity of the femur. When any pressurization technique is used the surgeon must be careful not to let the cement polymerize too far which would make insertion of the prosthesis almost im-possible. With such containment techniques the surgeon has less tactile feedback and must rely on a knowledge of the time and temperature setting qualities of the cement rather than his finger tips.

If the femur is narrow and distally plugged the femoral component should be inserted early into the cement because too firm a dough stage may prevent correct component placement. The com-ponent should *not* be inserted with hammer blows because of the hydraulic damper effect of bone and cement; a firm and prolonged thrust is more effective.

Pressurizing the cement reduces the thickness of the blood film at the interface and adequate pressurizing prevents capillary flow. Blood at the interface can be reduced by:

(a) Lavage;
(b) Irrigation with hydrogen peroxide acts as a haemostatic;
(c) Packing with gauze or other similar absorp-tive agents from distal to proximal.

On the acetabular side a flanged cup helps to enhance cement interdigitation with bone. Shelley shows that the flange on the Charnley cup enables some 20 mm mercury pressure to be maintained within the cement mantle prior to setting. This is because of the containment of the cement by the flange. When an ordinary cup is used cement extrudes around the edge of the cup and although modest pressure may be effective for a minute or two, it is not maintained during the time the cement takes to set; any reduction of pressure allows capillary flow of blood produce a film at the interface.

A similar effect is developed within the femur when a tapered femoral component is thrust into the cement. Maximal pressure is developed distally but is not uniform throughout the cavity.

Cemented acetabular component choice and insertion

With a 22 mm headed femoral component there is adequate thickness of the acetabular component in the average case to prevent excess stress developing in the cement. If a 32 mm headed component is used or smaller outer diameter sizes a metal backed component is recommended. The size should be predetermined by examination of radiographs and assessment with templates. An acetabular component should not have deep grooves for cement purchase. An adequate exposure of the acetabulum by removing the capsule and osteophytes is mandatory.

Adequate depth should be achieved in the acetabulum so that the largest component can be inserted maintaining adequate cover anteriorly, superiorly and posteriorly and yet allowing an adequate cement mantle of at least 3 mm. It should be flanged to maintain pressurization of the cement during polymerization, and to avoid bottoming out and an uneven cement mantle. The placement of the acetabular component is somewhat determined by the pathological anatomy of the arthritic hip. The 22 mm ID acetabular components are placed in neutral in the coronal plane, i.e. no anti- or retroversion and 45° to the horizontal, large ID sizes 28 mm should be slightly 10–15° anteverted. The O.G. cup of Charnley with its anterior flange allows a neutral placement (of the cup) where there is a deficient anterior acetabular wall yet it contains the cement and allows coverage of the ischial keyhole. This elegant implant can be shaped with scissors to accurately occlude the mouth of the acetabulum.

There is clinical evidence that three large keyholes produce less evidence of loosening than multiple small holes. Such large key holes should be perhaps 12–15 mm in diameter and depth. Ideally, to minimize cement stress concentration the edges of the hole should be bevelled and there should be some undercutting within the key holes.

There is much debate about whether the subchondral bone plate should be removed. Total removal of the subchondral bone plate with opening out of all trabecular bone can allow cement to intrude within the substance of the trabecular bone almost up to the inner pelvic table. Charnley [12] traditionally advocated leaving as much subchondral bone as possible consistent with adequate placement of the acetabular component. Multiple drill holes into good quality subchondral bone are utilized with a flanged acetabular cup to pressurize the cement. Long term advantages of any specific technique have not been reported.

Protrusio acetabuli

Physiological placement of the acetabular component is important to prevent the tendency for protrusion of the component into the pelvis. A flanged cup is used and bone grafting of the acetabular floor. Ordinary cement pressurization in such a case can be used. This author prefers a non cement porous coated acetabular component with a tight perimeter bearing placed to provide a physiological centre of rotation. Bone graft can be placed beneath before impaction.

Cemented femoral component design and technique

There is general agreement now that the femoral component stem should be straight and of even taper with no sharp edges. The size is predetermined with templates. An adequate range of implants is required. There is evidence that the femoral component of the implant should fill between some 70–80% of the canal but still allow for a 2–3 mm even cement mantle. There is no doubt that a slim femoral component with a lot of cement around it leads to premature failure.

Oversize rasps used with a plastic head as a trial are very useful for the trainee surgeon to assess soft tissue tension and stability.

The author believes that there should be no cement beyond the tip of the prosthesis, and even the tip of the prosthesis protruding for a millimetre or two beyond the tip of the cement mantle is advantageous. Whether the prosthesis should be polished to allow subsidence within an intact viscoelastic cement mantle or roughened or precoated to bond to the cement mantle is as yet unresolved.

Postoperative care and rehabilitation

The patient and nursing staff are advised about the postoperative care particularly if there is any risk of instability.

If there is a tenuous trochanteric reattachment or if the tissues are very slack, bed rest for 2 weeks after the operation is a justifiable postoperative plan to allow the soft tissues to firm up and prevent instability.

Intensive physiotherapy postoperatively is not required for most patients but advice about walking aids and how to tackle the simple aspects of daily life should be described to the patient by a physiotherapist.

There is no doubt that it is wise to advise the patient to limit impact activities and not to run or play any contact sports for the rest of their lives. Soft heeled shoes reduce shock waves during brisk walking.

What is not proven, however, is whether in younger patients total restriction of weight bearing with crutch walking for 3 months after cemented arthroplast is beneficial.

Complications of total hip replacement, incidence, aetiology, avoidance, identification and management

Since the more widespread use of total hip replacement for arthritis of the hip in the 1970s, published incidences of loosening have been reduced by refinement in surgical technique; and similarly local operative complications have been reduced by improved surgeon training. Perioperative fatality due to general systemic prob-

lems may be of the order of 1%. This figure will probably remain as the operation is increasingly being offered to more elderly patients with systemic disease.

The main medical complication that threatens our patients is thromboembolism with a reported fatality rate of 1–2%. Only recently, a large series has been published without any fatalities using prophylactic anticoagulation and a very low 0.8% (probably acceptable) bleeding complication rate.

Systemic operative complications of total hip replacement surgery

General medical assessment of patients preoperatively is essential to identify those patients at higher risk. There is an 8% incidence of coronary infarction in patients with pre-existing ischaemic heart disease even if there has been no recent infarct. Operation should not be undertaken if the patient has had a myocardial infarct in the last 6 months as the re-infarction rate in such patients is unacceptably high.

In patients with diabetes, coronary disease or a past history of thromboembolic disease it is necessary to institute measures to limit postoperative complications. Cervical spine instability in the rheumatoid patient or those with ankylosing spondylitis should be identified because of their anaesthetic risks.

There is no doubt that hypotensive anaesthesia cuts down blood loss during and in the early postoperative period by some two-thirds. Postoperative blood loss is generally equal to the operative loss. For surgical technical reasons hypotension is desirable to minimize blood film development at the cement bone interface.

Local complications

Vascular

Femoral artery damage is rare in primary hip replacement. More care is required with the anterior approach. Sharp Homan retractors should never be thrust into the tissues anteriorly to demonstrate the anterior acetabular margin. They should be insinuated gently between bone and soft tissues. Complications are rare with the posterior approach. Intrapelvic vessels occasionally have been damaged by sharp cutting instruments in the acetabulum. There should always be guards on keyhole cutting tools. It is the author's view that blunt drills are probably more dangerous than sharp. Providing power drills have a guard, i.e. end stop, they are satisfactory. 'Cheese grater' acetabular reamers are safe. The highest risk of intra pelvic damage arises in revision surgery where there has been cement intrusion into the pelvis. The fashioning of a Charnley central guide hole drilled right through into the pelvis is therefore inadvisable even if a cement retaining mesh is used.

Although thromboembolic complications are described later in this section, femoral vein occlusion can be demonstrated by venography when the hip is fully adducted and externally rotated, i.e. at dislocation with the anterior approach. The thromboembolic rate is much less with a posterior approach perhaps because of a different method of dislocation.

Neurological

More than 1% incidence of femoral or sciatic nerve damage in total hip replacement has been reported. The femoral nerve in the anterior approach is damaged less often than the sciatic nerve. In the posterior approach large retractors should not be forced around the posterior lip of the acetabulum and the sciatic nerve should be carefully identified and safeguarded before incising the posterior capsule with scissors. There is a risk of entrapping the sciatic nerve with any trochanteric attachment method that involves wire encirclement of the femoral shaft. Wroblewski suggests that a simple way of identifying this is to touch the encircling wire with a diathermy. If a sciatic nerve palsy is discovered postoperatively and the cause was not clearly identified intraoperatively, early exploration is advised. Early evacuation of haematoma may result in return of nerve function. An isolated apparently lateral popliteal nerve palsy may be localized by nerve conduction studies but it does appear that this section of the sciatic nerve is more vulnerable to local damage than the tibial nerve component of the sciatic nerve. Particular

care is required if significant limb lengthening is planned. The knee should be kept flexed during surgery to restrict intraoperative tension. Evoked cortical neurological potentials monitoring is recommended when significant limb lengthening is attempted during THR for dysplasia or CDH, to identify dangerous sciatic nerve tension.

Fracture

This is a real risk for inexperienced surgeons. It is more common in patients with osteoporosis caused either by age or rheumatoid arthritis. There are three stages of the operation when the femoral shaft is especially vulnerable.

(a) *Dislocation*; it is advised that only one surgeon manipulates the leg, and it is generally safer to lever on the head but adequate soft tissue release around the hip is also necessary. In an anterior approach any forceful demonstration of the proximal femur by an enthusiastic assistant before reaming may well result in a fracture of the lesser trochanter. Generous exposures produced by the modified McFarland's, posterior or trans-trochanteric approach reduces this complication.

(b) *Shaft penetration* by a 'T' handled or femoral reamer is similarly minimized by an adequate exposure. Femoral shaped reamers should never be hammered into the femur blindly without first identifying the general line of the shaft of the femur by the hand introduction of a taper pin reamer. A false passage can be created by this sharp instrument which should never be hammered into the shaft.

(c) *Rasp or trial impaction*; it almost goes without saying that careful choice of implants based upon preoperative measurement with templates reduces the risk when attempting to drive an over-size prosthesis into a femoral shaft. A trial prosthesis should always be used prior to final prosthetic insertion.

The current trend towards non-cement arthroplasty undoubtedly will lead to a much higher incidence of fractured femur. A blind assumption that all these fractures will heal because of the absence of cement is probably justified but no studies have been published on whether such patients go onto to have a pain free prosthesis.

Postoperative complications

Dislocation

Dislocation develops after 3% of total hip replacements. Charnley reports a 2% incidence of subluxation [12]. The incidence has little relationship to head size except with the posterior approach. Thus the 22 mm head size does not have a higher risk of dislocation. The component position in relationship to the approach is the most important factor. As might be expected, the posterior approach carries a higher likelihood of posterior dislocation and this increases when there is also a combination of retroversion of the components, slack soft tissues and a small head diameter. Care with patient positioning on the operation table, the use of a trial prosthesis to determine stability and soft tissue tension are vital. Reported incidences of early and late dislocation, are at variance. The author's experience is that early dislocation, if the prosthetic component looks satisfactory radiologically, can be treated successfully by reduction and immobilization to allow the soft tissues to heal. Late or recurrent dislocation if associated with a tech-

nical error of prosthetic insertion may need revision.

Revision arthroplasty itself has a much higher incidence of postoperative dislocation. The techniques that may be required to treat early dislocation are bed rest and traction for 3 weeks. The author has used successfully a pelvic abduction hinge orthosis. If operative revision is required, high speed cutting instruments to remove the prosthetic acetabular component from within its cement mantle are useful. The surgeon should not risk fracturing the acetabulum. It is easier to revise an acetabular component than a femoral. Soft tissue tension can often be taken up by more laterally placing an acetabular component, cementing with new cement into the old cement mantle. Special 22mm head anti-dislocation acetabular components are available. Similarly, soft tissue tension can be adjusted by correct reattachment of the trochanter if this is at fault.

Infection

The classic work of Charnley with ultra-clean air is reinforced by the recent Medical Research

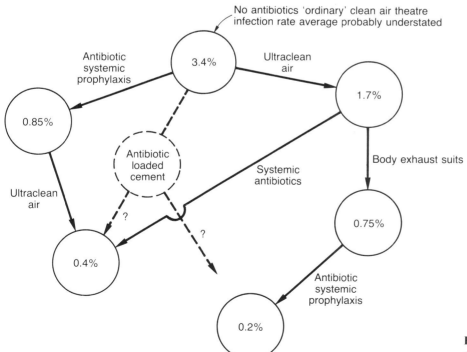

Fig. 18.12 MRC trial results in summary.

Council trial identified techniques that can minimize infection after hip arthroplasty [13] (Fig. 18.12).

Other principles of surgery should be followed. Any patient with active infection should have this treated. Body hair should be shaved with clippers rather than a razor as near to the time of surgery as possible. Whole body bathing with an antiseptic such as chlorhexidine gluconate can reduce dermal bacterial colonization. Skin preparation with either Povidone iodine or chlorhexidine in spirit for an adequate time, i.e. 1–2 minutes, exclusion of the skin edges, the use of double gloves and impervious gown sleeves or body exhaust suits are all factors that traditionally reduce infection.

High risk groups

These are rheumatoid arthritis 1.2% as compared with osteoarthritis 0.3%, diabetics 5.6%, psoriasis 5.5%, second operations 5% and males who have to be catheterized 6.6%

Bucholz has popularized the use of antibiotic loaded cement. Figures have been produced that are as low as those in the MRC trial when extra safety factors have been added. The general view is that in revision surgery or in patients with higher risks, antibiotic loaded cement is advised. The theoretical risk of late development of resistant organisms has not been reported. In any systemic study of infection after hip arthroplasty the following factors should be identified:

(a) Bacterial counts in settlement plates in the operating theatre and operative field.
(b) Bacterial counts in wound washings.
(c) Eventual infection rate bacteriologically identified.

A conventional operating theatre may have 500 colony forming particles per square metre. The ultra-clean air system with clothing impervious to bacteria or a total body exhaust system may limit the count to less than 1 per m^3. If fewer than 10 colony forming particles per m^3 is not achieved the theatre should really not be used for total joint replacement surgery. The addition of systemic antibiotics to the bone cement does not make up for deficient surgical environment. Down flow ultra clean air is advised with either side walls or high air velocity of at least 0.4 metres per second.

Thromboembolism

Fatal pulmonary embolism develops in between 0.5% (recent studies) and 3.0% (past studies) of patients without prophylaxis [14]. Calf vein thrombi occur in 50% of patients after total hip replacement. The peak incidences being on the 4th postoperative day with a second peak on the 14th day. There is a 6% pulmonary embolism rate. The relationship of calf vein thrombi to large vein potentially embolic thrombi is documented. Thus in any study where there is prophylaxis, isotopic assessment of calf vein thrombi probably can assess those methods of prophylaxis that could reduce this danger. Physical or pharmacological prophylactic methods are widely used.

Pharmacological prophylaxis has the hazard of excess bleeding. The surgeon must balance the risks and the benefits. A recent study [15] has demonstrated the effectiveness of dihydrogotamine and low molecular weight heparin in combination in reducing the incidence of calf vein thrombi from 50% in the placebo group to 25% in the prophylactically treated group. There are inadequate numbers to relate this statistically to a fatal pulmonary embolism rate. Recently the study described by Amstutz [16] with low dose warfarin has resulted in a nil rate of fatal pulmonary embolism, 3% of pulmonary embolism and a 0.8% of bleeding complications none of which was fatal in 2500 hip replacements. The incidence of bleeding complications is much higher in non-cement total hip replacements. The method used is to give 10 mg of warfarin the night of surgery (this is reduced if the patient's body weight is below 50 kg). The prothrombin time or the normalized international ratio is thereafter daily monitored. There is a preoperative control, and based on the prothrombin at postoperative day two the dose of warfarin is adjusted to a prothrombin time of 1.5 times control at a maximum. This level can be reached by postoperative day 4. To minimize the later risk of pulmonary embolism after discharge, the patient should be maintained on established low dose for at least 5 weeks.

Heterotopic ossification

The incidence is perhaps between 2% and 5%. Some cases are related to infection. The only known association is heterotopic ossification on a previous hip replacement. Statistically heterotopic ossification is much more common in a non-cement hip arthroplasty and ankylosing spondylitis. It may be associated with the extensive reaming. Although Indocid treatment has been used postoperatively, irradiation is the only method that has been proven to reduce the incidence of ossification. One thousand rads given in 5 divided doses in the first two weeks is the lowest dose that can give adequate control. The specific indication for this is a second side THR in a patient who on the opposite side had disabling ossification.

Loosening

The incidence is between 10% and 30% in long term follow-up depending on many variables. Two factors can be implicated in aseptic loosening:

(a) Inadequate strength of fixation.
(b) *biological factors*, including the abnormal host response to the implant primarily, which is rare, or the more common 'normal' biological response to wear debris from ground up cement or implant.

Implant fracture

Wroblewski described a high incidence of Charnley femoral implant fracture in heavy patients or those where there was inadequate proximal cement support for the prosthesis. It was almost exclusively in prosthesis of earlier design (flat backed Charnley). The incidence of stem failure is now virtually nil with the advent of high fatigue strength alloys. Acetabular component fracture is rare, the highest incidence being in thin walled high density polythene components and especially if there are deep cement retaining grooves. Higher incidences have been described in acetabular cups of the Muller design.

Assessment of results after total hip replacement

In the United Kingdom the most generally accepted method of assessment of results by clinical means is that of Charnley which was modified from d'Aubigne and Postel, although in the USA the method of Harris is preferred. The methods rely on a numerical scoring (see Fig. 18.13).

There are some studies which include in the assessment the activities of daily living. From such a comparative study it is evident that although the great majority of patients achieve almost total pain relief, the scatter of results in terms of hip movement, walking mobility and daily living postoperatively are more widely scattered, most patients moving up two grades. This study allows quantification of the benefit of total hip replacement in other than clinical terms.

Score	Range of hip movement	Pain	Mobility
1	0–30°	Severe spontaneous pain	Bedridden, or walks few yards with two sticks or crutches
2	31–60°	Prevents walking or severe on walking	Duration and distance very limited with or without sticks
3	61–100°	Tolerable with limited activity	Limited with one stick, difficult without sticks. Can stand for long periods
4	101–160°	Present only after activity; disappears quickly with rest	Long distance possible, but limited without aids
5	161–210°	Slight or intermittent, decreasing with activity	No aids required, but has a limp
6	210–260°	None	Normal

Fig. 18.13   Charnley hip score.

The results of total hip arthroplasty can be assessed by:

(a) Clinical follow-up based on a Charnley score indicating the percentage of patients that over a given period, say 10 years, have had a high score.
(b) Radiological follow-up with defined criteria for loosening.
(c) Absolute failure incidence as indicated by the revision rate.
(d) Statistical survival analysis.

For any study using any of the above methods the groups of patients, techniques and implants must be broadly comparable.

Cemented total hip replacement follow-up

The 15 year plus results have been described from the first era of cemented arthroplasty as described by Charnley and McKee with unsophisticated cement techniques. Eighty-five percent of survivors are painfree [17] (Fig. 18.14).

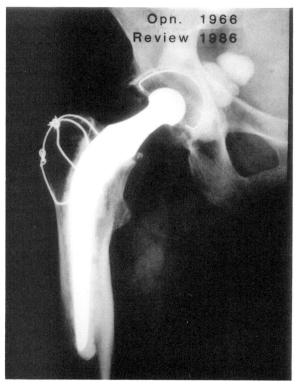

Fig. 18.14 Radiograph of successful asymptomatic 20 year follow up Charnley implant; note the femoral cortical hypertrophy (operation performed by the great man himself!).

Radiological follow-up demonstrates increasing evidence of cement bone lucencies and Charnley observed there were fewer flawless sockets than femoral components. Femoral components that are destined to fracture will do so within 10 years but high acetabular wear rates correlate with loosening due to impingement.

In the second era of cemented hip arthroplasty, post-1975, there remain a relatively low incidence of infection which has been reduced by the advent of systemic antibiotics, ultra-clean air enclosures and antibiotic incorporation into the cement. The dislocation rates are lower than in the first era probably due to increasing surgeon skill in the technical aspects of component placement. The factors in implant fracture have largely been identified and dealt with by the use of stronger materials. The techniques of bone preparation and cement insertion have developed and are described in previous sections.

The incidence of lucent lines at the cement bone interface with such techniques is greatly reduced and loosening rates are reported to be below 5% [18] in the 5–10 year follow-up.

Simple failure rate or loosening rate curves are not always comparable because they do not include those patients who have absconded from follow-up or those patients that have died. A statistical method of survivorship analysis that has long been used in cancer surgery has now been applied to follow-up of implants [19]. The American literature refers to Kaplan and Meier survivorship tables.

There are critical assumptions in the plotting of any survivorship curve for a group of patients who have had an identical implant. For the results to be meaningful there should be uniformity of implant, technique and age range. Publishing by authors of survivorship curves is to be deplored unless the calculation methods used by the authors are described. Dobbs [19] describes the assumptions that are made in the survivorship curves that he describes:

(1) It is assumed that withdrawals, i.e. patients not traced, are subject to the same probabilities as nonwithdrawals. If there is only a small loss of numbers for follow-up the induced error is small.

(2) It must be assumed that probabilities of implant removal remain reasonably constant, otherwise time life tables are difficult to interpret.

In the described method of calculation it must

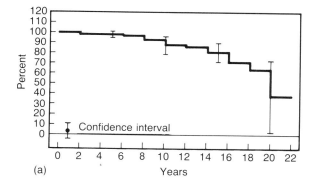

(a)

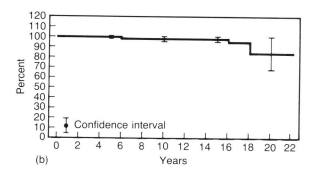

(b)

Fig. 18.15 (a) Survivorship analysis of first generation cemented Charnley acetabular components with revision for aseptic loosening or radiographic definite loosening as end point. (b) Survivorship analysis of first generation cemented Charnley femoral components using revision for aseptic loosening or definitive radiographic loosening as end point.

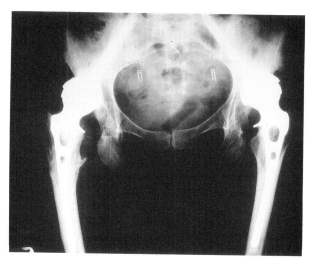

Fig. 18.16 Example of 20 year follow up of successful Ring early design metal on metal non cemented total hip arthoplasty. Note the complete absence of any significant radiolucent lines or osteolysis; note good bony condensation in the upper femur. The feature of note on the acetabular side is some proximal prosthetic migration.

be remembered that in any group of patients there may be some who suffer pain yet retain the prosthesis. Therefore the survivorship curve is a conservative estimate only of any failure rate, and do not include those without symptoms but with significant lucent lines. This method can be used to plot any particular defined aspect of failure. For example, combined results of aseptic revision rates and definite radiological loosening (Fig. 18.15).

Non-cement hip follow-up

Few non-cement arthroplasties have been followed up long enough to compile survivorship curves but the Ring Prosthesis has the longest follow-up (Fig. 18.16). Pain relief is probably inferior to cemented total hip arthroplasty but he

observes that low infection rates with ease of revision are desirable features and worth the additional burden of slight discomfort in noncement arthroplasty. If the results are satisfactory at 10 years with the metal/metal prosthesis later failure is rare.

The early results of the newer non cemented total hip replacement do not match those of cemented (2nd generation) arthroplasty. A 25% incidence of thigh pain at 5 years is recorded and a 30% incidence at 5 years of acetabular osteolysis in some series causes concern for the future.

Biomechanical aspects of implant design

Good cement penetration into trabecular bone can minimize shear and with a non-cement prosthesis suitable interdigitations have the same effect.

Even support for the prosthesis from proximal to distal with any method of fixation tends to reduce the prosthetic stress. Femoral implant failure in cemented hip arthroplasty is more likely if there is good distal support for the prosthesis and proximal loss of support. Such a maldistributlon of stress will tend to lead to a concentration at one point and it is at this point, particularly if there are associated implant defects in manufacture, that a fatigue failure will be initiated. With a non-cemented prosthesis a similar situation can arise, for example if there is a porous coat on the whole stem of the prosthesis, and the prosthesis becomes highly incorporated distally and yet proximally minimally incorporated. The stress concentration may lead to implant failure.

Mechanical analysis suggests that:

1. To reduced stem and interface stresses distally there should be a restriction of the length of the stem of the intramedullary prosthesis.
2. The proximal femoral stem should be as thick and as stiff as possible.
3. The distal stem should be relatively flexible as compared to the proximal stem.

Ideally, there should be a large load transferring area. Clearly even stress transfer from proximal to distal is required; therefore the prosthesis should be tapered. A defined step would tend to concentrate stresses. Requirement 3 is also fulfilled by a relatively slender distal femoral stem within a fairly thick cement mantle. An even cement mantle is desirable and a straight stem fulfils this better than a 'banana' stem. Clinical follow-up demonstrates that a straight stem produces fewer failures by loosening than curved stems.

To mechanically limit stresses in the cement the stem should have no sharp edges and to minimize implant stresses the stem should ideally be thicker laterally than medially. This is certainly so in a prosthesis that has a relatively high offset, i.e. physiological neck shaft angle. In a prosthesis with a much more valgoid disposition of the femoral neck, stresses within the implant stem will tend not to be concentrated laterally.

A more recent interesting means of reducing stresses at the interface between the metal shaft and the cement is to pre-coat the stem. Under laboratory conditions methacrylate is bonded onto the femoral stem. The methacrylate cement as used surgically bonds onto the pre-coat and whilst not a true adhesive the methacrylate mantle actually 'sticks' to the metal. Whilst theoretically desirable, such pre-coating may mean that it is virtually impossible to remove the prosthesis should the metal cement composite become loose within the bone.

Another potential complication of this method of enhancing the strength of the metal cement junction is that the metal stem will be less likely to slide within the cement mantle. Whilst no surgeon wishes the prosthesis to subside within a cement mantle, as many studies have shown this to correlate with clinical loosening, there is no doubt that with increasing age the medullary cavity increases in width and Charnley [12] and Ling have found that such settlement or subsidence can occur without there being a fracture within the cement and without there being clinical symptoms or signs of failure. There are two schools of thought on whether the capacity for controlled subsidence should be designed for!

The material composition of the femoral stem should generally be of a high fatigue resistance metal. Few other materials have the fatigue strength. Certainly this is true in a cemented prosthesis where because of the requirements to have an even cement mantle there are very definite limits on the thickness of the metal implant. The only metals that fulfil these requirements are forged, vacuum cast or isostatically pressed chrome cobalt, forged titanium aluminium vanadium alloy and high nitrite stainless steel. A polymer prosthesis for non-cement use is described as isoelastic, i.e. it is stated that its elastic modulus is similar to that of cortical bone. Whilst it is a composite structure in some senses in that it has a metal strengthener, it is not a composite in the sense bone is, with fibre bundles within a matrix. The polymer is isotropic whereas bone is anisotropic. Clinical studies demonstrate sclerosis of the proximal femur, but there are no very long term studies to show the fatigue resisting capabilities of the polymer prosthesis and particulate abrasion debris is likely to cause lucent areas.

Acetabular component

Studies of the acetabular components that have been removed from previously successful total hip replacements show that there is a great variation in the line of wear. A surprising 64% of wear was superolateral, 32% was vertical and only 3.4% was along the accepted line of resultant force R.

A conclusion from this must be that (and these studies were from a study of Charnley acetabular components with a relatively physiological neck shaft angle femoral component) stress analysis does not reveal certain mechanical factors that are induced by total joint replacement or that the abductor muscle force is in some way greatly reduced by the technique of hip operation. Such wear findings support the view of Bombelli that the acetabular component should be positioned relatively horizontal in the line of his 'sourcil'.

The acetabular bone forces are mostly compressive if the axial line of the acetabular component is along the line of the resultant force. To minimize peak stresses it is desireable that there is:'

(1) A large bone implant/cement interface provided this is consistent with a satisfactory placement of the acetabular component in bone of good quality with good cover of the component.

(2) A stiff implant, either thick plastic (Charnley's classic book describes his early photoelastic experiments on this [12]) or metal backing of the acetabular component. Clinical experience with thin cemented acetabular components shows that there is a high rate of failure.

(3) The external shape of the acetabular implant also contributes to the stress concentration. Hemispherical acetabular components have performed well cemented and non cemented. A tighter (more contact pressure) fit at the perimeter in non cemented components produces a more even stress distribution. More complex externally threaded screw designs have failed early with the exception of the original Ring long screwed metal cup. Acetabular components have irregularities on the external surface to key the cement into the plastic. The grooves in the acetabular components on the external surfaces should be no more than a millimetre or two and undercut grooves give the best fixation of the cup within the cement. Deepening or widening the grooves did not increase the bond strength. Slight prominences on the external surfaces of the cemented acetabular component, particularly if these are made of methacrylate, limit bottoming out of the prosthesis on the bone and help maintain an even cement mantle.

Mechanical attributes and tribological aspects of different head sizes can best be considered here.

Charnley [12] advocates a 22 mm head. The mechanical attributes of this are shown in Fig.

(a)

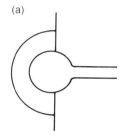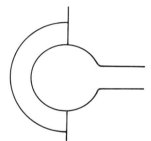

Small head
Less interface
Less frictional torque
More load/unit area
Less particulate debris
More penetrative wear

Large head
Larger interface
More frictional torque
Less load/unit area
More particulate debris
Less penetrative wear

(b)

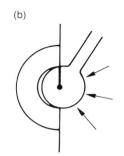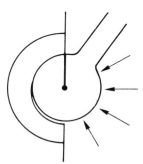

Impingement at less angle of movement
Less capsular stretch ∴ less force communication → socket interface **unless** deep penetrative wear

Greater arc of movement before impingement
More frictional torque communicated to socket

Fig. 18.17 Tribological characteristics of small and large head sizes.

18.17. (Tribology is the study of friction wear and lubrication.) Clearly with a small head there is a greater load per unit area and this affects penetrative wear – see later. The theory of tribology may be simple but in practice *in vitro* experiments and *in vivo* analyses are much more difficult to interpret.

1. *Friction*. Frictional torque is much less with a smaller head and socket and that between metal and high density polythene is much less than metal on metal. Theoretically, highly polished ceramic on ceramic should have the lowest frictional torque.

2. *Wear*. This can be considered as either wear in depth or volumetric wear. Volumetric wear is much greater with a large head and less with a

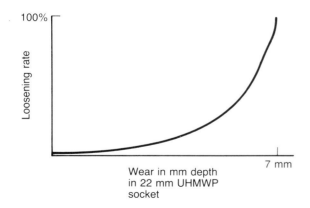

Fig. 18.18   Wear and loosening in patients under 40 years with Charnley THR.

small head, i.e. 22 mm. The wear in terms of depth is much increased with a small head. Wroblewski (Fig. 18.18) describes a high rate of wear in some very young active patients and this correlates in an almost exponential fashion with the loosening rate. Charnley [12] describes an average rate of wear of 0.022 mm per year (penetrative wear). An interesting point is that the wear rate in the second 5-year period of a 10-year follow-up is half that of the wear in the first 5-year period. This may be because of bedding in of the femoral head on the plastic. One factor that Charnley did not look at relates to both friction and wear and is the roughness of the femoral head and the socket of explanted prostheses (abrasive wear). The roughness of the prosthetic surface increases with time and at 5–10 years the surface finish is 0.05 microns, whereas the new implant surface finish is 0.01 microns. Wear is certainly increased if a third body is introduced, i.e. particulate cement 'valve grinding paste'.

3. *Lubrication*. The artificial hip is boundary lubricated, i.e. a layer of liquid adheres to the surfaces. Although lubrication factors can be studied in a laboratory, it is unlikely in the near future they will influence an artificial hip. This will not be considered further.

Implant fixation

The term 'implant loosening' has bedevilled the orthopaedic literature for lack of an agreed definition of the term 'loose'. In some ways it is easier to define what is adequate fixation. A working definition is that 'adequate fixation is present if the clinical result is within defined limits of success and that the result does not deteriorate with time nor is the fixation associated with increasing amplitude of interface movement with resultant pain or osteolysis or bone or implant debris accumulation'. The essential term in such a definition is progression, clinical or radiological.

Radiological progression may differ in cemented or non-cemented implants. The 'lucent line' around the cemented implant at the cement bone junction line is associated with implant failure particularly if 2 mm thick and if that lucent line progressively increases. Such loosening rates may differ on the acetabular and femoral sides of the total joint replacement. In a non-cemented implant progressively wide lucent lines similarly suggest imminent failure; Ring [20] has the longest experience of follow-up of non-cemented implants and describes that a lucent line of up to 2 mm thick in long term follow-up is not an indication of imminent failure of the joint replacement. In non-cement arthroplasty there may be adaptive changes that develop depending on the loading characteristics and the extent of porous coating fixation to bone. Areas of localized load transfer 'spot welding' can be radiologically identified. Adaptive changes can best be seen at junctional areas of porous coating and smooth uncoated stem.

In cemented hip arthroplasty there are radiological features that develop over some years that do not presage failure. An example of this may be increased bony density around the more distal femoral stem, indicating the load transfer to the more distal stem. If the material of the implant stem is strong enough to take the load imposed at the junctional area, fatigue failure is minimized.

Any implant system composed of materials of dissimilar characteristics will have movement, however slight, at the interfaces or junctional area between the components of the system.

Ling [21] details five basic facts of implant fixation.

1. The fixation of an implant system depends on the mechanical interlock created by the surgeon at the time of surgery. There is no doubt that this is true in cemented arthroplasty and the strength of fixation is maximal at the time of surgery but deteriorates with time. With a non-

cement arthroplasty it is likely that there is a less even stress distribution at the metal bone interface initially and a more even load transfer will develop in the course of time. There is no data on whether mechanical security improves with time in a non-cement arthroplasty.

2. Any implantation technique into the human skeleton produces a zone of bone death around the implant. The thickness of the zone of bone death is determined by the techniques of surgery and the materials used [22]. There is no doubt that the thicker the layer of bone death, the more likely that the implant is imperfectly fixed. The devitalized tissue can establish a new blood supply. It is at this critical time following implantation that the type of tissue forms (bone or fibrous tissue) dictated by the mechanical environment of the implant perhaps in the first 3 months post-implantation.

3. The absorption onto the implant surface of a thin film of glycoproteinaceous composition develops within seconds (the interface conversion film). The tissue attachment has to be via such a junctional material. Some materials have a more aggressive affinity for cellular material than others. An example is a recently developed material that appears to have positive tissue affinity is Bioglass. All alloys have an oxide, i.e. ceramic layer on the surface.

4. The bone of the hip deforms with load and the load is imposed by body weight and kinetic energy and by muscle forces.

5. The living tissue bone is constantly being remodelled by osteoblastic and osteoclastic activity. This bone turn over changes with the metabolic status of the patient. The medullary cavity probably increases in width with advancing years.

Ling suggests that there is a fundamental relationship between mechanical effects at a junctional area and its histological or ultrastructural make up.

Mechanical junctional factors

There is a fundamental difference between a cemented (methacrylate) metallic implant and a press-fit metallic implant (non-cemented). In the former there are two junctional areas to be considered: (1) implant cement and (2) cement bone.

The modulus of elasticity of cement is closer to that of cortical bone and therefore junctional stresses are highest between the metal and the cement. Taken overall, however the cement must effectively 'shock absorb' or attenuate stresses from metal to bone.

In the non-cement implant although surface coatings may modify this there are high junctional stresses between a metallic implant and the adjacent bone. The mechanical properties of the membrane in animals around an implant fixed with cement or without cement have the same physical characteristics. The material was Viscolastic and is structurally more capable of resisting compressive rather than shear stresses.

It is likely that it is the different loading characteristics of junctional tissues in a cement fixed acetabular or femoral component that determines the outcome where there are lucent lines, however fine, between the implant and bone. In the acetabular component the junctional tissues are mostly in compression and on the femoral component they are mostly in shear produced by axial or torsional loading. It is probably this that led Charnley in his earlier writing to suggest that there was a different clinical outcome in acetabular and femoral cemented components following the development of radiolucent lines at the bone cement interface.

Histological and ultrastructural features of junctional tissues

Charnley [12] showed in a classic study of retrieved specimens some years after successful cemented arthroplasty that there was a fundamental difference on the femoral and acetabular sides. On the femoral side, there was no thick continuous layer of cellular tissue at the cement bone interface. Live bone was close to the bone cement spheres and there was a thin layer of pale staining material at the interface. There were some cells similar to chondrocytes at the interface. Macrophages were rarely seen and only in association with thicker fibrous tissue and were more common in areas where cement was in contact with bone marrow. No granulomas were seen in successful hips. A characteristic is a scolloping of the junctional area where the bone cement is dissolved away in preparation. This demonstrates conclusively that there was no macro movement, otherwise the delicate bone cement spheres would have been abraded away.

On the acetabular side very different findings were seen. There was no direct bone contact and fibrous tissue of 0.5–1.5 mm thick was seen. This was often modified fibrous cartilage with occasional caseous material islands between bone and cement. There were many histiocytes and occasional granulomas with giant cells. The collagen bundles within the fibrous tissue were parallel to the surface of the acetabular component.

Linder [23], in an electron microscopic study, demonstrated that there could be a non-cellular membrane 0.3–7 microns thick between living bone and cement. This was considered to be uncalcified proteoglycan. Macrophages were seen but they were not associated with resorptive activity. Eng [24] has reported live bone implant contact without intervening fibrous tissue.

Osseointegration and microinterlock

Microinterlock is a description coined by Miller [25] describing an intimate interdigitation of bone cement into trabecular bone. The term can be applied in the interdigitation of bone between irregularities on a non-cemented implant. A working definition in structural terms might be that keyholes that are drilled by the surgeon in acetabular bone before introducing cement that may be from 5 mm to 15 mm could be termed macrointerlock, whereas the forcing of groups of spheres of bone cement between trabecular bone or a similar scale non-cement interface could be termed microinterlock. In the latter, non-cement category mechanical interdigitation of live bone into the roughened surface is rarely technically feasible. Bone marrow and fragmented trabecular bone as a slurry can be forced into the interdigitations. After insertion some osteoblasts will receive their nutrition by diffusion, remaining vital, and it is the surgeon's hope that microinterlock into a porous or roughened surface will take place.

There are few studies on the relationship of the mechanical environment at a non-cement roughened interface to the development of satisfactory bone ingrowth. Albrektsson's [22] classic study used a refined surgical technique with minimal tissue damage and these workers reported loosening of the implants only occurred where

loading was allowed before osseointegration had been achieved.

A definition of osseointegration is that 'normal living bone is in direct contact with the prosthesis'. With a non-cement implant it is the base material or oxide coating; with a cemented component it is the methacrylate that is in contact with the bone. The junctional tissues of both implants are in order: (a) demineralized living bone; (b) proteoglycan; (c) interface conversion film.

The interposition of cellular membranes, fibrous tissue or fibrocartilage by definition describes a state where osseointegration has not occurred.

Failure of implant fixation

If infection is excluded, mechanical or biological failure is the only possible mechanism producing implant failure (Fig. 18.19).

The techniques in cemented or non-cemented arthroplasty that may enhance long-term clinical survival are described in the appropriate sections. Long-term follow-ups of the newer techniques have not yet come to fruition, but it is useful to consider those parameters by which 'loosening' may be judged so that one's own clinical results can be reflected upon. Whilst clinical follow-up in gross terms provides the simplest method of determining patients' satisfaction, interpretation of fine radiological changes may lead to predictive likelihood of clinical failure, certainly in cemented arthroplasty. A study of implant loosening can incorporate: (a) membrane or 'lucent line' thickness; (b) subsidence; (c) migration.

Most observers would agree with Harris that definite loosening is evident by migration. Loosening is probable if there is a lucent line at the whole bone implant interface. The evidence of possible loosening is more arguable, Harris suggests that if more than half the interface has a lucent line possible loosening is likely. Localized osteolysis is more commonly seen with non cemented arthroplasty; infection can be responsible but if excluded the usual cause is a localized build up of particulate implant debris with consequent macrophage activity. Polyethylene debris with its microscopic birefringence even of submicron dimensions can be identified. Micro-

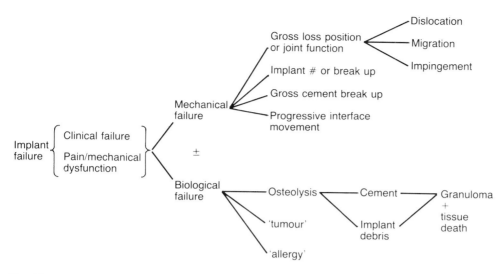

Fig. 18.19 Summary of factors involved in implant failure.

movement at polyethylene metal interfaces *that were not designed to fret or move* have been postulated as a source. Such particles have even been identified alongside the femoral stem of non cemented implants. There is much speculation about the means of transport and theories include joint and interface fluid pressure differences.

Critical objective measurement requires radiographs. The three methods in order of accuracy are:

(1) A standard radiograph of the individual hip with the beam centred at the centre of the hip.

(2) Standard grid radiograph as described by Amstutz. This simplified grid radiograph is simple to use and takes little time to reproduce. The reader is referred to the original article [26].

(3) Stereophotogrammetry as described by Ryd [27] involves a computer analysis of implants where metal ball markers have been incorporated in the bone at the time of surgery. X-rays are taken from a standard position and migration or subsidence of a prosthesis can be measured as accurately as 0.1 mm.

Current status of non-cement total hip arthroplasty including porous ingrowth

In the pre-cement era Thompson and Austin Moore designed implants that are the fore runners of what is used today. Ring in the UK published large series of total hip arthroplasty components fixed without cement. Charnley in his earliest experiments used a press fit.

The general trend towards non-cement arthroplasty is a natural development due to:

(a) The excessive loss of bone stock with failed cemented arthroplasty and the consequent difficulties of revision. There is no doubt that loose non-cement components produce less osteolysis provided particulate prosthetic debris does not develop.

(b) The possible increased susceptibility of cemented prosthesis to haematogenous sepsis.

(c) A possible reduction in the general infection rate in non-cement implant.

For any non-cement total hip replacement system to work there must be:

(a) Primary stability. To achieve this the design of prosthesis must enable there to be as wide as possible area of bone implant contact. The implant must be loaded onto bone of quality strong enough to take the load. To achieve this there must be a wide range of prostheses that fit accurately.

(b) The stress distribution from implant to bone must be of even gradient all around the implant and as low as possible. The design must minimize any tendency to relative movement at the interface. Non-physiological forces should be avoided to minimize bone resorption or loosening, stress transfer being maximal proximally. The force distribution should be such that bone remodelling potential is augmented. Ideally, the design and method of insertion should be such that necessary reparation of the bone close to the implant should be minimized. The technique of insertion should be with minimal bony tissue damage and devascularization, this may not be fulfilled with the extensive reaming necessary to 'fit and fill' suggested as necessary in inserting modern non-cement prostheses. The toxicity of the implant due to ionic insult from interface release or wear products should be minimal.

The factors above are interwoven.

(c) *Porous coating*. Pilliar and Eng [24] have utilized coatings in an attempt to enhance prosthetic fixation. There is no doubt that the condition of primary stability is vital and demands on any supplementary stabilization either cemented or porous coated being therefore minimized. For porous coatings to function and for it to be shown that bone ingrowth is demonstrated histologically in the coating, the following conditions must prevail:

(i) Primary mechanical stability, as above.
(ii) Pore size. For bone fixation the porous spaces must be more than l00 microns (fibrous tissue fixation takes place if there is less than 50 microns).
(iii) Bone implant apposition. The gap between the bone and implant must not be more than 2 mm.
(iv) Stress transfer. The proof of this function is to demonstrate that a porous coating actually carries load. Eng [24] describes cortical sclerosis at the junctional area between the smooth area distally and the proximal porous coated part of the AML prosthesis at 3 years. Trabecular bone orientation in response to loading induced by a microtextured surface is described. Fibrous tissue fibres also orientate to take the load from such a surface, as opposed to their parallel orientation along a smooth stem.

The author's stem design with proximal macrotexturing has shown no lucent lines in relationship to this surface suggesting bone incorporation. One of the unknown factors in the porous coat implants is the possibility of ionic release. The porous coating enhances the effective surface area of the metal to living tissue interface. Cobalt debris from simulated wear tests injected into experiment animals produced a high tumour incidence; not all authors have been able to repeat this. Sarcomatous lesions adjacent to metal on metal McKee implants have been reported.

The femoral medullary canal width increases with age and how such an expanding skeleton will respond to a non-cement implant is unknown.

Osseoconduction and Induction

It is considered the former is facilitated by the pores in porous coated prostheses filling with blood and bone slurry – the latter [28] is promoted if the surface is coated with a bone inducting agent for example, hydroxyapatite.

The problem of prosthetic retrieval should be considered in the design of an implant. The general view is that if a porous coating should be used at all it should be around the proximal end of the prosthesis and there should be some way of easily exposing the prosthetic bone interface should implant retrieval be necessary.

Eng [24] demonstrated that full length stem coating produced less thigh pain than just proximal coating – users of prostheses fully coated with hydroxyapatite have observed this.

Subsidence is an accurate index of the success or not of a non-cement implant coated as compared to non-coated. This can be assessed by the precise method of stereophotogrammetry.

There is no doubt that the trend is for a porous coating. Hydroxyapatite coatings have reduced subsidence as compared to a control series measured by stereophotogrammetry but the long term outcome is unknown.

There is some concern whether a porous coating applied to a stem reduces the fatigue resistance of the stem. The porous coating therefore should not be applied to a highly stressed area of the stem. Metallurgical studies show that diffusion weld bonding of titanium mesh pads affects substrate forged metal less than sintering chrome cobalt beads to a cast stem base. These findings have implications especially for the more slender prosthetic stems necessary in the narrow medullary cavity of the younger patient. If a stem that was coated throughout its length was to become securely fixed distally and proximal stress shielding was to occur and a distal stem fracture there would be extreme difficulty in removing the distal securely fixed segment of the fractured stem.

The long term benefits of an isoelastic stem are unknown. There is no doubt that proximal bony condensation occurs. Any polymer (with inevitably reduced abrasion resisting characteristics) adjacent to bone may give rise to build up of polymeric debris.

Long term survivorship studies on cemented acetabular components show much poorer performance compared to femoral components in the same study (Fig. 18.15).

Although the first non-cement threaded cups had a high failure rate – hemispherical porous coated metal backed acetabular components appear to perform well – initially they were fixed with screws and same size reamed when ingrowth was seen at the polar contact zone (close to the screw site) but more recent reports both laboratory and clinical suggest under reaming the acetabular by 2 m and impacting the cup giving perimeter contact and better stability and bone ingrowth produces excellent fixation.

There are some reports suggesting particulate debris can derive from a non rigidly held liner or the screws if any holding the cup in. This author's view is that the hemispherical non cemented cups have many advantages in primary and revisional surgery and if the surgeon has confidence in his fit especially in primary THR a factory fitted rigid bond (plastic-metal) acetabular component may be the answer.

On the femoral side the evidence is uncertain in terms of clinical success with pain relief and with less likelihood of microporous bone ingrowth and because of potential removal problems and anticipated stress remodelling changes it is probably desirable to use cemented femoral components in patients over 60 and non-cemented in very young patients.

References

1. Hackenbroch, M. H. *et al.* (1979) Radiological study of 976 arthritic hips, patients under mean age 42. *Arch. Orthop. Trauma Surg.*, **95**, 275–283.
2. Wroblewski, B. M. and Charnley, J. (1982) Classification of osteoarthritis of the hip based on X-ray morphology. *J. Bone Joint Surg.*, **64B**, 568.
3. Bombelli, R. (1983) *Osteoarthritis of the Hip*, 2nd edn. Springer, Berlin.
4. Paul, J. P. (1967) Institute of Mechanical Enginers, 181 (318).
5. English, T. (1978) British Orthopaedic Research Society, Bradford.
6. Rehn, 'Interposition arthroplasty of the hip'. 1930. *Arch. Clin. Chir.*
7. Maquet, P. (1979) Valgus osteotomy results for medial osteoarthritis. *J. Bone Joint Surg.*, **61B**, 424.
8. Morscher, E. W. (1980) Intertrochanteric osteotomy in osteo arthritis of the hip. In *The Hip . . . Proceedings of the Eighth Open Scientific Meeting of the Hip Society.* CV Mosby, St. Louis.
9. Osborne, G. (1986) The history of surgical access for hip replacement. *Current Orthopaedics*, I, 61–66.
10. Lee, A. J. C., Ling, R. S. M. and Vangala, S. S. (1978) Some clinically relevant variables affecting mechanical properties of cement. *Arch. Orthop. Trauma Surg.*, **92:1**.
11. Hallawa, M., Lee, A. J. C., Ling, R. S. M. and Vangala, S. S. (1978) Shear strength of trabecular bone and factors effecting. *Arch. Orthop. Trauma Surg.*, **92:19**.
12. Charnley, J. (1978) *Low Friction Arthroplasty of the Hip*. Springer, Berlin.
13. Lidwell, O. M., Lowburry, E. J. L. *et al.* (1982) Effects of ultra-clean air in operating rooms on deep surfaces after joint replacement. *Br. Med. J.*, 2, 10.
14. Salzman, E. W. and Harris, W. (1976) Pulmonary embolism fatality rate after total hip replacement surgery. *J. Bone Joint Surg.*, **58A**, 903.
15. Beisaw, N. *et al.* (1987) Dihydrogotamine/heparin prophylaxis of deep vein thrombosis in total hip replacement patients multiple centre trial. *Am. Acad. Orthop. Surg.*, **January**.
16. Amstutz, H. C., Karni, B., Dori, F., Friscia, D. and Yao, J. (1987) The prevention of fatal pulmonary embolism patients under going total hip replacement. *Am. Acad. Orthop. Surg.* **January**.
17. Wroblewski, B. M. (1986) 15–21 year results of Charnley low friction arthroplasty. *Clin. Orthop. Rel. Res.*, **211**, 30.
18. Harris, W. H., McCarthy, J. C. and O'Neill, D. A. (1982) Femoral component loosening using contemporary techniques of femoral cement fixation. *J. Bone Joint Surg.*, **64A**, 1063.
19. Dobbs, H. S. (1980) Survivorship of total hip replacements. *J. Bone Joint Surg.*, **62B**, 168.
20. Ring, P. (1986) Personal communication.
21. Ling, R. S. M. (1989) Mechanical Factors in Implant Fixation. *Current Orthopaedics*, **3**, 168–175.

22. Albrektsson, T., Branemark, P., Hansson, H. and Lindstrom, J. (1981) Osseointegrated titanium implants, requirements for ensuring a long lasting direct bone to implant anchorage in man. *Acta. Orthop. Scand.*, **15**, 155.

23. Linder, L., Hansson, H. A. (1983) Ultra structural aspects of the interface between bone and cement in man. *J. Bone Joint Surg.*, **65B**, 646–649.

24. Eng, C. H., Bobyn, J. D. and Glassman, A. H. (1977) Porous coated hip replacement – the factors growing bone ingrowth – stem shielding and clinical results. *J. Bone Joint Surg.*, **69B**, 95–99.

25. Miller, J., Kraus, W. R., Krug, W. H. and Kelebay, L. C. (1981) Low viscosity cement. *Orthop. Transact.*, **5**, 532.

26. Amstutz, H. *et al.* (1986) The grid X-ray in the follow-up of total hip replacements. *J. Bone Joint Surg.*, **68A**, 105.

27. Ryd, L. (1986) (220) A roentgen stereophotogrammetric analysis of tibial component fixation. *Acta. Orthop. Scand. Suppl.*

28. Furlong, R. J. and Osborn, B. F. (1991) Fixation of hip prostheses by hydroxyapatite coatings. *J. Bone Joint Surg.*, **73B**, 741–745.

29. Gallante (1971) *J. Bone Joint Surg.*, **53A.**, 101.

19

Management of unicompartmental arthritis of the knee

J. H. Newman

Many patients with unicompartmental arthritis of the knee require little in the way of treatment but Hernborg and Nilsson [1] have shown that, in most patients, the natural history of the condition is for a slow deterioration to occur, especially when the medial compartment is predominantly involved. Conservative treatment in the way of non-steroidal anti-inflammatory drugs and physiotherapy may help but many will eventually require invasive treatment. An intra-articular steroid injection can give pain relief, though Dieppe *et al.* [2] believe the improvement is short lived. Arthroscopy is coming to assume an important role, not only because it allows accurate assessment of the joint, but also because a temporary improvement can be obtained in a high proportion of joints treated by arthroscopic lavage alone [3].

When pain persists despite these measures, surgery has to be considered. If the arthritis is predominantly unicompartmental then the options lie between osteotomy, unicompartmental replacement and total joint replacement, with other possibilities such as arthrodesis, debridement [4] or allograft replacement [5] only rarely needing to be considered. Each of these three main procedures has its advocates.

Tibial osteotomy

Tibial osteotomy was first reported as a treatment of osteoarthritis by Jackson in 1958 [6]. Since that time many series have been published with a success rate that has varied from 97% at 2 years [7] to 56% [8]. Most of these series have been retrospective studies with variable criteria for defining success, so evaluation has been hard. It is now generally agreed that the procedure is more satisfactory in the treatment of varus than valgus deformities of the knee, possibly because tibial osteotomy for valgus deformity of the knee usually increases the tibial slope and the tibial spines prevent load transference to the relatively unaffected medial side; in addition, medial collateral ligament instability persists and over correction into varus can easily occur [9].

Theoretically a lower femoral osteotomy should overcome some of these problems with the valgus knee and give a better result. Satisfactory results have been reported [10–12] but the procedure is not widely practised.

In order to obtain a good result from a tibial osteotomy for a varus knee, accurate realignment must be achieved. In the past this has proved difficult and many cases have finished undercorrected; this, combined with other complications [13] has meant that the clinical result has been unpredictable. In addition, Insall [14] has demonstrated that the results of osteotomy deteriorate with time. In his series 97% had good results at 2 years but only 37% were painfree after 9 years. These problems, together with the improvement in the results of knee replacements, mean that there is a much greater need to reassess the indications for tibial osteotomy than was previously the case.

In 1973 Coventry [10] suggested that an upper

tibial osteotomy would do best when performed for early symptomatic unicompartmental arthritis and this has been confirmed by Tjornstrand *et al.* [15] It is now becoming accepted that advanced radiological changes or severe deformity make it hard to achieve a good result after osteotomy. Such cases should be considered for knee replacement.

Unicompartmental replacement

The concept of unicompartmental replacement is attractive because only abnormal surfaces are replaced and minimal bone is resected. Several reports have shown early good results following unicompartmental replacement [14,16–18] but others have been less encouraging [19,20]. Insall and Aglietti [21] presented a particularly worrying report in which initially satisfactory results deteriorated rapidly, and when followed up at 6 years 28% had been revised and only 36% were regarded as good or excellent. However, more than half the cases had undergone patellectomy and it was noted that the curvature of both components was critical so that incorrect positioning could result in binding and subsequent loosening. Both these factors would now be thought of as likely to lead to an unsatisfactory result.

Comparison of tibial osteotomy and unicompartmental replacement [22]

Early experience in Bristol of unicompartmental replacement using the St. Georg Sled prosthesis had been encouraging [23] but a longer term follow-up was clearly needed. Since the obvious alternative procedure was an upper tibial osteotomy, it was decided to carry out a retrospective

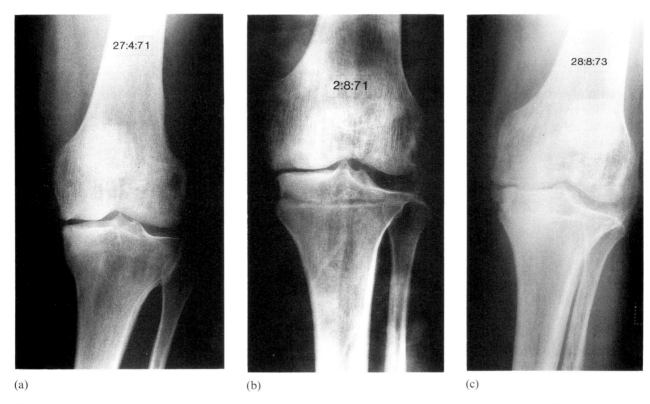

(a) (b) (c)

Fig. 19.1 (a, b) Pre- and postoperative radiographs of a 54-year-old female who underwent osteotomy for medial compartment disease. Postoperative alignment was 5° of valgus. (c) Two years later progressive arthritis of both medial and lateral compartments is occurring. Subsequently a knee replacement was performed.

study using the same assessment criteria for both groups. The object was to try to determine whether one procedure was superior to the other, both in terms of quality and longevity of result.

All patients treated in Bristol for osteoarthritis of the knee by unicompartmental replacement or tibial osteotomy between 1974 and 1979 were studied, giving a follow-up period of between 5 and 10 years. Forty-nine osteotomies were available for study and these were compared with 42 unicompartmental replacements. All osteotomies had been performed by resecting a wedge of bone above the tibial tubercle in order to correct the coronal tibio-femoral angle; the fibula was released in a variety of ways (Fig. 19.1). Post-operatively the knee was immobilized in plaster for 6 weeks.

The unicompartment replacements were all St. Georg Sled protheses, cemented in place with a deliberate effort being made minimally to under-correct the deformity.

The selection of the patients for the two procedures was purely determined by the pattern of referral from general practitioners. At that time the unicompartmental replacements were carried out by Mr R. A. J. Baily, the late Mr W. G. J. Hampson and their teams, while the tibial osteotomies were carried out by other Bristol surgeons. There was no evidence of cross referral. The preoperative parameters of the two groups were broadly similar (Table 19.1) and it was

therefore felt that retrospective comparison was justified.

All patients were assessed between 5 and 10 years after operation by history, examination and radiograph where possible. An objective assessment was made using the Baily knee score, which was adapted from that used by the Hospital for Special Surgery and has a maximum score of 50. A score of 35 or more is rated as good, 30–34 fair and less than 30 poor. The radiological features of arthritis were graded according to the system of Kellgren and Lawrence [24] and the coronal femoro-tibial angles were measured on long weight bearing films.

Results

Overall assessment

The unicompartmental replacements show significantly better results than the osteotomies (Table 19.2). Forty-three percent of the osteotomies had a result classified as good, whereas 76% of the unicompartmental replacement group were so classified ($p < 0.01$). Twenty percent of the osteotomies had been revised to a knee replacement whereas only 7% of the unicompartmental replacements had needed further surgery.

Table 19.2   Comparison of overall results in both groups

	Replacement	Osteotomy
Good	32	21
Fair	4	11
Poor	3	7
Revised	3	10

$p < 0.01$

Pain

Although pain represented 30% of the overall assessment, it is often considered the most important factor by the patient. It was therefore assessed separately. Of those patients who had not undergone further surgery, 67% of the unicompartmental replacement group had no pain, while only 26% of the osteotomy group were pain free.

Table 19.1   Comparison of preoperative condition of the unicompartmental replacement and osteotomy groups

	Replacement	Osteotomy
Average age	71 years	63 years
Sex F:M	31:11	38:11
Preoperative deformity:		
Varus	36	33
Valgus	6	16
Average deviation from coronal tibio-femoral angle of 7° valgus	10.2°	9.9°
Average Kellgren–Lawrence score in:		
affected compartment	3.2	3.3
unaffected compartment	1.9	2.0
patello-femoral joint	2.0	2.4

Table 19.3 Incidence of radiological deterioration in compartments

Compartment	Replacement		Osteotomy	
	Deterioration	*No deterioration*	*Deterioration*	*No deterioration*
Affected	—	—	2	15
Unaffected	2	18	12	5
Patello-femoral joint	3	16	8	8

Radiological changes

Not all cases had adequate radiographs to allow full assessment but it can be seen from Table 9.3 that following tibial osteotomy the affected compartment rarely deteriorated but the loaded compartment usually did and the patello-femoral joint deteriorated in 50% of cases. Following unicompartmental replacement with deliberate slight undercorrection, radiological deterioration in the opposite or patello-femoral compartments was unusual (Fig. 19.2).

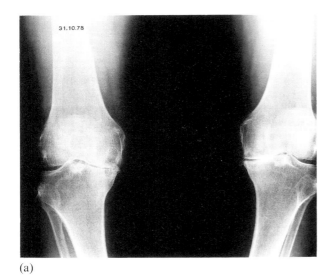

(a)

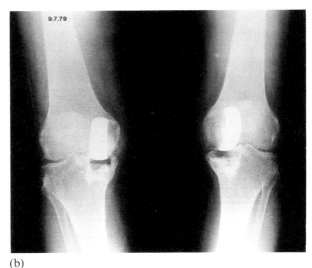

(b)

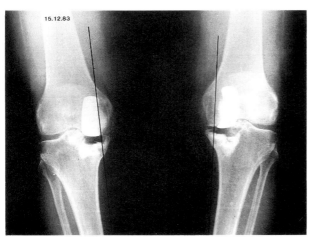

(c)

Fig. 19.2 (a) Preoperative radiograph demonstrating bilateral varus osteoarthritis. (b) Standing radiographs taken 6 months after unicompartmental replacement with St. Georg Sled prostheses. (c) Five years postoperatively there is no evidence of loosening or progressive arthritis. Note the weightbearing line showing undercorrection of the varus deformity.

Thus on the criteria studied, the unicompartmental group appeared to do better when reviewed between 5 and 10 years. The study is open to criticism because it was retrospective and also because the average follow-up of the osteotomies was slightly longer. However, this did not appear to affect the results and in Bristol it seems that patients get a better quality of result and are less likely to need further surgery within 10 years following unicompartmental replacement than upper tibial osteotomy. A more recent review of these patients has demonstrated that the superior results of unicompartmental replacement are maintained at 12 to 17 year follow-up [25].

Although the outcome of the unicompartmental replacements was encouraging, better results can probably be achieved by better patient selection and more accurate component positioning with modern jigs. The choice of prosthesis is also crucial since polyethylene quality and prosthetic design are critical. Possibly longer term survival will be achieved by cementless fixation.

Total knee replacement

Because some of the early reports of unicompartmental replacement were discouraging, some surgeons have not considered the procedure. Such individuals have carried out a total knee replacement when the patient did not appear suitable for an osteotomy. The results of total knee replacement have improved markedly in recent years and good results with a 10-year follow-up have now been reported [26].

With better techniques it is likely that the results will improve still further so that total knee replacement becomes an increasingly attractive option for patients with unicompartmental arthritis. The question that will have to be answered is whether total knee replacement gives better immediate or long term results than unicompartmental replacement.

A comparison of unicompartmental and total knee replacement

When the total knee replacements performed in Bristol during 1974–1979 are compared with the unicompartment St. Georg Sled replacements, it is found that the latter gave 76% good results

between 5 and 10 years compared with 50% good results for the total knee replacement group. However, it should be noted that at the time the predominant total knee replacement being used was a Sheehan arthroplasty and the situation may well be different now that a more modern resurfacing type of arthroplasty is being performed.

Using a standard knee replacement assessment form with a maximum score of 100, the results of resurfacing total knee replacements and unicompartmental replacement have been compared at 2 years. The average score for the total knee replacement group rose from a preoperative figure of 44 to 80, while that for the unicompartmental group rose from 55 to 86. It therefore seems that in Bristol patients undergoing unicompartmental replacement fare slightly better at 2 years than those who have a total knee replacement, but they were a less severely damaged group in the first place.

The only conclusive way to establish the merits of these three procedures is by a prospective trial. The short term results of such a study have shown a slight advantage for unicompartmental replacement in appropriate cases but the long term follow-up is still awaited [27].

Conclusion

Tibial osteotomy is a relatively unpredictable procedure that is not without complications and needs accurate realignment of the knee. It should probably be reserved for younger patients who have early medial compartment arthritis and intact ligaments (Fig. 19.3). For patients with marked unicompartmental arthritis, unicompartment replacement can give good results which do not deteriorate rapidly. However, patient selection is important and the arthritis should be truly unicompartmental [28]. Møller *et al.* [29] have suggested from cadaveric studies that an intact anterior cruciate ligament is necessary for long term survival of an unconstrained implant and recently Goodfellow and O'Connor [30] have presented clinical data to support this theory. In addition, it has been stressed that a flat tibial prosthesis is needed and that over-correction must definitely be avoided in order to prevent deterioration of the opposite compartment. Provided these criteria are met, a predictably good

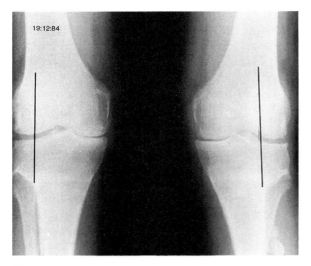

(a)

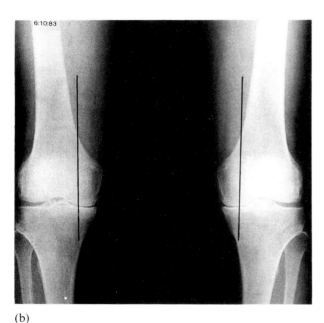

(b)

Fig. 19.3   (a, b) Standing radiographs showing early medial compartment osteoarthritis suitable for an upper tibial osteotomy. The weightbearing line has been transferred from the medial to the lateral compartments (perhaps insufficiently on the left).

result can be expected from the procedure which resects minimal bone, is technically straightforward and which can be easily revised should the need arise [31]. For cases in which the liga-

ments are damaged, or more than one compartment is involved, a resurfacing total knee replacement is probably preferable.

References

1. Hernborg, J. S. and Nilsson, B. E. (1977) The natural course of untreated osteoarthritis of the knee. *Clin. Orthop. Rel. Res.*, **123**, 130–137.
2. Dieppe, P. A., Sathapatayavongs, B., Jones, H. E. *et al.* (1980) Intra-articular steroids in osteoarthritis. *Rheumatol. Rehab*, **19**, 212–217.
3. Jackson, R. W. and Abe, I. (1972) The role of arthroscopy in the management of disorders of the knee. *J. Bone Joint Surg.*, **54B**, 310–322.
4. Isserlin, B. (1950) Joint debridement for osteoarthritis of the knee. *J. Bone Joint Surg.*, **32B**, 302–306.
5. Locht, R. C., Gross, A. E. and Langer, F. (1984) Late osteochondral allograft resurfacing for tibial plateau fractures. *J. Bone Joint Surg.*, **66A**, 328–335.
6. Jackson, J. P. (1958) Osteotomy for osteoarthritis of the knee. *J. Bone Joint Surg.*, **40B**, 826.
7. Insall, J. N., Joseph, D. M. and Msika, C. (1984) High tibial osteotomy for varus gonarthrosis. *J. Bone Joint Surg.*, **66A**, 1040–1048.
8. Harding, M. L. (1976) A fresh appraisal of tibial osteotomy for osteoarthritis of the knee. *Clin. Orthop. Rel. Res.*, **114**, 223–234.
9. Shojl, H. and Insall, J. (1973) High tibial osteotomy for osteoarthritis of the knee with valgus deformity. *J. Bone Joint Surg.*, **55A**, 963–973.
10. Coventry, M. B. (1973) Osteotomy about the knee for degenerative and rheumatoid arthritis. *J. Bone Joint Surg.*, **55A**, 23–48.
11. Maquet, P. G. J. (1980) Osteotomy. In *Arthritis of the Knee* (ed. M. A. R. Freeman), Springer, Berlin, Heidelberg, New York, pp. 149–183.
12. Tasker, T. P. B. and Harding, M. L. (1985) Supracondylar osteotomy for valgus arthritis knees. *J. Bone Joint Surg.*, **67B**, 158.
13. Jackson, J. P. and Waugh, W. (1974) The technique and complications of upper tibial osteotomy. *J. Bone Joint Surg.*, **56B**, 236–245.
14. Inglis, G. S. (1984) Unicompartmental arthroplasty of the knee. *J. Bone Joint Surg.*, **66B**, 682–684.
15. Tjornstrand, B. A. E., Egund, N. and Hagstedt, B. V. (1981) High tibial osteotomy. *Clin. Orthop. Rel. Res.*, **160**, 124–136.
16. Marmor, L. (1979) Marmor modular knee in unicompartmental disease. *J. Bone Joint Surg.*, **61A**, 347–353.

17. Scott, R. D. and Santore, R. F. (1981) Unicondylar unicompartmental replacement for osteoarthritis of the knee. *J. Bone Joint Surg.*, **63A**, 536–544.

18. Thornhill, T. S. (1986) Unicompartmental knee arthroplasty. *Clin. Orthop. Rel. Res.*, **205**, 121–131.

19. Cameron, H. D., Hunter, G. A., Welsh, R. P. and Baily, W. H. (1987) Unicompartmental knee replacement. *Clin. Orthop. Rel. Res.*, **160**, 109–113.

20. Laskin, R. S. (1978) Unicompartmental tibio femoral resurfacing arthroplasty. *J. Bone Joint Surg.*, **60A**, 182–185.

21. Insall, J. N. and Aglietti, P. A. (1980) A five to seven year follow-up of unicondylar arthroplasty. *J. Bone Joint Surg.*, **62A**, 1329–1337.

22. Broughton, N. S., Newman, J. H. and Baily, R. A. J. (1986) Unicompartmental replacement and high tibial osteotomy for osteoarthritis of the knee. *J. Bone Joint Surg.*, **68B**, 447–452.

23. Staniforth, P. and Baily, R. A. J. (1982) St. Georg 'Sledge' resurfacing of the tibio femoral joint. *J. Bone Joint Surg.*, **64B**, 246.

24. Kellgren, J. H. and Lawrence, J. S. (1957) Radiological assessment of osteoarthritis. *Ann. Rheum. Dis.*, **16**, 494–502.

25. Weale, A. E. and Newman, J. H. (1994) Unicompartmental arthroplasty and high tibial osteotomy for osteoarthrosis of the knee. A comparative study with a 12–17 year follow up period. *Clin. Orthop. Rel. Res.*, **302**, 134–137.

26. Insall, J. N. and Kelly, M. (1986) The total condylar prosthesis. *Clin. Orthop. Rel. Res.*, **205**, 43–48.

27. Newman, J. H., Acroyd, C. E. and Ahmed, S. R. (1994) The early results of a prospective randomised trial of unicompartmental or total knee replacement. *J. Bone Joint Surg.*, **76B**, 5.

28. Sarangi, P. P., Jackson, M., Karachalios, T. and Newman, J. H. (1994) Patterns of failure of unicondylar knee replacement. *Revue de Chir. Orthop.*, **80**, 217–222.

29. Møller, J. T., Weeth, R. E., Keller, J. O. and Nielsen, S. (1985) Unicompartmental arthroplasty of the knee. *Acta Orthop. Scand.*, **56**, 120–123.

30. Goodfellow, J. W. and O'Connor, J. (1986) Clinical results of the Oxford knee. *Clin. Orthop. Rel. Res.*, **205**, 21–42.

31. Jackson, M., Sarangi, P. P. and Newman, J. H. (1994) Revision Knee Replacement. Comparison of outcome of primary proximal tibial osteotomy or unicompartmental arthroplasty. *J. Arthroplasty*, **9**, 539–542.

20

Mechanical and degenerative disorders of the lumbar spine

J. S. Denton

Introduction

Back pain is a problem of epidemic proportions. It ranks with headache and tiredness as the commonest symptom of which the general public complain and it causes around half of the population to seek advice from their general practitioners at some time. The cost of back pain in sickness benefit is enormous.

The subject is plagued by the twin difficulties of correctly identifying the source of pain and of finding an effective treatment even for those patients in whom the pain source has been confidently defined. Fortunately, the majority of patients with back pain improve regardless of treatment and only a very few become 'back cripples'.

Classification of back pain

Back pain, like abdominal pain or headache, is but a symptom. It is not a diagnosis. The poor reputation that back pain has among the general public arises largely from the failure to make a diagnosis. Even with the most meticulous enquiry about the history, a detailed examination of the patient and sophisticated investigation, there are occasions when the exact site and source of the pain cannot be identified. Many patients, even though severely incapacitated by their complaint, will be satisfied by an explanation of the nature of their condition and simple advice on how best to come to terms with it in order to minimize the disruption which it causes to their lives.

A rational analysis of the many syndromes of back pain requires a knowledge of anatomy, an understanding of the physiology of pain and some comprehension of the biomechanics of the spine. The chosen classification of back pain is that suggested by Macnab.

Viscerogenic back pain

Backs have fronts. Back pain may thus be derived from any of a number of structures lying in the retroperitoneal space. Common sources of viscerogenic back pain include the kidneys, pancreas, duodenum, malignant infiltration or secondary deposits from remote disease. It is uncommon for back pain to be the only complaint in those patients with visceral pathology. It follows that no assessment of a patient complaining of back pain is complete without an enquiry into the patient's general health, particularly his respiratory, genito-urinary and digestive functions. A careful abdominal and rectal examination is mandatory, as also is an examination of the vascular supply of the lower limbs. Viscerogenic back pain is typically not relieved by rest or aggravated by activity, although occasionally a patient with a posterior duodenal or gastric ulcer penetrating the pancreas may report exacerbation of the pain by stooping or exercise and relief by lying down. On occasion, the complaint of back pain may override the digestive symp-

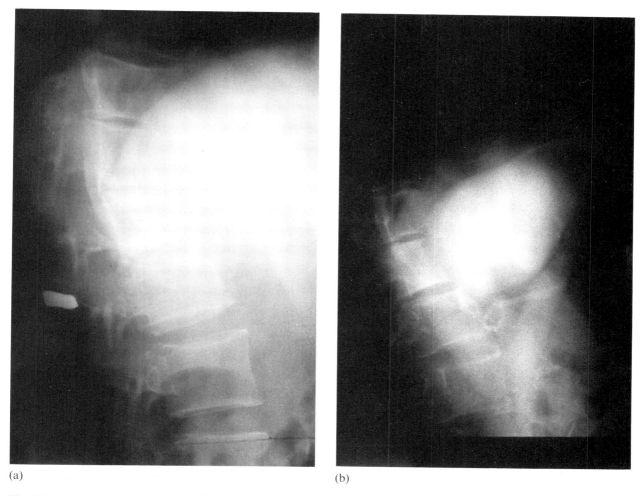

(a)   (b)

Fig. 20.1   Abdominal aneurysm: scalloping of the anterior borders of vertebral bodies and calcification in the wall of the aneurysm.

toms to such a degree that the primary problem may escape the attention of the physician unless the appropriate inquiries are made.

Vascular back pain

An aortic aneurysm may cause severe deep seated boring back pain and abdominal examination may reveal a pulsatile and easily palpable mass. Aneurysmal dilatation of the aorta will not in itself lead to the disappearance of the distal pulses, but such patients may have occlusive vascular disease as well as a propensity for aneurysm formation. The femoral pulses may therefore be reduced in volume or absent. The presence of a thrill or bruit over the femoral artery is a further sign of circulatory disturbance. A scalloped appearance of the anterior borders of the vertebral bodies is often present on the plain lateral radiograph as well as calcification in the wall of the aneurysm (Fig. 20.1).

Neurogenic back pain

The thalamus relays and may record sensory stimuli. Occasionally, a lesion of the thalamus such as a tumour or more commonly an infarct in a hypertensive patient may cause pain in the leg. The pain has a typically bizarre nature which the patient finds difficult to describe. Severe hyperaesthesia may be present, provoked by light touch but not by firm touch such as grasping the limb. Other causes of neurogenic back pain include primary or secondary tumours invading from the vertebrae or arising *de novo* in the meninges, spinal cord or cauda equina. Thus ependymomata, neurilemmomata and neurofibromata are rare but possible causes of neurogenic pain. Occasionally, the syndrome may be clinically indistinguishable from that produced by a prolapsed intervertebral disc with nerve root entrapment. Finally, in childhood, an intraspinal tumour must be suspected.

Psychogenic back pain

True psychogenic back pain is rare but the problem of somatism is not unique to back pain and may dominate the clinical picture. It requires time, patience and a certain expertise to recognize this problem and the management may be outside the province of many surgeons.

Spondylogenic back pain

This category, comprising those causes of back pain arising as a result of pathology in the spinal or paraspinal structures, accounts for the vast majority of patients presenting with a complaint of backache. The pain may arise from bone, joint or soft tissue, the latter being the commonest source. The commoner causes of spondylogenic back pain are discussed in detail in the sections below.

The anatomy of low back pain

The design of the spine arises from a compromise between conflicting requirements. The structure must be capable of withstanding enormous loads yet allow sufficient mobility to perform many activities. Failure of one or more components of the spine will result in one of the recognizable clinical syndromes of backache.

The design of the vertebral column

The cervical, thoracic and lumbar vertebrae articulate with their neighbours by means of synovial facet joints and intervertebral discs. Stability is conferred to the spine by these articulations and their ligaments and associated muscles. A smooth kyphotic configuration in fetal life is transformed by lordotic curves in the cervical and lumbar regions as soon as the upright posture is established.

The intervertebral disc

The disc is a complex structure attached firmly to the hyaline end plates on the adjacent surfaces of the vertebral bodies and within it the nucleus pulposus, a remnant of the notochord, lies towards the posterior half. The tough annulus fibrosus surrounds the nucleus.

In the fetus and during the first years of life, the nucleus pulposus has a blood supply. This diminishes rapidly within a few months of birth and by the age of 8 has virtually disappeared so that the adult nucleus is entirely avascular. Its nutrition is obtained by diffusion of metabolites from the marrow spaces of the neighbouring vertebrae via the end plates and to a lesser extent by a similar process of diffusion through the annulus. The nucleus is composed mainly of ground substances, which consist of a variety of macromolecules held in colloidal suspension. The substances present include glycoproteins and proteoglycans. The latter are strongly hydrophilic and as a result, the water content of the nucleus is high. The diffusion of water into the nucleus gives rise to a hydrostatic pressure within the disc which is resisted by the surrounding annulus fibrosus. As a result, the fibres of the annulus come to lie under tension rather in the manner of the walls of a pressure vessel. The organic content of the nucleus is produced by the cells which lie enmeshed within a loose network of collagen fibrils. Most of the ground substances and collagen are produced by those cells which lie close to the junction of nucleus and annulus. With ageing, the water content and proteoglycan content of the nucleus diminish. This is related to a tendency to fibrosis of the nucleus with simultaneous diminution in cellular activity at the junctional zone.

The annulus fibrosus consists mainly of sheets of collagen fibrils lying in laminae of differing orientations, rather akin to the walls of a tyre. At their ends, they are firmly attached to the cartilaginous endplates of the vertebrae. The orientation of successive sheets of fibrils varies but most lie at an angle of 60° to their neighbours and to the axis of the spine. In this way, they are most favourably disposed to withstand the shear stresses to which they are subjected during load bearing.

The anterior longitudinal ligament is a condensation of the annulus lying along the anterior aspect of the disc and is attached to the endplate. It continues over the anterior aspect of the vertebral body but is easily separated from it. The fibrils of collagen in the ligament are aligned with the long axis of the spine.

The posterior longitudinal ligament by contrast is less robust. It lies in the midline over the posterior aspect of the vertebrae and discs to which it is loosely attached.

The nerve supply of the disc is scanty. Free nerve endings are seen in discs of infants and young children but they degenerate in adolescence, leaving nerve fibres which penetrate only a short distance into the outer layers of the annulus. The main source of nerve endings lies in the fibroelastic tissue attaching the posterior longitudinal ligament to the annulus of the disc. They are likely to be stimulated in a central disc prolapse but not in the more common lateral disc herniation.

Facet joints

The facet joints in the upper part of the lumbar spine lie in the sagittal plane, but lower down the orientation of the facet joints progressively rotates so that at lumbosacral level they lie in the coronal plane.

The role of the facet joint as a cause of back pain has for long been a matter of dispute. Recent imaging techniques have demonstrated pathological changes in these structures so that their importance is more evident.

A concentric articulation is achieved by a convex upper and a concave lower surface though asymmetry is common and may lead to degenerative changes when subject to load bearing. The main movement at the facet joints is gliding to allow flexion and extension. Asymmetric sliding allows lateral flexion. Rotation is limited in the lumbar spine but is brought about by distraction of the facet on the side to which

bending occurs, combined with compression and anterior sliding of the opposite facet; the compressed facet acting as a fulcrum.

Constraints to movement depend not only upon the shape of the facets but also upon the surrounding ligaments and the joint capsules. There are recesses at the upper and lower limits of the joint capsule where multifidus muscle fibres are attached presumably to prevent entrapment of the synovial lining during movement.

Ligaments

The ligamentum flavum is a thick fibroelastic structure which extends from the anterior aspect of the inferior surface of the lamina above to the upper surface of the lamina below. It provides a smooth posterior border of the spinal canal. In flexion it is tight but in extension it tends to buckle so narrowing the anteroposterior diameter of the spinal canal and thus becoming a potential contributing factor to spinal stenosis. It is a bifid structure with a median raphe allowing for easy midline fenestration when the spinous process has been removed. Its attachment to the anterior surface of the upper lamina may interfere with the passage of sublaminar wires.

The interspinous ligament is segmental and is a strong constraint in flexion of the spine.

The innervation of the spine

The innervation of spinal and paraspinal structures follows a complex and variable pattern. The earlier theory that pain was produced by overstimulation of a variety of different receptors has been abandoned since the recognition of specific nociceptive nerve endings. Such receptors have been identified in most tissues of the spine. They are represented by unmyelinated plexiform nerve fibres with free endings ramifying throughout the skin, subcutaneous fat, fasciae, ligaments, bone, periosteum, joint capsules, dura and adventitia of blood vessels.

The neurological anatomy of the lumbar spine has been clarified by the studies of Wyke [1], Paris [2] and Bogduk *et al.* [3]; a pattern has emerged. The ventral and dorsal roots within the central canal are bathed in cerebrospinal fluid and join to form a mixed spinal nerve in the root canal just distal to the dorsal root ganglion but still within the evagination of the dural sheath. As the mixed nerve emerges from the root canal, a branch arises which joins with another from the ramus communicans to form the recurrent sinuvertebral nerve of Luschke. The latter re-enters the spinal canal via the foramen and giving off branches which supply the posterior longitudinal ligament, the fibroelastic tissue attaching the ligament to the disc, the meninges, particularly the anterior surface of the dura, the nerve root sleeves, the ligamentum flavum and the facet joints. The mixed spinal nerve then divides almost immediately into anterior and posterior primary rami. Most of the fibres in the anterior primary ramus are destined to form the lumbar and sacral plexuses. Branches arise which innervate the immediate surrounding tissues of the postero-lateral and lateral aspects of the disc, though with only minimal penetration into the annulus.

The posterior primary ramus innervates the paravertebral muscles and overlying skin as well as the facet joints at adjacent levels. Further branches innervate the interspinous, supra-spinous and intertransverse ligaments. In addition, the posterior primary rami of L4, L5 and S1 send branches to the sacroiliac joints. This simple description belies the wide innervation of spinal structures. Virtually every tissue in the spine is innervated by at least three spinal nerves by virtue of their ascending and descending branches. As a result, referred pain fails to conform to the exact and expected dermatome, which may prove misleading when attempting to identify the level of the source of pain.

Pain pathways in the spine

When nociceptive receptors are stimulated, the nerve impulses are carried in small diameter unmyelinated fibres to the dorsal root ganglion. From here, the fibres enter the cord via the dorsal root travelling in its anterior ramus. The posterior ramus carries large diameter fibres conveying sensations such as proprioception, light touch and vibration sense. As the pain fibres enter the cord, ascending and descending branches are given off which typically span one or two segments. The main fibres and their branches then enter the grey matter of the posterior horn of the cord where they form a synapse with inter-

mediate neurones. From these neurones, most fibres can be traced across the cord where they enter the contralateral anterolateral ascending tract to be conveyed to the brain. Other fibres, via a series of intermediate synaptic connections, project to the motor neurone pools of the muscles of the back and lower limbs. These circuits probably account for the peculiarities of gait and posture which are seen in many patients with back pain.

The gate theory

Within the spinal cord, mechanisms exist for the modulation of pain. Certain of the larger diameter fibres entering the cord through the posterior ramus of the dorsal root relay with neurones within the substantia gelatinosa – a lightly staining area which caps the dorsal horn. These neurones relay with the presynaptic fibres of the nociceptive neurones and inhibit the transmission of pain stimuli across the neighbouring synapses. This is the basis of the 'gate theory'. The application of non-noxious stimuli such as rubbing the skin, gentle heat or even moving the affected source of pain, may be sufficient to reduce the level of perceived pain. The theory may also explain the severity of pain in post-herpetic neuralgia. The destruction of the larger diameter fibres removes their moderating influence on the onward transmission of pain and a more profound painful stimulus thus arrives at the brain.

The gate theory, while still valid, has been modified by better understanding of the modulating influence on pain of descending tracts from the brain. These are conveyed via the reticular formation from the frontal and paracentral regions of the brain. The descending tracts exert their influence via a series of intermediate neurones in the dorsal horns and inhibit the onward transmission of pain impulses in a similar manner to that operating in the classical gate theory.

The anterolateral tract transmits the pain impulses to the brain. Formerly known as the spino-thalamic tract, it is now named according to its position in the cord as recent work has revealed that fewer than one third of its fibres actually terminate in the thalamus. Most of the fibres relay within the reticular formation or other brain stem nuclei; others re-enter the grey matter of the cord to form a synapse with neurones therein. Those with synaptic connections within the thalamus are generally of larger diameter and are myelinated. They project to cortical sensory area 'One' and are chiefly concerned with the location, intellectual perception and recognition of the quality of the painful stimulus.

The frontal area relates to the emotive response and subjective sensation of unpleasantness; the temporal region is concerned with the memory of previous painful stimuli and the hypothalamus regulates the viscerohumoral response to pain, including the changes which occur in the gastrointestinal and cardiovascular systems as well as various hormonal responses.

Communication between these components is achieved by a complex system of association fibres. One component may be modified independently of the rest and there is thus no direct correlation between one and the other. Attempts to quantify pain by measuring visceral responses in a laboratory are unreliable and the best solution is to rely on the well tried method of being a good listener and attending to the patient's complaints and their effect on the quality of life.

Soft tissue injuries of the spine

As with articulated structures elsewhere in the body, the muscles, ligaments and joints associated with the spine are liable to injury. A number of syndromes are described, though it must be admitted at the outset that there is often considerable difficulty attached to the identification of the specific structure which has been damaged.

The acute back strain

The acute back strain is occasioned by activities such as injudicious lifting, falling or other externally applied violence to the soft tissues of the spine. Muscles, ligaments and joints may be torn as the soft tissues tighten to prevent damage to the osseous and neural components of the spine. The patient experiences severe pain in the back, often with ill-defined radiation to the buttocks and thighs. Any attempt to move the injured

structures in the acute stage is confounded by intense muscle spasm, resulting in rigidity of the lumbar spine together with a limp and sometimes profound disturbances in posture. In the absence of symptoms or signs suggestive of a prolapsed intervertebral disc, there is little point in attempting to identify the exact site of the pathology. The treatment is simple. Bed rest is indicated until the worst of the pain has subsided and the patient has begun to mobilize. Adequate analgesia must be provided. Regardless of what treatment if any is applied, the vast majority of patients will make a full recovery from the acute episode in a matter of a few weeks.

Many will benefit from a short course of non-steroidal anti-inflammatory drugs and from a muscle relaxant such as diazepam. If it is possible to locate an area of particularly acute tenderness, infiltration of the region with 0.5% bupivicaine in a dose of around 10 ml may provide instantaneous if short-lived relief. Such manoeuvres probably do not affect the speed of resolution of the pathology, but can bring welcome relief to the patient and encourage him in the belief that his back will eventually recover.

Physiotherapy has little part to play in the earliest phase of the illness. If recovery is prolonged or if the patient is unable or unwilling to go to bed until the symptoms have abated, some form of external splintage must be provided, perhaps in the form of a plaster jacket. It is rarely necessary to continue such treatment for longer than 2 weeks. After this time, efforts should be directed to restoring mobility to the spine and to recovering muscle tone. At this stage when soft tissue healing is under way and the initial hyperaemia and oedema have subsided, a course of physiotherapy may be of benefit, although the great majority of patients will not in fact require it. Local heat, ultrasound, short wave diathermy and megapulse treatment may be applied in conjunction with gentle stretching exercises aimed at breaking down any adhesions which may have formed. The damaged soft tissues will inevitably repair by scar tissue. As long as this scar is prevented from adhering to adjacent structures of different mobility and is protected from further damage by adequate paraspinal musculature, it is reasonable to expect a smooth and rapid convalescence with uneventful return to former activities. Prior to discharge, the patient should be counselled regarding lifting activities at work and taught how to protect his back against further episodes.

The chronic back strain

Some patients do not recover well from an acute back strain. This may be due to inappropriate or inadequate initial treatment, to attempts on the part of the patient to return to strenuous activity too soon or to a lack of resolve on the part of the patient to overcome the illness and rehabilitate himself to what may be seen as an unpalatable if not overtly hostile working environment. Patients who are involved in litigation because of an accident at work which may have precipitated their symptoms can be particularly difficult to manage and it can take a great deal of persuasion that an early return to former activities is what is required in order to rehabilitate their back most effectively.

Much reassurance is needed that the experience of back pain does not equate with progressive structural damage to the spine. The active role of the patient in any treatment programme must be emphasized and it should be made clear that a firm commitment is called for in order to ensure recovery. The patient is not merely a passive onlooker in this scenario. The responsibility for recovery is his as much as the surgeon's.

The long term outlook for patients with a chronic back strain is not good. Very few of those who have been off work for longer than 1 year will return to their former employment and virtually none who have been absent for 2 years or more. The key to prevention of this undesirable situation is the effective treatment of the acute condition.

The prolapsed intervertebral disc

It was not until 1932 that Barr of Boston recognized the existence of prolapse of the intervertebral disc as a cause of back pain. The material which he had removed from his patient's spinal canal had been labelled as chondroma by the pathologist – a common report to obtain from such specimens in that era. In 1934, Barr and Mixter [4] suggested that sciatic pain could be produced from the encroachment of prolapsed intervertebral disc material upon a lumbar nerve root. At first received with scepticism, this concept rapidly gained wide acceptance and it was not long before the intervertebral disc was incriminated as the cause of back pain in the majority of such patients presenting to the orthopaedic surgeon. The balance has now hopefully been restored to a more realistic level and the prolapsed disc has taken its rightful place as a prominent but by no means the sole cause of back pain and sciatica.

Pathology

The changes of ageing in the normal disc do not in themselves cause back pain but render the disc more vulnerable to damage when challenged with loads that a healthy disc in a younger patient would withstand. The stresses required to bring about failure of the disc are debatable but simple compressive loading of the spine will not induce disc failure. The more likely outcome in such a situation is that the vertebral endplate will fail, leading to herniation of disc material into the body of the vertebra and the subsequent appearance on the radiograph of the so-called 'Schmorl's node' (Fig. 20.2). Even when a longitudinal incision is made in the annulus in its posterolateral portion (the most frequent site of annular tears in the patient with the prolapsed

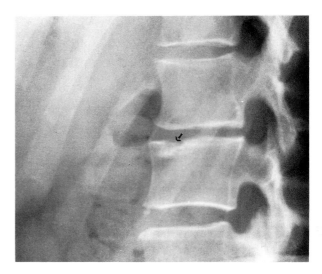

Fig. 20.2   Schmorl's node: herniation of disc material through the vertebral end-plate.

disc), the disc will still herniate into the vertebral body when direct compression is applied rather than fail by a rupture through the annulus [5]. The load required to bring about endplate failure is quoted as between 1800 Newtons and 5300 Newtons by different authors. It is instructive to compare these figures with the normal loads experienced by the disc in everyday activities. Nachemson and co-workers [6] measured the intradiscal pressure in volunteers performing various activities. The L3 disc carries about 60% of the body weight above it – typically 420 Newtons. Sitting or standing in 20° of flexion increases the load in this disc to over 200% of body weight. Forward flexion of 5° alone will increase the load on the disc by 25%.

Compression is certainly of importance in bringing about failure of the annulus but it must be combined with loading in other modalities if other structures are not to fail first. Hickey and Hukins [7] suggest that the combination of compression and rotation is of importance while Adams and Hutton [8] indicate flexion of the compressed disc as being the more likely mode of failure. It is most likely that all three factors are involved. The amount of rotation required to produce failure of the annular fibres of the disc is of the order of 4° [9]. It is unlikely that this can be achieved in the erect normal spine because of the restraint offered by the facet joints. If, however, the spine is flexed, the facet joints will now allow further rotation to occur and the integrity of the annulus will be jeopardized. Reflex protective mechanisms are invoked to prevent such an occurrence. These take the form of involuntary muscle contractions which resist the tendency for the spine to flex and rotate. The application of an unexpected load to the spine in the form of a fall or grabbing at a heavy load to prevent its escaping may, however, overcome these protective mechanisms and expose the disc to loads which can bring about an annular rupture and prolapse of the intradiscal material.

The most common site for the intervertebral disc to fail is just lateral to the posterior longitudinal ligament. It is here that the annulus is thinnest and therefore most vulnerable. A very common clinical finding is the reporting of intermittent backache for some months or even years prior to the sudden onset of severe back pain and sciatica. A possible explanation of this phenomenon is the existence of a small tear in the

annulus of the disc prior to the release of the disc material into the canal. The paucity of innervation of the annulus casts some doubt upon this as the true explanation for this phenomenon. The resolution of this difficulty may lie in the invasion of damaged areas of the disc by granulation tissue which carries with it small diameter nerve fibres which could indeed act as nociceptors in the damaged disc. The tears described are generally radially disposed. They arise at the posterolateral corner of the disc, where the annulus experiences its greatest load and occur most commonly in the lower lumbar spine. The concave shape of the posterior border of the vertebral bodies and disc in this region leads to stress concentration at the posterolateral corner of the disc [10]. Furthermore, the lumbar discs, particularly that at the lumbosacral junction, are wedge shaped and carry a greater fraction of the body weight than do discs at higher levels. It is this combination of factors that is thought to predispose the lower lumbar discs to preferential failure given the appropriate mechanical challenge. The radial tear starts centrally and progresses towards the outer margin of the annulus. As progression occurs it may be accompanied by bulging of the disc along the line of the tear but at this stage no communication exists between the nucleus and the spinal canal. This represents a disc protrusion – that is an early prolapse of disc material where the nucleus is still shielded from the spinal canal by layers of intact annulus. Once the tear has reached the periphery of the annulus, the way is clear for the contents of the nucleus to be exuded into the canal – in other words, for the disc to rupture. This may occur slowly or with great rapidity depending upon the mechanical properties of the individual disc and the loading patterns to which it is subjected. Once disc material can be found outside the margins of the annulus, a disc extrusion is said to exist. Initially there is still continuity between the extruded material and the nuclear remnants within the disc. If, however, the extruded fragment becomes separated from the nucleus and lies free within the canal, a sequestration of the disc is said to have occurred. Such free disc fragments may migrate in a cephalad or caudal direction and may give rise to misleading signs when an attempt is made to localize the level of the lesion.

The mechanisms involved in the production of radicular pain are not straightforward. According to Macnab [11], direct pressure on a normal nerve root produces paraesthesiae rather than pain. This observation correlates well with the common clinical finding of lower limb paraesthesiae accompanying back pain in the early stages of a disc herniation, rather than pain. It appears that the nerve root must be inflamed for pain to be produced by direct pressure from the disc. With a longstanding disc prolapse, such inflammation does in fact occur. The herniated disc material irritates the surrounding tissues and an inflammatory reaction is set up with oedema and hyperaemia of the dural sheath of the root. Subsequently, dense adhesions may develop around the root and give rise to clinical features suggestive of nerve root tethering. The cause of the inflammatory reaction is unresolved. It is likely that owing to the avascularity of the disc, the latter occupies an immunologically privileged position and that exposure of the body's immune mechanisms to ruptured disc material may therefore initiate a form of autoimmune reaction. Attractive though this concept is, it awaits rigorous confirmation.

The precise direction in which the herniation occurs is of importance in determining the clinical features of the condition. Occasionally a central disc prolapse is found wherein the disc bursts through the posterior longitudinal ligament. This usually arises very acutely and may be precipitated by trauma. The diagnosis is a matter of great urgency, for there is a severe risk of cauda equina compression developing with subsequent paralysis and loss of sphincter control. The lower limbs are affected bilaterally. Weakness and numbness in the legs are accompanied by loss of perineal sensation and loss of sphincter tone. Unless the situation is remedied by urgent decompression within a few hours, the patient may not recover normal sphincter function and may be left with a residual paraparesis. This type of disc rupture most commonly occurs at the L4–L5 level.

More commonly, the herniation occurs more peripherally, just lateral to the posterior longitudinal ligament. The disc material comes to lie under the root, which is displaced either medially or, in the case of a so-called paramedian disc protrusion, laterally. Characteristically, the root involved is that corresponding to the spinal segment below which the prolapse occurs. Thus, at the lumbosacral level, it is the S1 root which is most commonly affected and at the L4–L5 level, the L5 root is at greatest risk. Atypical patterns of root involvement are well recognized. With a large herniation of the disc two roots may be involved, with disc material impinging upon the root emerging at the level of the prolapse as well as upon that emerging below. Variations in the anatomy of the sacral plexus can give rise to further confusion. It is not uncommon for the fifth lumbar root to accompany the first sacral root and to emerge via the first sacral foramen. Clearly, both roots will be at risk in the event of a lumbosacral disc prolapse.

In the event of the rupture occurring further laterally, the root emerging at the same level may be affected in its extradural course – thus with a lumbosacral disc prolapse, the fifth lumbar root may occasionally be involved rather than the first sacral.

Finally, a sequestered disc fragment may migrate in a cephalad or caudal direction to embarrass nerve roots at other levels or alternatively may become lodged in a root canal, giving rise to a severe local inflammatory response with nerve root tethering. Such fragments may be difficult to detect at surgical exploration unless an assiduous attempt is made to follow the root far out into its canal until it is seen to be completely free.

Clinical presentation

A disc prolapse may occur at any age. Those arising in young patients have special features; an acute prolapse is most common between the ages of 20 and 40 years.

Acute onset

This is often associated with radicular pain and precipitated by lifting a heavy weight. Initially, there may be numbness or paraesthesiae in the distribution of a nerve root with a dull ache in the buttock and thigh. If, for example, the first sacral root is affected, the patient will complain of pain and numbness over the outer aspect of the foot. The pain will be exacerbated by any activity which increases the pressure within the disc such as bending, sneezing or straining at stool. Pain patterns vary and some patients may have minimal backache but severe radicular pain.

Urinary incontinence

Urinary incontinence is serious and indicates that there is pressure on the cauda equina.

Frequently, the acute symptoms subside with rest to a sufficient degree to allow the patient to return to work perhaps with some residual discomfort. Any recurrence of the acute pain may be more severe and take longer to settle down than the first attack; residual symptoms tend to be more pronounced and prolonged.

Motor symptoms are not so frequent and other causes such as multiple sclerosis or an intraspinal tumour have to be considered and excluded.

Physical examination

Posture

In the acute phase there will be paravertebral spasm, loss of the normal lordotic curve and limited spinal movements. The patient may stand with a tilt to one side which disappears on lying down. The explanation for this 'sciatic scoliosis' is not entirely clear. It was formerly thought to be connected in some way with the anatomical relationship of the disc prolapse to the nerve root. Thus, it was said that with a disc prolapse lateral to the root, the patient tended to lean away from the side of the prolapse in order to gain relief from his symptoms; conversely, with a prolapse medial to the root, leaning towards the side of the pain brought relief. This is a highly simplistic and incorrect explanation of a complex phenomenon and in practice, the operative findings often disagree with one's prediction of the exact site of the prolapse. It is likely that the true explanation of this phenomenon involves derangements in the finely tuned postural reflexes which exist at cord level, rather than an obvious mechanical explanation. The matter awaits further clarification. The presence of a sciatic scoliosis is however highly suggestive of the presence of a disc prolapse and in this respect remains an invaluable physical sign.

Straight leg raise

Any increase in tension on an already stretched nerve root will provoke further pain in the dis-

tribution of the affected root. The straight leg raise test is most evident in the presence of a disc prolapse affecting the fourth or fifth lumbar or the first sacral nerve roots. Limitation of straight leg raising to 45° or less is positive [12] but there is also variation within the healthy population. A difference between the two sides is more significant, ranging from 15° [12] to 30° [13]. The production of radicular pain in the affected leg when a straight leg raise is performed on the 'healthy' side (the crossed straight leg raise test) is an important sign which gives unequivocal evidence of nerve root tension and is often associated with the presence of a sequestered disc fragment.

The bowstring test

This is another test for nerve root tension. The straight leg raising test is performed to the point where the patient complains of pain. The hip is maintained in this position while the knee is flexed by 5°. This should relieve the patient of pain. Pressure is then applied behind the knee. If this evokes a similar pain to that experienced with straight leg raising, the test is positive.

Likewise, with the straight leg raise being performed just to the point of pain production, forced dorsiflexion of the ankle, internal rotation of the hip or even flexion of the neck may produce a similar positive response.

With a disc prolapse in the upper lumbar region, the sacral nerve roots are unaffected and the straight leg raise and its qualifying tests are normal. However, an equivalent test (the femoral nerve stretch test) is available to test for tension in the upper lumbar roots. The test is performed with the patient lying prone. The hip is passively extended and the knee passively flexed. If pain in a radicular distribution is evoked, the test is positive.

Neurological examination

Neurological symptoms appear at an earlier stage than neurological signs. Consequently, the significance of a normal neurological examination depends to a certain extent upon the duration and severity of the symptoms. The tendon reflexes, muscle tone and skin sensibility

Table 20.1 Typical patterns of neurological abnormality in patients with acute lumbar disc herniation

Level of disc prolapse	Nerve root involvement	Sensory loss	Motor weakness	Disturbance of reflex
L5/S1	S1	Outer border of foot	Calf muscles	Ankle jerk absent or depressed
L4/L5	L5	Outer side of calf and medial border of foot	Extensor hallucis	E.H.L. jerk absent or depressed
L3/L4	L4	Medial side of calf	Quadriceps	Knee jerk absent or depressed
L2/L3	L3	Anterior aspect of knee	Quadriceps	Knee jerk absent or depressed
Central disc prolapse	Cauda equina	Variable pattern in legs; often perineal loss	Variable; may be profound; usually asymmetrical; loss of sphincter control	Variable; corresponds with loss of motor function

Not all patients will display all features for a disc herniation at any given level. Patterns of sensory disturbance, in particular sensory symptoms as opposed to sensory signs may vary somewhat. Patients often find difficulty in localizing sensory symptoms and variations occur in the anatomy of the lumbosacral plexus. In addition, a disc herniation at any given level may affect the exiting root at that level rather than, or in addition to, the traversing root, leading for example to the presence of L5 root signs in a L5/S1 disc herniation.

must be recorded and compared with the normal side. A general neurological examination must be performed in order to exclude either central or widespread disease. A typical abnormal pattern may emerge depending upon which nerve root is affected (Table 20.1).

McCulloch [14] lists five criteria which may be found in the patient with a disc prolapse, of which at least three should be present if a confident clinical diagnosis is to be made. These are:

1. Unilateral leg pain in a sciatic distribution including pain below the level of the knee.
2. Specific neurological symptoms of numbness, paraesthesiae or weakness which can be attributed to the involvement of a single nerve root.
3. Limitation of straight leg raising by at least 50% of normal.
4. At least two neurological signs which may include muscle wasting, weakness, sensory deficit or reduction or absence of a tendon reflex.
5. Myelographic evidence of a disc prolapse. This could nowadays be extended to include computerized tomography or magnetic resonance imaging.

Intervertebral disc lesions in childhood

Most of the clinical features of a prolapsed intervertebral disc in childhood are similar to those seen in the adult. The patient presents with back pain of variable severity which may be of acute or gradual onset. There is sometimes a history of trauma preceding the appearance of symptoms. Leg pain is very common and is not infrequently bilateral. Numbness and paraesthesiae are less prominent than in the adult and motor weakness is an unusual complaint.

The child often presents with a bizarre gait, avoiding the swing through phase of walking by circumduction of the pelvis or by shuffling in those patients with bilateral leg pain in an attempt to reduce nerve root tension by avoiding traction on the sacral plexus. Local cord reflexes may also be involved in the production of this type of gait. The posture may be equally bizarre with marked spasm of the erector spinae muscles and a pronounced list to one side.

Nerve root tension signs are often more striking in the child than in the adult and severe limitation of straight leg raising is the rule. Sensory changes are uncommon but may be present. Usually there are no abnormal motor signs and reflexes are similarly well preserved.

In childhood as in adult life, intraspinal tumours may mimic a prolapse of the intervertebral disc. In the young patient however, such lesions are at least as common as prolapsed discs and every patient with such a presentation must therefore be considered to have an intraspinal tumour until proved otherwise.

Investigation of the patient with a prolapsed disc

The diagnosis of prolapse of an intervertebral disc can usually be made with some confidence from the history and physical examination alone. The purpose of investigations is to exclude other causes of the patient's symptoms, such as an intraspinal tumour and to identify the level of the prolapse in those patients who require surgery.

In the presence of a disc prolapse, haematological and biochemical investigations will be normal though a full blood count, sedimentation rate and alkaline phosphatase should be obtained in order to assist in the exclusion of more sinister pathology.

Radiography

Plain radiographs of the spine are completely unhelpful in making a positive diagnosis of prolapsed intervertebral disc but are essential investigations in order to rule out other pathology. The radiograph will confirm the alterations in the sagittal and coronal contours of the spine found on physical examination. Depending on the length of time which has elapsed since the acute episode, there may be some narrowing of a disc space though this is insufficient to identify the level of the prolapse with any confidence. Degenerative changes in the lumbar spine on plain radiography are a common normal finding and may be completely coincidental, appearing at a different level from the prolapse, or may be widespread throughout the lumbar spine.

Radiculography

In patients who are to be subjected to surgery, identification of the level of the disc prolapse is important. Water soluble radiculography is still the commonest procedure undertaken for this purpose. It is an accurate method with a true positive rate of over 90%. False positives can occur in cases where there is poor root sleeve filling and false negatives are sometimes produced in cases with a prolapse which is situated

far laterally. Radiculography is not without its complications. Headache, nausea and vomiting are all common complaints following the procedure. Myoclonic spasms, fever, back pain, psychomotor disturbances and chemical arachnoiditis have also been reported. The latter was a much more important consideration in the days of oil based radiography dyes than with modern water soluble agents. The investigation is unpleasant for the patient not only because of the lumbar puncture involved but also because of the considerable manoeuvring of the subject required to achieve adequate visualization of the nerve roots.

The radiological features seen in the presence of a disc prolapse include extradural indentation of the dural sac, usually with a failure of the affected root sleeve to fill with contrast and in the case of a disc prolapse of substantial size, deviation of the nerve root from its normal course (Fig. 20.3). With a disc prolapse situated far

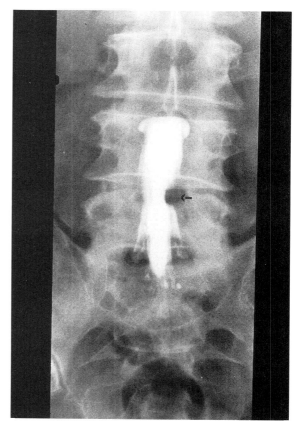

Fig. 20.3 Indentation of the dural sac and obliteration of the nerve root sleeve.

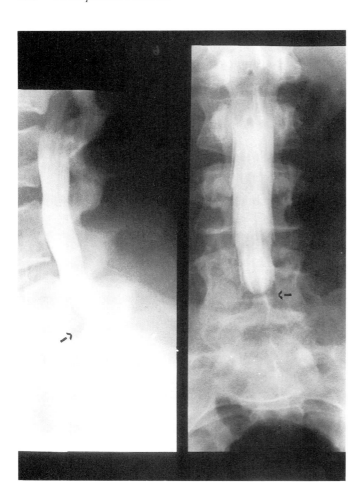

Fig. 20.4   Complete block of contrast medium in a cauda equina syndrome.

laterally, deviation of the affected root or amputation of the root sleeve may be the only changes seen on radiculography. In the event of a massive central disc prolapse resulting in a cauda equina syndrome, a complete block may be seen (Fig. 20.4).

Computerized tomography

The accuracy and increasing availability of computerized tomography has led to its replacing radiculography to some extent. It is non-invasive and lacks complications. The sensitivity of the method is about equal to that of radiculography in detecting prolapse of an intervertebral disc. Certain drawbacks must be recognized. The resolution of the method is less than that of radiculography. The levels at which examination is required must be specified. Migration of sequestered fragments of disc material or choice of incorrect level may lead to false negative results. Enhanced computerized tomography with contrast material introduced into the canal as a prior procedure improves the sensitivity of the method. Computerized tomography is more sensitive than radiculography in identification of lateral disc prolapse and in posterior disc prolapse in the presence of a wide epidural space (Fig. 20.5).

Magnetic resonance imaging

Magnetic resonance imaging is a more recent development which is proving to be the most sensitive technique currently available for the detection of degenerative disc disease (Fig. 20.6). Unlike computerized tomography, it is capable of distinguishing nuclear from annular material. It is thus possible to distinguish between disc

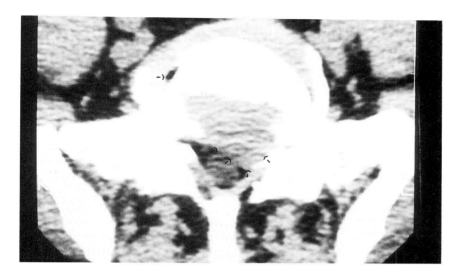

Fig. 20.5 CT scan showing postero-lateral disc herniation.

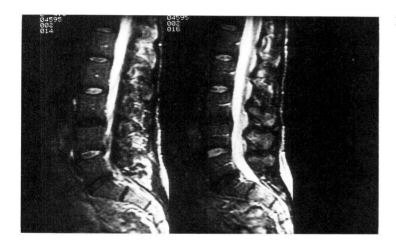

Fig. 20.6 MRI scan showing disc degeneration.

protrusion, disc extrusion and disc sequestration by identifying the relationship of the annulus to the nuclear material under suspicion (Fig. 20.7). This is an important distinction as failure of a patient to respond to chemonucleolysis may result from application of the technique in the presence of sequestrated disc material.

Discography

Discography is seldom performed purely as a diagnostic procedure in cases of suspected prolapsed intervertebral disc. In certain situations where the diagnosis is still in doubt after investigation by radiculography and computerized tomography it may be a useful tool. In addition to the provocation of the patient's symptoms by the procedure, the radiological appearance of the discogram itself may be diagnostic. In a typical case contrast is seen extruding through the annular tear into the epidural space. Discography in conjunction with computerized tomography is particularly useful in visualizing more laterally placed disc prolapses.

The 'investigation of choice' in a patient with a prolapsed disc depends upon the availability of the investigative techniques and upon the degree of confidence with which the level of the prolapse has been identified clinically.

At present, the main limiting factor with magnetic resonance imaging is its lack of availability

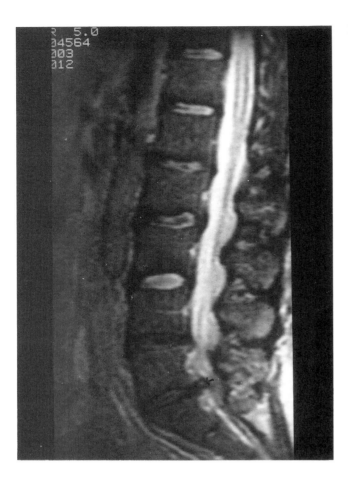

Fig. 20.7   MRI scan showing disc degeneration.

in most hospitals. As it becomes more freely available, it will probably supersede other imaging methods for the study of the prolapsed disc.

If the level of the prolapse can be predicted with any confidence, then computerized tomography is normally the investigation of first choice. If, however, the level of the prolapse is uncertain, radiculography is likely to be more productive, simply because it allows the visualization of several levels in the spine.

Treatment

Most patients with a prolapsed intervertebral disc improve without an operation. In the initial phase, a few days bed-rest, supplemented by analgesia, anti-inflammatory agents and muscle relaxants is beneficial. This treatment should not be prolonged. Patients who have lingered in bed for several weeks following a disc prolapse de-

velop stiff backs, lose muscle tone and most important, they lose motivation. They are extremely difficult to rehabilitate.

Traction gives variable benefit. In order to exert any mechanical effect on the disc, traction of one third of the patient's body weight must be applied. Patients cannot tolerate this and any effect which traction normally exerts is attributable to the enforced bed-rest, relaxation of muscles and to a placebo effect. As with straightforward bed-rest there is no point in continuing this treatment for more than a few days.

As soon as the most acute symptoms have settled, normally within a few days, the patient should be mobilized. A lumbosacral support is often helpful. A course of physiotherapy designed to restore mobility to the spine and to improve muscle tone is the single most useful treatment which can be offered at this stage, a useful adjunct to treatment.

The patient must be given appropriate advice

about sitting posture and avoidance of heavy lifting with reassurance that the symptoms are likely to remain in abeyance as long as the patient continues to treat his back with reasonable respect and avoids activities which are likely to provoke a further prolapse.

Epidural injection

In those patients with persistent but not distressing sciatica and only minor abnormalities on neurological examination, an epidural steroid and local anaesthetic injection is often effective in relieving pain.

The route of administration is either via the L2–3 interspace or via the sacral hiatus. A fine gauge spinal needle is used after preliminary infiltration of the skin with local anaesthetic.

Complications include puncture of the dura, headache, transitory muscle weakness and very occasionally infection.

There is little unequivocal evidence to indicate that patients undergoing epidural injection fare better in the long term than others. Dilke [15] however, in a double blind trial, found that return to work was quicker, reported pain levels were lower and referrals for surgery were fewer in the treated group than in controls and most surgeons would agree that epidural injection is a useful technique in selected patients.

Chemonucleolysis

Chymopapain is a proteolytic enzyme derived from the papaya fruit. It is capable of hydrolysing the protein component of glycosaminoglycans in the disc, as a result of which the disc loses its water-binding capacity and subsequently shrinks. It was isolated in 1941 by Jansen and Balls and was first used in human subjects in 1964. Since that time, it has had a rather chequered history and its use remains sporadic.

The indications for the use of chymopapain are similar to those for discectomy. It is useful in the patient with sciatica secondary to a prolapsed intervertebral disc, which is not settling on adequate conservative treatment. It should not be used in patients with a serious or rapidly progressive neurological deficit, where surgery is to be preferred. It is ineffective in the treatment of

sequestered disc fragments. No patient should ever receive more than one chymopapain injection because of the great danger of a severe allergic response.

The technique of injection is similar to that for discography and indeed a preliminary discogram is a useful step in the procedure, allowing as it does confirmation that the needle placement and disc level are correct. The procedure must be performed under sterile conditions with adequate radiographic control and preferably twin image intensifiers so that simultaneous biplanar visualization of the needle can be achieved.

The injection should be performed under local anaesthesia with the patient sedated but sufficiently aware so that he can communicate with the surgeon. An anaesthetist should be present, however, to control the level of sedation and in case the patient should suffer an anaphylactic reaction to the injection. The latter is the most serious complication of the technique. Other complications include incorrect placement of the injection, infection, thrombophlebitis, radiculopathy, total paralysis, post-injection back pain and headache. Inadvertent intrathecal injection of chymopapain, in addition to being ineffective in relieving the patient's symptoms, has been reported to lead to the development of a Guillain–Barré like syndrome in a number of cases. Puncture of a nerve root during introduction of the needle is a well recognized complication and is probably more common than is generally realized. Although uncomfortable for the conscious patient, this does not seem to give rise to unwanted side effects.

Discectomy

Persistence of sciatic pain after a full trial of conservative treatment is the principle indication for discectomy. Other indications include progressive neurological symptoms, particularly when there is sphincter disturbance, in which case surgical intervention is a matter of great urgency.

The aim of discectomy is to free the patient of sciatic pain and associated radicular symptoms by decompression of the affected nerve root. Before surgery is undertaken, the patient should be warned that the operation will not necessarily cure his back pain. It is often the case that back pain is substantially reduced by discectomy but this is a difficult outcome to predict and surgery should therefore be reserved for those patients in whom the major symptoms are those of sciatic pain, numbness, paraesthesiae or dysaesthesiae in a radicular distribution.

In such circumstances, the results of surgery are good in around 80% of patients as judged by their ability to return to their former employment without disabling symptoms. Sensory blunting in the distribution of the affected root will usually disappear after surgery but motor weakness may not resolve completely and an absent ankle jerk frequently does not return.

Operative technique

The disc is extraordinarily susceptible to infection and for this reason, some surgeons advocate the use of prophylactic antibiotics (typically cefuroxime 1.5 g at induction, followed by two doses of 750 mg 8 and 16 h postoperatively).

For a simple discectomy, the patient is placed prone in the knee elbow jack-knife position. A midline incision is usually employed, though a paramedian muscle splitting approach or transverse incision are equally acceptable. The incision is centred over the offending disc space, a length of about 10 cm giving adequate exposure in the midline approach. The muscles on the affected side are stripped from bone with diathermy in order to expose the spinous process and lamina on the affected side. At this stage, a check radiograph is a useful procedure in order to confirm that the level of exploration is correct. This is normally unnecessary at the lumbosacral level but elsewhere is a very wise precaution. The commonest mistake in surgery for the prolapsed disc is to operate at the wrong level. This is a difficult situation to defend medicolegally, quite apart from the failure to improve the patient by performing the wrong operation.

Occasionally removal of the caudal lip of the lamina of the upper vertebra assists in exposure of the ligamentum flavum. This is, however rarely necessary. A window is created in the ligamentum flavum with a knife and is then enlarged with a fine punch. Deep to the ligamentum flavum, a layer of fat will be encountered with the epidural plexus of veins coursing through it. These veins are often engorged at the site of the prolapse and can cause troublesome bleeding, so

care should be taken to preserve them. Diathermy coagulation should be avoided.

The nerve root lying stretched over the prolapsed disc will then be encountered. The root should be retracted gently to one side in order to allow free access to the disc, taking great care to avoid excessive tension. The bulging disc is then incised. Its consistency is much softer than that of a normal disc and entry to its substance is easily gained by the creation of a small circular window in the most prominent part of the bulge. The disc is evacuated with a combination of punches and curettes, leaving the annulus intact throughout. Great care should be taken not to perforate the disc anteriorly. It is important not to leave any loose fragments of disc in the wound as they are the cause of a vigorous inflammatory response and may migrate into the root canal, causing a recurrence of symptoms. Disagreement exists about how much of the nucleus should be removed. There is no proven advantage in removing the whole of the nucleus and indeed this is normally impossible as remnants will virtually always remain even after meticulous attempts at disc clearance. It is probably sufficient to remove sequestered fragments, bulging disc material and any obviously loose or degenerate fragments of disc which yield themselves easily to the exploring instrument. More assiduous attempts at disc clearance are probably counterproductive.

Following removal of the disc, the root should glide freely throughout its course. A probe should be passed along the side of the root into the intervertebral foramen in order to ensure that there is no stenosis of the root canal. In such circumstances an undercutting facetectomy must be performed, removing enough of the medial lip of the facet joint to ensure complete freedom of the root. The probe should also be passed medially deep to the dura to check for the medial extent of the prolapse and upward and downward to search for sequestered fragments.

If no prolapse is encountered, there should be no hesitation in exploring adjoining levels until definite pathology is found. Puncture of the dura during exploration should be repaired using a fine monofilament suture.

A free fat graft is applied to the window in the ligamentum flavum in order to prevent ingrowth of scar tissue into the spinal canal following muscle stripping. The wound is closed in layers.

Wound drainage is not mandatory but we prefer to use a single superficial vacuum drain led to the site of removal of the fat graft in order to minimise the chance of wound haematoma.

Postoperative care

Immediate relief of radicular pain following surgery is common. The recurrence of radicular pain is frequently due to tethering of the root by scar tissue. The patient should therefore be encouraged to perform straight leg raising exercises from the earliest stages in order to ensure that the mobility of the freed root is maintained. Passive straight leg raising is facilitated by a system of beams and pulleys over the bed.

Postoperative retention of urine is a common complication but is only very rarely due to peroperative neurological damage. If he is unable to void in the supine position, the patient may be stood with assistance. Should this prove unsuccessful, it may be necessary to pass a Foley catheter which should be of fine bore and retained for only 24 h. Voiding is normally successful after removal of the catheter.

It is safe to mobilize the patient following removal of the vacuum drain 48 h postoperatively. Sitting, including the adoption of a sitting posture during activities such as getting in and out of bed, should be discouraged for the first few days. Following this, sitting on a high stool is allowed. Walking is encouraged, though some postural reeducation by the physiotherapist may be required.

The patient is allowed home following wound healing with a programme of exercises and with a lightweight canvas lumbosacral support without paravertebral steels. Normal sitting is allowed at 2 weeks, car travel at 4 weeks and resumption of car driving at around 6 weeks. Patients undertaking clerical or office work may be expected to resume their employment at around 4–6 weeks postoperatively. Those with heavier occupations are likely to remain off work for about 3 months.

Results of surgery

The great majority of patients are relieved of leg pain by surgery and achieve a rapid improvement in their mobility. They must, however, be warned that full recovery of lost neurological function cannot be guaranteed. Some will be disappointed by the persistence of motor symptoms such as foot drop or by the failure of a sensory deficit to resolve. Neither is the relief of back pain assured, though many patients do in fact improve in this respect. Most sedentary workers will return to their former employment but manual workers fare less well. Only around 60% of patients are able to resume their former occupation, and over 20% remain totally and permanently incapacitated. It is important when considering these figures to remember that the most important factor in the outcome is patient selection for surgery. Performing an inappropriate operation on an inappropriately selected patient will inevitably lead to poor results.

In the long term, there is little evidence that patients undergoing discectomy do better as a group than those treated conservatively. The aim of surgery in the patient with a prolapsed intervertebral disc is therefore to achieve a more rapid resolution of radicular pain with a swifter return to work and quicker social rehabilitation than would be the case if conservative treatment alone were pursued. With careful patient selection, confident identification of pathology and meticulous surgical technique, this seemingly modest aim is achievable.

Minimal intervention discectomy

Discectomy can be accomplished by less traumatic surgery than the conventional operation described above. The operation of 'Microdiscectomy' is undertaken via a 2–3 cm incision directly over the affected level. 'Micro' in this context refers to the size of the incision. An operating microscope is used in this operation but its main advantage is to provide illumination into the depths of the wound rather than magnification. Equally good illumination is achievable by the use of specially designed nerve root retractors which carry fibreoptic light into the wound and are also available with a suction tip. The identification of the correct level is obviously more difficult with such a small incision and X-ray control with image intensification is mandatory. Operating table design is obviously an important factor in this context and it is advisable to perform the procedure using a specially designed table attachment. The procedure allows for the removal of sequestered disc fragments and for undercutting of the facet joint should this prove to be necessary. The advantages of the operation are the quicker rehabilitation of the patient and shorter hospital stay. The long term advantages over the conventional operation, if any, have yet to be defined.

An even less invasive procedure involves the introduction of a fine trocar into the disc under radiographic control with removal of the disc by fine rongeurs or by suction. This procedure is normally undertaken under local anaesthetic with the patient sedated. It allows for the removal of only a small quantity of disc material and it is not possible to identify or remove sequestered disc fragments. Rehabilitation, however, is very rapid and short term results in correctly selected patients seem good.

Other recent developments include removal of the disc under endoscopic control by means of a laser. Once again, the technique involves minimal intervention but its long term results await evaluation.

Discectomy and spinal fusion

In simple discectomy undertaken for sciatic pain secondary to a prolapsed intervertebral disc, there is no place for spinal fusion. Attractive though the concept is of fusing the diseased motion segment in order to relieve back pain, the results of such procedures do not justify the added complications and longer recovery rate. Under certain circumstances, spinal fusion may indeed be indicated. These are:

1. Patients in whom there is an element of segmental instability which may have contributed to their symptomatology prior to surgery (for example patients with a spondylolisthesis).
2. Those in whom instability may have been created at the time of operation by the enforced removal of large amounts of bone in order to effectively decompress the root.
3. Those with advanced arthritic change in the facet joints at the level of the discectomy.
4. Those in whom there is a requirement to return to heavy manual work which they were previously unable to perform because of recurrent episodes of incapacitating back pain superimposed upon sciatic symptoms.

Spondylolysis and spondylolisthesis

The term spondylolisthesis indicates a forward slipping of one vertebra upon that below it. The first account has been attributed to Herbineaux in 1782, an obstetrician who described the presence of a bony prominence anterior to the sacrum which could present an obstruction to normal labour. This could have been a spondyloptosis or complete spondylolisthesis. Kilian [16] recognized the abnormal displacement of the fifth lumbar vertebra upon the sacrum and attributed it to a gradual subluxation of the facet joints. He was the first to coin the term spondylolisthesis. The condition is graded according to the degree of slip which has occurred. Based on the lateral radiograph of the lumbosacral spine, a forward slip of up to 25% is grade one, 25–50% grade two, 50–75% grade three and 75–100% grade four. A slip of greater magnitude than this, in which the bodies of the two adjacent vertebrae have lost all contact, is referred to as a spondyloptosis or grade five. It is significant that the area of contact remaining between the two vertebrae in question is not accurately reflected in the system of grading. For example, a slip with 50% forward displacement will leave only 38% of the apposing surfaces of the vertebral bodies in contact. This loss of contact contributes to the continuing tendency for the slip to increase.

Classification

The classification of spondylolisthesis generally adopted is that of Wiltse *et al.* [17]. Five types are described:

1. Congenital or dysplastic, associated with a defect in the lumbosacral articulation and in the neural arch of the sacrum.
2. Isthmic, associated with a defect or attenuation of the pars interarticularis.
3. Degenerative, arising as a result of degenerative changes in the facet joints and intervertebral disc.
4. Traumatic, following severe injury which results in an unstable fracture dislocation of the spine.
5. Pathological, occurring as a result of tumour, infection or other destructive processes compromising the stability of the spine.

Dysplastic spondylolisthesis

This is characterized by a congenital deficiency of the upper sacrum including the articular processes and an extensive spina bifida occulta of the neural arch of the sacrum. The fifth lumbar vertebra is subjected to large shear forces during weight bearing. As a result of the deficient posterior articulations, the lumbosacral junction is unable to resist these forces and the fifth lumbar vertebra slips forward on the sacrum carrying the remainder of the lumbar spine with it. Eventually, the spinous process of the fifth lumbar vertebra comes to lie against the defect in the neural arch of the upper sacrum. Further forward slip does not normally occur but the anteroposterior diameter of the spinal canal may be severely narrowed by this movement, giving rise to compression of the cauda equina. As a secondary feature, a defect or attenuation of the pars interarticularis of L5 may arise allowing a greater degree of slip to occur, similar to that which takes place in the isthmic type 2 spondylolisthesis. The congenital type of spondylolisthesis is commoner in women by a ratio of two to one. Despite the presence of the dysplastic lumbosacral articulation at birth, it is not until the child starts to weight bear that forward displacement of the fifth lumbar vertebra normally occurs. Even then, the slip is usually very gradual and it is uncommon for the diagnosis to be made before the age of 6 years.

Isthmic spondylolisthesis

This type of spondylolisthesis is associated with a fibrous or cartilaginous defect in the pars interarticularis, i.e. a spondylolysis. It is the commonest cause of spondylolisthesis in patients before middle age. The origin of the defect is debatable but most accept that it arises as a result of a stress fracture. Troup [18] has demonstrated that the pars interarticularis is subject to high shear stresses during spinal hyperextension and suggests that a stress fracture may occur as a result of repetitive loading during activities such as gymnastics. Those who indulge in such forms of athletic activity certainly demonstrate a high incidence of spondylolysis. Other authors have proposed a genetically determined cause for the defect. Certain races such as the Eskimos demonstrate a high incidence of isthmic spondylolisthesis, though whether this is purely genetic in origin or whether it is partly behavioural is open to debate. It is probable that the defect arises as a result of the development of a stress fracture in individuals who for whatever reason have some intrinsic weakness or hypoplasia of the pars interarticularis. The secondary development of an isthmic lesion in the dysplastic type of spondylolisthesis (type 1) suggests that the pars interarticularis may be a vulnerable structure when it is subjected to abnormal loads and lends support to the stress fracture theory of spondylolysis. On the other hand, it is by no means uncommon to find some minor degree of dysplasia of the neural arch of the sacrum or of the lumbosacral articulations during surgery for what appears to be a purely isthmic type of spondylolisthesis. The possibility therefore arises that the two types described are no more than the opposite ends of a continuum. Within this spectrum, varying degrees of dysplasia of any part of the posterior arch of the lumbosacral region may give rise to a spondylolisthesis because of mechanical failure of one of the elements involved in the stabilization of the spine. Failure of one element may lead to failure of another, with further slip occurring. The situation is further confused by the presence of a continuous remodelling process with growth which may alter the morphology and orientation of the facet joints or the pars according to the disposition of the loads on the system. Most commonly, the slip occurs as a result of a lytic defect in the pars interarticularis of the fifth lumbar vertebra (90% of cases) thus causing a forward movement of L5 on the sacrum. In almost all other cases, the slip is between L4 and L5 with a defect in the pars of L4.

Degenerative spondylolisthesis

Degenerative spondylolisthesis is uncommon before middle age. It is frequently asymptomatic and is a common finding on lateral radiographs of the spine taken as a part of the investigation of totally separate pathology. The spondylolisthesis arises as a result of degenerative changes in the facet joints and discs with advancing age. These structures then lose their ability to restrain the

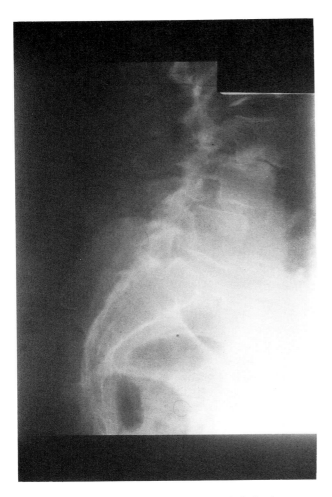

Fig. 20.8 Spinal stenosis due to spondylolisthesis.

tribute to the evolution of the condition include obesity and poor paraspinal and abdominal muscle tone. Patients presenting with symptoms attributable to degenerative spondylolisthesis generally do so at around the age of 60. The condition is more common in women by a factor of approximately four to one. The symptoms can take three forms. Firstly, those of segmental instability, with either fatigue pain or momentary subluxation pain predominating; secondly, radicular pain due to nerve root entrapment, usually the L5 root as it rolls over the bulging degenerate L4–L5 disc or the L4 root in the root canal; thirdly, symptoms suggestive of spinal stenosis due to narrowing of the spinal canal at the level of the spondylolisthesis (Fig. 20.8).

Traumatic spondylolisthesis

Traumatic spondylolisthesis may occur as a feature of a major spinal injury, most commonly a fracture-dislocation involving the thoracolumbar junction. Its management follows that of all the major spinal injuries and it is doubtful whether such conditions should properly be classified with the other forms of spondylolisthesis. Rarely, a patient may be seen following an acute hyperextension injury to the spine where the radiographic findings are those of a spondylolytic spondylolisthesis. It may be virtually impossible in such circumstances to be certain as to whether or not there was a pre-existing pars defect which has undergone an acute disruption in the injury, or whether the neural arch was previously normal. Occasionally, such acute lesions may be observed to heal following immobilization in a plaster jacket, suggesting that the true origin of the defect was the specific injury in question rather than a pre-existing lysis.

spine from undergoing abnormal movements and a gradual slip occurs. Unlike the dysplastic and isthmic types, the level most commonly involved is L4–L5, though it is by no means unusual for several levels to be affected. There is often a discernible degree of osteoporosis present in such patients. This is thought to contribute to the instability of the spine by means of collapse of the subchondral bone in the region of the facet joints, thereby disturbing the normal anatomy of the articulation and allowing subluxation of the joints. Individuals in whom the facet joints are orientated in a more sagittal plane than normal are particularly prone to developing degenerative spondylolisthesis. Other factors which can con-

Pathological spondylolisthesis

This may occur in a number of conditions in which the mechanical strength of bone is compromised. Examples are Paget's disease, osteogenesis imperfecta, tumour and infection. An attenuation of any part of the neural arch may develop allowing the slip to occur.

Clinical features

Spondylolisthesis may be totally asymptomatic, even in the presence of an advanced degree of slip. Indeed, such absence of symptoms is the rule rather than the exception in the young child.

The isthmic type of spondylolisthesis characteristically presents in early adolescence with ill-defined low back pain radiating over the buttocks and posterior aspect of the thighs. Frequently, there is a history that a previously athletic child has had to curtail his or her sporting activities because of exacerbation of the symptoms with physical exertion. At this stage, a marked degree of slip may already have taken place. The physical signs are variable. In the presence of an advanced slip, there may be an exaggeration of the lumbar lordosis with shortening of the trunk and an obvious skin crease in the flanks. Palpation of the spinous processes will reveal a step between the fourth and the fifth lumbar vertebrae – the spinous process of L5 is left in its normal position with respect to the sacrum whilst the whole of L4 is carried forward with the body of L5. Some limitation of movement of the lumbosacral spine is present almost universally and there is sometimes localized tenderness at the level of the slip. One characteristic finding is of hamstring tightness with limitation of straight leg raising and a peculiar waddling gait. Typically, the child will walk with a rotatory movement of the pelvis with flexed hips and knees rather than with the normal swing-through gait. Neurological signs are the exception rather than the rule.

Spondylolysis may exist in the absence of a spondylolisthesis. Again, this is frequently totally asymptomatic. Usually, the presentation is of intermittent episodes of mild aching low back pain exacerbated by exercise and relieved by rest. This pattern of symptoms may continue into adult life without ever giving rise to major disability. The age of presentation is therefore highly variable but frequently the patient first presents in early adolescence. As with the isthmic spondylolisthesis, some limitation of movement of the lumbosacral spine is often present, together with an exaggeration of the lumbar lordosis, though to a much lesser degree. Hamstring tightness is much less marked and the gait is usually normal.

The dysplastic or congenital type of spondylolisthesis tends to present with a more acute history than the isthmic type though this is by no means always the case. The age of the patient tends to be somewhat greater, typically middle or late adolescence. The findings on physical examination are generally similar with lumbosacral stiffness and tenderness, hamstring tightness with limitation of straight leg raising and disturbance of gait, exaggerated lumbar lordosis and a step on palpation of the spinous processes. In this case, however, the step will be between L5 and the sacrum, as the whole of the fifth lumbar vertebra is involved in the slip. With the more acute history, spasm of the hamstring and paravertebral muscles may be very marked. The degree of slip tends to be somewhat less than in the isthmic variety so that trunk shortening and skin creases in the flanks are less marked. However, the contents of the spinal canal are more at risk and it is by no means unusual to detect neurological signs of root compression or to elicit a history of sphincter disturbance.

Radiological features

The diagnosis is often revealed on plain radiographs of the spine but oblique views should be taken in order to give a clear demonstration of a lytic defect in the pars. The so-called 'Scottie dog sign' is present in this situation (Fig. 20.9). In the presence of a spondylolysis without a spondylolisthesis, the dog can be seen to be wearing a collar. Once a slip of appreciable degree has occurred, the dog appears to be decapitated.

In the lateral view, the degree of forward slip and hence the grade of the spondylolisthesis is established. The defect in the pars is usually visible though it may not be easy to detect in early cases. In advanced cases, a bony buttress may be visible extending from the anterior border of the sacrum under the anterior longitudinal ligament to the body of L5. In the extreme case, bony ankylosis may occur between the fifth lumbar vertebra and the sacrum and the inferior facets of L4 may abut onto the upper sacrum.

The anteroposterior view usually adds relatively little information. In the presence of a spondyloptosis, the characteristic 'Napoleon's hat sign' is seen (Fig. 20.10).

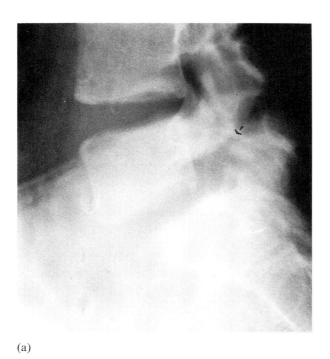

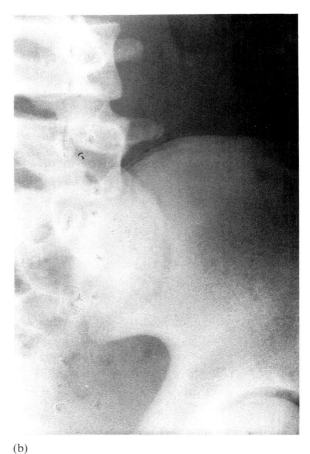

(a)

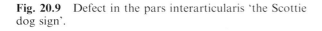

Fig. 20.9   Defect in the pars interarticularis 'the Scottie dog sign'.

(b)

Myelography will give objective evidence of the degree of spinal canal stenosis and nerve root compression. The myelogram may show alarming appearances with marked deformity of the dural sac in spite of minimal clinical symptoms and signs. Often, there is a complete block at the lumbosacral level. Abnormal myelographic appearances are not in themselves an indication for any active intervention in spondylolisthesis, though if surgery is contemplated it should always be preceded by this investigation or, if available, by MRI scanning.

Treatment

Frequently, the symptoms attributable to the spondylolisthesis are so slight that no treatment is indicated. There is a poor correlation between the degree of slip and the severity of symptoms, but as a generalization, slips of lesser degree are associated with less pain. Frequently, mild and intermittent symptoms in childhood and early adolescence can be controlled adequately by the provision of a lumbosacral support and moderation of physical exercise. A course of hamstring stretching exercises is often beneficial. It is essential however, that children presenting with a spondylolysis or spondylolysthesis should be monitored carefully until late adolescence lest the slip should progress.

If the slip continues to increase or if the pain proves intractable in spite of adequate conservative treatment, there should be no hesitation in recommending surgery. The procedure of choice in most cases is a posterolateral fusion *in situ*. If there is evidence of neurological involvement, the procedure must be combined with an adequate decompression of the compromised spinal canal. There is disagreement about the desirability of attempting to reduce the spondylolisthesis at the time of surgery in order to re-establish a normal

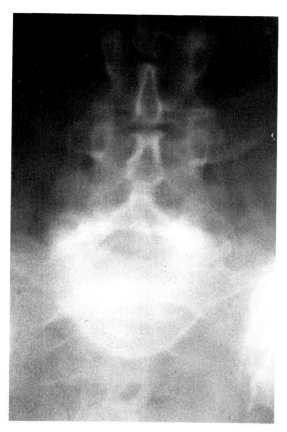

Fig. 20.10 Anteroposterior view of spondylolisthesis 'the Napoleon hat sign'.

anatomical alignment in the spine. In the presence of a severe slip, a combined anterior and posterolateral fusion may be required.

For study of the numerous operative techniques available in this somewhat controversial field further consultation is recommended in the detailed surgical literature.

Spinal stenosis

The term spinal stenosis encompasses a group of conditions in which limitation of space within the vertebral canal contributes to the symptomatology of the disease. Several different clinical syndromes are recognizable within this broad based definition.

The existence of the syndrome classically regarded as representative of spinal stenosis was recognized in 1911 by DeJerine [19], who coined the term 'claudication of the spinal cord'. Verbiest [20] was the first to recognize the association of this clinical syndrome with structural narrowing of the spinal canal. Blau and Logue [21], described six patients with disc protrusions who had exercise related pain and paraesthesiae. They ascribed the mechanism of pain production as compression of the blood vessels to the cauda equina, that is, a form of ischaemic neuritis. Epstein [22] proposed that the pathology lay at nerve root level and described what has become known as the lateral recess syndrome.

Anatomical considerations

There is considerable diversity of shape and size of the normal spinal canal, both between individuals and throughout the length of the canal in any particular spine. The upper lumbar canal is normally circular in cross-section. The sacral canal is triangular. There is a transitional zone within the lumbar spine between these two limits, where the canal may assume a deltoid or trefoil shape. The trefoil shape has well defined apical and lateral recesses, the latter serving to accentuate the length of the root canal. The lateral recess is defined as that part of the central vertebral canal at the pedicular level anterior to the medial aspect of the superior apophyseal joint. It is only the trefoil shaped canal which may be considered to have a lateral recess. The more common dome-shaped canal has a continuous concave posterior surface to the canal and thus the lateral recess does not exist in this configuration.

Various anatomical parameters are measurable in the vertebral canal. The central diameter of the canal in the sagittal plane tends to be widest at the level of the first lumbar vertebra, reducing in size to a minimum at L4 and increasing again at L5. The interpedicular distance is fairly constant from L1 to L3 and then widens progressively over the fourth and fifth lumbar levels. The cross-sectional area of the canal as measured at the level of the pedicles becomes progressively smaller from L1 to L4 but then increases substantially again at the L5 level, to attain a size comparable to that at L1. There is, however, considerable variation between individuals as regards the precise dimensions of the canal at any specified level. This variability is particularly marked at L5. The wide range of cross-sectional areas in the lower lumbar spine is accounted for by variations in the shape of the canal, the trefoil configuration serving to significantly reduce the area as compared to that found in the more usual dome-shaped canal.

The size of the canal in terms of the central sagittal diameter and interpedicular distance is determined by the age of 10 years. This presumably comes about as a requirement for the canal to accommodate its neural contents. The shape of the canal however, may change after this time and thus changes in the cross-sectional area may occur later in life. The trefoil configuration is not seen in young children and if it is to develop, it occurs gradually during adolescence.

The variable size and shape of the vertebral canal is not sufficient in itself to account for the various syndromes of spinal stenosis. Other changes of a degenerative nature are required to produce symptoms. However, such changes, which include bulging of degenerate discs, arthritic lipping of the facet joints, instability secondary to degenerative changes in the disc and facet joints and finally disc prolapse, will all tend to exert their effects on the neural structures within the canal more readily if there is less space available than if the canal is capacious. Other factors can also serve to reduce the area available within the canal. Osteophytes on the cranial lip of the lamina, thickening of the ligamentum flavum with buckling of this structure into the posterior aspect of the canal, particularly during extension of the lumbar spine and iatrogenic scarring following previous exploration are examples of such factors.

Classification

Verbiest [23] described the various subdivisions of spinal stenosis:

> Congenital – due to disturbed foetal development.
> Developmental – due to properties of the neural arch.
> Acquired – due to degenerative changes in the spine.

The classical example of congenital spinal stenosis is achondroplasia. There is impairment of end plate and epiphyseal growth but increased appositional growth. Thus broad, squat vertebrae with short, heavy pedicles and thick, broad laminae are seen. The dorsal surfaces of the vertebral bodies are concave and the discs bulge prominently. The neural contents of the canal are of normal size and as a result of their being accommodated in a canal of small size, may suffer compression over a wide area.

Developmental stenosis implies the presence of a narrow canal with broad, squat pedicles and medially situated posterior joints producing a flattening and stenosis of the exit canals disproportionate to the anteroposterior diameter of the central canal. The articular pillars and laminae may be massive. A typical trefoil shaped canal may ensue. Such patients are initially asymptomatic but problems may develop in later life because of the development of degenerative changes superimposed upon the pre-existing abnormal configuration of the canal.

Clinical features

Any condition which is brought about in whole or in part by the encroachment on the canal of a space occupying lesion will be more likely to produce symptoms if the space within the canal is already limited. Thus, a central disc herniation is more likely to impinge upon the cauda equina if the sagittal diameter of the vertebral canal is reduced. Equally, a posterolateral disc prolapse more readily involves the nerve root in the root canal in the presence of a trefoil configuration. The two classical syndromes in which restriction of space within the canal plays a major part are neurogenic claudication resulting from central canal stenosis and the lateral recess syndrome resulting from nerve root entrapment in the constricted lateral recess.

Neurogenic claudication

The syndrome usually affects men over the age of 50. The presenting complaint is of pain in the buttocks and lower extremities precipitated by walking. The pain is relieved by rest, particularly if the patient sits or leans forward upon a stick. The explanation for this postural effect is the increase in cross-sectional area of the lumbar canal during flexion as compared to extension.

During extension of the spine, buckling of the ligamentum flavum into the canal occurs, whereas when the spine is flexed this structure tightens and does not impinge upon the space within. This postural effect lies at the basis of certain other features of the syndrome. For example, it is often said that the patient can walk uphill for long distances because he tends to bend forwards when climbing a gradient. When coming downhill, however, the spine is extended and the symptoms of neurogenic claudication are more readily precipitated. If present, this symptom serves as a useful feature in distinguishing neurogenic from vascular claudication. Perhaps of more use in this respect is the cycling test. Here, the patient is asked to cycle on an exercise bicycle with the spine in an extended position until the symptoms of neurogenic claudication cause him to stop. After a suitable interval, the test is repeated, the exercise being carried out this time with the spine flexed. A significant increase in the exercise tolerance when the second position is adopted may be expected if the pain is true neurogenic claudication but not if peripheral vascular disease is responsible for the symptoms. In severe cases, the pain may be provoked by simple extension of the spine while standing.

There is often a long history of low back discomfort prior to the onset of leg symptoms. Sometimes there may have been previous surgery to the back, which should raise the possibility of iatrogenic spinal stenosis, particularly if a fusion has been carried out.

Some patients complain not so much of pain as of paraesthesiae or hypoaesthesiae in the legs, again characteristically provoked by exercise. Others complain of a variety of dysaesthetic symptoms in the limbs, on occasion quite bizarre. The sensation may, for example, be described as like having the legs wrapped in cotton wool, like cold water running down the legs or simply as deadness of the legs.

Differentiation of the syndrome from vascular claudication is the most important distinction to be made. The presence of a normal peripheral circulation with good foot pulses excludes the diagnosis of intermittent claudication attributable to peripheral vascular disease. Occasionally, however, the foot pulses may be coincidentally absent and the distinction between the two conditions can then become difficult. Doppler pressure studies may be helpful in this situation. Occasionally it is necessary to perform angiography in order to establish the state of the peripheral vascular tree beyond doubt.

There are a number of conditions arising from the spine itself which may produce leg pain exacerbated by activity. Referred pain from degenerative disease of the disc and facet joints is occasionally felt to be worse on exercise, presumably due to the motion of the diseased spinal segments during walking. Disc herniation can also produce pain which is increased by exercise but the pain is likely to affect only one leg and other features in the history and examination will normally clarify the matter.

Physical examination of the patient may be remarkably normal. A frequent finding, however, is the adoption of a forward flexed posture by the patient – the so-called simian stance. The patient can normally correct this stance when asked to do so but subsequently readopts it as soon as his attention wanders. Flexion of the lumbar spine is usually unrestricted. There is usually, however, significant limitation of extension and this manoeuvre is likely to be painful. It may cause the appearance of leg pain in severe cases if the posture is maintained for more than a very short period. Straight leg raising is normally unimpaired and it is unusual to find any neurological abnormality.

Lateral recess syndrome

Entrapment of the nerve root in the lateral recess may occur as a result of bone or soft tissue impingement within the root canal. The distribution of pain resembles that of sciatica due to a prolapsed intervertebral disc. Usually, however, it is more severe and is rarely relieved by resting flat on a firm surface. Unlike the pain associated with a herniated disc, it is not made worse if the patient coughs or sneezes. The patient finds it impossible to stand or sit for long periods because of the pain and may have to get up and walk around in order to gain some temporary respite. In others, the pain is made worse by walking.

Many patients have a long history of back complaints. Some will have suffered a previous acute disc prolapse with sciatic pain which subsequently resolved, perhaps leaving a minor degree of backache. Others give a history suggestive of longstanding degenerative disc disease without sciatica and still others have never previously been aware of any problem in their backs. The symptoms which a disc prolapse evokes are dependent in part upon the capacity of the vertebral canal. In patients with capacious canals, even a disc prolapse of substantial size may not cause any embarrassment to the nerve root. With the passage of time, the prolapse is likely to resolve and settling of the disc space may occur. Secondary degenerative changes in the facet joint with osteophytic lipping impinging upon the root canal may then compromise the nerve root and result in the emergence of radicular pain.

The pain of which such patients complain is highly variable in its periodicity and severity. Some victims are tormented by unremitting pain while others carry on for months or years with only minor intermittent discomfort before seeking help.

Clinical examination is equally variable. Straight leg raising is impaired in around one third of patients. In the remainder, it is likely that performing the straight leg raising test relieves the nerve root entrapment by virtue of the passive flexion of the spine which the test produces. Such a manoeuvre serves to open up the intervertebral foramina and lateral recesses and allows more room for the nerve in its course through the root canal. Spinal movements, except for extension, are generally well preserved. Neurological examination is also usually normal.

Pathology

A disturbance of the circulation to the cauda equina or nerve root is thought to be the underlying cause of the various clinical syndromes of spinal stenosis. The mechanism by which such a disturbance operates is purely speculative at present. Either the arterial or the venous side of the microcirculation could be at fault and it may be that either factor can be responsible in a particular situation. Such a circulatory disturbance could be precipitated by a variety of triggers. Restriction of space within the canal arising as a result of degenerative changes within an already stenotic area, the effects of fibrotic scarring from past disease and atherosclerotic changes in the vessels supplying the contents of the canal may combine to bring about these ischaemic changes.

The symptoms of claudication which result probably arise for a number of reasons. The most important of these is the further physical restriction of space within the canal brought about by spinal motion during exercise. In addition, there is an increase in the metabolic demands of the cauda equina during exercise. This may be impossible to meet because of the already compromised blood supply. Finally, the increased venous return from the legs during exercise results in an engorgement of Batson's plexus and further reduces the space available within the canal. Other factors which could play a part in the production of symptoms include intraosseous shunting of blood and disturbances in the circulation of the cerebrospinal fluid. The latter comes about as a result of narrowing of the dural sac and impairment of the free flow of CSF, so preventing the removal of metabolites from the affected area. The adoption of a flexed position allows the flow of cerebrospinal fluid to return to a more normal pattern and thereby brings about relief of the symptoms.

Investigation

Plain radiographs of the spine are of limited use but should nevertheless always be obtained. Measurement of the interpedicular distance in cases of suspected neurogenic claudication is a useless exercise owing to the poor correlation between reduction in this parameter and the presence of symptoms of the condition. Evidence can sometimes be seen on the anteroposterior view of subluxation of the facet joints, particularly in the presence of a lateral recess syndrome. This may help to identify a level in localized disease but is also a normal variation in the ageing spine and more detailed investigation is required before a definitive radiological diagnosis can be made. A common finding on the lateral radiograph is the presence of a degenerative spondylolisthesis. This is seen in up to half of the patients presenting with neurogenic claudication. Again, this finding can be of use in helping to decide which level is involved in localized disease but must not be relied upon without further investigations. Attempts to measure the sagittal diameter of the vertebral canal on plain radiographs are fraught with difficulty. Aside from the difficulties involved in performing the measurement, the technique takes no account of soft tissue structures such as the ligamentum flavum which may be impinging on the canal and is now discredited as a significant aid to investigation.

Some surgeons advocate the use of ultrasound to measure the canal diameter. Porter *et al.* [24] point out that a canal of wide sagittal diameter is incompatible with a diagnosis of neurogenic claudication and that there is a good correlation between the presence of a narrow sagittal diameter as measured by ultrasound and the syndrome of neurogenic claudication. The technique is however difficult to perform accurately and is subject to considerable observer error.

Myelography is invaluable in confirming the clinical diagnosis and in assessing the extent of the disease. It should always be performed if surgery is contemplated. The myelographic findings are variable. Congenital stenosis is often associated with a thin pencil-like column of contrast throughout the affected area. This is also seen in developmental stenoses but is then usually associated with 'waisting' of the column of contrast at several levels over areas corresponding to the discs and facet joints. In degenerative stenosis, the pattern varies according to the direction from which the canal is compromised. Thus, posterior indentation of the column may be seen at several levels corresponding to buckling of the ligamentum flavum. This is always pathological. Anterior defects in the column represent bulging degenerate discs and posterior osteophytes from the margins of the vertebral bodies. Some indentation of the contrast column on its anterior

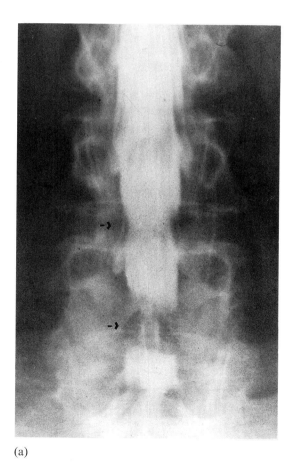

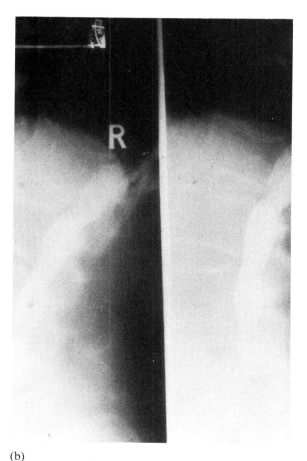

(a) (b)

Fig. 20.11 Considerable deformity of the column of contrast.

aspect is a normal finding in the ageing spine and the appearance may thus not be significant. Posterolateral filling defects correspond to hypertrophy and osteophytic lipping of the inferior facets. The width of the column of contrast is variable but is generally considerably reduced compared to the normal width of at least 15 mm. There may be a complete block of contrast in cases of severe stenosis (Fig. 20.11). It is very important to obtain dynamic studies when performing myelography. Of particular value in this respect are erect films and flexion extension views. The latter may serve to demonstrate the existence of a posturally dependent block in the contrast column. The interpretation of the myelogram in patients who have had previous spinal surgery is particularly difficult. It is important, however, that the investigation be performed in order to exclude conditions such as arachnoiditis which may cause similar symptoms.

CT scanning is a useful technique in that it allows accurate assessment of the canal dimensions and demonstrates the presence of soft tissue intrusion into the canal. The presence of the trefoil configuration, the anatomy of the lateral recesses and their contents and the cranial and caudal extent of the disease are all well demonstrated.

Magnetic resonance imaging appears to hold great promise in the assessment of spinal stenosis. It is as accurate as myelography or CT scanning and is of great value in demonstrating bony and soft tissue encroachment on the canal and lateral recess.

Treatment

Patients with neurogenic claudication may be helped by a programme of physiotherapy including postural advice and by the provision of a lumbosacral support. Such measures generally do not produce a dramatic improvement and the decision must then be made as to whether the patient is to live with his symptoms, with the appropriate modification of activities that this entails or whether he should be offered surgery.

If surgery is undertaken for neurogenic claudication, it is in the form of a spinal decompression. The results are generally very gratifying and there should be no hesitation in recommending surgery to those patients with intractable symptoms. A dramatic improvement in walking distance often occurs, although some back discomfort may remain. The improvement in the quality of life for such patients is considerable. Some patients will relapse after a period of months or years and start to claudicate again. This is usually due either to arachnoiditis following surgical intervention or to encroachment upon the canal of scar tissue from the posterior surgery. A free fat graft placed over the decompressed dura at the time of surgery reduces the chances of such postoperative scarring developing. If it does occur, a further attempt at decompression may be worthwhile.

If surgical decompression is undertaken, it must be adequate in extent. Hence preoperative investigation must be thorough in order to establish the extent of the disease. By adequate decompression is meant that a free flow of cerebrospinal fluid must be re-established within the affected area. In order to achieve this, the decompression must extend rostrally and caudally until a canal of normal dimensions is encountered. In a typical localised stenosis, this may involve removing the spinous processes and laminae of three vertebrae. Usually it is not necessary to remove the facet articulations to achieve adequate decompression and the risk of postoperative iatrogenic instability is thereby avoided. This is of particular importance in those patients in whom degenerative spondylolisthesis is contributing to the stenosis. Even in such cases, however, the risk of inadequate decompression outweighs the chance of creating further instability and the first priority is to ensure that the decompression is adequate. Occasionally, in order to provide adequate decompression, a large quantity of bone must be removed from the area of the facet joints. The possibility of iatrogenic instability is then very real and serious consideration must be given to performing a fusion of the spine at the same operation in order to prevent this.

In those patients with the lateral recess syndrome, a trial of conservative treatment is worthwhile. As the impingement upon the nerve root is often bony, improvement in the symptoms by expectant treatment may not be as rewarding as in the case of leg pain secondary to a disc herniation. Physiotherapy and a back support help some patients, though the results of such measures are unpredictable. Epidural injections are often very helpful in this condition and non-steroidal anti-inflammatory medications are also worth a trial. Many patients will settle to an extent over the course of time, though a substantial number will continue to complain of some radicular symptoms.

Surgery in this condition is indicated when the pain fails to settle to tolerable levels following adequate conservative therapy. Accurate preoperative identification of the root involved is mandatory. An adequate decompression of the root throughout its course in the lateral recess and root canal should then be undertaken. This often involves considerable undercutting of the lamina and an undercutting facetectomy which should be continued until there is no doubt that the nerve is freely mobile throughout its course. Most patients are relieved of their leg pain by such measures although in a substantial number the relief is incomplete and many continue to complain of low back discomfort.

Fusion of the affected segment is not usually indicated at the time of decompression. Some authors, however, feel that the additional procedure is beneficial in that it eliminates the degenerate facet joints as a potential pain source and thereby reduces subsequent low back pain. Fusion without decompression, however, has no place to play in the treatment of either of the two syndromes of spinal stenosis.

Finally, a small number of patients who present with clinical features of spinal stenosis are shown to have Paget's disease of the lumbar vertebrae. It is thought that a 'vascular steal' phenomenon may operate in this situation which contributes to the patient's symptoms by causing ischaemia of the cauda equina. Such patients may respond to the administration of calcitonin or diphosphonates.

Segmental instability

The term segmental instability implies that there is excessive or unnatural movement between adjacent vertebrae during spinal motion. The spine normally moves in a coordinated manner. In the presence of disturbances in the intervertebral articulations, it is possible that abnormal motion may occur beyond the limits normally set by the restraints of facet joints and soft tissues. Such motion may occur in any of the three axes of rotation of the spine. Anteroposterior instability

produces a spondylolisthesis or retrolisthesis. Lateral instability may be seen in scoliosis. Rotatory instability may occur if there is more pronounced instability on one side than the other.

The question of the definition of instability is a vexed one. The nature and degree of movements seen in the normal spine is very variable between different subjects and between different levels in the same subject and the appearance of what might seem to be abnormal spinal movement does not correlate well with the patient's symptoms. White and Panjabi [25] offer a definition of 'Clinical instability': 'The loss of the ability of the spine under physiological loads to maintain relationships between vertebrae in such a way that there is neither damage nor subsequent irritation to the spinal cord or nerve roots and in addition, there is no development of incapacitating deformity or pain due to structural changes.'

The restraints to motion in the normal spine (facet joints, disc, muscles and ligaments) are strong and considerable disturbance to these structures is required before appreciable instability can develop. Such damage may be produced by trauma to the spine, by degenerative change, or by surgery.

Clinical features

Even gross displacement of vertebrae may produce no symptoms for many years. Complaints of back pain or sciatica are indeed more common in the presence of such vertebral displacement but may be caused by the disease process underlying the displacement rather than by the instability itself.

Two distinct clinical presentations of segmental instability are recognized. The first of these is a reflection of fatigue in those structures which normally limit spinal mobility. The paravertebral muscles and associated ligaments are the principle structures involved. Such patients complain of low back pain, occasionally with radiation to the buttocks and thighs. The pain is characteristically worse after prolonged activity, particularly if this involves stooping forwards for long periods. Thus, such activities as bed making or gardening become impossible. Prolonged standing can also provoke the symptoms whereas lying down produces relief. Obesity or pregnancy exacerbate the problem.

Other patients complain of symptoms primarily while changing position. Rising from a sitting or stooping position is accompanied by a momentary sharp pain in the back. The victim has to use the arms of a chair to assist him in standing up and may be observed to 'climb up his legs' with his hands while standing upright from a forward flexed position. Trick movements may be adopted to achieve an upright posture, such as circumduction of the spine midway through the movement of extension. The presence of such movements on physical examination is a useful clue to the underlying pathology. The pain is caused by momentary subluxation of one vertebra upon its neighbour during the change of posture.

Both types of pain may coexist in the same patient. Other pain patterns may also appear, such as sciatica or symptoms suggestive of spinal stenosis. These, however, are reflections of the underlying disease or of secondary changes brought about in part by the abnormal vertebral motion rather than manifestations of segmental instability *per se*.

Clinical examination is likely to be relatively normal. Hypertrophy of the paraspinal muscles is a frequent finding but may be a normal variant. It is a difficult sign to assess objectively and may in any case be masked as many of these patients are obese. In patients with pain of momentary subluxation, difficulty in regaining the erect posture from a forward flexed position may be noted. Movements of the lumbar spine are often slightly restricted but not grossly so. Straight leg raising is normal and signs of neurological involvement are absent.

Radiological findings

Radiographs of the spine often reveal the presence of a spondylolisthesis or retrolisthesis. In gross instability, there may be lateral displacement of the vertebrae on the A-P film. Traction spurs indicating the unstable segment are a frequent finding. The disc space may be narrowed and accompanying arthritic changes in the facet joints might also be seen, these latter two signs being indicative of the underlying degenerative process. Flexion extension views of the lumbar spine are usually unhelpful. If forward displacement is seen, its degree does not correlate well with the level of pain.

On computerized tomography, gas may be visible in the disc (Knuttson's sign) (Fig. 20.5). This is often associated with instability of the motion segment.

All of the above radiological signs are frequent findings in subjects with no pain. Nevertheless, they may serve as useful reassurance that the diagnosis is correct providing that the history is sufficiently convincing.

Treatment

Many patients can be managed with simple measures such as reassurance that the problem is unlikely to progress relentlessly combined with advice on weight reduction and modification of activities, postural exercises and the provision of a lumbosacral support.

For those patients who fail to improve, consideration must be given to surgical intervention. This will usually take the form of a fusion aimed at restoring stability to the spine. It is particularly important in this situation to be certain that the diagnosis is correct and further investigation may be warranted. Myelography is usually normal in the absence of complicating factors such as secondary spinal stenosis. Magnetic resonance imaging will demonstrate degenerative changes in the disc at the unstable level. In addition, it will hopefully confirm that the disc above is healthy. This is an important consideration as if a fusion is undertaken below an already degenerate segment, a recurrence of the patient's symptoms will almost inevitably occur as a result of the increased loads to which the articulation at this level will be subjected. A normal MRI scan is a useful reassurance that this complication is unlikely to develop. Discography is an alternative useful investigation. A normal discogram will effectively exclude the presence of instability at the level of the investigation. The demonstration of a degenerate disc is useful confirmatory evidence but it is essential to remember that the finding of this abnormality does not guarantee that instability at this level is the cause of the pain. The diagnosis is essentially clinical and the ancillary investigations merely serve to confirm one's clinical suspicions. As with MRI scanning, discography is able to demonstrate the presence of degenerative changes in the disc above the level of the proposed fusion.

The operation offered will usually be in the form of a posterolateral fusion extending out sufficiently far lateral to include the transverse processes. If more than one segment is to be spanned by the fusion, there is undoubtedly a higher incidence of pseudarthrosis. Many surgeons would therefore advocate supplementing the fusion by an implant to stabilize the spine and promote fusion. It is important in such situations to maintain the lumbar lordosis over the fused segment. Failure to achieve this will result in a compensatory increase in the lordosis above or below the level of the fusion and may predispose to the further degenerative changes. Distraction methods, such as Harrington instrumentation, are therefore to be avoided in favour of Knodt compression rods, segmental methods of fixation, such as the Hartshill rectangle which can be contoured to the sagittal curve of the spine or fixation by means of contoured plates attached to the spine by screws passed along the pedicles into the vertebral bodies.

Anterior interbody fusion is also advocated by some authors, although the postoperative complications of ileus, urinary retention and impotence are greater. O'Brien [26] advocates a combined anterior and posterior fusion for gross instability such as in the post-laminectomy syndrome.

The degenerate lumbar spine

Many patients seek help from the surgeon because of symptoms arising from pathological changes directly attributable to the ageing processes of the motion segment. The lateral recess syndrome, central canal stenosis and segmental instability are manifestations of this pathology. Other patients with chronic back pain, however, do not fall into any of these categories.

Typically such patients present with a long history of low back ache which is frequently accompanied by referred pain in the thighs. Their pain is characterized by exacerbations often precipitated by some injudicious activity such as heavy lifting or gardening. Long periods of remission may occur during which the patient may be virtually asymptomatic although mild backache is not uncommon during these intervals. The initial insult to the back often takes the form of an acute disc prolapse with all the typical features thereof. The acute symptoms settle with the course of time and the radicular pain is lost. Thereafter, however, the pattern of chronic grumbling backache interspersed with frequent severe remissions of pain may persist for years.

Physical examination of these patients in between their acute attacks does not reveal very much of value. There is often some restriction of lumbar spinal movement. Straight leg raising is unimpaired and neurological examination is normal. Tenderness over the lower lumbar spine is a frequent finding.

Repeated attacks may leave the patient very apprehensive about his back. Some will restrict their activities for fear of a further attack and as a result may find increasing difficulty in pursuing their occupations and leisure activities.

It is in this group of patients that there is particular difficulty in establishing the pain source. Extensive efforts have been made to categorize the various syndromes of chronic low back pain in the hope of rationalising the management of the individual patient. Thus the concepts of the 'facet syndrome' due to disease of the facet joints, the degenerate disc syndrome etc. have arisen. The more closely one examines these so-called syndromes, however, the more apparent it is that no particular clinical picture is especially characteristic of degenerative disease in one structure of the spine as opposed to another. The attempt to subdivide these patients into such groups is flawed from the outset because so closely are the facet joints, intervertebral disc, ligaments and muscles associated, that dysfunction in one eventually will inevitably lead to equivalent changes in the others. Most patients with low back pain who present to the orthopaedic surgeon will fall into this group. These patients cannot be cured but almost all of them can be helped.

Investigation and treatment

Plain radiographs of the lumbar spine must always be obtained, chiefly for the purposes of excluding other more sinister pathology. Aside from these and routine haematological and biochemical tests such as full blood count, eryth-rocyte sedimentation rate and alkaline phos-phatase, further investigation is usually not in-dicated unless serious consideration is being given to surgery.

The great majority of patients can be managed with advice regarding general back care, a pro-gramme of physiotherapy and occasionally a back support. The active role of the patient in his physiotherapy must be emphasized. It is wrong to reassure the patient that any of these measures will automatically cause the pain to disappear. The patient must be told at the outset that none of the available treatments can reverse the changes that the passage of the years has brought about in his spine. At the same time, he must be reassured that help is available and that while it may not be possible to abolish the pain com-pletely, it should nevertheless be feasible to reduce symptoms to a tolerable level and to go some way towards preventing the severe exacer-bations which characterise many of these patients' complaints.

The role of surgery

Occasionally a patient with low back pain uncomplicated by radicular pain, spinal stenosis or instability will be encountered, who despite the best efforts of the surgeon, physiotherapist and orthotist is still severely handicapped by his com-plaint. The question of surgery must then be given serious consideration. The selection of such patients is a matter of the greatest difficulty. Most of the bad results of back surgery arise as a result of operating on patients without clear indications to do so, in the vague hope that exploration and fusion of the lumbar spine will somehow abolish the patient's complaints. Such a blunderbuss approach has nothing to recommend it. Instead, a painstaking appraisal of the situation must be made, taking into account the psychosocial aspects of the problem as well as the pathological basis of the patient's complaints.

The patient must display a genuine and deter-mined desire to get better. This is by no means always the case. Many patients become locked into patterns of behaviour which provide a form of secondary gain from their symptoms. In such patients, the benefits of the care, attention and

sympathy which they reap from their family and friends, the avoidance of unwanted sexual atten-tions of a partner or the possibility of escape from an unpleasant working environment may outweigh the disadvantages of their backache. Such behaviour may well seem inappropriate to the surgeon, though from the point of view of the patient, it may well offer the least objectionable of the various options with which he is con-fronted. This neurosis is seldom consciously embraced by the patient but is nevertheless a very real and not uncommon phenomenon and one which will inevitably lead to failure of any sur-gical measures which may be undertaken. These patients may derive help from the ministrations of a psychiatrist but are unlikely to do well in the hands of an orthopaedic surgeon. Various tools are at the disposal of the surgeon to assist him in his selection of the patient for surgery. Psycho-logical testing of the patient is highly regarded in some circles, the most widely accepted method being the Minnesota Multiphasic Personality Inventory (MMPI). This is a complex and cum-bersome questionnaire which is designed to be answered by the patient. There is a high failure rate with the method, many patients having great difficulty in understanding and completing it. Various other attempts have been made to devise simpler systems of psychological assessment, none of which has proved wholly satisfactory and all of which require the expertise of a clinical psychologist in their interpretation. Nevertheless, if it possible to establish with certainty the organic basis of a patient's complaints and if the lesion is potentially remediable by surgery, then psychological testing in one form or other may be a useful addition to the surgeon's armamen-tarium in arriving at a decision as to whether surgery should be offered.

Surgery in this context means fusion of the painful motion segment. The role of fusion in this situation is the most controversial subject in the whole of spinal surgery and there is very little evidence to indicate that in the long term, patients with this type of low back pain fare any better if they are subjected to surgery than if they are treated conservatively.

If fusion is to be contemplated, there must be no doubt as to the level at which the pathology lies. This is a far from straightforward matter. In certain cases, plain radiological assessment may suggest that a particular motion segment is responsible for the patient's pain; computerized tomography excels at displaying degenerative changes in the facet joints whereas magnetic resonance imaging may show equivalent changes in the intervertebral discs. All such changes, however, may be regarded as part of the normal ageing process of the spine and are therefore insufficient to allow the incrimination of the motion segment under suspicion as the pain source. Provocative tests are, however, available which can greatly enhance the confidence of the surgeon in his clinical diagnosis. Essentially, such tests involve the injection of the facet joints or intervertebral disc under suspicion with hypertonic saline. The injection is undertaken under radiological control. It should accurately reproduce the patient's symptoms, which should subsequently be abolished by injection of local anaesthetic. At the same time as the injection is undertaken, it is useful to obtain contrast studies in the form of a discogram or facet arthrogram, although it must be emphasized that the demonstration of degenerative changes in the disc or facet joint are of less importance than the provocative aspects of the investigation.

If the pain source has been identified with confidence, if the motion segments above this level are demonstrably normal and above all if the patient has been selected with sufficient care, then it is reasonable in certain cases to offer fusion. The operation is most likely to succeed if only one segment is to be fused. Instrumentation may reduce the pseudarthrosis rate and allow more rapid mobilization of the patient. Most commonly, a posterolateral fusion will be undertaken although some surgeons advocate anterior fusion in certain situations or even a combination of anterior and posterior fusion.

Fortunately, very few such patients will come to surgery and the great majority will find that their symptoms can be reduced to a tolerable level by the application of the simple conservative measures outlined above.

Acknowledgement

Figures 20.1 and 20.7 reproduced by kind permission of Professor G. Whitehouse, Department of Radiodiagnosis, University of Liverpool.

References

1. Wyke, B. D. (1969) In *Principles of General Neurology*. Elsevier, Amsterdam, London.
2. Paris, S. V. (1983) Anatomy as related to function and pain. *Orthop. Clin. North Am.*, **14**, 475.
3. Bogduk, N., Tynan, W. and Wilson, A. S. (1981) The nerve supply to the human lumbar intervertebral discs. *J. Anat.*, **132**, 39.
4. Mixter, W. J. and Barr, J. S. (1934) Rupture of intervertebral disc with involvement of spinal canal. *New Eng. J. Med.*, **211**, 210–215.
5. Markolf, K. L. and Morris, J. M. (1974) Structural components of the intervertebral disc. *J. Bone Joint Surg.*, **56A**, 675.
6. Nachemson, A. and Morris, J. M. (1964) *In vivo* measurements of intradiscal pressure. *J. Bone Joint Surg.*, **46A**, 1077.
7. Hickey, D. S. and Hukins, D. W. L. (1980) Relation between the structure of the annulus fibrosus and the function and failure of the disc. *Spine*, **5**, 106.
8. Adams, M. A. and Hutton, W. C. (1981) Prolapsed intervertebral disc – a hyperflexion injury. *Spine*, **7**, 184.
9. Klein, J. A., Hickey, D. S. and Hukins, D. W. L. (1982) Computer graphics illustrations of the operation of the intervertebral disc. *Eng. Med.*, **11**, 11.
10. Farfan, H. F. and Sullivan, J. B. (1967) The relation of facet orientation to intervertebral disc failure. *Can. J. Surg.*, **10**, 179.
11. Macnab, I. (1977) In *Backache*. Williams & Wilkins: Baltimore.
12. Troup, J. D. G. (1981) Straight leg raising and the qualifying tests for increased root tension. *Spine*, **6**, 61.
13. Blower, P. W. (1981) Neurological patterns in unilateral sciatica: a prospective study of one hundred new cases. *Spine*, **6**, 175.
14. McCulloch, J. A. (1977) Chemonucleolysis. *J. Bone Joint Surg.*, **59B**, 45.
15. Dilke, T. W. F., Burry, H. C. and Grahame, R. (1973) Extradural corticosteroid injection in management of lumbar nerve root compression. *Br. Med. J*, **2**, 635.
16. Kilian, H. F. (1854) Schilderungen Neuer Beckenformen und ihres Verhalterns im Lebem. Basserman und Mathy, Mannheim.
17. Wiltse, L. L., Newman, P. H. and Macnab, I. (1976) Classification of spondylolysis and spondylolisthesis. *Clin. Orthop.*, **117**, 23.
18. Troup, J. D. G. (1975) Mechanical factors in spondylolisthesis and spondylolysis. *Clin. Orthop. Rel. Res.*, **117**, 59.

19. De Jerine, T. and Baudouin, A. (1911) La pathologie radiculaire, *Paris Med.*, 386–391.

20. Verbiest, H. (1954) A radicular narrowing from developmental narrowing of the lumbar vertebral canal. *J. Bone Joint Surg.*, **36B**, 230.

21. Blau, J. N. and Logue, V. (1961) Intermittent claudication of the cauda equina. An unusual syndrome resulting from central protrusion of a lumbar disc. *Lancet*, **1**, 1081.

22. Epstein, J. A., Epstein, B. S. and Lavine, L. (1962) Nerve root compression with narrowing of the lumbar spinal canal. *J. Neurol. Neurosurg. Psychiatry*, **25**, 165.

23. Verbiest, H. (1977) Results of surgical treatment of idiopathic developmental stenosis of the lumbar vertebral canal. A review of twenty-seven years' experience. *J. Bone Joint Surg.*, **59B**, 181.

24. Porter, R. W., Wicks, M. and Ottewell, D. (1978) Measurement of the spinal canal diameter by diagnostic ultrasound. *J. Bone Joint Surg.*, **60B**, 481.

25. White, A. A. and Panjabi, M. M. (1978) The problem of instability in the human spine: A systematic approach. In *Clinical Biomechanics of the Spine*. J. B. Lippincott, Philadelphia, Toronto, p. 192.

26. O'Brien, J. P. (1983) The role of fusion for chronic low back pain. *Orthop. Clin. North Am.*, **14**, 475.

21

Surgical management of the cervical spine in rheumatoid arthritis

P. M. Yeoman

The concept that most patients with rheumatoid arthritis involving the cervical spine require surgical treatment is fortunately not correct. There are indications for an active surgical approach but most are confined to those patients who are in need of in-patient care as a result of their disease. Occasionally, young patients may require surgical decompression of the cervical spinal cord but the majority of candidates for surgical treatment have been afflicted by the disease for not less than 5 years; most on average developed the disease between 10 and 15 years before the onset of more serious problems in the cervical spine.

Pathology

Only a few tissues in the body are immune from attack by rheumatoid arthritis but some are more susceptible than others.

Synovial tissue is the first to be affected, and in the cervical spine this is located (1) in the articular facet joints (2) on the posterolateral aspects of the vertebral bodies (3) between the odontoid peg of the axis and the anterior arch of the atlas (4) between the posterior aspect of the odontoid and the transverse ligament of the atlas.

The initial inflammatory process gives rise to swelling of the synovium due to an increased blood flow and oedema. This in turn will cause pain by increasing the tissue pressure or by direct stimulation of nerve endings. Further swelling may encroach on surrounding structures, in particular nerve roots which lie in confined spaces adjacent to articular joints. This elementary introduction forms the basis for a clinical picture and sets the scene for future more serious problems.

Ligaments are also affected more by adjacent inflammation than any direct attack. They become slack and consequently their main function of restraint is diminished thus allowing abnormal movement and possible subluxation of a joint.

Articular cartilage is eroded not only by direct enzyme attack but by deprivation of its nutrition from synovial fluid by a covering of inflammatory pannus, similar to granulation tissue, but extending from the synovium. The pannus may itself cause pressure on nerve tissue or indeed on the spinal cord [1]. It is not uncommon to find plaques of this abnormal tissue embedded between the vertebral laminae. The effect of articular cartilage destruction is simply a mechanical disruption of a joint. It is well established that rheumatoid arthritis initially affects the more mobile and stressed joints, which accounts for the early signs of the disease in the wrist of the dominant limb before affecting other joints. Similarly in the cervical spine the occipito-atlanto-axial complex and later the C5/6 areas are the prime sites for the earliest phase of the disease.

Bone may be eroded by abnormal pressure or destroyed by active resorption. Invariably the bone is softer than normal due to a combination of hyperaemia, active rheumatoid granulation and osteoporosis, which combined with articular destruction and ligamentous laxity will give rise to rapid instability of the vertebral column. Conversely, the opposite affect may obtain if abnormal forces are eliminated so that spontaneous fusion is achieved.

Symptoms

Pain is the predominant concern. It may be localized to the neck; aggravated by movement and related to involvement of the articular joints. Pain may be referred to the occipital area of the scalp from pressure on the posterior primary rami of a cervical nerve and particularly the second or greater occipital nerve. Further spread of pain across the vertex to the frontal area of the scalp mimics the pain of a cervical disc lesion or spondylosis at the level of C5/6, but the pathway is obscure. Peripheral radiation of pain is usually localized to a nerve root distribution and is most common in the upper limbs, but can be confused with the symptoms of a carpal tunnel syndrome which is a frequent manifestation of rheumatoid disease.

Stiffness of the neck is more commonly found on clinical examination than as a complaint, although it can be a distressing problem in juvenile arthritis.

Weakness, loss of balance, paraesthesiae and numbness are all related to spinal cord compression, and when superimposed on the pain, instability, stiffness and deformity on peripheral joints it is very difficult to isolate the true cause of the problem. The onset of these further symptoms is the clue to their more sinister origin because clinical examination may not be helpful. For example, spasticity, clonus or a positive Babinski response are impossible to unravel in patients with stiff and painful joints [2].

Investigations

Radiographic examination of the cervical spine is still the first and most important investigation. The site and possibly extent of the lesion will be revealed and it is still obligatory to obtain lateral views in flexion and extension before embarking on operations requiring general anaesthesia in order to determine any instability of the spine [3].

The occipito-atlanto-axial area and the cervico-thoracic junction are still a problem beyond the compass of conventional radiography.

Nuclear magnetic imaging is undoubtedly the most effective and accurate method of assessment of the structure of the spine, which includes the bone and soft tissues, with a minimal invasive threat to the patient. Soft tissue swelling from rheumatoid pannus may be revealed as a cause of compression of the spinal cord which might have been missed in the past. Multiple levels of disease causing destruction and instability are defined accurately so that surgical intervention can be planned with an increased expectancy of recovery. Almost the entire pathological picture can be displayed, which in turn may confuse and distort the surgical judgement.

Bone scan produces a more refined image of bone structure without all the important soft tissues. It therefore lacks the vital assessment of much of the rheumatoid disease process which can so easily cause spinal cord compression. The introduction of water soluble contrast medium can provide an excellent image of soft tissue infringement, but it involves a more invasive technique for the patient and indeed for the radiologist.

Treatment

Occipito-atlanto-axial level

The joints between the occiput and atlas allow flexion and extension of the head as well as a small range of lateral flexion, but they have been denied any significant study because they are so inaccessible; that is by conventional radiography or surgery. Lateral views of that area are shrouded by the thick mastoid process of the temporal bones. It is not uncommon to find at autopsy a spontaneous fusion of the joints, but it may not occur simultaneously which would account for an oblique range of painful movement of the head. Forward or anterior displacement of the skull may occur depending on the destruction of the joints and this in turn may cause impingement of the posterior arch of the atlas on the overlying occiput; and associated compression may lead to upward migration of the odontoid process of the axis. Atlanto-

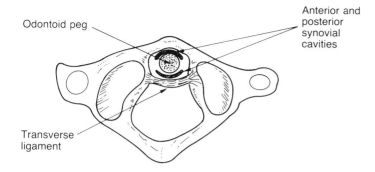

Odontoid peg

Anterior and posterior synovial cavities

Transverse ligament

Fig. 21.1   Horizontal section through odonto-atlantal articulation.

occipital fusion is rarely a practical or indeed necessary surgical procedure.

The axis by contrast is a very real site for problems; mainly related to its odontoid peg and the associated instability between it and the atlas. The odontoid process may become eroded (Fig. 21.1), occasionally it fractures (Fig. 21.2), but in either case it aggravates any instability resulting from laxity of the supporting ligaments (Fig. 21.3). The range of rotation and exaggerated stress from flexion and extension when the

atlanto-occipital joints are fused provides the exact conditions for the deterioration in rheumatoid disease. Hence the reputation that the occipito-atlanto-axial is the prime site for rheumatoid disease of the cervical spine.

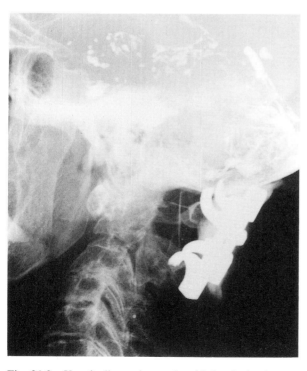

Fig. 21.2   Knodt distraction rods with hooks in the occiput and posterior arch of the axis used for vertical subluxation of the odontoid peg through the foramen magnum.

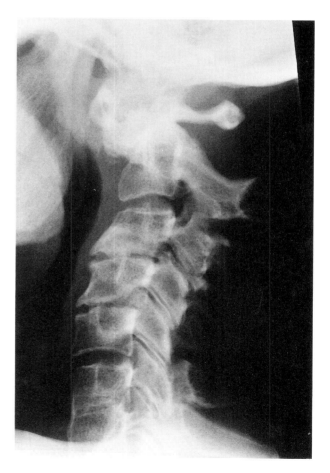

Fig. 21.3   Erosion of the odontoid peg causing horizontal subluxation of C1 and 2.

Indications for surgical treatment

(1) Presence of spinal cord compression.
(2) Failure to control pain and/or symptoms by wearing a supporting collar.
(3) Failure to achieve stability by wearing a collar [4].

Methods available

(1) Posterior fusion with or without decompression of the spinal cord. The extent of fusion would depend on the area of displacement or instability but generally the occiput is fused to the atlanto-axial complex [5]. Cancellous bone graft is laid on the finely decorticated occiput, posterior arch of the atlas and the laminae of the axis.

Internal fixation is achieved with wires threaded through fine drill holes in the occiput and encircling the posterior arch of the atlas and laminae of the axis [6]. The potentially precarious fixation can be augmented with acrylic cement (Fig. 21.4) [7,8].

(2) Anterior decompression and posterior fusion. This method has the distinct advantage of removing the cause of spinal cord compression which has been identified by an image intensifier; namely the odontoid process. It is a major procedure for a frail old patient and much care is required in the selection.

Cephalic subluxation of the odontoid process

This is undoubtedly associated with destruction of the atlanto-occipital process and deserves special mention in spite of its comparative rarity [9,10]. The odontoid peg can be demonstrated in its elevated position within the foramen magnum (Fig. 21.5). The symptoms are usually those of

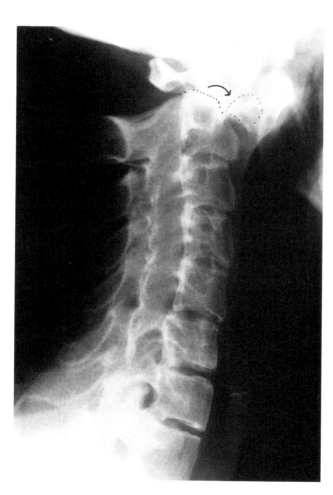

Fig. 21.4 Fracture of the odontoid peg causing horizontal subluxation of C1 and 2.

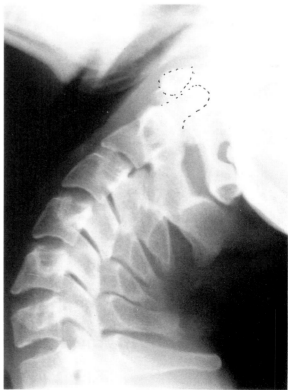

Fig. 21.5 Odontoid peg in extension of the spine.

cord compression with variable signs of an upper motor neurone lesion but with an additional, and often missed, physical sign which is numbness over the side of the face.

Decompression can be achieved by careful resection of the posterior margin of the foramen magnum or by distraction between the occiput and the posterior arch of the axis. The author has used two small Knodt rods as a successful method of distraction; one hook is inserted into a groove made with a burr in the occiput and the other rests on the upper surface of the thick lamina of the axis bone (Fig. 21.2).

Cervical 5/6

Instability may arise at this level either *de novo* or because it has become a junctional area between two fused segments of the cervical spine. The degree of instability will depend on the extent of bone destruction (Fig. 21.6).

Fusion usually involves two vertebrae above

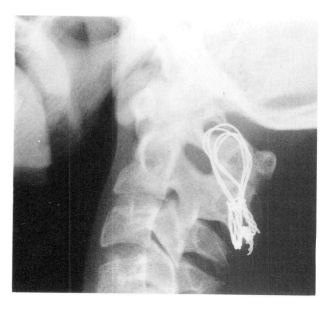

Fig. 21.7 Posterior fusion of C1 and 2 using encircling wires and cancellous bone graft.

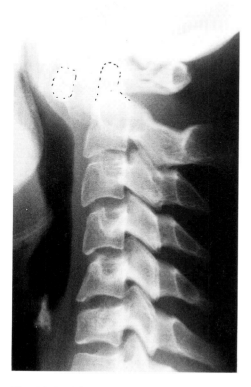

Fig. 21.6 Odontoid peg with subluxation in flexion of the spine.

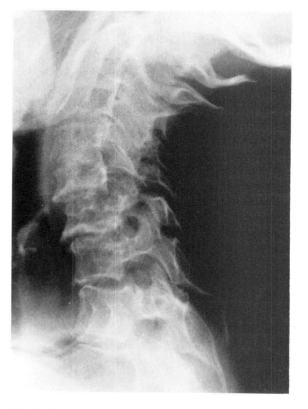

Fig. 21.8 Considerable bone erosion with instability at C5/6 and 'pencil-sharpening' of the spinous process.

and two below the unstable area; and cancellous bone is packed round the decorticated laminae and secured with wire encircling the spinous process (Fig. 21.7).

Decompression of the spinal canal will render the spine more unstable and firm internal fixation is more difficult to achieve; again, the use of distraction rods can provide better fixation than encircling wires but they require transverse holding rods to reduce rotation strain. Acrylic cement may also augment firm fixation (Fig. 21.8) [11].

Multiple levels

Instability and associated compression of the spinal cord may occur at more than one level [12]. In the past this was difficult to identify by myelography unless the contrast medium was introduced both in the cervical and lumbar cisterns (Fig. 21.9). Wide and extensive decompression is required but at the expense of stability, and this is

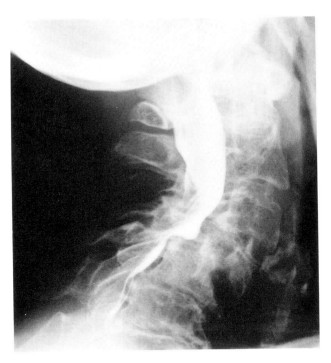

Fig. 21.10   Hartshill rectangle used after wide decompression for multiple level spinal cord compression.

very difficult to achieve by any internal method (Fig. 21.10). Longer holding distraction rods, bone graft and cement are the main components. Anterior fusion is rarely used in these extreme conditions because the vertebral bodies are soft and will not hold any cortical bone graft.

External fixation

It is not sufficient to rely on internal fixation even in a relatively simple two body fusion when a supporting collar is required for at least 3 months.

Block leather or plastic collars with extended vest pieces will provide firmer support and are widely used, but in the frail, aged or grossly unstable necks it is better to rely on the halo-chest fixator [13]. It is tolerated surprisingly well in the most unlikely and unpromising patients. Occasionally it has been used as a most effective single form of management in patients considered to be too ill or frail to withstand a major operation (Fig. 21.11).

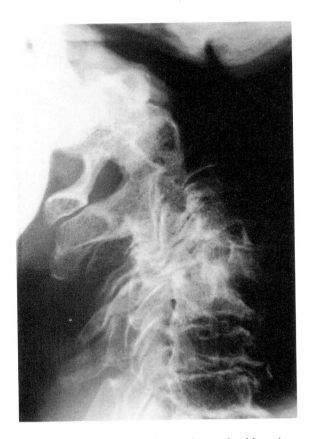

Fig. 21.9   Multiple level destruction and subluxation.

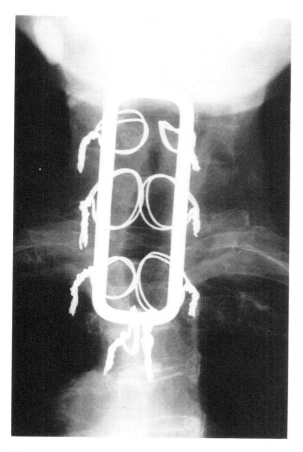

Fig. 21.11 Contrast medium introduced at the basal cistern reveals considerable block at C5/6 but failed to reveal block at lower level.

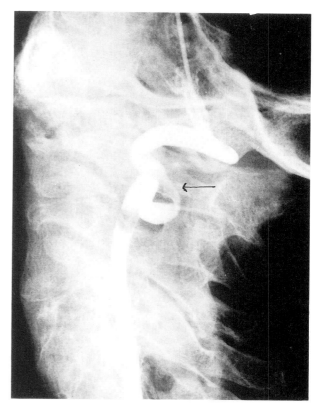

Fig. 21.12 Vertebral artery occluded at base of skull in extension (specimen prepared and artery injected at autopsy).

Conclusion

The hazardous problems of the effects of rheumatoid arthritis of the cervical spine have been outlined. There are reasonably simple solutions for most patients and they are successful. A few have such widespread destruction and osteoporosis that they may be deemed inoperable. It is those patients who are also aged that the halo-chest fixator has been effective; which suggests that perhaps others would be equally helped without operation. Recovery from spinal cord compression is not absolute in spite of apparent successful decompression and there may be a vascular complication in some of the older patients (Fig. 21.12). Spinal artery thrombosis is a difficult enough diagnosis to determine without rheumatoid disease, but it is the most likely reason for some who fail to recover. Finally, the effect of spinal cord compression leads to an unpleasant lingering death and every attempt must be made avoid it.

References

1. Crockhard, H. A., Essigman, W. K., Stevens, J. M. *et al.* (1985) Surgical treatment of cervical cord compression in rheumatoid arthritis. *Ann. Rheum. Dis.*, **44**, 809–816.
2. Christophidis, N. and Huskisson, E. C. (1982) Misleading symptoms and signs of cervical spine subluxation in rheumatoid arthritis. *Br. Med. Jr.*, **285**, 364–366.
3. Ornilla, E., Ansell, B. M. and Swannell, A. J. (1972) Cervical spine involvement in patients with chronic arthritis undergoing orthopaedic surgery. *Ann. Rheum. Dis.*, **31**, 364–366.
4. Althoff, B. and Goldie, I. F. (1980) Cervical

collars in rheumatoid atlanto-axial subluxation: a radiographic comparison. *Ann. Rheum. Dis.*, **39**, 485–489.

5. Heywood, A. W. B., Learmonth, I. D. and Thomas, M. (1988) Internal fixation for occipito-cervical fusion. *J. Bone Joint Surg.*, **70B 5**, 708–711.

6. Brattstrom, H. and Granholm, L. (1976) Atlanto-axial fusion in rheumatoid arthritis: a new method of fixation with wire and bone cement. *Acta Orthop. Scand.*, **47**, 619–628.

7. Bonney, G. and Williams, J. P. R. (1985) Trans-oral approach to the upper cervical spine. *J. Bone Joint Surg.*, **67B 5**, 691–698.

8. Crockard, H. A., Pozo, J. L., Ransford, A. G. *et al.* (1986) Transoral decompression and posterior fusion for rheumatoid atlanto-axial subluxation. *J. Bone Joint Surg.*, **68B 3**, 350–356.

9. Swinson, D. R., Hamilton, E. B. D., Mathews, J. A. *et al.* (1972) Vertical subluxation of the axis in rheumatoid arthritis. *Ann. Rheum. Dis.*, **31**, 359–363.

10. Redlund-Johnell, I. and Pettersson, H. (1984) Vertical dislocation of the C1 and C2 vertebrae in rheumatoid arthritis. *Acta Radiol. Diag.*, **25**, 133–141.

11. Clark, C. R., Keggi, K. J. and Panjabi, M. M. (1988) Methylmethacrylate stabilisation of the cervical spine. *J. Bone Joint Surg.*, **66A 1**, 40–46.

12. Zoma, A., Sturrock, R. D., Fisher, W. D. *et al.* (1987) Surgical stabilisation of the rheumatoid cervical spine. *J. Bone Joint Surg.*, **69B 1**, 8–12.

13. Wang, G. J., Moskal, J. T., Albert, T. *et al.* (1988) The effect of halo-vest length on stability of the cervical spine. *J. Bone Joint Surg.*, **70A 3**, 357–360.

22

Surgical treatment of rheumatoid arthritis of the shoulder

P. J. M. Morrison

Introduction

Symptoms in the shoulder joint are common in rheumatoid disease. Occasionally they are a presenting feature and in hospitalized patients over 50% will admit to symptoms.

Such symptoms are a serious concern to rheumatoid patients. Pain may render life miserable and sleep impossible. Loss of function may make the most mundane tasks of daily living such as dressing, eating and attending to personal hygiene, distressing. Loss of shoulder power may make rehabilitation from other joint surgery more prolonged and difficult. The use of crutches can present a particular problem.

The shoulder complex

Movement of the upper limb involves motion in the joint complex comprising the main glenohumeral joint, the acromioclavicular and sternoclavicular joints and the smooth gliding of the tissues in the subacromial bursa. All these structures may be involved by rheumatoid disease.

Acromioclavicular joint

Local pain, tenderness and occasional swelling of this surface joint suggests involvement, and radiographs (Fig. 22.1) may show erosions and occasionally subluxation of the joint.

Injection with steroid and local anaesthetic may not only determine the proportion of pain arising at this site, but will often settle early symptoms.

Persistent pain is best treated by excision of the outer centimetre of the clavicle but this is seldom

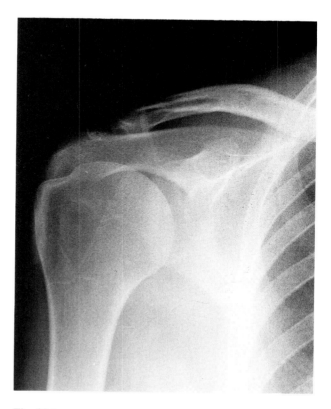

Fig. 22.1

necessary in the author's experience, as an isolated procedure.

The sternoclavicular joint

This joint is relatively infrequently involved. It can usually be settled by instillation of steroid, and only rarely are procedures such as synovectomy or excision of the inner 1 cm of the clavicle (a quite hazardous procedure because of the proximity of the great vessels) needed.

The subacromial bursa

This is commonly affected in rheumatoid disease. Occasionally, it may produce a massive swelling of the shoulder and may occur in isolation or with associated glenohumeral disease.

Affliction of the bursa will usually respond to aspiration and injection of steroid. Occasionally, excision of the bursa is required but this can be an extensive and difficult operation which may damage the deltoid muscle. Associated removal of the acromion must be avoided, but sometimes trimming of the anterior edge of it, if it is specifically impinging on the rotator cuff, may be desirable.

The glenohumeral joint

With involvement of the true shoulder joint, the patient's disability becomes more apparent. The actual onset may be insidious, being masked by an acute flare in the general disease process. Only when this settles does the loss of shoulder function become apparent to the patient and his doctor.

The presenting features are pain and loss of movement. The pain is usually felt all around the shoulder, but often radiates to the root of the neck and onto the outer aspect of the arm; so that the origin of the pain may be mistaken. If there is tenderness, it is usually anteriorly, over the joint.

The loss of function may be slow. The shoulder possesses such a large range of movement in all directions, that the loss of 50% of any modality may produce only minor disabilities, such as difficulty reaching a high cupboard.

However, as motion is progressively lost, there

rapidly comes a point where simple tasks of daily living, such as combing the back of the hair, or washing the neck, become impossible. Almost without warning, the patient is grossly disabled.

Radiographic changes

Early changes may present radiologically as simple osteoporosis. As the disease progresses, erosions can be noted around the neck of the humerus and under the insertion of the supraspinatus tendon (Fig. 22.2). Loss of the joint space and damage to the subchondral plate follow (Fig. 22.3), and ultimately there is destruction of the bony surfaces of the humeral head and glenoid with eventual loss of the normal bone architecture (Fig. 22.4). These changes may progress to secondary osteoarthritis with sclerosis of the bone surfaces.

Usually, the humeral head migrates upwards and this signifies loss of a functional rotator cuff

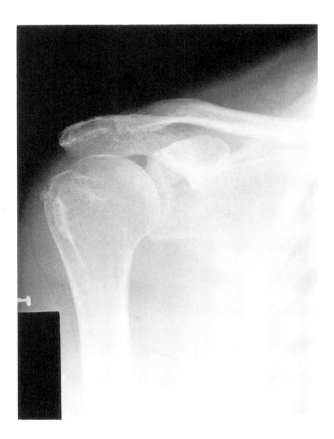

Fig. 22.2

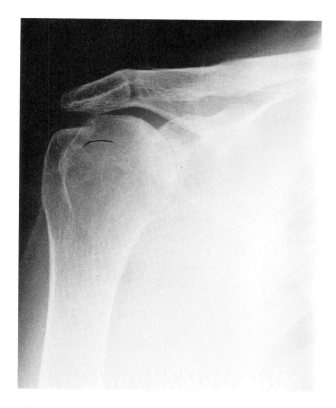

Fig. 22.3

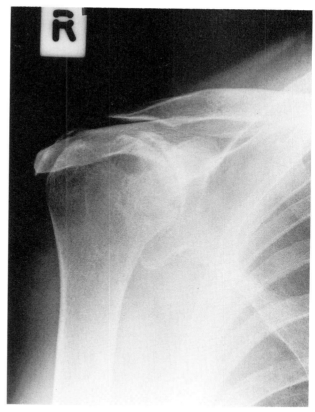

Fig. 22.5

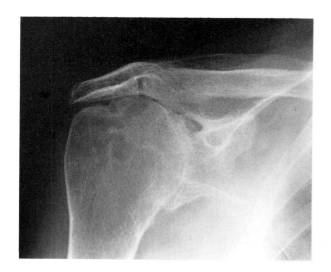

Fig. 22.4

and rupture of the supraspinatus tendon. If the cuff is lost (Fig. 22.5), the dome of the humeral head will articulate with the under surface of the acromion and the root of the coracoid. These surfaces become eburnated.

The glenoid becomes progressively eroded, occasionally allowing the neck of the flattened humerus to articulate with its inferior margin, producing an extraordinary scallop of the humeral neck. The loss of glenoid bone stock may render its eventual replacement difficult because adequate fixation of a scapular component becomes impossible (Fig. 22.6).

The correlation of these radiographic changes and the patient's clinical features and function is quite a close one [1]. The changes were graded I–V in 100 shoulders: it was only when loss of the glenohumeral joint space was apparent (grade IV) that the patient had significant pain and loss of function. Distortion of the humeral head (V) tended to correlate with severe pain and impairment of function.

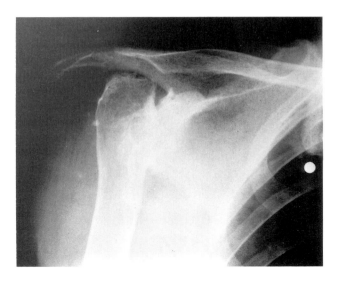

Fig. 22.6

Treatment of glenohumeral joint disease

In the early stages, injection of steroid into the joint cavity (as opposed to the subacromial bursa) may produce dramatic remission of the local inflammation and pain.

However, with persistent pain, and when function is reduced to a level no longer acceptable to the patient, a surgical approach may be advised. The following surgical treatments are available: synovectomy; double osteotomy; glenoidectomy; arthrodesis; interpositional arthroplasty; joint replacement – either half of total.

Synovectomy

This is a neglected operation. It is clear from the writings of Pahle [2] that with good patient selection, a sensible surgical approach, meticulous clearance of the joint and a careful postoperative regime, not only good but long lasting pain relief can be obtained.

In a series of 54 shoulders, only six had required total joint replacement later in a mean follow-up of 5.3 years. The best results are obtained in early cases. A standard anterior

approach was used in the later cases, allowing early postoperative mobilization.

As in all series of synovectomies, whatever the joint, a prophylactic procedure in a disease with variable progression is very difficult to evaluate. The earlier the operation is carried out, the more difficult it is to know whether a spontaneous remission could have occurred.

None the less, the pain relief and maintenance of function are impressive.

Double osteotomy

Benjamin [3] has advocated this operation at several joints and published his results on the shoulder as long ago as 1974. They are undoubtedly impressive.

The operation, consisting of osteotomy of the surgical neck of the humerus and the glenoid $\frac{1}{4}$ inch medial to the glenoid fossa, through an anterior approach, is, according to Benjamin, simple. The posterior cortices of both bones are left intact and the osteotomies are not displaced. The arm is supported in a sling and active shoulder exercises are started on the 10th postoperative day.

Twelve patients with rheumatoid arthritis were treated. The abduction range was increased by an average of 50° 'probably due to relief of pain and muscle spasm' Benjamin states. There was no increase in glenohumeral movement observed. Pain relief was very impressive, with 13 of 16 patients (with all forms of arthritis) having no pain, or slight pain only postoperatively. There were no serious complications.

Despite these results, however, the operation is not widely practised, which suggests that the results were not uniformly reproducible.

Glenoidectomy

Wainwright [4] and Gariepy [5] have both written about and advocated this operation.

Wainwright described six patients operated on by a posterior approach removing $\frac{1}{2} - \frac{3}{4}$ inch of the glenoid and maintaining the arm on an abduction splint for 3 or 4 weeks postoperatively.

Pain relief was pleasing: glenohumeral function was poor but because of the pain relief, overall shoulder function was improved. Increased internal rotational movement, however, was very valuable to these disabled patients.

Wainwright reserved this operation for totally disorganized joints with intractable pain.

Gariepy described 12 cases: an anterior approach was used and 7 or 8 mm of the glenoid were removed.

Full removal of the pannus was carried out, the capsule was left open and subscapularis was not overlapped. No postoperative fixation was used and a sling only was worn for 48 hours.

The follow-up was between 1 and 13 years. Relief of pain had been satisfactory in all cases; the range of movement had been improved except where there was severe deformity of the humeral head. Gariepy suggested, therefore, that the operation was best carried out in undeformed joints, where the systemic disease was not too severe and the muscles were good, in other words, early cases.

Although Gariepy says that the operation does not preclude prosthetic surgery in the future, it must surely make such surgery exceedingly difficult and render the fixation of a scapular component of a total shoulder replacement, well nigh impossible.

The author regards this operation, therefore, as a minor salvage procedure for intractable pain and stiffness. As such, it still has a place and he can confirm its usefulness.

Arthrodesis

This operation has been condemned by many authors over the last 30 years. Various reasons have been given but the two main criticisms are, firstly, the fear that the period of immobilization of the upper limb postoperatively will lead to loss of function in all other joints in that limb, and secondly, that the loss of rotation resulting from arthrodesis will greatly restrict simple but important functions of personal hygiene. This is particularly true, it is said, in patients whose other shoulders may be partially restricted.

However, the operation has its advocates and there is no doubt, if well performed, that it can offer great benefit in terms of pain relief and thereby an increase in shoulder girdle function.

The hazards of the operation may have been exaggerated. Arthrodesis is a reliable operation and in a Finnish series the results were remark-

able. Raunio [6] describes a simple three-screw technique and achieved bone union in 90% of patients (37/41). Even in the non-unions, there was sufficient fibrous union to abolish shoulder pain.

All the patients had an increased range of motion – an average total flexion and abduction of 100° before operation and 160° afterwards. But, most remarkably, all patients were able to use the operated limb for eating, combing the hair and were able to take care of their own personal hygiene. Ninety-five percent of the patients were satisfied with their operations.

The technique used involved an anterior approach, removal of all synovial tissue and all remaining cartilage from the head, the undersurface of the acromion and the glenoid. The denuded surfaces are approximated and held with two compression screws passed through the humeral head into the glenoid and one screw passed through the acromion downwards into the humeral head, with osteotomy of the acromion if necessary.

The position of the arm is very important. The aim was to obtain 55° abduction, 25° flexion and 20° internal rotation – an easy hand to mouth position. Postoperatively, a light custom-made thoracobrachial splint was worn for about 10 weeks. The splint allowed exercise of the elbow and hand which is so important to the end result of the operation.

A technique using an extensive compression device has been described. This avoids the need for a splint postoperatively but clearly such a technique is not feasible in many of the osteoporotic damaged shoulders that are encountered in rheumatoid disease.

Thus, there is dispute about the place of arthrodesis of the shoulder.

It should probably be reserved for cases where total joint replacement is contraindicated, or has failed [7]. Nevertheless, the author has been impressed by the confidence and comfort that patients with an arthrodesis seem to exhibit.

Arthroplasty

Interposition with silastic

In 1980 Varion [8] reported a clinical trial of 28 patients with rheumatoid arthritis who had a silastic cup slipped between the humeral head and the glenoid through an anterior approach without removing any bone.

The early results of this seemingly simple procedure were most encouraging with pain relief in all but two patients at a mean 14-month review. A small personal series was also favourable.

However, it seems that in the longer term, the improvement is not maintained. The cups eroded, slipped out of position and fragmented with consequent return of symptoms.

Varion originally stated that the operation was reversible: certainly as at the hip, interposition is an attractive idea if an ideal material could be found to remain in good condition, or if a material could be developed that provoked good quality fibrous cover for the eroded joint surfaces.

Glenohumeral joint replacement

There is no doubt that this surgical procedure should have most to offer the disabled rheumatoid patient. However, even after more than 20 years of evolution its expectations are strictly limited and they are in no way on a par with those achievable at the hip or other major joints. Thus, careful selection and preparation of the patient is vital, if the limited goals and patient satisfaction are to be obtained.

Design considerations

The rheumatoid shoulder presents particular paradoxes to the designer.

1. Absent or poorly functioning rotator cuff musculature makes it difficult for the rheumatoid patient to stabilize an unconstrained implant in elevation and thus achieve good function.

2. Any constrained implant will rely on the fixation of one component in the scapula. The normal human scapula is a thin, light structure. It has been estimated that lifting one's arm carries forces equivalent to the body weight through the articulation. Only at the glenoid and neck of the scapula is there sufficient bone stock to carry such loads and yet in rheumatoid patients, particularly in those patients being referred for shoulder surgery, the bone stock is often grossly eroded and excavated.

3. The space between the humerus and the scapula is extremely limited. Any mechanism inserted must retain the same centre of rotation, otherwise the greater tuberosity will foul the acromion during abduction.

The mean distance between the centre of rotation of the humeral head and the centre of the glenoid dish is only 24 mm.

This awkwardness has led to some radical redesigning of the shoulder mechanism.

4. A normal human shoulder has a remarkable range of movement and this is achieved, to some extent, by a wandering fulcrum of movement. Allowing the fulcrum to move would obviously also reduce the load and torque being carried by the components in a constrained joint. Yet, control of this wandering fulcrum requires muscle balance and strength is often sorely lacking in the patient with rheumatoid arthritis.

5. The shoulder is used mainly in compression but it is sometimes distracted in normal use and a prosthesis must remain stable under all conditions. These considerations have led to the evolution of a number of different designs, none of which has achieved the ideal.

Evolution

As long ago as 1953, Neer [9] produced a hemiarthroplasty replacing the humeral head in a group of patients with fracture dislocations of the shoulder. Hidden within this group, there are patients with secondary avascular necrosis and one patient with primary osteoarthritis.

Neer himself experimented with fixed fulcrum prostheses but in the early 1970s had found them disappointing and returned in 1973 to a redesigned head component and introduced a polythene glenoid surface replacement. This design aimed to provide 'near normal anatomical design'.

Meanwhile, a series of fascinating alternatives were tried, including a group of joints where the anatomy was reversed. This allowed the centre of rotation to be retained by burying the cup (the most difficult component to fix) within the humeral head. The ball was fixed to the scapula. Some of these joints were truly constrained using the principle of the captive ball.

Post [10] of Chicago, introduced two types of prostheses between 1973 and 1977. Forty-three replacements were performed; a few were in rheumatoid arthritis. However, more than half of the first series of prostheses broke or had to be revised. Nearly all his patients had absent rotator cuff function and he regarded his operation by 1980, as a salvage procedure in judiciously selected patients.

Beddow [11] designed a reversed prosthesis where the glenoid ball component was fixed into the lateral border of the scapula, whilst Kessel [12] introduced a simple reversed prosthesis with the ball screwed into the glenoid using a single strong self-tapping screw. The majority of his patients were rheumatoid patients and his early results were most encouraging. In the long term, however, the scapular fixation is bound to be in jeopardy; loosening and breakage of this prosthesis has been seen by the author.

The Stanmore prosthesis, a semi-captive ball and socket implanted in the normal anatomical relationship, provided a stable fulcrum also but in at least eight of 34 patients with rheumatoid arthritis (i.e. almost a quarter), the cup became loose within the period of follow-up.

Lettin in a later article [13] confirmed that patients suffering from rheumatoid arthritis would almost certainly benefit from total shoulder replacement. However, comparisons of different prostheses are few; most reviews being a little coloured by the enthusiasm of the author/designer. Bodey and Yeoman [14] compared 3 prostheses (Stanmore, Kessel and Neer) in 18 patients with rheumatoid arthritis and although the numbers are very small, it is interesting that the Neer hemiarthroplasty performed almost as well as the other two prostheses.

Inevitably, therefore, it is Neer's work that carries the greatest conviction and authority.

A series published in 1982 [15] contained no less than 273 total shoulder replacements, of which 65 were for rheumatoid arthritis. The special difficulties in dealing with this group of patients are detailed, with particular attention to the rotator cuff and its repair. The surgical technique is carefully explained; the follow-up is quite short.

Surgical technique

A deltopectoral approach is used with care being taken to spare the anterior fibres of deltoid. Only

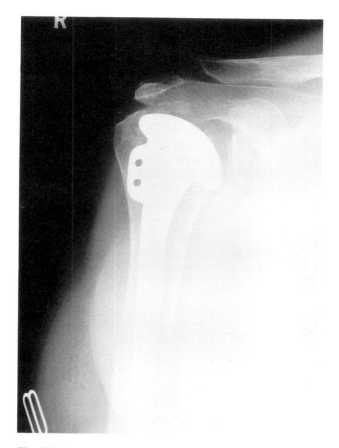

Fig. 22.7

subscapularis is divided. Rotator cuff tears are repaired and great attention is paid to correct tensioning and alignment of the prosthesis.

Difficulties of correctly aligning the glenoid in an eroded bone are discussed and special glenoid components are sometimes used.

Anterior acromioplasty and acromioclavicular arthroplasty are sometimes performed if indicated.

Postoperatively, the arm is placed in a sling and body bandage in normal cases, but an abduction brace should be used if the rotator cuff repair demands it.

Neer has a detailed postoperative rehabilitation programme (Fig. 22.7).

Results

Neer himself reviewed 50 shoulders with rheumatoid arthritis, finding the results to be excellent in

28 and satisfactory in 12, with considerable gains in function and satisfactory relief of pain. Fourteen of these patients had complete rotator cuff tears repaired.

However, Cofield [16] reviewing 77 Neer arthroplasties, of which 29 were for rheumatoid arthritis, reached rather different conclusions. Whilst Neer reported no clinical or definite radiological loosening of the glenoid component, Cofield found eight components definitely loose and 80% of shoulder replacements with a lucent line at the cement bone interface of the scapula. Some of these lucent lines were thought to be significant. Cofield also suggested that the glenoid component needed an improved design. His results were otherwise similar to Neer's.

More recently, Barratt *et al.* [17] have confirmed Cofield's results, finding 10% of radiologically loose glenoid components after $3\frac{1}{2}$ years. They emphasize that osseous support of the glenoid component and functional repair of the rotator cuff are important if glenoid loosening is to be minimized.

Kelly *et al.* [18] deal specifically with rheumatoid arthritis having 42 patients in their series. They note the good relief of pain emphasized in the previous series, 88% of patients had no significant pain. But, for this group, the gains in movement were much more moderate. Elevation was improved by an average of 20°. However, the patients achieved good gains in rotation, leading to an improvement in overall function.

They dispute the significance of the lucent line, that they have also found in 80% of their glenoid components and they were encouraged by the lack of clinical loosening. They expressed doubts about the durability of the glenoid in the long term, however.

The conclusion of all these authors is that non-constrained shoulder arthroplasty merits a place alongside other joint replacements in the surgical management of rheumatoid arthritis. It seems that the 'near anatomical design' of Neer is the one that has proved the most satisfactory in the medium term. There are no cases of humeral component loosening in the series quoted.

Occasionally, cases are mentioned where it has been impossible to implant a glenoid component, but to the author's knowledge, there is no published series of hemiarthroplasties performed for rheumatoid arthritis. Correctly performed, this procedure might have many advantages.

Overall, the objective gains mentioned in series of glenohumeral joint replacements may be small: but all series point out the high patient satisfaction rate.

Recently, the author saw a patient who had undergone shoulder replacement 2 years previously. She was requesting that the other shoulder be similarly treated: a recommendation in itself. The range of movement in the two joints was not dissimilar, however. Certainly the gain from surgery would not have been regarded as statistically significant. The patient, however, had no doubts 'What I can do with the operated arm, I can do comfortably. It makes so much difference', she said.

At present, it is on this limited basis that shoulder replacement surgery should be offered to patients suffering from rheumatoid arthritis.

References

1. Crossan, J. F. and Vallance, R. (1980) Clinical and radiological features of the shoulder joint in rheumatoid disease. *J. Bone Joint Surg.*, **62**, 116.
2. Pahle, J. A. (1981) The shoulder joint in rheumatoid arthritis: synovectomy. *Reconstr. Surg. Traumatol.*, **18**, 33–47.
3. Benjamin, A. (1974) Double osteotomy of the shoulder. *Scand. J. Rheumatol.*, **3**, 65.
4. Wainwright, D. (1974) Glenoidectomy. A method of treating the painful shoulder in rheumatoid arthritis. *Ann. Rheum. Dis.*, **33**, 10.
5. Gariepy, R. (1977) Glenoidectomy in the repair of the rheumatoid shoulder. *J. Bone Joint Surg.*, **59**, 122.
6. Raunio, P. (1981) Arthodesis of the shoulder joint in rheumatoid arthritis. *Reconstr. Surg. Traumatol.*, **18**, 48–54.
7. Neer, C. S. and Kirby, R. M. (1982) Revision of humeral head and shoulder arthroplasties. *Clin. Orthop.*, **170**, 189–195.
8. Varian, J. P. W. (1980) Interposition silastic cup arthroplasty of the shoulder. *J. Bone Joint Surg.*, **62**, 116–117.
9. Neer, C. S. (1955) Articular replacement for the humeral head. *J. Bone Joint Surg.*, **37**, 215.
10. Post, M., Haskell, S. E. and Jablon, M. (1982) Total shoulder replacement with a constrained prosthesis. *J. Bone Joint Surg.*, **62**, 327–335.
11. Beddow, F. H. and Elloy, M. A. (1977) *The Liverpool Total Replacement for the Gleno-Humeral Joint.* Mech. Eng. Publications pp. 21–25.

12. Kessel, L. and Bayley, I. (1979) Prosthetic replacement of the shoulder joint. *J. R. Soc. Med.*, **72**, 748.
13. Lettin, A. (1981) Shoulder replacement in rheumatoid arthritis. *Reconstr. Surg. Traumatol.*, **18**, 55–62.
14. Bodey, W. N. and Yeoman, P. M. (1983) Prosthetic arthroplasty of the shoulder. *Acta Orthop. Scand.*, **54**, 900–903.
15. Neer, C. S. (1982) Recent experience in total shoulder replacement. *J. Bone Joint Surg.*, **64A**, 319–337.
16. Cofield, R. H. (1984) Total shoulder arthroplasty with the Neer prosthesis. *J. Bone Joint Surg.*, **66A**, 899.
17. Barrett, W. P. *et al.* (1987) Total shoulder arthroplasty. *J. Bone Joint Surg.*, **69A**, 865.
18. Kelly, I. G., Foster, R. S. and Fisher, W. D. (1987) Neer total shoulder replacement in rheumatoid arthritis. *J. Bone Joint Surg.*, **69B**, 723.

23

Rheumatoid arthritis of the elbow

P. M. Yeoman

Rheumatoid arthritis is a generalized disease affecting almost all the tissues in the body, and so it should not come as any surprise that the elbow is affected in more than 50% of patients. That does not mean that all require treatment and indeed only a relatively few of the total come to surgery. It is only during the last 15 years that arthroplasty of the elbow has been developed; before the start of this era only a fairly limited number of operations was available and some are still performed with success.

The aim of treatment for patients with rheumatoid arthritis is directed towards the relief of pain; sadly, it is not yet possible to provide a cure by any means. Surgical treatment has to be incorporated into the management of the patient as a whole and is thus regarded as a milestone within the overall medical care. Pain relief by surgical methods is naturally an important aim, but it is not the prime achievement because that can only be guaranteed by robbing the patient of function. In other words, pain could be relieved by an arthrodesis which theoretically would abolish the pain, but in practice it could be a very difficult procedure, fraught with problems and would not contribute to the function of the limb; indeed the patient's existence would be converted from one crippled life to a worse one.

The aims of surgical treatment for the rheumatoid elbow are to provide movement and stability – pain relief will be a bonus.

Movement

The main function of the elbow is to enable the hand to be placed at the optimum position for the patient's use which might be at an angle less than 90° when eating or greater when writing at a desk. Rotation of the forearm has to accompany the range of flexion and extension of the elbow. There are therefore two planes of movement to be considered [1].

Stability

If bone at the elbow is removed either at operation or by disease then the joint will become unstable because the articular surfaces are so designed to provide inherent stability, the surrounding ligaments support the joint but are better served to act as checks against excessive movement. The degree of instability not only depends on the site of bone destruction but its extent. The joint can be transposed into a flail structure, lacking in any direction and resulting in severe loss of function.

Elbow movement and stability related to the entire upper limb

It would be a relatively easy exercise to plan surgical reconstruction of the elbow as an isolated joint, but there are severe restraints on elbow function depending on the shoulder, wrist and hand. For example, a stiff and painful shoulder would mean that rotary movements of the limb would be transferred to the elbow; similarly, a fixed deformity of the forearm or wrist would have the same undesirable effect. In either case the resulting rotary stress imposed on the elbow might hasten the demise of any arthroplasty. It is therefore of importance to restore some part or all of the original function of the elbow without introducing another. Rotary function of the upper limb is just as important as any other but it has to be restored at the wrist, shoulder or both.

Surgical procedures at the elbow

Excision of the olecranon bursa

This is not just a simple little operation because almost invariably the bursa communicates with the joint, and somewhere in the history there may have been some minor infection. The patient may have been gently coerced into agreeing to this minor event as a day case, but the bursa is full of black ingratitude not only for the surgeon but for the patient who may have to endure a long period of repeated dressings because of a sinus; antibiotic cover is essential and the whole affair may result in endless delay for a proposed arthroplasty.

Resection of the head of radius

The indications for this procedure should be confined to those patients with painful restriction of rotation of the forearm, tenderness over the head of radius and only minor erosions on the radiographs. The operation can combine a limited synovectomy from a lateral approach but it must be emphasized that it is unwise to embark on this operation if the disease displays a destructive process in other joints, because it will

progress relentlessly in the elbow and rapidly convert it into a useless unstable joint. The early reports of this operation were good, but alas the joints tended to deteriorate after 4 or 5 years [2], and it is only used as a short term palliative procedure.

Arthroplasty

Assessment of the patient's needs are paramount and the important factors are described by Dunkerley in his chapter on the treatment of the wrist and hand; those factors apply to the elbow. The most difficult decision relates to weight-bearing, either at the first consultation with the patient or in the future depending on the activity of the disease. Most of the essential needs of the patient can be restored by an arthroplasty, and these will include feeding, washing, management at the lavatory and gentle housework; all of which are necessary for an independent life.

Moderate weight-bearing may be required to rise out of a chair but a spring loaded seat will ease this burden. Similarly, the patient's needs are better assessed by an expert who is either a physiotherapist or an occupational therapist.

Heavy weight-bearing is the real problem. Walking with the aid of one stick implies that only a small fraction of the body weight is transferred through the upper limb, but the need for two sticks or crutches will throw a great strain on the elbows. It is questionable whether any prosthesis will last the course if the body weight has to be taken regularly through the elbow because the demands upon it and the bone interface would lead to early loosening.

Interposition arthroplasty

This is the prototype of most arthroplasties and has a long history. Many materials have been used to cover the roughened articular surfaces varying from relatively inert gold foil to living triceps muscle. The author reported a series using silastic sheeting; the early results were encouraging but after 3 years the silastic sheet became brittle and tended to fragment. The method was abandoned but not before admiring the better results obtained by using a thicker piece of plastic designed by Helal [4].

Unconstrained prosthesis

The pioneer work by Lowe and later by Roper [5] produced a relatively simple prosthesis with minimal bone resection, but it was soon evident that a stem was necessary for either the ulnar or humeral component because of loosening. The early results were very good but either they were used when the bone stock was poor or the disease progressed and only about 50% success could be secured. This type of prosthesis is still an excellent method for the relief of pain in those patients with good bone stock and no obvious destructive traits in the disease.

Semi-constrained prosthesis

The various designs of semi-constrained prostheses have built-in mobility not only in the lateral but also in the rotary plane [6]. Greater emphasis on the importance of the medial collateral ligament is made by Souter, who considers that rotary forces are checked by this ligament, thus reducing the enormous stress imposed on any prosthesis when heavy objects are being lifted. The ligaments must be restored and this is very necessary if the surgical approach involves detachment of the ligament from the bone. Similarly, if bone is resected then the tension in the ligaments has to be readjusted after insertion of the prosthesis. These principles may appear elementary but have been founded on the causes for loosening.

Ulnar nerve entrapment is an occasional complication of the rheumatoid elbow due to pressure from the tense synovium, but there is a surprisingly high incidence of ulnar nerve lesions resulting from arthroplasty [7]. The author invariably dissects out the nerve as one of the important initial procedures and the nerve should be protected during the entire operation.

The Souter–Strathclyde prosthesis has been in use for nearly 13 years and the results are impressive. This prosthesis has varying sizes for left and right sides, also various lengths of stem and snap-fit components for use when there has been extensive bone loss and instability.

The tri-axial prosthesis has been used with success by the author for mildly unstable elbows resulting from extensive articular cartilage erosions. The snap-fit connection provides immediate stability and at least 60° of movement can be guaranteed. Rotation of the forearm is not always so successful and it may be necessary to resect the lower end of the ulna in order to restore a useful 90° range of rotation.

Hinge prosthesis

The idea of a straight or even an offset hinge mechanism to replace the elbow is contrary to the accepted movements of the joint. The shearing strains imposed on the prosthesis will undoubtedly cause loosening of one or both components; but this is not the only failure. If the stem and/or cement interface revolve within the bone this will lead to serious loss of bone stock. The stem may penetrate the softened cortical bone or a fracture may develop; these consequences are tragic when they arise in patients who are already severely handicapped by the disease and the results of revision arthroplasty are not particularly inviting [8]. This complication can be avoided by a careful assessment of the patient's disease process, their needs and proper selection of prosthesis. The hinge does not fulfil the requirements.

The stiff shoulder

It is quite apparent that a patient with a stiff painful shoulder has to transfer much of the rotation strains on to the elbow in order to achieve any reasonable function in the upper limb. The best solution is to proceed with an arthroplasty of the shoulder and reassess the function at a later date.

References

1. Torzilli, P. A. (1982) Biomechanics of the elbow. Am. Acad. Orthop. Surg. *Symposium on Total Joint Replacement of the Upper Extremity*. C. V. Mosby, New York, p. 150.
2. Summers, G. D., Webley, W. and Taylor, A. R. (1987) Synovectomy and excision of the radial head in rheumatoid arthritis: a short term palliative procedure. *Clin. Exp. Rheumatol.*, **5**. (Suppl. 2), 115.

3. Yeoman, P. M. (1979) Arthroplasty of the elbow in rheumatoid arthritis using a silastic sheet insert. *J. Bone Joint Surg.*, **61B**, 123.

4. Coates, C. J., Bolton-Maggs, B. G. and Helal, B. H. (1990) Interpositional arthroplasty in the management of rheumatoid arthritis of the elbow. *Rheumatology*, **15(8)**, 1.

5. Roper, B. A., Tuke, M., O'Riordan, S. M. and Bulstrode, C. J. (1986) A new unconstrained elbow. *J. Bone Joint Surg.*, **68B 4**, 566.

6. Inglis, A. E. (1982) Tri-axial elbow replacement: indications, surgical techniques and results. Am. Acad. Orthop. Surg. *Symposium on Total Joint Replacement of the Upper Extremity*. C. V. Mosby, New York, p. 100.

7. Souter, W. A. (1988) In *Surgical Management of Rheumatoid Arthritis*. Wright, London, p. 69.

8. Morrey, B. F. and Bryan, R. S. (1987) Revision total elbow arthroplasty. *J. Bone Joint Surg.*, **69A 4**, 523.

24

Rheumatoid arthritis of the wrist and hand

D. R. Dunkerley

This is a difficult field of hand surgery. Any or all of the many articulations of the hand and wrist, and of the tendons and muscles, may be involved in the disease process. Certain patterns of deformity are seen; the surgeon must be familiar with the patho-mechanics of these deformities. Greater than usual care is required in the selection of patients for surgery, the performance of the operations and the postoperative management.

For each patient the following factors must be assessed:

1. The state of the joints and the function of both upper limbs.
2. The function of both lower limbs. Are the hands required to assist in walking?
3. Timing. While it is not technically wrong to operate while the patient is undergoing a 'flare-up' of his arthritis, it can be unkind, in that the patient may feel unwell either from the arthritis or the treatment. Hand surgery is best deferred if lower limb surgery is contemplated, since crutches or a frame may be required postoperatively.

While hand and wrist operations can be performed under regional nerve block, general anaesthesia is occasionally necessary, for which the anaesthetist must be assured of cervical spine stability. Cervical spine stabilization may therefore need to take precedence, especially if long tract signs are present. The introduction of laryngeal mask airway has, however, greatly reduced the hazards of operating on patients with stiff necks.

4. The patient's ambitions and determination. One needs to know what the patient wants to be able to do, and whether he has the determination to go through with an exacting programme of operations and postoperative therapy.

All this takes time: time to get to know the patient and to give him confidence. Patients with rheumatoid disease are often very trusting of their doctors, and are inclined to accept advice uncritically. This means that the surgeon has an extra responsibility to explain honestly the advantages and disadvantages of surgery.

5. Examination of the hand and wrist. The examination should be more than a catalogue of joint movements or deformities. The mechanism of deformity should be in the examiner's mind and thus govern which features he looks for. It is convenient to examine the following sequence: wrist and inferior radio-ulnar joint, extensor tendons, metacarpophalangeal joints, interphalangeal joints, thumb, flexor tendons. The fingers should be examined for evidence of digital arteritis (Fig. 24.1), a contraindication to hand surgery. The stage of the disease should be noted.

A full assessment must include radiographs, particularly when surgery is contemplated.

6. The patient's manual function. Pain, deformity and functional loss are not always related. It is helpful to have a detailed assessment by an occupational therapist. Great care must be taken to ensure that surgery does not impair function already present.

The hand must be considered as a whole but in the following sections the patho-mechanics of

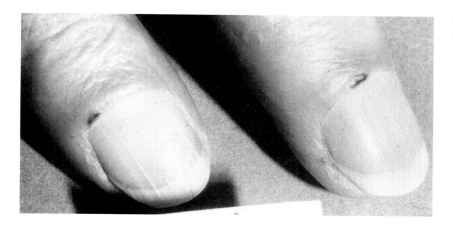

Fig. 24.1   Nail-fold lesions in digital arteritis.

deformity and surgical treatment of each part are, for convenience, considered separately.

The wrist, inferior radio-ulnar joint and extensor tendons

Rheumatoid synovitis may first appear in either the radiocarpal joint or the inferior radio-ulnar joint; sometimes in both at once. Early radiographic changes may be seen as areas of subchondral rarefaction appearing at the inferior radio-ulnar joint and at the insertions of the radiocarpal ligaments on the scaphoid and triquetrum (Fig. 24.2). Later, attenuation of ligaments and loss of bone height, due to articular cartilage loss and bone compression, results in joint laxity. The tendon sheath of extensor carpi ulnaris is often affected, allowing the tendon to displace forwards until it comes to lie anterior to the axis of wrist flexion.

A series of deformities then develops. The carpus translocates in an ulnar direction on the radius. It often also rotates into radial deviation because of the loss of the stabilizing power of the extensor carpi ulnaris (Fig. 24.3). For the same reason the ulnar side of the carpus drops forwards. Thus, the carpus supinates on the radius. This, coupled with dorsal subluxation of the head of the ulna, produces a hollow distal to the ulnar head (Fig. 24.4). Pronation and supination become restricted and painful. Passive anteroposterior movement of the head of the ulna, the so-called piano-key sign, is painful.

In later stages the anterior part of the radial articular surface erodes. The carpus subluxates anteriorly and proximally (Fig. 24.5). Radiographs may also show a collapse of the mid-carpal joint: usually the volar intercalated segment instability (VISI) deformity in which the proximal row of the carpus tilts into flexion and the distal row hyperextends (Fig. 24.6). Hodgson *et al.* [1] have described a staging of the disease based on radiographs.

Stage 1: Peri-articular rarefaction with early erosions. The architecture of the wrist remains well preserved but there may be a little rotatory instability of the scaphoid.

Stage 2: While the mid-carpal and radio-scaphoid joints are well preserved one or more of the following deformities may be present:

a. ulnar translocation
b. palmar flexion of the lunate
c. flexion deformity of the scaphoid
d. deterioration of the radio-lunate joint

Stage 3: The mid-carpal joint shows evidence of degeneration. There is degeneration in the radio-scaphoid joint. The carpus subluxes forward on the radius and there may be pseudo cyst formation of the volar lip of the radius.

Stage 4: There is erosion of the volar edge of the distal radius and bone loss in the region of the inferior radio-ulnar joint.

Synovitis of the digital extensor tendons is common in the region of the extensor retinaculum. The synovium may bulge distally and proximally; the distal edge of the bulge can be seen to move as the fingers are flexed and extended.

Rupture of the extensor tendons, including

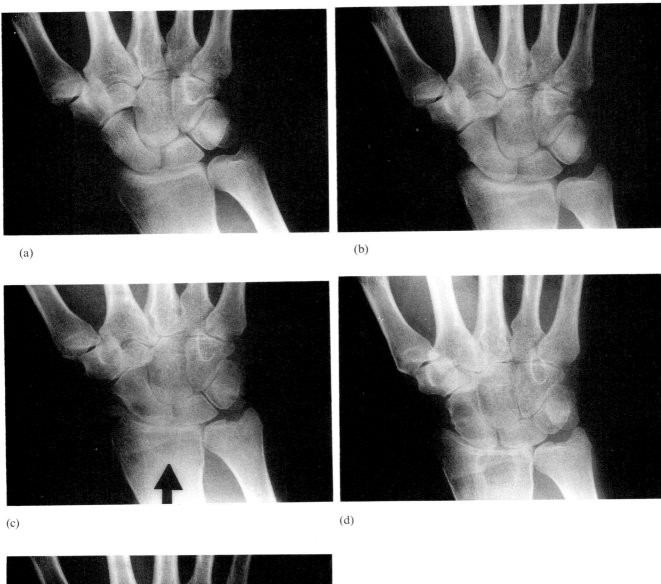

(a)

(b)

(c)

(d)

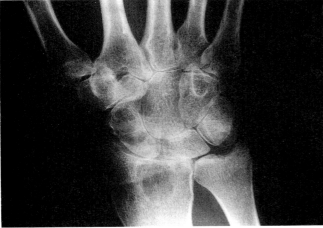

(e)

Fig. 24.2 (a–g) Radiographs taken at 1-year intervals to show progression of rheumatoid disease in the wrist. (a) Normal, (b) early rarefaction of scaphoid-lunate and inferior radio-ulnar joint surfaces, (c) more obvious lesions of scaphoid, radial styloid, radial articular surface and lunate, (d) loss of joint space in radiocarpal joint, erosion of radial surface of scaphoid, early ulnar shift of carpus, (e), (f), (g) rapid progression.

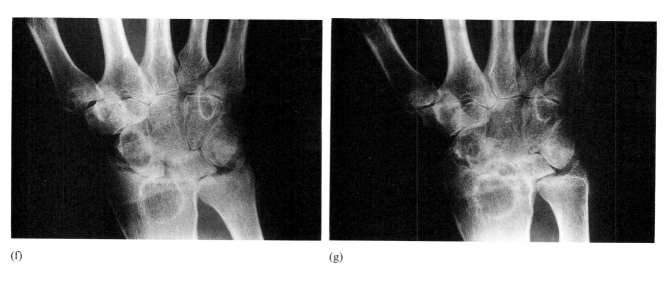

(f)   (g)

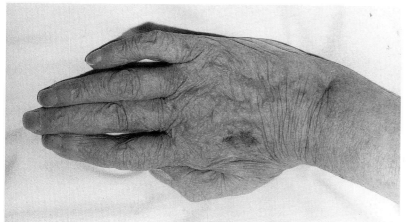

Fig. 24.3   Radial deviation deformity of the wrist.

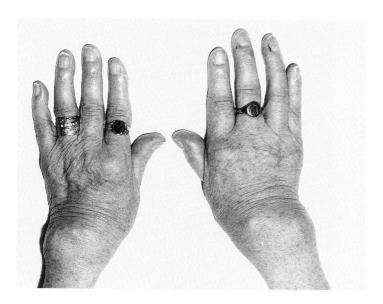

Fig. 24.4   Hollow distal to ulnar head due to carpal supination on the radius.

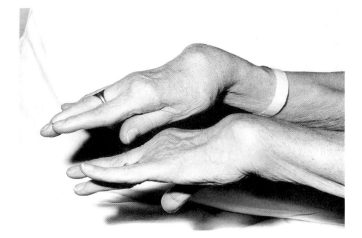

Fig. 24.5 Anterior subluxation of carpus on radius.

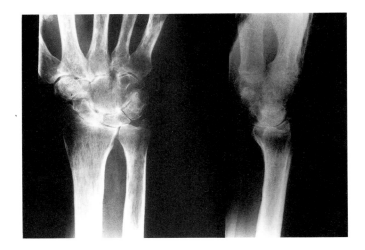

Fig. 24.6 VISI deformity of carpus.

Fig. 24.7 Rupture of extensor tendons to thumb, ring and little fingers.

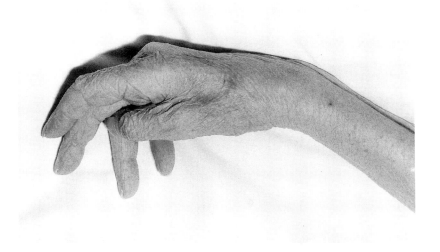

extensor pollicis longus, may occur. Usually, in the fingers, the little finger tendons rupture first, followed at intervals by the others in order. Rupture is often painless (Fig. 24.7).

There are several causes of rupture. It may be due to attrition of the tendons on spikes of bone arising from the eroded ulnar head or radius. The tendons may be invaded by rheumatoid synovium. Ischaemia due to pressure of the mass of synovium under the retinaculum may play a part. Sometimes the two ends of a ruptured tendon are found at operation to be joined by a narrow tube of paratenon.

Surgical treatment

There is a standard surgical approach which gives good access to all these areas. A straight longitudinal incision is made over the midline of the dorsum of the wrist. A straight incision produces less wound healing problems than a sinuous incision. It is deepened down to the extensor retinaculum, preserving the dorsal branches of the radial nerve and ligating as few veins as possible. By gauze dissection the flaps can be reflected at the level between the superficial fascia and retinaculum. The retinaculum is reflected as a flap, usually from ulnar to radial side, and is left attached to the radius between the extensor carpi radialis longus and extensor pollicis brevis tendons. A tongue of the extensor retinaculum can be fashioned on the ulnar side during the reflection. During closure this tongue can be looped round the tendon of the extensor carpi ulnaris to maintain its dorsal position.

Extensor tendons

If the tendons are intact, synovectomy is all that may be required. A very thorough synovectomy may weaken or devascularise the tendons; the synovitis in any case will regress after decompression.

Replacing the retinaculum deep to the tendons decompresses them, protects them from attrition on rough bony edges and diminishes the risk of adhesions.

Ruptured tendons cannot usually be repaired end to end. Tendon transfer or suture of the distal stump to an intact neighbouring tendon is

Table 24.1 Restoration of extensor tendon function

Extensor tendon rupture	Tendon transfer
Little, ring or middle finger alone	Extensor indicis proprius (EIP) transfer
Little and ring fingers	EIP to little finger Attach ring to middle finger tendon
Little, ring and middle fingers	EIP to little Flexor digitorum superficialis (ring) to ring and middle
All four fingers	Flexor digitorum superficialis (ring and middle)
Extensor pollicis longus	EIP or extensor carpi radialis longus

required. A useful plan of treatment is given in Table 24.1.

Tendon transfers from the flexor to the extensor surfaces may be difficult. The flexor digitorum superficialis to the ring finger is most directly routed through a large defect created in the interosseous membrane; some advocate a subcutaneous route via the radial border of the wrist.

Following the operation the MCP joints should be immobilized in extension (with the PIP joints free) for 3 weeks, after which an outrigger splint should be fitted for several weeks.

Inferior radio-ulnar joint

Excision of the lower end of the ulna is one of the most useful and successful procedures in this condition.

Indications for the operation are:

(i) painful subluxation of the head of the ulna,
(ii) severe painful synovitis of the inferior radio-ulnar joint,
(iii) pain or restriction of movement on pronation and supination,
(iv) rupture of one or more extensor tendons.

It is easiest to transect the shaft with a power saw first, about 1.5 cm from the ulnar styloid. The distal stump can be held in a clamp and the soft tissues dissected off the bone.

If this operation alone is performed, post-operative immobilization is unnecessary.

Swanson advocates capping the ulna with a silicone rubber ulnar head prosthesis. Many authors, including the present one, do not find that this procedure confers any benefit and it carries some risk of complications such as dislocation.

Radiocarpal and intercarpal joints

A large number of procedures have been described for the treatment of these joints in rheumatoid disease. Not all have stood the test of time. The following can be recommended:

   (i) Synovectomy
   (ii) Radio-lunate fusion
   (iii) Arthrodesis
   (iv) Prosthetic replacement

Synovectomy

Straub and Ranawat [2] described this operation as dorsal wrist stabilisation: essentially a dorsal synovectomy with modifications. The aim of the procedure is a stable, painless, mobile fibrous union.

Extensor tendon and dorsal wrist synovectomy are performed as far as possible. The capsule is carefully repaired and if there is instability crossed k-wires are inserted. The ulnar head is excised. The operation may need to be augmented by transferring the extensor carpi radialis longus tendon to the ulnar side of the hand to restore balance. Plaster support is maintained for 6 weeks; the wires, if used, are removed at 4 weeks. Good results are reported in a long term survey by the originators [3].

The operation is indicated in Stage 1 of the disease. More severely diseased wrists are not suitable for this procedure and arthrodesis or arthroplasty should be considered. Particular contra-indications are fixed deformity, radio-carpal subluxation and a flail joint.

Ishikawa *et al.* [4] have shown that 88% of patients achieve pain relief but there is an increased incidence of ulnar translocation of the carpus.

Radio-lunate fusion

In stage 2 of the disease affecting chiefly the radio-lunate articulation and often accompanied by an ulnar translocation, radio-lunate fusion will confer stability while permitting some movement at the mid-carpal joint. (Chamay *et al.* [5], Stanley and Boot [6] and Ishikawa *et al.* [7]).

Arthrodesis

As in other joints, arthrodesis provides a stable, painless joint without the possibility of future complications. Arthrodesis of the wrist has two further advantages. The wrist functions chiefly in its middle range. Brumfield and Champoux [8] have shown that in normal adults the range of wrist movements required for the activities of daily living is between 35° extension and 10° flexion. Arthrodesis does not, therefore, cause serious loss of function. The other advantage is

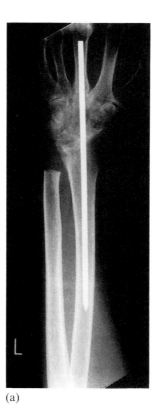 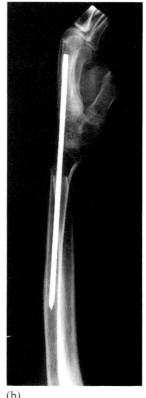

(a)   (b)

Fig. 24.8 Arthrodesis of the wrist using countersunk pin through 3rd metacarpal.

that stabilization of the wrist greatly improves function of the fingers and thumb.

The position in which the wrist should be fused has been the subject of much discussion. The author agrees with Clayton and Ferlic [9] who give good reasons for placing the wrist in a position of 10° of ulnar deviation with neutral flexion-extension.

The technique [10] involves exposing the dorsum of the joints, excising the remains of the articular cartilage, and correcting any collapse of the mid-carpal joint in order to maintain the length. The wrist is then transfixed with a Steinmann's pin driven down the shaft of the third metacarpal and across the wrist into the shaft of the radius (Fig. 24.8). The pin is countersunk into the metacarpal. If any rotational instability remains, a staple or oblique K-wire can be added. To achieve ulnar deviation it may be necessary to put the pin through the radial side of the third metacarpal shaft or between the bases of the second and third metacarpals (Fig. 24.9). Plaster

immobilization for 4–6 weeks is only required if there is still some joint mobility at the end of the operation.

Replacement arthroplasty

This operation is designed to combine pain relief with limited wrist motion. The best results are obtained in the relatively less damaged wrists. The operation is contraindicated in patients who will put heavy stress on the wrists, for example when walking with crutches, in wrists where the bone stock is inadequate to support the prosthesis or where there is severe deformity, especially fixed flexion and subluxation. A particular contraindication to wrist arthroplasty is rupture of the wrist extensor tendons.

Three prostheses have been in use long enough for long-term follow-up reviews to become available. The Volz and Meuli prostheses are true arthroplasties with their respective components cemented into the radius and metacarpus. Swanson [11] developed a one-piece flexible Silastic® implant designed to be a spacer (Fig. 24.10).

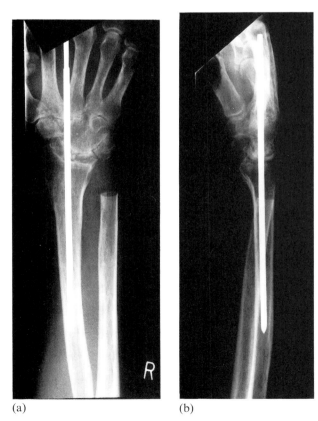

(a)   (b)

Fig. 24.9 Arthrodesis of the wrist using pin between 2nd and 3rd metacarpals.

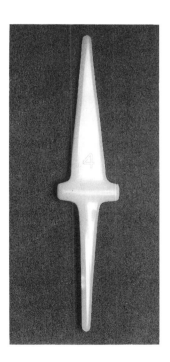

Fig. 24.10 Swanson Silastic® flexible wrist implant.

The Silastic® is soft which protects the bone; on the other hand it is, itself, susceptible to damage from the bone edges and recently Swanson has introduced metal grommets to protect the prosthesis. So far long term studies of this effect are not available.

All these operations are difficult; they require meticulous attention to the positioning of the prosthesis, tendon balance and post-operative care. On the published evidence the Swanson prosthesis, which is the most widely used, leads to fewer complications. The results of all three deteriorate in time.

Advising a patient between arthroplasty and arthrodesis is not always easy. Where arthroplasty and arthrodesis have been compared (sometimes in the same patient) arthroplasty tends to have the advantage in terms of patient acceptability and objective examination.

In planning treatment it can be said that in mild cases of rheumatoid disease with synovitis, the dorsal stabilization is indicated. In more severe cases, where the contraindications to arthroplasty enumerated above do not exist, either arthrodesis or arthroplasty may be chosen, but a successsful arthroplasty is better. Where arthroplasty is clearly contraindicated, arthrodesis is required.

Where both wrists require treatment the best procedure, if possible, is to perform an arthroplasty of the dominant wrist and arthrodesis of the other. The subject is well reviewed by Vicar and Burton [12].

Metacarpophalangeal joints

Synovitis in its early stages can be severe and painful; later the characteristic deformities of ulnar deviation and palmar subluxation occur. A simple staging of the deformities is a follows:

Stage 1: Early ulnar drift alone.
Stage 2: Ulnar drift with palmar subluxation but an intact joint.
Stage 3: Ulnar drift with palmar subluxation and joint damage.

While the primary cause of these problems is attenuation of the ligaments and joint damage, the deformities are produced by unbalanced forces. These may be summarized as follows:

Normal anatomy

The metacarpophalangeal joints have considerable mobility when in extension, allowing sideways and rotary movements. The radial collateral ligaments are longer than the ulnar. In the index and middle finger metacarpals, the slope of the articular surfaces allows more ulnar than radial deviation, and in these fingers the line of the long flexor and extensor tendons means that they tend to pull to the ulnar side.

It has been shown that when the radial and ulnar interossei are stimulated equally the pull of the ulnar inserted muscles is stronger. The arrangement in the little finger means that the powerful abductor digiti minimi muscle is opposed only by the weak third palmar interosseus.

Normal use

In lateral pinch grip the thumb forces the fingers into ulnar deviation. As the radial collateral ligament weakens, the fingers are deviated more. When a tight fist is made, the little and ring fingers become ulnar deviated as the fourth and fifth metacarpals are flexed.

Pathological changes

The radial side of the extensor hood is thinner than the ulnar, and more easily stretched by the synovial proliferation. The extensor tendon is thus allowed to deviate to the ulnar side, and in its extreme position comes to lie in the valley between the metacarpal heads. Adaptive shortening or adhesion of the ulnar intrinsics may occur.

As the joint deviates, the volar plate/transverse metacarpal ligament complex moves ulnarwards, carrying the entrance to the fibrous flexor sheath with it. The flexor tendons then accentuate the ulnar pull. As the extensor apparatus weakens and displaces, the powerful flexors, obtaining a greater moment of force as they are distanced from the metacarpal head, add to the palmar subluxation.

It has been postulated that an external force acting on the metacarpophalangeal joints is the effect produced by radial deviation of the wrist (Fig. 24.11). The metacarpal may be regarded as

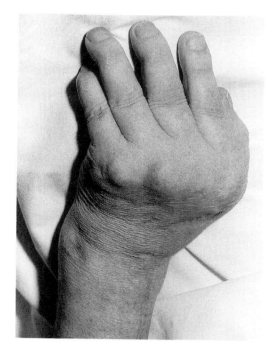

Fig. 24.11 Radial deviation of wrist associated with ulnar deviation of metacarpophalangeal joints.

an intercalated bone in a chain of bones controlled by the long tendons. Once a sideways collapse is permitted at one joint, a zigzag reaction occurs. Thus radial wrist deviation contributes to the opposite, ulnar, deviation force at the metacarpophalangeal joint. However, it is possible that patients hold the wrist in radial deviation to bring the ulnar deviated fingers into line with the forearm.

Surgical treatment

Arthrodesis is never indicated here. The aim is to provide mobile, stable, painless joints. As with many operations for this disease a compromise must be accepted between mobility and stability, and it is rare to achieve 90° of movement with complete stability.

Stage 1. Early ulnar drift alone

Since the joint is intact and there is no palmar subluxation, the aim of surgery is to realign the forces acting on the joint. Synovectomy alone

will render the joint more comfortable and increase mobility but it does not correct the ulnar drift or prevent the progression of the disease in the long term.

A mid-line longitudinal dorsal skin incision is deepened through the radial extensor hood. The extensor expansion is reflected off the capsule, which is opened. Synovectomy should be thorough with particular attention paid to removing synovium from between the collateral ligaments and metacarpal head, and from the dorsal lip of the base of the proximal phalanx. It is often difficult to preserve the capsule.

After synovectomy the extensor tendon is centred over the metacarpal head by plicating the radial hood over the dorsum of the tendon. The intrinsic tendons on the ulnar side, including abductor digiti minimi, should be released.

A stronger correction can be provided by crossed intrinsic transfer in which the detached ulnar intrinsic wing is sutured into the radial intrinsic wing of the adjoining finger.

Stage 2. Ulnar drift and palmar subluxation with an intact joint

The procedures for stage 1 can be augmented by the extensor loop operation [13] in which a strip from the centre of the extensor tendon is passed through a drill hole in the dorsal lip of the base of the proximal phalanx and sutured back on itself (Fig. 24.12).

Stage 3. Ulnar drift with palmar subluxation and joint damage

Arthroplasty is required here. The various excision arthroplasties favoured in the 1960s have been replaced by implant arthroplasties. The silicone prostheses of Swanson or Niebauer have emerged as superior to hinged prostheses for this joint. The silicone prostheses are essentially spacers permitting flexion and extension and conferring limited lateral stability. Alone, they do not prevent recurrence of the deformities. Original articles should be consulted for operative details [14,15].

Good functional and cosmetic results can be obtained and late complications are uncommon. However, to achieve good results meticulous

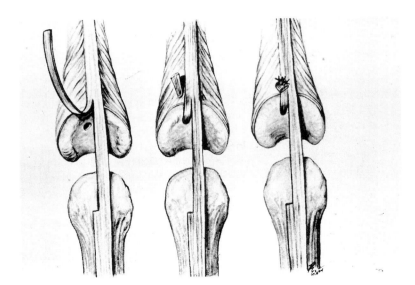

Fig. 24.12 Harrison extensor loop operation. (From Harrison S. H. (1971) *Br. J. Plast. Surg.,* **24**, 307.)

attention to detail is required, both in the performance of the operation and in the postoperative management.

Interphalangeal joints

Two main deformities are common in rheumatoid disease, swan-neck (Fig. 24.13) and fixed flexion. Both may occur in the same hand.

Swan-neck deformity

The primary causes of the deformity are,with one exception, found in the proximal interphalangeal joint. Hyperextension develops as a result of one or more factors. In normal individuals, hyperextension may occur if congenital joint laxity is present, or after division or excision of the flexor digitorum superficialis tendon. Either of these make swan-neck deformity more likely in a patient with rheumatoid disease. The rheumatoid process can weaken the volar plate and accessory collateral ligaments, and may itself cause dysfunction of flexor digitorum superficialis.

   External forces may then accentuate the deformity. Intrinsic tendon tightness is found in a proportion of swan-neck digits, usually secondary to metacarpophalangeal joint disease with ulnar deviation and palmar subluxation. Shapiro [16] points out that loss of length at the wrist, due to a combination of true loss of carpal height and

proximal erosion of the radial articular surface, causes the long flexors and extensors to become less efficient, producing an 'extrinsic-minus' effect.

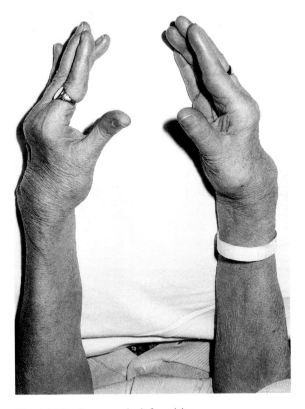

Fig. 24.13 Swan-neck deformities.

Mallet finger is the one exception to the statement that PIP joint disease is the first cause of the deformity. In non-rheumatoid patients with familial joint laxity, mallet finger can produce a secondary swan-neck deformity. This can also happen in rheumatoid disease where the PIP joint is weakened. The loss of tension in the distal extensor tendon allows maximum force to be exerted through the central slip. At the same time, the oblique retinacular ligament is relaxed, and the normal flexion sequence thus broken.

As the deformity progresses the transverse retinacular ligaments stretch, permitting the lateral bands of the extensor apparatus to migrate dorsally until they come to lie dorsal to the axis of rotation of the PIP joint when the joint is extended. They later lose the ability to move in a palmar direction during active finger flexion. In the hyperextended position of the PIP joint the lateral slips are relaxed allowing the DIP joint to droop. With a greater degree of PIP hyperextension the oblique retinacular ligaments come to lie dorsal to the axis of the PIP joint, which finally destroys the flexion sequence of the finger.

When the finger is examined, therefore, the condition of the wrist, MCP joint, long flexor and extensor tendons and intrinsic tendons should be noted. Nalebuff and Millender [17] have described four stages or types of the deformity; their classification is particularly useful because it relates to functional loss (Table 24.2).

Table 24.2   Classification of swan-neck deformity [13]

Type 1:   The PIP joint is flexible in all positions of the MCP joint. The MCP joint is usually not seriously affected. Functional loss is slight.
Type 2:   PIP flexion is limited when the MCP joint is held in extension or radial deviation, due to a tight ulnar intrinsic. This may follow untreated type 1 deformity or be secondary to MCP joint subluxation.
Type 3:   PIP joint flexion is limited in all positions of the MCP joint, but the PIP joint is well preserved on X-ray. Here functional loss is more severe: tip to tip pinch is impossible and the patient develops the 'long pinch' with thumb and fingers extended.
Type 4:   PIP joint stiffness with radiological intra-articular damage.

Treatment depends on the stage at which the deformity is seen. Nalebuff and Millender [17] described a series of operations for each type of deformity, but this has been simplified by Souter [18].

The aim of treatment in types 1–3 is to restore active controlled PIP flexion where possible. This can easily be achieved in types 1 and 2 but is more difficult in type 3. The basic operation is a tenodesis on the volar surface of the finger to prevent hyperextension; this can be achieved by either a retinacular ligament reconstruction [19] or a tethering using a slip of flexor digitorum superficialis.

In type 1 the tenodesis alone is sufficient. If the primary cause is a mallet finger, the DIP joint should be fused.

Where the metacarpophalangeal pathology is contributory to the type 2 deformity it should be treated as described above. During this procedure the tight ulnar intrinsic will be released. Tenodesis of the PIP joint will also be required.

Difficulties arise in type 3 because the joint is fixed in hyperextension. This is due to a combination of tight dorsal skin, adherent extensor expansion and tight collateral ligaments. Nalebuff and Millender [17] described a technique for releasing the skin by leaving an oblique incision open on the dorsum of the middle phalanx and allowing it to heal without skin graft. The expansion should be mobilized and the lateral bands allowed to displace volarwards. The central slip may need to be lengthened and the collateral ligaments mobilized. By gentle manipulation flexion can be restored.

Of the two procedures for effecting a tenodesis, the Littler is easier but weaker than the technique utilising a slip of flexor digitorum superficialis. In the Littler technique a strip is mobilized from the lateral edge of one lateral slip. It is left attached distally; the other end is passed volar to Cleland's ligament. Two incisions are made in the flexor sheath at the proximal phalanx level, the strip is passed through them and sutured to itself with the joint held in 45° of flexion. This may seem excessive at the time but stretching of the tenodesis will occur.

The alternative is to mobilize a distally attached strip of flexor digitorum superficialis, taking care that one slip remains intact and the vinculum brevis is not damaged. The strip is passed through a drill hole in the proximal phalanx. After either procedure, the joint is splinted for 4–6 weeks. An extension block splint is used, permitting flexion but restricting extension to 45°.

In type 4, arthrodesis of the PIP joint is the treatment of choice. This may be effected using a Harrison–Nicolle intramedullary peg [20].

Fixed flexion deformity (Boutonnière)

The problem always lies in the PIP joint where synovitis leads to stretching or rupture of the central slip of the extensor tendon. As the PIP joint falls into flexion, hyperextension of the DIP joint occurs. At first this is a secondary effect due to tendon imbalance, but shortening and adhesion of the lateral slips leads to a fixed hyperextension deformity. Initially the patient can oppose to the thumb; later, functional loss occurs because the finger is too flexed to oppose and cannot be extended to grasp.

In the first stage the patient develops an extensor lag at the PIP joint which is often swollen. The lag can be passively corrected. Functional loss, if any, is caused by inability to flex the DIP joint actively. although passive flexion is possible.

In stage 2, the PIP joint deformity worsens and the DIP hyperextension becomes fixed. Finally, the PIP joint becomes fixed in 70–90° of flexion. As the deformity progresses, compensatory hyperextension of the MCP joint develops.

Examination is therefore directed to noting the degree of synovitis of the PIP joint, the degree of active and passive loss of the PIP and DIP joint movements and the actual functional loss. The PIP joint should be radiographed.

In the early stages treatment may be nonsurgical. Steroid injection of the PIP joint should be undertaken with the aims of correcting deformity and restoring active movement. The multiplicity of operation described for this deformity in non-rheumatoid patients testifies to the difficulties of achieving a good result. The difficulties are not less in rheumatoid disease.

The steps of the operation are to remove the synovium, tighten or reconstruct the central slip and relocate the lateral bands dorsal to the PIP joint axis. It may be necessary to lengthen or divide the extensor tendon over the middle phalanx to permit active flexion of the DIP joint.

The exact technique will need to be adapted to the findings at operation. Most surgeons use a basic operation, with appropriate variations, and the present author finds Rothwell's [21] operation effective.

When there is joint or irreparable soft tissue damage, arthrodesis of the PIP joint in 30° flexion is an excellent salvage procedure. The extensor tendon should be divided over the middle phalanx to restore active flexion of the distal joint.

The thumb

The problems caused by finger deformities are compounded when the thumb is diseased. A recent survey showed that 60% of thumbs examined were abnormal.

All three joints should be examined, clinically and radiologically, paying attention to the function of the long tendons and intrinsic muscles.

The patterns of thumb deformity in rheumatoid disease have been worked out [22]. These can be simplified by classifying deformities according to the state of the metacarpophalangeal joint.

Flexion deformity at the metacarpophalangeal joint

This is the most commonly seen deformity (Fig. 24.14). At first the deformity is mobile; the joint may be subluxated. Because of the alteration in the pull of the intrinsics the interphalangeal joint

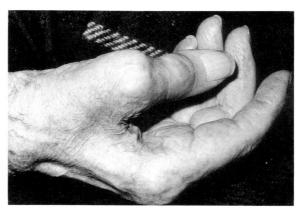

Fig. 24.14   Thumb: type 1: flexion deformity.

becomes hyperextended and after a while the ability to flex this joint is lost.

If, however, the examiner holds the metacarpophalangeal joint in extension, active interphalangeal flexion is at once restored. If it is not, a rupture of the flexor pollicis longus tendon should be considered.

At a later stage both joints become fixed. Before deciding on treatment the function of the carpometacarpal joint must be noted.

Hyperextension deformity of the metacarpophalangeal joint

Here, the deformity of the metacarpophalangeal joint is secondary to a flexed and adducted posture of the first metacarpal caused by disease in

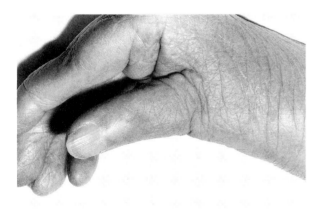

Fig. 24.15   Thumb: type 2: hyperextension deformity.

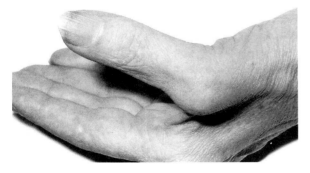

Fig. 24.16   Thumb: type 3: unstable metacarpophalangeal joint.

the carpometacarpal joint. As in swan-neck deformity of the fingers, the terminal interphalangeal joint adopts a flexed position (Fig. 24.15).

Instability of the metacarpophalangeal joint

The whole joint may become loose; laxity of the ulnar collateral ligament is particularly disabling. The interphalangeal joint is also prone to become flail, either alone or as well as the metacarpophalangeal joint (Fig. 24.16).

Surgery

The aim of surgery is to provide a firm post to which the fingers can oppose; of course the fingers may also need surgery to achieve this. One should aim to retain mobility of at least one joint, which ideally should be the carpometacarpal joint. Provided this joint moves, fusion of the other joints is compatible with good function.

Flexion deformity at the metacarpophalangeal joint

Where the deformity is mobile and the joint well preserved the operation described by Nalebuff [23] can be used. The tendon of extensor pollicis longus is passed through the insertion of extensor pollicis brevis and tightened until the deformity is corrected. In more advanced cases with fixed deformity or joint damage, arthrodesis is indicated.

If the interphalangeal joint has become fixed in hyperextension it will need to be fused in 10–20° of flexion.

Hyperextension deformity of the metacarpophalangeal joint

Since disease at the carpometacarpal joint is the primary source of the deformity, this joint should be tackled first. It must not be arthrodesed; arthroplasty with correction of the first web contracture is required. The contracture can usually be released by incising the dorsal aponeurosis over the web, parallel to the first metacarpal. A Z-plasty of the skin of the web may be required.

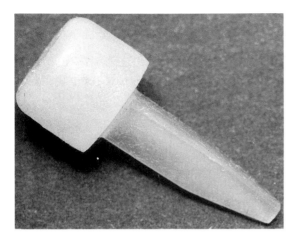

Fig. 24.17 Swanson Silastic trapezium implant.

The choice of arthroplasty may be difficult. The Swanson Silastic® trapezium implant is designed to articulate with the scaphoid (Fig. 24.17). In rheumatoid disease the scaphoid may be severely damaged, or have been partly resected for a wrist implant. Alternative procedures are to insert a rolled-up tendon, usually palmaris longus, or to use a Swanson convex condylar implant.

Arthrodesis of the other joints of the thumb may be needed to give pulp to pulp opposition.

Instability of the metacarpophalangeal joint

A ruptured ulnar collateral ligament can be reconstructed using a strip of extensor pollicis brevis passed through appropriate drill holes in the bones. However, a degree of rheumatoid invasion sufficient to cause laxity of the ligament usually damages the joint surfaces, and arthrodesis is required.

Flexor tendons

Rheumatoid involvement of the flexor tendons occurs at the site of the synovial coverings. Synovitis may produce restricted movement due to pain, adhesions, triggering and rupture of tendons. In the carpal tunnel the swelling may lead to median nerve compression. Barnes and Currey [24] found that 53% of 45 patients with rheuma-

toid arthritis had clinical evidence of carpal tunnel syndrome, and a further 16% had impairment of nerve conduction without clinical manifestations.

The carpal tunnel, palm and digits should be examined for swelling and tenderness. The active range of finger flexion may be less than the passive range, which is pathognomonic of flexor synovitis. Digital flexor synovitis may cause the interphalangeal joints to be held in flexion, and the joints can develop fixed deformity due to secondary changes in the periarticular structures. Triggering, if present, is due to nodules catching either at the entrance to the fibrous flexor sheath, limiting flexor digitorum superficialis excursion, or at the superficialis decussation, limiting profundus excursion. Gross digital synovitis stretches the fibrous flexor sheath.

Tendon ruptures may occur, usually in the carpal tunnel or in the palm. They may be clinically disguised by matting of tendons to one another or by the much reduced excursion of all the tendons. The possible causes of rupture have been enumerated by Mannerfelt and Norman [25] as:

   (i) granulomatous invasion along the vincula;
  (ii) infarction of the vincula;
 (iii) attrition due to bony spurs;
 (iv) pressure of the flexor retinaculum on weakened tendons;
  (v) weakening following steroid injections.

The usual site of bony spurs in the carpal tunnel is the trapezio-scaphoid joint; the most commonly affected tendons are flexor pollicis longus and the flexors to the index finger.

The first line of treatment for flexor synovitis is steroid injection, which can be given into the carpal tunnel or digital sheath. There is probably a small increased liability to tendon rupture after repeated injections.

The diagnosis of carpal tunnel syndrome is an indication for urgent surgical decompression if a steroid injection fails to give relief. The condition is easily relieved if treated early; if neglected the patient has numbness added to the patient's already considerable disabilities.

When should flexor synovectomy be undertaken? The main indications are (i) persistent pain and restriction of movement which has failed to respond to steroid injection, (ii) carpal tunnel syndrome, (iii) triggering and (iv) tendon rupture. Surgery should be undertaken early rather than late [26].

The surgical approach is through a longitudinal incision over the carpal tunnel, with a Z component at the wrist to avoid scar contracture and damage to the palmar branch of the median nerve. In the fingers, zigzag incisions give a wide exposure and excellent scars. The thinner portions of the fibrous flexor sheath may be excised but pulleys should be left at the entrance to the sheath, and over the proximal and middle phalanges. Careful synovectomy is performed; intratendinous lesions can be shelled out but the split in the tendon should be repaired where possible. If there is an obstruction at the decussation of the superficialis tendon one half may be excised back to the palm. The other half should be retained to prevent swan-neck deformity.

Harrison, Ansell and Hall [27] point out that if palmar and proximal subluxation of the base of the proximal phalanx has occurred, the scarring following flexor tendon surgery may make future passive correction of the deformity impossible; this is, therefore, a contraindication to flexor tendon surgery.

Flexor tendon rupture may present problems of management. Direct repair is seldom possible. Tendon grafting is difficult in the rheumatoid hand though some claim good results [28]. The best results are obtained by tendon transfer or appropriate joint fusion. Rupture of flexor pollicis longus or an isolated finger profundus tendon should be treated by arthrodesis of the distal joint. If both flexor tendons to a finger are ruptured the superficialis is excised, leaving one slip. An intact superficialis is then transferred from another finger to the ruptured profundus.

All such surgery will fail unless the greatest attention is paid to postoperative therapy. After synovectomy active movements are started at 5 days. If necessary, extensor assist splints or static splints localizing active movements to certain joints may be used. Therapy needs to be continued for up to 8 weeks.

Provided the postoperative treatment is properly carried out, good results can be obtained in the majority of patients. Unfortunately, recurrence of synovitis may occur. Reports mention figures of 29% [18] and 37% [29] although the recurrence is rarely sufficient to require surgery.

Planning for treatment

While the above account deals with individual parts of the hand the surgeon is faced with a patient whose hands may have many problems. A sequence of operations may be required. Although some advocate combining several major procedures at one sitting [30], it is probably better not to overburden the patient by attempting too much at once. The following are guidelines only and there will be many exceptions. For example, the thumb may be the worst affected digit and need to be treated before the fingers. Decompression of the median nerve for carpal tunnel syndrome takes absolute precedence.

1. Operate on one hand at a time. Occasionally, bilateral wrist surgery may be performed if immediate use of the fingers can be permitted.
2. Operate on proximal joints before distal. Stabilization of the wrist, excision of the distal end of the ulna and extensor tendon surgery, where indicated, should be undertaken first.
3. Flexor synovectomy should usually precede digital joint surgery, and therefore comes next. But, where palmar and proximal subluxation of the metacarpophalangeal joint is present, joint replacement should be carried out first.
4. The metacarpophalangeal joints should be treated before correction of swan-neck deformities. However, an uncorrected severe boutonnière deformity may put a hyperextension stress on a metacarpophalangeal joint arthroplasty and should be dealt with first.
5. Stabilization of the thumb can be combined with any of the other procedures, but if it is left to the last the thumb can be placed in the best position to oppose to the previously operated fingers.

References

1. Hodgson, S. P., Stanley, J. K. and Muirhead, A. (1989) The Wrightington classification of rheumatoid wrist X-rays: a guide to surgical management. *J. Hand Surg.*, **14B**, 451–455.
2. Straub, L. R. and Ranawat, C. S. (1969) The wrist in rheumatoid arthritis: surgical treatment and results. *J. Bone Joint Surg.*, **51A**, 1–20.
3. Kulick, R. G., De Fiore, J. C., Straub, L. R. and Ranawat, C. S. (1981) Long term results of dorsal stabilisation in the rheumatoid wrist. *J. Hand*

Surg., **6**, 272–280.

4. Ishikawa, H., Hanyu, T. and Tajima, T. (1992) Rheumatoid wrists treated with synovectomy of the extensor tendons and the wrist joint combined with a Darrach procedure. *J. Hand Surg.*, **17A**, 1109–1117.

5. Chamay, A., Della Santa, D. and Vilaseca, A. (1983) Radiolunate arthrodesis, factor of stability for the rheumatoid wrist. *Ann. Chir. de la Main*, **2**, 5–17.

6. Stanley, J. K. and Boot, D. A. (1989) Radio-lunate arthrodesis. *J. Hand Surg.*, **14B**, 283–287.

7. Ishikawa, H., Hanyu, T., Saito, H. and Takahashi, H. (1992) Limited arthrodesis for the rheumatoid wrist. *J. Hand Surg.*, **17A**, 1103–1109.

8. Brumfield, R. H. and Champoux, J. A. (1984) A biomechanical study of normal functional wrist motion. *Clin. Orthop.*, **187**, 23–25.

9. Clayton, M. L. and Ferlic, D. C. (1984) Arthrodesis of the arthritic wrist. *Clin. Orthop.*, **187**, 89–93.

10. Millender, L. H. and Nalebuff, E. A. (1973) Arthrodesis of the rheumatoid wrist. An evaluation of sixty patients and a description of a different surgical technique. *J. Bone Joint Surg.*, **55A**, 1026–1034.

11. Swanson, A. B. (1973) *Flexible Implant Resection Arthroplasty in the Hand and Extremities*. Mosby, St Louis, pp. 254–264.

12. Vicar, A. J. and Burton, R. I. (1986) Surgical management of the rheumatoid wrist – fusion or arthroplasty. *J. Hand Surg.*, **11A**, 790–797.

13. Harrison, S. H. (1971) Reconstructive arthroplasty of the metacarpophalangeal joints, using the extensor loop operation. *Br. J. Plast. Surg.*, **24**, 307–309.

14. Swanson, A. B. (1972) Flexible implant arthroplasty for arthritic finger joints: rationale, technique and results of treatment. *J. Bone Joint Surg.*, **54A**, 435–455.

15. Goldner, J. L., Gould, J. S., Urbaniak, J. R. and McCollom, D. E. (1977) Metacarpophalangeal joint arthroplasty with silicone-Dacron prostheses (Niebauer type): six and a half years' experience. *J. Hand Surg.*, **2**, 200–211.

16. Shapiro, J. S. (1982) Wrist involvement in rheumatoid swan-neck deformity. *J. Hand Surg.*, **7**, 484–491.

17. Nalebuff, E. A. and Millender, L. H. (1975) The surgical treatment of swan-neck deformity in rheumatoid arthritis. *Orthop. Clin. North Am.*, **6**, 733–752.

18. Souter, W. A. (1984) The rheumatoid hand. In *Operative Surgery* (eds H. Dudley and D. Carter) Butterworth, London, pp. 363–443.

19. Littler, J. W. and Cooley, S. G. E. (1965) Restoration of the retinacular system in hyperextension deformity of the proximal interphalangeal joint. *J. Bone Joint Surg.*, **47A**, 637.

20. Harrison, S. H. (1974) The Harrison–Nicolle intramedullary peg: follow-up study of 100 cases. *Hand*, **6**, 304–307.

21. Rothwell, A. G. (1978) Repair of established post-traumatic boutonnière deformity. *Hand*, **10**, 241–245.

22. Nalebuff, E. A. and Philips, C. A. (1984) The rheumatoid thumb. In *Rehabilitation of the Hand* (eds J. M. Hunter, L. H. Schneider, E. J. Mackin and A. D. Callahan), 2nd Edition, Mosby, St Louis, pp. 681–694.

23. Nalebuff, E. A. (1969) Extensor pollicis re-routing in the rheumatoid thumb – a new operative approach. *J. Bone Joint Surg.*, **51A**, 790.

24. Barnes, C. G. and Currey, H. L. F. (1967) Carpal tunnel syndrome in rheumatoid arthritis. *Ann. Rheum. Dis.*, **26**, 226–233.

25. Mannerfelt, L. and Norman, O. (1969) Attrition ruptures of flexor tendons in rheumatoid arthritis caused by bony spurs in the carpal tunnel. *J. Bone Joint Surg.*, **51B**, 270–277.

26. Nalebuff, E. A. (1969) Surgical treatment of rheumatoid tenosynovitis in the hand. *Surg. Clin. North Am.*, **49**, 799-809.

27. Harrison, S. H. Ansell, B. and Hall, M. A. (1976) Flexor synovectomy in the rheumatoid hand. *Hand*, **8**, 13–16.

28. Moberg, E. (1965) Tendon grafting and tendon suture in rheumatoid arthritis. *Am. J. Surg.*, **109**, 375–376.

29. Dahl, E., Mikkelsen, O. A. and Sorensen, J. U. (1976) Flexor tendon synovectomy of the hand in rheumatoid arthritis. *Scand. J. Rheumatol.*, **5**, 103–107.

30. Stanley, J. K. and Hullin, M. G. (1986) Wrist arthrodesis as part of composite surgery of the hand. *J. Hand Surg.*, **11B**, 243–244.

25

Surgical treatment of rheumatoid arthritis of the knee

P. Bliss

The mechanics of the knee joint with high load and long leverages make the joint vulnerable to progressive changes either from trauma or inflammation.

Rheumatoid disease produces progressive changes in the knee, initially in the surrounding soft tissues but later in the joint surfaces. In the early stages capillary dilatation occurs in the synovium and is more evident than in a comparable stage in osteoarthritis. By contrast, in the capsule the capillaries are only slightly dilated and they run a straight course when viewed by a magnifying arthroscope, but are not adequately seen with an ordinary arthroscope. Subsequent hypertrophy of the synovium with increasing excretion of fluid produces the early clinical picture of a warm swollen joint. Precipitation of fibrin and necrosis of synovial villi arises as a result of cyclical remission and recurrence of the acute inflammation in rheumatoid arthritis. At this stage there is no apparent change in the articular cartilage, but later a progressive and destructive pannus arises which spreads across the articular surface. It may undermine the margins of the articular cartilage before covering the surface, and small erosions may be revealed on the radiographs (Fig.25.1).

The natural history of the disease in juvenile rheumatoid arthritis shows a spontaneous remission in nearly two-thirds of the patients [1], but progression can occur relentlessly or in a series of peaks, often related to physical or emotional stress. The resulting swelling, effusion and pain are together serious problems which may lead to instability, varus or valgus de-formity, contracture and further destruction of articular cartilage. If this stage is not controlled by medication and suitable rest and splints, then synovectomy should be considered.

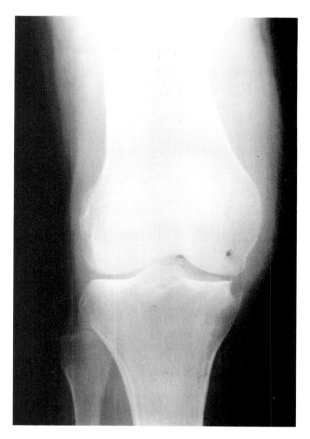

Fig. 25.1 Erosion of the medial tibial condyle in the early stages of rheumatoid arthritis.

Synovectomy

Synovectomy was first performed by Volkmann in 1877 for tuberculosis but in 1900 Mignon reported the operation for rheumatoid arthritis.

Indications

In patients complaining of pain associated with joint swelling due to synovial inflammation, and when free fluid cannot be withdrawn by aspiration due to fibrin deposition. Radiographs should reveal well preserved joint spaces and minimal marginal articular erosion, but there may be some loss of bone density. A steadily rising plasma viscosity is a contraindication to synovectomy but a stable elevated viscosity is not. A more advanced stage of the disease associated with quite definite articular erosions, some fixed deformity and a contracted capsule resulting from 'chemical sympathectomy' are all less favourable indications for synovectomy.

Operation

In essence this is a sub-total excision of knee joint synovium which includes the suprapatellar pouch, medial, lateral and intercondylar recesses with some posterior synovium. A retained area in the proximal part of the suprapatellar region may reduce the tendency for quadriceps adhesions. Degenerate or torn fragments of menisci are also removed. Haemostasis is important, particularly in those fairly active inflammatory joints, and due attention must be paid to the geniculate vessels.

Postoperative care

This is confined to static exercises until the wound has healed; thereafter graduated flexion exercises in the pool or with a continuous passive motion machine are supervised by the physiotherapy team. Manipulation is rarely necessary. Synovectomy carried out arthroscopically either using an electric resectoscope or a mechanical shaver has advantages over open operation but direct articular trauma from repetitive instrumentation is a hazard in inexperienced hands.

Results

A good functional result may be achieved in those patients with monoarthritis in whom the plasma viscosity is stable but elevated, and where there are only minimal radiographic changes. If the resultant good function is maintained for 3 years then there is every chance that it will continue indefinitely. However, although recent surveys [2,3] show promising long term results, the quality diminishes progressively if there are advanced articular erosions at operation.

Juvenile chronic arthritis

This condition introduces other problems including cessation of bone growth or stiffness of joints from a non-cooperative young patient. A review of synovectomy in this young age group

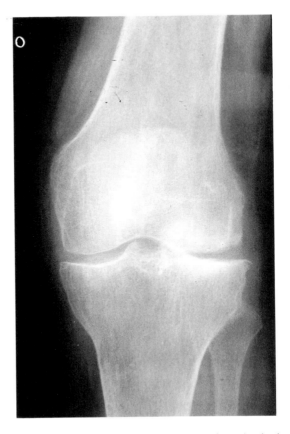

Fig. 25.2 Destruction of articular surfaces in the lateral compartment will not be halted by synovectomy at this stage of the disease.

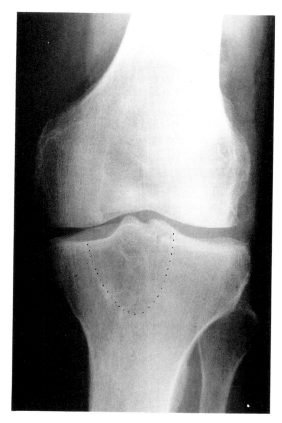

Fig. 25.3 A large bone cyst in the mid-part of the tibia which is a potential hazard.

[4] outlines these extra hazards but in making the decision to perform a synovectomy it is known that cessation of epiphyseal activity and joint stiffness are real complications of the disease. If the child can be relieved of pain, then there is a fair chance that early arthroplasty can be delayed or even avoided. The older the child at the onset of the disease the worse the outlook after synovectomy, and recurrent synovitis is more frequent when the disease is very active particularly in those with polyarthritis.

Finally, synovectomy does not halt the progression of destructive articular damage and indeed these changes may develop in spite of synovectomy but arise in patients with polyarthritis (Fig. 25.2). Progression of the disease not only destroys articular cartilage but causes attenuation of the medial and cruciate ligaments. Bone cysts and destruction of articular surfaces give rise to increasing deformity and disability (Fig. 25.3).

Arthroplasty

The combination of poor bone density and muscle wasting with valgus or varus deformity precludes successful high tibial or low femoral osteotomy to correct alignment and should not be performed for patients with rheumatoid disease although occasional acceptable results are still reported.

Stabilizing the knee joint with collateral ligaments under tension by adequate prosthetic design is the obvious method of management of the more severely damaged knee joint.

In varus deformity the use of a hemi-arthroplasty has been variously reported but it should be noted that in rheumatoid knees the bone density could be questionable and the prosthesis may be unstable and difficult to position. Marmor [5] reports good and excellent results in 106 patients in a series of 137 patients with rheumatoid disease, the better results being in young patients with joint surface destruction. Contra-indications include severe fixed deformities and marked osteoporosis. It is also noted that hemi-arthroplasty used as a bicompartmental implant produced good pain relief but not in patients with angular deformity not correctable by passive stress testing. Unicompartmental replacement tends to be followed by second side degeneration.

A flexion contracture can be corrected by posterior capsular release and excision of osteophytes to stop bony impingement; contractures over 35° require more bone resection.

Correction of valgus deformity is by lateral release from the femur, taking particular care to identify and protect the peroneal nerve; varus deformity is corrected by medial soft tissue release from the tibia to allow realignment of the limb.

Knee prosthetics can be either ligament sparing or ligament resecting and may be constrained, semi-constrained or unconstrained. The patella may or may not be resurfaced.

The meticulous attention to surgical technique in the implantation of knee prosthetics with the correct alignment of the components and adequate fixation reduces the failure rate which in most series is still high. The careful handling of all tissues is essential in order to reduce the incidence of tissue necrosis which is a major cause of wound breakdown. It is recommended that a mid-line or medial curved incision with regard to

Langer's lines is employed. Careful wound closure in layers without tension at the end of the operation, combined with diligent haemostasis and drainage, aim to reduce the incidence of postoperative haemarthrosis and wound haematoma. Recent research has shown that oxygen tensions in the lateral skin flap are significantly reduced in the immediate postoperative period and this relative deficiency is made worse if the knee joint is flexed more than 40° during the first 4 days. The oxygen tension in the skin flaps can be considerably enhanced by supplemental nasal oxygen during this critical time.

The question of perioperative anticoagulant therapy is raised by the incidence of deep vein thrombosis. With serial monitoring of patients using venography and lung scanning, the incidence of vein occlusion is higher than clinically appreciated and appears to be raised with bilateral two stage arthroplasty during the same hospitalisation as opposed to bilateral arthroplasty under the same anaesthetic. Other studies [6] show no difference between bilateral and unilateral arthroplasties, but there appears to be a slightly higher infection rate if second side arthroplasty is performed at a second operation during the same hospitalization or at a later hospitalization.

Assessment of knee function [7] shows that the range of knee movement required for a swing phase of gait is 67° but it requires 83° of knee movement to enable the patient to climb stairs. Slightly more flexion, to 90°, is required to descend stairs and 93° required to rise from a sitting position in a chair provided the femoral axis is parallel with the ground.

Bicompartmental knee joint resurfacing using unlinked femoral and tibial components show, on long term review, that although the success rate was 66%, the failures were due to instability in 13% with component loosening in 7% and infection 3%. Patellar femoral joint pain occurred in 4%.

Deformity of the polyethylene tibial component is a major cause of loosening of tibial elements. This can be resolved in the cementless fixation [1,7] of the tibial component by using a component of adequate thickness to prevent deformation; or by altering the sheer stresses exerted on the tibial component by using a metal plate, possibly with a duocondylar prosthesis

with intercondylar stabilization. Thus in the Oxford knee a non-congruent fit allows slippage between component parts which reduces the sheer stress at the prosthetic/bone interface.

Early reports of arthroplasty of the knee using an endoprosthesis suggested major changes in the management of rheumatoid disease in the knee but also contained warnings of the potential complications. Uniaxial hinges with restrictions built into the prosthesis with metal stops to restrict flexion and extension will produce the familiar click [8] and high impact loads transmitted to the prosthetic medullary stems; thus leading to loosening, particularly in the porotic rheumatoid bone. The experience of the Walldius arthroplasty over prolonged usage bears out this complication.

Selecting a prosthesis

The number of prosthetic implants on the market gives rise to concern. A selection is recorded to illustrate the difficulty in making a suitable choice.

The *Stanmore* modification of the simple hinge, by production of a polyethylene bush and introduction of a femoral tibial angle together with long stems improved the clinical results, although retropatellar problems arose and were a major cause for concern. Early good results at 1 year were maintained for ten years. Further review showed that two thirds of patients had pain relief, four fifths of patients had stable flexion to 90°, but one third complained of retropatellar pain.

The *Kinematic* rotating modification of a simple hinge on review [9,10] in use in rheumatoid disease showed approximately 72% excellent or good results but still problems with infection, implant breakage, patella instability and wound healing. Incomplete non-progressive radiolucent lines of less than 1 mm at the tibial bone interface were considered insignificant, clinically, at 2–4 years postoperatively; but there was some progression of the lucent lines in a review of over 1000 Kinematic knees. There were significant complications: infection in 7%, wound healing problems in 5.5%, peroneal palsy in 3.1% and patella instability in 2.2%.

The *Attenborough* stabilized gliding prosthesis showed good functional results in 92% but there were also wound healing problems and serious prosthetic patellar instability.

The *Geupar* arthroplasty [11] carried an infection rate of over 9%.

Thus the hinged prostheses, incorporating modifications to reduce torque forces, still have a high incidence of loosening and infection.

The *Spherocentric* knee allows 15° of internal and external tibial rotation together with 120° range of knee flexion. It is used in grossly unstable knees with severe fixed deformities or metaphyseal bone loss to give improved ambulation in 92% of patients, whilst avoiding many of the problems of a uniaxial hinge replacement arthroplasty. With total condylar knee replacement it was noted that knees with preoperative flexion of more than 100° lost flexion, whilst knees with less than 100° preoperative flexion gained flexion. A preoperative flexion contracture of more than 10° could be corrected at operation but, on retrospective assessment, the longer rehabilitation took to regain flexion the less was the correction of the preoperative flexion contracture.

Bone lysis

Investigations of bone cement interface activity and bone lysis [12] have identified the histological and histochemical characteristics of the tissue layer between the bone and cement. Synovial like cells adjacent to the cement layer, and cell culture of the membrane contain stellate cells which are similar to those found in cell culture of normal and rheumatoid synovial tissue. It suggests that the membrane has the capacity to produce large amounts of prostaglandin E2 and collagenase which may explain the progressive lysis of bone.

As a result of the problems with fixation of the unrestrained components, development towards cementless fixation utilizing bone ingrowth into the implant has continued and the porous coated anatomical total knee [13] and polypropylene finned pegs are now being used. However, these methods of fixation are unsatisfactory when used within insufficient bone stock, or in severely osteoporotic bone or even in dense sclerotic bone where biological ingrowth is inhibited.

Complications

Prosthetic failure [14]

This can be due to obesity of the patient which has to be regarded as a patient failure. By contrast, joint or primary systemic failure may be due to progressive bone weakness, osteopenia or osteonecrosis resulting from steroid therapy.

Patella displacement

The problems which occur with the patellar femoral compartment vary in different reported series from 5% to 30% and do not appear to be specifically related to implant design. Patellarfemoral lateral tracking problems are higher in constrained hinge prostheses. The greater the valgus angle the higher is the tendency to lateral tracking and subluxation [14].

Lateral tracking should be eliminated at operation. If the patella tends to track laterally with the knee flexed to 90° before closure of the extensor expansion, a lateral release should be performed.

Patella dislocation after knee replacement may be due to trauma, incorrect tracking or malrotation of the tibia and should be treated by proximal realignment, lateral release or revision of the components [15].

Malalignment

The mechanical complexities of knee prostheses carry an inevitable failure rate, and varus malalignment, in particular, is perhaps the worst.

Axial rotation malalignment, if left uncorrected, results in a magnitude of increased sheer stresses at the prosthetic/bone interface beneath the tibial component. It will inevitably approach values equivalent to the body weight and result in loosening [16].

Flexion deformity

It is known that a flexion deformity in rheumatoid arthritis is present in over 60% of knees preoperatively, reduced to 17% postoperatively and in only 21% of prostheses requiring revision.

A second procedure results in reduction of flexion deformity to only 8%. Against this is the relief of pain and reduced need for revision found in those patients with the most serious deformities. It is in the light of their multiple problems which are so great that the relief after a successful knee replacement is not outweighed by their limited but hopefully renewed activity.

Aseptic loosening

The management of aseptic loosening of the total knee replacement [11] using intramedullary stems and metal back tibial component has a high success rate for the relief of pain and flexion to 90° with 80% being able to walk for more than 30 min.

Prosthetic infection

The most serious problem for a surgeon is the management of the infected knee prosthesis. Careful tissue handling at operation cannot be over emphasized as well as antibiotic cover and ideal theatre conditions, in order to minimize primary prosthetic infection. It has been shown [17] that micrococci and diphtheroids are frequent causes of operating theatre infections. Late infections due to haematogenous spread should be reduced again by prophylaxis with pre- and postoperative antibiotics for 48 or 72 h. Subsequently all dental procedures [18] likely to cause gingival bleeding should be covered with penicillin or appropriate antibiotics. Similarly, antibiotic cover is essential for all genitourinary and gastrointestinal procedures and particularly drainage of abscesses.

Reviews of knee prostheses [10,19,20,21] have reported that the rate of infections vary between 1.7% and 16%, but stemmed constrained implants have a higher infection rate particularly in rheumatoid arthritic patients. It is reported [20] that superficial infections of the wound with erythema and delayed healing, when aggressively treated, do not present a major problem with regard to prosthetic infection.

All reviews record that revision arthroplasty for aseptic loosening or malposition carry a higher infection rate by a factor of between 2 and 4.

Primary one-stage exchange arthroplasty requires gentamicin impregnated cement and antibiotic therapy initially by intravenous administration followed by oral therapy for at least 3 months. The antibiotic is designed after appropriate operative specimens have been obtained. This method can give a 60% success rate if used in cases of unconstrained knee revision but without impregnated cement and antibiotic cover the success rate falls to only 35%.

Failure to eliminate prosthetic infection [22] leads to the possibility of resection arthroplasty with excision of all necrotic material, particularly the bone cement and bone cement membrane. After excision the patient remains in a long leg non weight bearing cast for 6 months, after which both active assisted and passive assisted exercises are programmed before weight bearing can be contemplated. A knee brace may be necessary to reduce the inevitable feeling of instability.

Arthodesis

The alternative to resection arthroplasty is to attempt an arthrodesis. Three types of arthrodesis techniques have been used most frequently for salvaging a failed total knee implant, namely, external fixation, internal fixation and intramedullary fixation. Care must be exercised to avoid thin skin flaps. Wide exposure with extensive subperiosteal elevation of tissue adherent to the distal femur and proximal tibia is needed to allow adequate mobilization of the femur and tibia. The debridement of necrotic tissue and prostheses removal should avoid fracturing the bone and preserve the maximum bone stock. The previous wide dissection helps the exposure of the prostheses, and pulsatile irrigation is useful in assisting removal of loose acrylic cement from the intramedullary canals and soft tissues. Accurate apposition of bone ends may be aided by the original prosthetic alignment jigs, and it may be necessary to excise the fibula head to allow the femur and tibia to be closely approximated. A short limb is inevitable.

The fusion technique to be employed is selected and the fixation applied. Proper angulation and rotational alignment can be assisted by using small Kirschner wires in the femur and tibia orientated using the original prosthetic jigs.

Flexion must be secure and rigid and any supplemental bone graft, if used, should be applied around the outside of the bone rather than in the medullary cavity where it is liable to form a series of sequestra.

If skin closure is difficult, delayed primary or secondary closure may be carried out.

External fixation

The use of an external fixator may be difficult if the fusion of two hollow tubes or cortical bone is being attempted. But it should be used where rigid fixation can be achieved and when an adequate quantity of cancellous bone is present such as in failed bicompartmental or unconstrained devices.

Internal fixation

The application of internal fixation plates can be more difficult than external fixation. The more extensive exposure required may warrant the application of more than one plate. They can be applied after removal of stemmed hinged or semiconstrained prostheses have resulted in two hollow cortical tubes. The length of time to obtain fusions, up to 12 months, precludes external fixation with its certainty of retrograde pin track sepsis and loss of rigid fixation. The disadvantage of rigid two plate fixation is that remodelling of the bone after fusion may be inhibited and predispose to fracture at the ends of the plate. Thus, after fusion, the plates should be removed.

Intramedullary fixation

The use of a long pre-bent intramedullary nail can be successfully employed on occasions. The technique utilizes the relatively normal bone in the proximal femur and mid tibia to achieve adequate fixation. Careful planning preoperatively is required so that rods of appropriate length and curve are available.

All attempts at fusion must be covered with appropriate antibiotics for at least 3 months.

Failure to control infection either by exchange

of implant, resection arthroplasty or fusion leads to a distressing and disabling discharge from the operation site which, if not controlled, may become life threatening. Reports of failures of knee arthroplasty [19,20] contain a small number of mid thigh amputations. The use of amputation may be in the patient's best interest from the aspect of pain relief, absence of a chronic discharge and a mobile lower limb prosthesis with knee flexion, but the energy requirements and physical muscle power needed to mobilize independently with an artificial limb may well not be possible in a rheumatoid arthritic patient with multiple joint involvement. Consequently, amputation most frequently results in the patient being confined to a wheelchair for the remainder of their life.

References

1. Laaksonen, A-L. (1966) A prognostic study of juvenile arthritis, analysis of 544 cases. *Acta Pediatr. Scand.*, Suppl. 166.
2. Brattstrom, H. (1985) Co-ordinating E.R.A.S.S. long term results after synovectomy for adult rheumatoid arthritis. *Clin. Rheumatol.*, **4**, 19–22.
3. Ishikawa, H., Ohnd, O. and Hirohata, K. (1986) Long term results of synovectomy in rheumatoid arthritis. *J. Bone Joint Surg.*, **68A**, 198–205.
4. Rydholm, U., Elborgh, R., Ranstam, J. *et al.* (1986) Synovectomy of the knee in juvenile chronic arthritis. *J. Bone Joint Surg.*, **68B**, 223–228.
5. Marmor, L. (1982) The Marmor knee replacement. *Orthop. Clin. North Am.*, **13(1)**, 55–64.
6. Morrey, B. E., Adams, R. A., Ilstrup, D. M. and Bryan, R. S. (1987) Complications and mortality association with bilateral or unilateral total knee arthroplasty. *J. Bone Joint Surg.*, **69A**, 484–488.
7. Laubenthal, K. N., Smidt, G. L. and Kettlekamp, D. B. (1972) A quantitative analysis of knee motion during the activities of daily living. *Phys. Ther.*, **52**, 34–42.
8. Matthews, L. S. and Kaufer, H. (1982) The spherocentric knee: a perspective of 7 years clinical experience. *Orthop. Clin. North Am.*, **13(1)**, 173–186.
9. Ewald, F. C., Jawbs, M. A., Miegel, R. E. *et al.* (1984) Kinematic total knee replacement. *J. Bone Joint Surg.*, **66A**, 1032–1048.
10. Rand, J. A., Chad, E. Y. S. and Stauffer, R. N. (1987) Kinematic rotating hinge total knee replacement. *J. Bone Joint Surg.*, **69A**, 489–497.
11. Bertin, K. C., Freeman, M. A. R., Samuelson,

K. M. *et al.* (1985) Stemmed revision arthroplasty for aseptic loosening of total knee replacement. *J. Bone Joint Surg.*, **67B**, 242–248.

12. Goldring, S. R., Schiller, A. L., Roelke, M. *et al.* (1983) Synovial like membrane at bone cement interface in loose total hip replacement and its role in bone lysis. *J. Bone Joint Surg.*, **65A**, 575–584.

13. Hungerford, D. S., Kenna, R. V. and Krackow, K. A. (1982) Porous coated anatomic total knee. *Orthop. Clin. North Am.*, **13, 1**, 103–122.

14. Matthews, L. S. and Goldstein, B. (1986) Biomechanical causes and prevention of failed joint replacement. *Curr. Orthop.*, **1**, 1.

15. Merkow, R. I., Soudry, M. and Insall, J. N. (1985) Patella dislocation after total knee replacement. *J. Bone Joint Surg.*, **67A**, 1321–1327.

16. Kagan, A. II (1977) Mechanical causes of loosening of knee joint replacement. *J. Biomech.*, **10**, 387–391.

17. Bechtol, C. O. (1979) Environmental bacteriology in a unidirectional (vertical) operating room. *Arch, Surg.*, **114**, 784–788.

18. Irvine, R., Johnson, B. L. and Amstutz, H. C. (1974) Relationship with genitourinary procedures and deep sepsis after total hip replacement. *Surg. Gynaecol. Obst.*, **139**, 701–706.

19. Grogan, T. J., Dorey, F., Rollins, I. and Amstutz, H. C. (1981) Deep sepsis following total knee arthroplasty. *J. Bone Joint Surg.*, **68A**, 226–234.

20. Johnson, D. P. and Bannister, G. C. (1986) The outcome of infected arthroplasty of the knee. *J. Bone Joint Surg.*, **68B**, 289–291.

21. Schurman, D. J. (1981) Functional outcome of Guepar hinge knee arthroplasty evaluated with Aramis. *Clin. Orthop.*, **155**, 118–132.

22. Stulberg, S. D. (1982) Arthrodesis in failed total knee replacement. *Orthop. Clin. North Am.*, **13** (1), 213–224.

26

Rheumatoid arthritis of the ankle and foot

J. R. Kirkup

Treatment for the painful rheumatoid foot is a challenge which demands both assessment of current pathology and an appreciation of future changes based on the natural history of a disease process which can involve some 25 closely related joints. Thus the severely disabled foot presents: (i) multiple joint damage, often at different stages of evolution and asymmetrically distributed between the two feet (Fig.26.1), (ii) a commonly progressive yet often erratic pathology which renders the feet elusive targets for considered surgical opinion, and also (iii) problems in management priorities posed by proximal disability especially at the knee.

Clinically it is useful to separate the hindfoot from the forefoot; the former embraces the ankle, subtaloid, mid-tarsal, naviculo-cuneiform, inter-cuneiform and tarso-metatarsal joints, and the latter the metatarso-phalangeal and toe joints. Hindfoot pathology dictates the attitude and stability of the foot, that is whether it is valgus, varus, equinus or calcaneus. Forefoot pathology leads to severe disorganization with dislocation of the toes and callosity problems due to shoe containment and weight-bearing pressures. Whilst both areas may be attacked simultaneously or consecutively, in practice either hindfoot or forefoot disease predominates at any one time.

In a survey of 200 consecutive rheumatoid patients admitted to the Bristol Royal Infirmary and the Royal National Hospital for Rheumatic Diseases in Bath, 104 were noted to have pain or deformity involving the feet, this being second only to the knee as a source of symptoms [1]. Of 204 feet analysed, radiological changes were seen in 176 forefeet (metatarso-phalangeal and toe joints) and 133 hindfeet (124 mid tarsal, 64 sub-taloid and 52 ankle joints); additionally, erosion

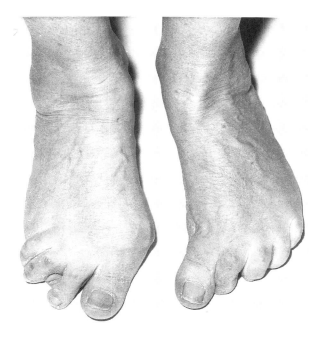

Fig. 26.1 Asymmetrical changes in rheumatoid arthritis. The right foot shows classical hallux valgus with dorsal dislocations of the lesser toes except the fifth which underlies its fellows in a varus position. The left foot shows unusual varus of all the toes and severe flexion of the lesser toes. The right hindfoot is valgus and the left cavo-varus.

of the os calcis was observed in 11 feet, whilst 55 feet assumed a valgus and 2 feet a varus heel profile, It was clear that disease of the metatarso-phalangeal and inter-tarsal joints commonly co-existed, whilst the ankle joint often remained intact. Further, unlike the other joints, 55% of radiologically damaged inter-tarsal joints were not a source of complaint at the time of examination. As we will demonstrate shortly, the inter-tarsal joints often ankylose and fuse spontaneously.

Proximal joint disease and the foot

Fixed flexion deformity at the hip and particularly at the knee induces a dorsi-flexed attitude of the foot under load. If fixed flexion persists, a diseased ankle may lose plantar-flexion yet maintain dorsi-flexion. On the other hand, if the knees are straight, fixed equinus at the ankle may result and is a hindrance to walking without a raised heel; such equinus then overloads the forefoot joints.

Valgus of the knee compounds or is compounded by valgus of the foot and may compromise treatment. Generally knee valgus is painful and unstable whereas foot valgus may be pain free and can be stabilized by apparatus. Unless foot valgus is severe and associated with skin breakdown, the knee takes operative precedence. However, severe forefoot disorganization with plantar callosities uncontrolled by suitable shoes, or associated with skin breakdown, takes precedence over both knee and hip disability.

The hindfoot

Natural history

We examined 150 consecutive adult patients attending the Foot Clinic of the Royal National

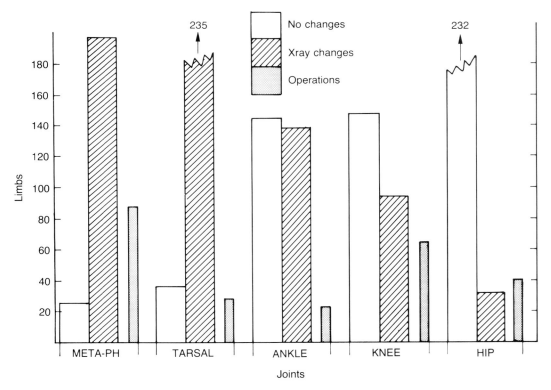

Fig. 26.2 Survey of 150 patients complaining of the hindfoot: radiographic changes and surgical operations due to rheumatoid in 300 lower limbs.

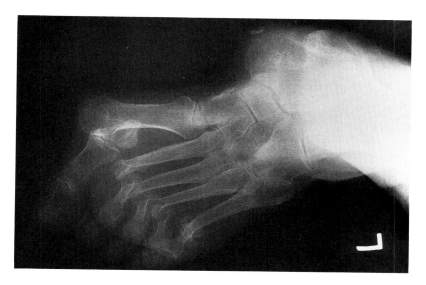

Fig. 26.3 Talo-navicular dislocation with minimal bone destruction: the opacity medial to the weight-bearing talar head was sited in sloughing skin and tendon. The forefoot shows classical destructive changes with dislocation of the hallux.

Hospital for Rheumatic Diseases complaining of the hindfoot, usually bilaterally. All had attended the Clinic for at least 1 year and had proven rheumatoid arthritis present from 2 to 47 years, an average of 15 years. A radiographic survey of the 300 lower limbs (Fig. 26.2) demonstrated joint pathology or previous operation in: (i) 92% of the forefeet, (ii) 88% of the inter-tarsal joints, (iii) 52% of the ankles, (iv) 51% of the knees and (v) 23% of the hips.

As the figure indicates, although the hip was often spared disease, the chance of surgical intervention relative to pathological damage was high. By contrast, surgery for the knee and forefoot was less likely, whilst surgery for the hindfoot was least likely, despite a high incidence of pathology.

Of the 300 feet, almost two-thirds presented a valgus attitude, principally due to inter-tarsal joint subluxation but also due to tilting of the talus in the ankle mortise, or both. Standing radiographs were necessary to measure valgus or varus at the ankle joint. Varus and equinus was uncommon, the latter being associated with ankle joint pathology.

What is understood by radiographic change? Clearly many hindfeet joints manifested narrowing and erosions, leading to joint destruction and often spontaneous ankylosis or arthrodesis. However some inter-tarsal joints without these articular changes were pathologically subluxated and occasionally dislocated (Fig. 26.3). Observation of weight-bearing serial radiographs of individual ankle joints confirmed that changes were often minimal or indeed absent before significant tilting of the talus promoted bone destruction (Fig. 26.4). Fusion was common especially between the joints of the os calcis, talus, navicular, cuboid and cuneiforms. The ankle joint rarely fused and then usually in chair-bound patients; nevertheless, this joint frequently stiffened and developed secondary osteophytosis.

Of 247 surgical procedures performed on these 300 lower limbs, 45 operations (19%) involved the hindfoot and included 28 inter-tarsal and ankle arthrodeses, five osteotomies, two ankle synovectomies combined with tarsal arthrodeses and ten total ankle replacements.

This analysis of 150 patients, supported by more extensive experience, suggested the following:

(i) If the ankle joint is diseased then the tarsal joints are already or will shortly be affected. By contrast, if the tarsal joints are diseased then the ankle joint may escape.

(ii) The tarsal joints commonly ankylose and fuse spontaneously, the ankle joint only rarely.

(iii) Valgus deformity of the foot is common either with or without tarsal ankylosis. Severe valgus and tarsal ankylosis is often associated with subluxation of the ankle joint. Severe valgus and hypermobility sometimes leads to talo-navicular subluxation and occasionally frank dislocation.

(iv) Extreme valgus stresses, distorts and fractures the fibula; even the tibia may undergo stress fracture (Fig. 26.5).

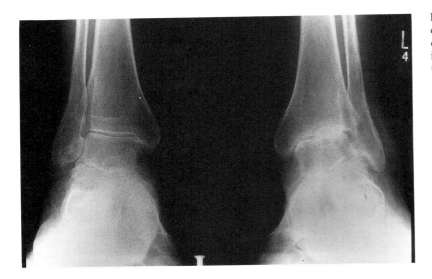

Fig. 26.4 Standing radiographs demonstrating subtalar valgus deformity on the left associated with valgus tilting in the ankle mortise and collapse of the tibia laterally.

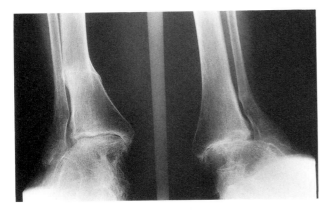

Fig. 26.5 Severe hindfoot disease with bilateral total tarsal ankylosis, in extreme valgus, aggravating ankle disease to cause fibular and tibial stress fractures.

(v) Extreme valgus generates painful weight-bearing callouses opposite the navicular and head of the talus which often progress to skin necrosis.

(vi) Most patients can be treated conservatively.

Hindfoot movements [2]

Accurate measurement of ankle joint movement is only possible by radiological means, for clinical separation from inter-tarsal movement is impossible unless the tarsus is fused. If the tarsus is mobile then significant plantar-flexion of the foot is possible at the mid tarsal joint. It is a practical compromise to measure dorsi-flexion and plantar-flexion actively with the assistance of the clinician passively, when the knees are extended on a couch, using the sole of the foot as an indicator in relation to the shin. Thus if there is fixed equinus of the mid-tarsal joint with mobility in the ankle, the above technique will indicate whether the sole of the foot can achieve a plantigrade position or not, at least when barefoot. Separate movements of the subtaloid, mid-tarsal and other inter-tarsal joints cannot be estimated accurately and the global peritalar movements of foot pronation and supination are a better assessment of foot function, again using the sole of the foot as an indicator.

The theoretical movements of eversion and abduction and of inversion and adduction are considered to equal pronation and supination, respectively. Such movements do not necessarily disappear if the tarsus is fused for they may develop in a painfree mobile ankle. In summary, it is more realistic to determine movement of the foot as a whole in relation to the leg rather than individual joint movements.

The ankle joint

Clinical

This joint is the least likely to be involved in the adult foot. However, in juvenile polyarthritis [3] the ankle is initially the most involved joint, although at a later date the ankle often recovers and the inter-tarsal joints become major targets. Ankle pain is felt diffusely around the joint between the malleoli and should be distinguishable from subtaloid pain, usually felt beneath the lateral malleolus, and talo-navicular pain somewhat distal to the medial malleolus. It is important to ask the patient to indicate with one finger the site of pain when walking.

Admittedly, pain location may be difficult, especially if both ankle and subtaloid joints are active. Even a pain relieving injection may prove uncertain because connections between the ankle and subtaloid joints via tendon sheaths have been demonstrated [4]. Early pain is associated with swelling in the joint itself and frequently the tendon sheaths of the peronei, tibialis posterior and tibialis anterior. Severe pain and swelling are associated with loss of dorsi-flexion and the foot may assume an equinus position. Repeated attacks lead to radiological changes and increasing stiffness. In the later stages tendon swelling often diminishes and both dorsi- and plantar-flexion are lost. A few patients giving a history of an ankle fracture prior to the onset of arthritis find this ankle becomes a target joint and a source of early disability.

Radiology

In the survey of Vidigal *et al.* [1] clinical symptoms and signs were present in 97 ankles yet only 52 developed radiological changes. Persistent disease, however, leads to joint narrowing, followed by subcortical cysts, collapse and joint destruction, stress fractures and secondary osteophytes (Fig. 26. 5) but spontaneous fusion is rare. If the tarsus is ankylosed and in valgus or varus, undue concentration of pressure at the points of contact of the talus in the mortice produces distinct acceleration of destructive disease and disability.

Radiological changes may remain unilateral or if bilateral appear contemporaneously or consecutively.

Conservative treatment

In addition to general treatment, acute flare-ups may require bed-rest and plaster of Paris casts.

Local injections of steroid via an antero-lateral portal [4] often help to keep the patient mobile and can be repeated depending on the general condition, but are best avoided if surgery is being contemplated. When less acute, a cosmetic caliper, an ankle-foot brace or formal below-knee double steels with boots or bootees may assist weight-bearing mobility, especially where there is a correctable valgus or varus posture. However, apparatus is less likely to help when fixed changes develop.

Surgical treatment

If disability persists despite conservative measures and the patient has adequate arterial circulation, surgical relief must be debated. The procedures available are synovectomy, surgical decompression of the lateral compartment of the joint, arthrodesis or replacement arthroplasty.

Synovectomy is mainly directed to adjacent tendon sheaths and can be undertaken as an adjunct to tarsal fusion if synovial swelling does not respond to injection therapy. Good results have been reported in early cases [5].

A valgus foot may cause pain limited to the lateral malleolus by impingement against the calcaneum [6], and resection of the distal fibula to decompress the adjacent talar facet, with local synovectomy, is simple and often provides relief.

In more advanced cases, arthrodesis may be the best option, especially if disability is unilateral, if the peritalar joints remain mobile and if the patient is a large male still employed in moderately heavy work. An antero-lateral approach dividing the fibula at the level of the joint is recommended, which gives ready access and permits correction of deformity if present. When good contact is achieved the position is maintained using staples with the foot in neutral; if the joint is fused in equinus this stresses the forefoot and the knees. However, if there is fixed flexion of the knees, then ankle fusion in slight dorsi-flexion may be required. Unfortunately fusion takes time and requires the patient to be non-weight-bearing for 6 weeks or so and at least 6 further weeks in a walking cast. In our experience, rheumatoid patients do not cope well with compression clamps which often damage the fragile skin of the other leg and can become loose in the os calcis.

Ankle replacement

If severe disability involves both ankles, the question of joint replacement arises because the alternative of bilateral ankle arthrodesis in the presence of previous bilateral tarsal ankylosis and fixed great toes, results in the knees being the most distal mobile joints, a severe handicap when attempting to rise from a chair or lavatory seat [7]. For these patients ankle joint replacement, at least unilaterally, offers significant advantages and moreover a relatively quick return to weight-bearing, unlike arthrodesis.

It is not pretended that ankle replacement has achieved the success of hip replacement and indeed some reports recommend that the ankle prostheses now available are not satisfactory for rheumatoid patients [8]. The I.C.L.H. prosthesis [9] and several other prostheses are constrained and aim to provide dorsi- and plantar-flexion only. We believe that a 'ball and socket' prosthesis is advantageous in the ankle to permit polyaxial movement. The rationale for utilizing a 'ball and socket' or sphero-centric joint is derived from the observation that children with congenital tarsal fusion often have a 'ball and socket' configuration of the ankle with universal motion of the foot, that is the ankle assumes additional subtaloid and mid-tarsal function. If the peritalar joints are fixed, the ankle is subject to pronatory and supinatory strains and thus it is logical to opt for an unconstrained prosthesis with the possibility of polyaxial motion. As with total hip arthroplasty, surgical placement of a polyaxial ankle prosthesis is less critical than that of a uniaxial prosthesis.

No incision is ideal for ankle replacement. Access includes a trans-fibular approach allowing partial subluxation of the joint and a posterior approach [6] detaching the insertion of the Achilles tendon with a block of the os calcis. Bone division, however, retards early weight-bearing, or may result in delayed union and slow rehabilitation. Thus an anterior approach between extensor hallucis longus and extensor digitorum is recommended, taking the vessels medially; this is minimally invasive, provides satisfactory exposure of both malleoli and allows early weight-bearing. Unlike hip and knee replacement procedures, the ankle is not dislocated and therefore, the insertion of the talar component is assisted by os calcis pin traction, to avoid impacting acrylic cement into the posterior compartment of the joint. Careful handling of the skin is also vital as it is often thin and prone to slow cicitrization in patients on steroids.

In 1979, Demottaz *et al.* [10] studied 21 total ankle replacements of which 16 were for rheumatoid arthritis, at an average follow-up of 14.7 months. The follow-up was very comprehensive and included gait analysis and electromyographic studies. Pain relief was considered complete in only four instances, whilst radiolucent lines were present in 19 joints of which two were loose. Seven of the joints were Smith or similar multiple-axis joints whilst the remainder were single-axis articulations principally of the Mayo design. In this small series of short follow-up, no significant difference between the two groups was observed. They concluded that ankle arthrodesis was the operation of choice except for elderly patients with limited mid-tarsal motion. In 1985, Bolton-Maggs *et al.* [8] followed up 41 of 62 uniaxially designed I.C.L.H. ankle prostheses inserted between 1972 and 1981 (mean follow-up 5.5 years), during which the prosthesis was modified several times and both anterior and posterior approaches were used. Of 34 arthroplasties for rheumatoid arthritis, seven were lost to follow-up, five were arthrodesed for loosening and 22 were reviewed. Pain was absent in seven, mild in seven, moderate in five and severe in three. The average range of movement changed from 18° to 23° and walking ability generally was improved. Only six rheumatoid arthroplasties were considered fully satisfactory and it was concluded that total ankle replacement could not be recommended as a long term solution; however, they also observed that arthrodesis in rheumatoid arthritis might be less satisfactory than for osteoarthritis.

Other reports have been more optimistic. In 1982, Herberts *et al.* [11], reporting on 18 I.C.L.H. prostheses at a mean of 36 months and of which 13 were for rheumatoid arthritis, concluded that ankle arthroplasty has a definite place in the treatment of severe arthritis in rheumatoid patients; they considered the osteoarthritic ankle did less well and found a high incidence of loosening and radiolucent zones. In 1984, Lachiewicz *et al.* [12], reporting on 15 uniaxial arthroplasties (14 being of the Mayo type) all for rheumatoid arthritis, at a mean of 39 months, noted gratifying pain relief and rated

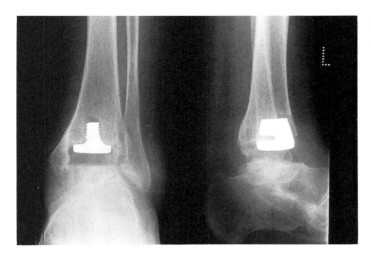

Fig. 26.6 Richard Smith ankle arthroplasty. Note absence of barium in the cement and that the medial malleolus underwent stress fracture following surgery. Joint still functioning at 12 years.

seven ankles excellent and eight good; nevertheless, 11 ankles developed radiolucent lines and six components showed evidence of subsidence.

Our own experience supports the view that arthroplasty benefits the severely disabled rheumatoid with bilateral hindfoot disease. Of 20 polyaxial Smith prostheses (Fig. 26.6) inserted for rheumatoid arthritis in 17 patients between 1975 and 1979, 15 were reviewed at a mean of 7 years; six components were undoubtedly loose mainly in the tibia, yet the patients continued walking, whilst nine had no or little pain although two of these had no movement [13]. This experience suggested that whilst the polyaxial design was safe and not prone to dislocation, the single thickness design restricted choice in accommodating variations of vertical joint space, despite a standard bone resection, due to differing ligamentous tensions between patients. We therefore designed a prosthesis with a polyethylene tibial implant which can be trimmed to size in the antero-posterior plane and is cemented *in situ* under pressure with a special clamp, and steel talar implants of 2, 3, 4, 5, and 6 mm thickness inserted using pin traction (Fig. 26.7). A preliminary report [14] on 25 arthroplasties in 20 patients at a minimum follow-up of 3 years was encouraging; it was noteworthy that having undergone one arthroplasty, several patients asked for surgery on the opposite ankle. A fuller account was presented to the College Internationale de Podologie meeting in 1987, when 24 Smith joints (1975–79) and 66 Bath joints (1980–85) were surveyed. Of the 90 arthro-

plasties, 77 were for rheumatoid arthritis including ten patients with bilateral replacements.

Late infection occurred at 1, 7 and 8 years respectively. No osteoarthritic patients had wound problems. At follow-up, seven patients had died and two limbs were amputated, all for reasons unconnected with their ankle surgery. Ten joints were removed for infection and loosening. Of 71 joints available for follow-up, 47 had no pain or minor pain and only one had severe pain associated with ischaemia. The gain in ankle movement was modest and 12 ankles were stiffer. Of the Smith joints followed for a mean of 10 years 55% were intact; of the Bath joints followed for a mean of 4.2 years 74% remained intact.

If these results cannot compare favourably with current hip and knee total replacement arthroplasties, they resemble the sequelae of hip arthroplasty at its inception and of knee arthroplasty some 15 years ago. Recent innovations including three-part prostheses, two-stage procedures and uncemented components raise expectations that second generation techniques will parallel the evolution of knee replacement.

The intertarsal joints

Clinical

Pain, stiffness and deformity are the principal complaints; more rarely severe varus can produce instability and severe valgus ulceration over the

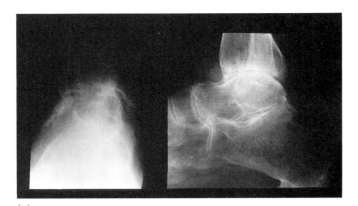

(a)

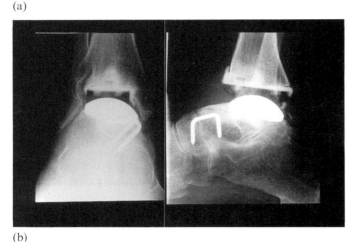

(b)

Fig. 26.7 Bath and Wessex ankle joint. The talar component is 3 mm in height. At operation the talo-navicular joint was found to be slightly mobile and a staple was inserted. Joint still functioning well at 7 years.

medial aspect of the foot (Fig. 26.3); severe valgus may also be associated with rupture of the tendon of tibialis posterior. The intertarsal joints often ankylose spontaneously either in neutral or deformity. If fixed in valgus whilst the ankle joint remains mobile, the fibula distorts or even undergoes stress fracture (Fig. 26.5), causing temporary pain.

The talo-navicular joint can be the first to cause symptoms but generally the patient presents with pain sited beneath the lateral malleolus arising in the subtaloid joint. Frequently this pain is minimal or moderate, or overshadowed by more acute pain in the forefoot, ankle or other joints, and it may subside as the joints quietly ankylose.

Radiology

Despite pain and swelling radiological changes are often minimal. Ultimately joint narrowing, erosions and cysts appear often commencing in the talo-navicular joint. Spontaneous ankylosis is not infrequent and sometimes the whole tarsus becomes a single osseous entity. Patients with a propensity to subluxation and dislocation develop extreme valgus deformity (see Fig. 26.3).

Conservative treatment

Localized pain in the talo-navicular or subtaloid joints often responds to local injections of steroid and may need to be repeated before eventual ankylosis. More persistent pain is relieved by a below-knee plaster cast but this is not practical when the symptoms are bilateral. Fusion may follow repeated plaster immobilization if the foot can be held in neutral position More chronic pain, especially that associated with mobile valgus deformity, benefits from splintage, either a polyethylene cosmetic splint or steel calipers.

Surgical treatment

The absolute indications for surgery are persistent pain, foot instability and skin necrosis. Stiffness and deformity are not primary indications in themselves and the surgeon is cautioned against believing that complete correction of valgus deformity is a long term possibility, as this often proves illusory (Fig.26.8).

If signs are localized to the subtaloid joint, fusion of this joint alone is recommended. This will prevent pro-supination but preserve dorsiplantarflexion at the mid-tarsal joint. A lateral approach gives adequate access; to correct minor valgus, bone chips from the malleolus or os calcis can be packed into the joint; more obvious valgus may need iliac crest bone in the sinus tarsi.

When symptoms are localized to the talonavicular joint, fusion of this joint alone is required, utilizing a short medial incision to excise minimal bone from the articular surfaces and hold with staples or a screw. This blocks all movement in the peritalar joints and causes the undamaged joints to ankylose quietly.

Damage to all the intertarsal joints may result in severe valgus and uncovering of the talar head; for this two incisions are best, one to remove a wedge of bone medially from the talo-navicular joint and the other to excise the calcaneo-cuboid and subtaloid joints. Bone from the talar head and/or the iliac crest can be packed in laterally to aid correction; os calcis osteotomy is sometimes necessary. Full correction of the valgus may

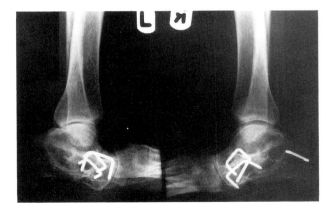

Fig. 26.8 Bilateral tarsal fusions with corrective osteotomy of the right os calcis. Standing lateral radiographs after successful fusions demonstrate valgus recurring distal to the fused segment, at the naviculo-cuneiform joints.

result in supination of the forefoot which must be avoided. Thus a valgus attitude often remains and even after solid fusion in a corrected position, a valgus attitude can recur either in the distal tarsus (Fig. 26.8) or by tilting of the talus in the ankle mortise (see Fig. 26.4).

Nevertheless, tarsal fusions are very successful in resolving pain [15] and would be undertaken more willingly if these did not demand 5–6 weeks non-weight-bearing and up to a total of 12 weeks in plaster.

The forefoot

As indicated above, the forefoot is the most commonly attacked segment of the foot and also rivals the hand in presenting the earliest evidence of rheumatoid disease.

A mobile, painfree forefoot enables the toes to function as a platform for push-off in walking and also contributes to the balance, especially when standing still; if the hallux plays a dominant role, the remaining toes make a significant contribution and therefore it is important to view the forefoot as a single functional unit. Nevertheless, the pathomechanics of rheumatoid damage of the first ray as against the lesser rays is distinct and these differences will be emphasized.

Natural history

In a survey of 100 patients with foot symptoms, we identified deformity of the hallux in 93 patients of which 70 had bilateral changes [16]. This survey demonstrated that at the first metatarso-phalangeal joint, the commonest deformity was valgus and involved 60% of the feet, whilst hallux rigidus (dorsi-flexion 20° or less) involved 28% and hallux elevatus (absence of plantar-flexion) involved 10%. These deformities often overlapped and thus some two-thirds of rigid and elevated toes were also in valgus. Rigidus is equated with considerable intra-articular damage often leading to spontaneous fusion, even in a valgus position in some instances, and also hyperextension of the inter-phalangeal joint which, if extreme, forces the toe nail to cut through the upper of the shoe, the so-called 'chisel toe'. Elevatus is associated with inability of the hallux to take weight and also 'chisel toe'

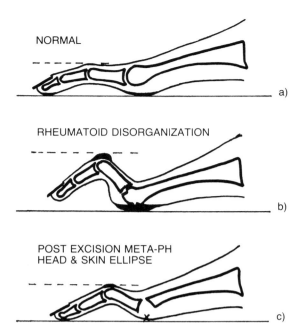

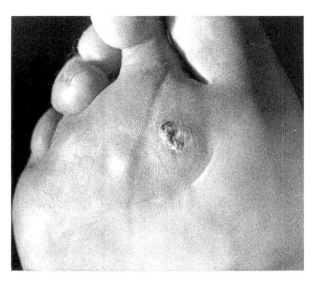

Fig. 26.10 Rheumatoid toe dislocations, metatarsal head callosities and skin necrosis overlying second metatarsal.

Fig. 26.9 Diagram of lesser toe and metatarsal: (a) normal, to demonstrate vertical clearance necessary for toe; (b) rheumatoid dislocation with secondary toe hammering and increased vertical clearance; (c) following excision of metatarsal head and plantar skin ellipse.

deformity; overall, the latter deformity involved 22% of the feet. Only one foot displayed hallux varus whilst three first metatarso-phalangeal joints were truly dislocated.

In another survey [17] we noted that severe valgus deformity precedes dislocation of the proximal phalanx laterally between the first and the second metatarsal heads (Fig. 26.3); dislocation of the phalanx medially and into flexion is very rare but we observed three great toes dislocated dorsally. By contrast, at the metatarso-phalangeal joints of the second, third, fourth and to a variable extent the fifth toe, dorsal dislocation is the commonest deformity promoting excess pressure on the metatarsal heads (Fig. 26.9). At times the lesser toes drift into valgus without dislocating dorsally.

The metatarso-phalangeal joints

Clinical

Swelling of these joints leads to a complaint of tight shoes and with progression of the disease,

bunion pressure and plantar pain with callosities, especially opposite the second and third metatarsal heads; this metatarsalgia is often described by the patient as 'walking on stones'. Increasing deformity and unsuitable shoes may result in skin breakdown and ulceration of the callosities, sometimes leading to deep infection and bone destruction. The bunion area does not normally develop a bony exostosis, and is simply painful as a result of severe valgus and accompanying metatarsus primus varus; the overlying skin may also break down (Fig. 26.10). Valgus is only one component of a three-dimensional deformity and is associated with tortus, that is medial torsion of the toe, which may exceed 60° in severe cases [17] and cause a painful callosity on the medial aspect of the inter-phalangeal joint. In many patients, all these problems co-exist.

Radiology

Standing antero-posterior and lateral radiographs should be obtained whenever possible to assess deformity of the hallux and especially metatarsus primus varus which can exceed 20°. Note that the sesamoids remain in constant relationship to the base of the proximal phalanx even when the latter is severely subluxated or dislocated (Fig. 26.3). The considerable strength of the ligaments and tendons connecting the sesamoids to the phalanx prevents dislocation of the hallux more readily.

Standard radiographs display lesser toe dislocation somewhat imperfectly due to overlap, and a tangential view of the metatarsal heads is useful; this highlights the prominence of the heads and demonstrates their destruction to spike-like remnants in severe cases.

Conservative treatment

In the first instance, wider shoes with a lower heel and a simple metatarsal neck support may suffice. If a single joint is persistently swollen, an intra-articular injection of steroid may help. More serious deformity, especially when the toes dislocate, requires the manufacture of special lightweight shoes from plaster casts; such shoes provide increased depth to accommodate the toes and cushioning to relieve metatarsal head pain [18]. Many patients do not require any other measures.

Surgical treatment

Synovectomy of metatarso-phalangeal joints has been advocated but is best undertaken before deformity arises; very few patients are prepared to accept such surgery when local injections and suitable shoes are easier alternatives.

Helal [19] and others recommend tread-levelling osteotomies by oblique section through the distal metatarsal shaft combined with a Wilson osteotomy of the first metatarsal to correct hallux valgus. If the toes are totally dislocated, operative elevation of the metatarsal heads also elevates the toes and hence they remain functionless and special shoes are required to accommodate them. Nevertheless, in early cases with minor toe subluxation, multiple Helal osteotomies can be very successful.

Radical surgery includes excision arthroplasty of all the metatarso-phalangeal joints; experience has shown that removing one or two prominent metatarsal heads is unsatisfactory, for the patient soon returns with callosities beneath the remaining metatarsals. This procedure was first suggested by Hoffmann in 1912, since when it has undergone various modifications. Fowler [20] ad-

vised a dorsal approach to remove the metatarsal heads and bases of the proximal phalanges combined with removal of a plantar ellipse of skin. Kates *et al.* [21] advised a plantar approach to remove the metatarsal heads and their necks leaving the phalanges intact, removing skin from the sole and the insertion of a stabilizing wire into the first ray. If sufficient bone is removed, both these procedures relieve pain and improve the appearance of the foot. In our experience the Fowler procedure leaves the toes rather floppy and weak, whereas the Kates procedure ensures better control of the toes presumably because the attachments to the proximal phalanx are not disturbed. The results of excision arthroplasty of the metatarsal heads are mostly excellent in relieving metatarsal head pain and in improving function generally (Fig. 26.11). Often patients can buy commercial shoes and remain comfortable. However, hallux valgus may recur, for which reason some surgeons fuse the first metatarso-phalangeal joint and claim better long term results. Recurrent metatarsal pain may be the consequence of leaving a metatarsal shaft too long, of a tender scar or to the formation of rheumatoid nodules [22].

Regnauld [23] has advocated removal of the metatarsal heads and implantation on the metatarsal shafts of homograft metatarsal heads and claims these incorporate well. This is a highly skilled and time-consuming procedure and also may be limited by the supply of suitable metatarsal heads. Cracchiolo [24] has advised multiple joint replacements with Swanson silastic implants. This too is time-consuming and also difficult, especially for the smaller toes. Gould [25] recommends silastic replacement of the first metatarso-phalangeal joint and excision arthroplasty of the remaining metatarsals and has achieved good results.

The inter-phalangeal joints

The problems of the lesser toes are generally secondary to their dislocation on the metatarsals, leading to muscle imbalance and flexion or hammering of the inter-phalangeal joints. Severe hallux valgus can induce further deformity by pressure against the lesser toes or by under or over-riding the second and sometimes the third toes.

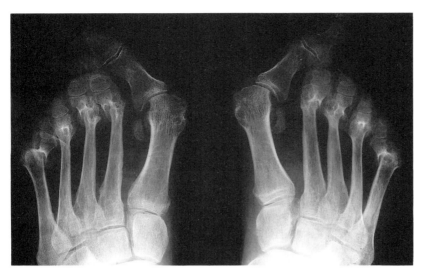

(a)

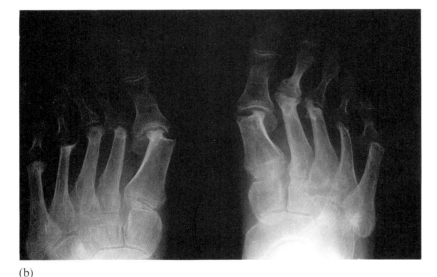

(b)

Fig. 26.11 Severely disorganized forefeet, before and after Kates–Kessel metatarsal head and neck excisions. The right first metatarsal has been over-shortened causing prominence of the second. Note the rounding of the metatarsal stumps; the patient was pleased at 5 years.

Treatment is largely that required for the primary deformity. If inter-phalangeal joint fusions are undertaken alone, full correction of metatarso-phalangeal deformity by tenotomy and capsulotomy is necessary to achieve a plantigrade toe. Partial proximal phalangectomy, sparing the base, is another alternative. Osteotomy of the proximal phalanx can also be applied usefully to re-align toes.

The inter-phalangeal joint of the hallux may present marked valgus or severe hyperextension causing painful callouses whilst the metatarso-phalangeal joint remains normal; arthrodesis of the joint in neutral is best although we have experienced failure when joint destruction has been severe and in retrospect this would have been helped by a cancellous bone graft.

Postoperative care

One penalty of severe forefoot destruction is failure of the toes to take weight, reducing the foot to a static platform whose function ceases at the metatarsal heads. In order to improve toe function, it is essential to alert the patient before surgery that vigorous postoperative toe exercises, especially plantar-flexion, are vital to a good result. These exercises should start during the anaesthetic recovery and be encouraged by all staff. As patients with bilateral plantar incisions cannot take weight until their wounds heal, they have every opportunity to obtain control and power in the toes before walking. Critics of excision arthroplasty rightly observe that it shortens the foot; however, whilst anatomically shorter, the foot proves to be physiologically longer. Indeed the patient who exercises conscientiously can ultimately stand on tip-toe unsupported, despite the absence of all metatarsal heads.

References

1. Vidigal, E., Jacoby, R. K., Dixon, A. St J. *et al.* (1975) The foot in chronic rheumatoid arthritis. *Ann. Rheum. Dis.*, **34**, 292–297.
2. Kirkup, J. R. (1988) *Terminology.* In *The Foot: Disorders and Management* (eds B. Helal, and D. W. Wilson) Churchill Livingstone, London.
3. Arden, G. P. and Ansell, B. M. (1978) *The Surgical Management of Juvenile Chronic Polyarthritis.* Academic Press, London.
4. Dixon, A. St J. and Graber, J. (1981) *Local Injection Therapy.* E.U.L.A.R. Publishers, Basel.
5. Tillmann, K. (1979) *The Rheumatoid Foot.* Thieme, Stuttgart.
6. Benjamin, A. and Helal, B. (1980) *Surgical Repair and Reconstruction in Rheumatoid Disease*, Macmillan, London, p. 204.
7. Kirkup, J. R. (1974) Ankle and tarsal joints in rheumatoid arthritis. *Scand. J. Rheumatol.*, **3**, 50–52.
8. Bolton-Maggs, B. G., Sudlow, R. A. and Freeman, M. A. R. (1985) Total ankle arthroplasty: a long-term review of the London Hospital experience. *J. Bone Joint Surg.*, **67B**, 785–790.
9. Samuelson, K. M., Freeman, M. A. R. and Tuke, M. A. (1982) Development and evolution of the I.C.L.H. ankle replacement. *Foot and Ankle*, **3**, 32–36.
10. Demottaz, J. D., Mazur, J. M., Thomas, W. H. *et al.* (1979) Clinical study of total ankle replacement with gait analysis. *J. Bone Joint Surg.*, **61A**, 976–988.
11. Herberts, P., Goldie, I. F., Korner, L. *et al.* (1982) Endoprosthetic arthroplasty of the ankle joint: a clinical and radiological follow-up. *Acta Orthop. Scand.*, **53**, 687–696.
12. Lachiewicz, P. F., Inglis, A. E. and Ranawat, C. S. (1984) Total ankle replacement in rheumatoid arthritis. *J. Bone Joint Surg.*, **66A**, 340–343.
13. Kirkup, J. R. (1985) Richard Smith ankle arthroplasty. *J. R. Soc. Med.*, **78**, 301–304.
14. Marsh, C. H., Kirkup, J. R. and Regan, M. W. (1987) The Bath and Wessex ankle arthroplasty. Proceedings report. *J. Bone Joint Surg.*, **69B**, 153.
15. Vahvanen, V. A. J. (1967) Rheumatoid arthritis in the pantalar joints. *Acta Orthop. Scand.*, **Suppl.**, **107**, 1–157.
16. Kirkup, J. R. Vidigal, E. and Jacoby, R. K. (1977) The hallux and rheumatoid arthritis. *Acta Orthop. Scand.*, **48**, 527–544.
17. Kirkup, J. R. (1978) Dislocation of the hallux in rheumatoid arthritis. *Chirurg. del Piede*, **2**, 87–93.
18. Dixon, A. St J. (1970) Medical aspects of the rheumatoid foot. *Proc. R. Soc. Med.*, **63**, 677–679.
19. Helal, B. (1975) Metatarsal osteotomy for metatarsalgia, *J. Bone Joint Surg.*, **57B**, 187–192.
20. Fowler, A. W. (1959) A method of forefoot reconstruction. *J. Bone Joint Surg.*, **41B**, 507–513.
21. Kates, A., Kessel, L. and Kay, A. (1967) Arthroplasty of the forefoot. *J. Bone Joint Surg.*, **49B**, 552–557.
22. Morrison, P. (1974) Complications of forefoot operations in rheumatoid arthritis. *Proc. R. Soc. Med.*, **67**, 110–111.
23. Regnauld, B. (1974) *Techniques Chirurgicales du Pied.* Masson, Paris, p. 81.
24. Cracchiolo, A. (1982) Management of the arthritic forefoot. *Foot and Ankle*, **3**, 17–23.
25. Gould, N. (1982) Surgery of the forepart of the foot in rheumatoid arthritis. *Foot and Ankle*, **3**, 173–180.

27

Correction of posture in ankylosing spondylitis

P. M. Yeoman

The flexed posture caused by ankylosing spondylitis is one of the more distressing complaints amongst young adults (Fig. 27.1). It is difficult enough to adapt to a life when the spine is rigid even if that problem develops insidiously, but when the forward vision is restricted to only a few paces ahead the quality of life is seriously impaired. The era is past when rest, firm support, radiotherapy and an assortment of analgesics

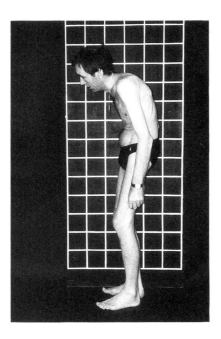

Fig. 27.1 Typical flexed posture with limited forward vision.

were common practice but it left behind a number of patients who have severely flexed and rigid spines. It has been superseded by a regime of exercises and anti-inflammatory drugs backed up by a trained experienced team who can assess and compare the results of their courses of management, which in turn is of benefit to the patient. The diagnosis is made earlier in the course of the disease, and backache in teenage girls may well be the first indication of ankylosing spondylitis. A diagnosis rarely considered 20 years ago for a condition which was thought to be predominantly affecting young men. Ankylosing spondylitis occurs equally between the sexes.

The B27 antigen study has revealed a greater incidence of ankylosing spondylitis among those patients who possess this antigen [1]. There can be peripheral joint changes almost identical with those seen in rheumatoid arthritis and yet it lies within the sero-negative arthropathies [2].

Ulcerative colitis and occasionally Crohn's disease is linked with ankylosing spondylitis [3,4], and either condition can seriously impair the general health of the patient and render them unfit for major surgery. Intestinal low-grade infection from the Klebsiella organism has been incriminated [5] but appropriate treatment has failed to provide more than a brief improvement in the spinal condition.

Pain is foremost in the patient's mind and is the responsibility of the rheumatologist who can employ a variety of anti-inflammatory drugs to good effect. Steroids are rarely used but occasionally ACTH is indicated. Pain developing after a

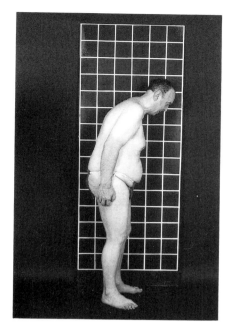

Fig. 27.2 Flexed posture suitable for correction in lumbar spine.

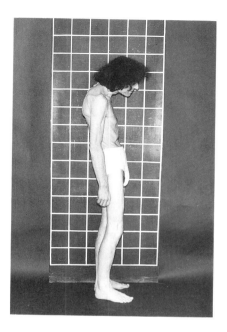

Fig. 27.3 Flexed posture suitable for correction in cervical spine.

reasonably long quiescent period may well be associated with posture and this may not respond to the conservative management.

The flexed posture

The three sites of deformity may be in: the hips, lumbar spine (Fig. 27.2), cervical spine (Fig. 27.3) or a combination of the three. Assessment by the team in hospital includes specially trained physiotherapists who can detect and measure the prime cause of the flexed posture, and thus determine a baseline for the graduated course of exercises. Progress or relapse between these courses can be assessed but most require in-patient supervision on an annual basis, or less depending on the severity of the disease.

Hips

A flexion contracture of both hips in ankylosing spondylitis is not easy to assess with accuracy owing to the rigidity of the lumbar spine. Clinical examination of the patient in the supine position is not possible, which rules out the classical

Thomas' test for demonstrating any flexion contracture in the hips. The patient has to be examined on their side. In the early stages of the disease it should be possible not only to detect but to prevent contractures of the hips [6].

Physiotherapy

Gentle passive movements by the physiotherapist and instruction of the patient to lie face downwards for at least part of the day and night may reduce and even prevent flexion contractures of the hips. The patient's relative should also be instructed on the method of passive stretching of the hips.

Arthroplasty of the hip

This is a well established surgical procedure and both hips can be replaced under the one anaesthetic. The author does not recommend a simultaneous bilateral hip replacement using two surgeons and assistants because of the hazards of blood loss, apart from the obvious technical difficulties. It is better carefully to assess the patient and blood loss after the first operation and only proceed with the second if all is well. In the postoperative period it is essential for the physiotherapist to continue with passive extension exercises of the hips and the patient is encouraged to lie prone for at least two periods during each day for at least 3 months. Heterotopic bone formation and subsequent ankylosis was a particular hazard in the Smith–Petersen era of mould arthroplasty but a recent review in 56 hip replacements [7] has revealed the importance not only of good quality physio- and hydrotherapy but the distance between the acetabulum and the greater trochanter will determine future stiffness and even ankylosis. A small gap between these two points is less likely to succeed.

Indocid has been recommended as a means of reducing heterotopic new bone formation; diphosphonate has not been successful [8].

Osteotomy of the lumbar spine

At first this would appear a formidable task but there are two essential criteria for success: first, not to attempt too great a correction; second, to obtain sound internal fixation (Figs 27.4, 27.5).

The author has always taken an active part in the preliminary scene not only in the anaesthetic room but also in positioning the patient on the operating table. Details can include the correct height of pillows under the chest to allow clearance for abdominal respiration and thus avoid venous congestion in the operating site; suitable padding under the pressure points at the knees and chin; and a check that the table is suitably adapted for breaking in order to accommodate the rigid flexed posture and adjustments for obtaining the proposed correction. A transverse incision in the mid-lumbar area would appear to be the optimum approach because of the clean healing without tension after the correction. In practice, this did not provide the necessary access above and below the osteotomy for applying the internal fixation; a midline longitudinal incision was preferable. The bone was surprisingly soft to resect except on occasions when it was dense and hard around the pedicles, and this called for slow arduous dissection in order to obtain precise clearance for the emerging nerve roots. A chevron shaped osteotomy resection gave the most stable closure, with the axis anterior to the cauda equina [9]. Internal fixation is obligatory, not only to avoid a long period in a corrective

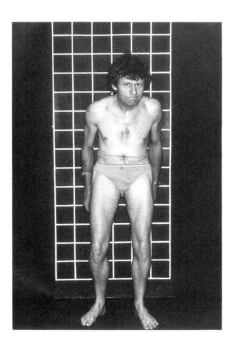

Fig. 27.4   Posture before correction.

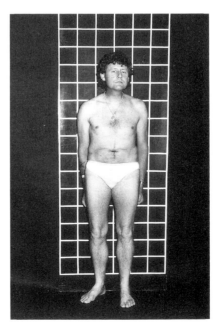

Fig. 27.5   One year after lumbar osteotomy.

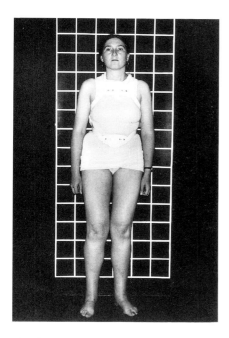

Fig. 27.6 Lightweight spinal brace worn for second period of 6 months.

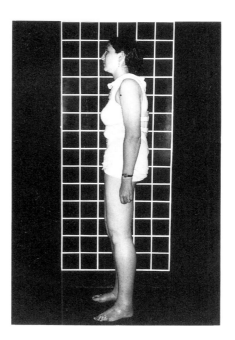

Fig. 27.7 Lightweight spinal brace worn for second period of 6 months.

plaster bed but to achieve stability thus preventing loss of correction or worse, the fatal damage to the cauda equina. Many methods were used [10] and by far the best fixation was obtained by transpedicular screws and interconnecting cables [11]. There is bound to be some loss of correction by any method but in the final group of 17 patients out of a total of 37, there was an average loss of only 6° by the pedicular screws and cable fixation.

In the postoperative period a corrective or supporting corset was worn for 6 months (Figs 27.6, 27.7).

Cervical osteotomy

This can be a formidable task [12]. The bone texture is invariably soft, the cervical canal has less accommodation than in the lumbar area, and there has to be more reliance on external fixation than in the previous account of internal fixation in the lumbar osteotomy. The advice is similar – overcorrection may lead to disaster (Figs 27.8, 27.9).

External fixation is obligatory and halo-vest is the chosen method because it provides safe and reliable external stability and allows the patient to be mobile and return home (Figs 27.10, 27.11).

After the induction of anaesthesia the application of the halo is the first part of the operation. Thereafter it is necessary to position the patient prone on the operating table which has a separate adjustable head piece. A transverse incision may be acceptable and it heals better than a midline longitudinal approach. Sadly the bone texture is relatively soft which makes resection easier but fixation unreliable. The meningeal covering of the spinal cord and emerging nerve roots has to be widely exposed at the site of the osteotomy, which is usually at the level of C5/6 or 7. Closure of the osteotomy is performed as a combined procedure with the surgeon manipulating the patient's towelled head and the anaesthetist on the table controls. Internal fixation is not adequate and consists of encircling wire around the laminae and spinous processes. Occasionally a small metal jaw fixation plate has been used. The halo-vest support may be required for at least 6 months and a collar for a further 6 months. The results reveal a satisfactory angle of correction which has been maintained.

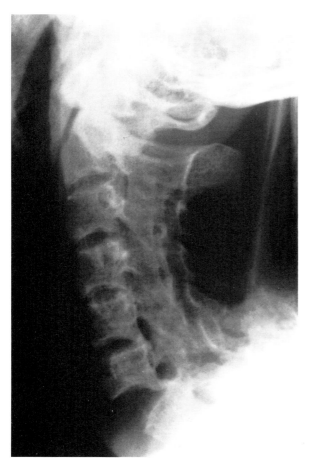

Fig. 27.8   Cervical osteotomy at C6/7 level (maximum correction).

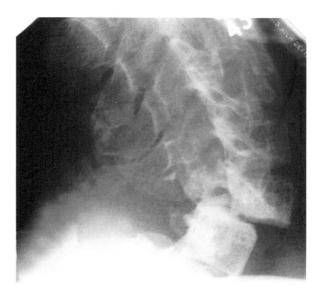

Fig. 27.9   Overcorrection resulting in instability; requiring revision.

Anaesthesia

Perhaps the most important development in anaesthetic technique has been unfairly relegated but there is no doubt that the flexible fibreoptic bronchoscope has made an immense difference; it has transformed a definite hazardous procedure of intubation in patients with ankylosing spondylitis to one of relative safety and reliability. It could be stated that intubation in the past was a hit and miss affair with all the dangers of a failed procedure before embarking on the operation which carried a high morbidity and mortality in itself. Preoperative assessment by the anaesthetist is obligatory not only for appraisal of the rigid neck deformity but to gain the confidence of the patient if it has been decided to perform an 'awake' intubation [13].

Correction without operation

Elderly and others who are unfit candidates for such a major event can be corrected by using an external fixator alone. The halo-vest technique has to incorporate turnbuckle screws with universal joints to allow a slow but steady correction of a few degrees each day. The patients are better in hospital, but not in bed, because problems arise with the apparatus which requires daily adjustment and almost hourly supervision. Some elderly patients develop respiratory problems not only as a result of a rigid rib cage but from the flexed cervical spine; even to the extent of developing a pressure sore between the chin and the chest. Successful correction was obtained without an operation in a select group of five elderly patients. Younger patients who do not have osteoporosis or a recent fracture are not suitable for this method; their spines are unyielding.

Fractures of the spine in ankylosing spondylitis

These patients are as likely to be involved in automobile accidents as any other person but

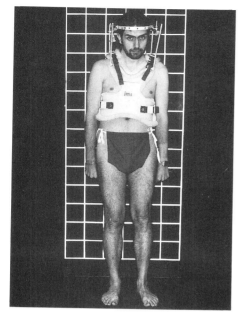

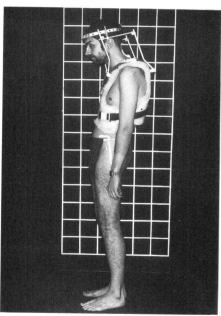

Figs. 27.10 & 27.11   Halo-vest apparatus allows the patient to return home.

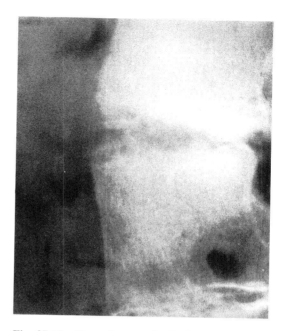

Fig. 27.12   Stress fracture in the lumbar area resembles a chronic infection.

they are more at risk if they have a rigid cervical spine [14]. Older patients with quiescent ankylosing spondylitis may suffer a fracture of the cervical spine as a result of trivial trauma, such as a fall from a chair. The opportunity to correct the flexed posture must not be missed. An external fixator with suitable turnbuckle attachments is indicated. Unfortunately in practice this is not often achieved because time is wasted in making a diagnosis. A fracture is most common at the cervico-thoracic junction, a site which is often obscured on the lateral radiographs by the shoulders, and the fracture is missed. Any patient who develops pain in the neck after a period of remission is deemed to have a fracture until proved otherwise [15].

A stress fracture (Fig. 27.12) may mimic a low-grade chronic infection on the radiographs, and indeed clinically [16]. Brucellosis may be suspected and time is wasted unnecessarily. A bone scan or MRI screening will reveal the site and diagnosis.

Conclusion

The future lies not only in determining the cause of ankylosing spondylitis but in active management to ensure minimal deformity of posture. Already the need for surgical correction of these terrible deformities has diminished and should be confined to special centres.

References

1. James, D. C. O. (1983) HLA-B27 in clinical medicine. *Br. J. Rheumatol.*, **22 (suppl. 2)**, 20–24.
2. Miehle, W., Schattenkirchner, M., Albert, D. and Bunge, M. (1985) HLA-DR4 in ankylosing spondylitis with different patterns of joint involvement. *Ann. Rheum. Dis.*, **44**, 39–44.
3. Moll, J. M. H. (1983) Pathogenetic mechanisms in B27 associated diseases. *Br. J. Rheumatol.*, **22 (suppl. 2)**, 93–103.
4. Hickling, P., Bird-Stewart, J. A., Young, J. D. and Wright, V. (1983) Crohn's spondylitis: a family study. *Ann. Rheumat. Dis.*, **42**, 106–107.
5. Ebringer, A. (1983) The cross-tolerance hypothesis HLA-B27 and ankylosing spondylitis. *Br. J. Rheumatol.*, **22 (suppl. 2)**, 53–66.
6. Bulstrode, S. J., Barefoot, J., Harrison, R. A. and Clarke, A. K. (1987) The role of passive stretching in the treatment of ankylosing spondylitis. *Br. J. Rheumatol.*, **26**, 40–42.
7. May, P. C. and Yeoman, P. M. (1990) Primary total hip arthroplasty in ankylosing spondylitis. *Rheumatology*, **13**, 223–227.
8. Thomas, B. J. and Amstutz, H. C. (1985) Results of the administration of diphosphonate for the prevention of heterotopic ossification after total hip arthroplasty. *J. Bone Joint Surg.*, **67A(3)**, 400–403.
9. McMaster, M. J. and Coventry, M. B. (1973) Spinal osteotomy in ankylosing spondylitis. *Mayo Clin. Proc.*, **48 (7)**, 476–486.
10. Fidler, M. W. (1986) Posterior instrumentation of the spine: an experimental comparison of various possible techniques. *Spine*, **11.4**, 367–372.
11. Weale, A. E., Marsh, C. H. and Yeoman, P. M. (1995) The secure fixation of lumber osteotomy. In press.
12. Simmons, E. H. (1972) The surgical correction of flexion deformity of the cervical spine in ankylosing spondylitis. *Clin. Orthop. Rel. Res.*, **86**, 132–143.
13. Sinclair, J. R. and Mason, R. A. (1984) Ankylosing spondylitis: the case for awake intubation. *Anaesthesia*, **39**, 3–11.
14. Wordsworth, B. P. and Mowat, A. G. (1986) A review of 100 patients with ankylosing spondylitis with particular reference to socio-economic effects. *Br. J. Rheumatol.*, **25**, 175–180.
15. Marsh, C. H. (1985) Internal fixation for stress fracture of the ankylosed spine. *J. R. Soc. Med.*, **78**, 377–379.
16. Yau, A. and Chan, R. (1974) Stress fracture of the fused lumbo-dorsal spine in ankylosing spondylitis. *J. Bone Joint Surg.*, **56B(4)**, 681–687.

28

Musculoskeletal sepsis: current concepts in treatment

R. H. Fitzgerald

Although the incidence of musculoskeletal sepsis has been reduced, septic complications of traumatic and elective surgery of the musculoskeletal system continue to be devastating to the patient. The most efficient treatment of musculoskeletal infections remains prevention of septic complications following the surgical treatment of traumatic injuries and elective reconstructive surgery. Fortunately, there have been numerous improvements, initiated by orthopaedic surgeons, which have the capability of reducing the incidence of postoperative surgical sepsis. Osteomyelitis of haematogenous origin in the child, once a dreaded disease, rapidly responds to specific antimicrobial therapy if diagnosed early. Most adult patients who are afflicted with osteomyelitis sustained a traumatic injury which was complicated by sepsis. Septic complications of total joint arthroplasty have become one of the major complications of total joint arthroplasty. Currently, there are several different approaches to the treatment of the patient with an infected total joint arthroplasty. Unfortunately, none of these approaches has universally resolved the process and preserved the arthroplasty. An infection of the spinal column has been referred to as 'the greatest masquerader', as it can mimic so many other clinical syndromes. Earlier diagnosis necessitates that all physicians become conversant with the initial clinical manifestations.

Prevention of postoperative sepsis

Prevention of septic complications following musculoskeletal surgery includes careful preoperative evaluation of the patient, the selective and appropriate utilization of prophylactic antimicrobial agents, and the use of ultra-clean operating rooms. Many of the elderly patients seeking reconstructive musculoskeletal surgery are malnourished. Jenson and co-workers have found that 10–15% of patients scheduled for total hip arthroplasty are severely malnourished and have evidence of immunodepression. Since protein depletion can adversely influence wound healing and impair humoral and cell-mediated immunity, such patients need to be identified preoperatively to permit nutritional therapy. Identification of such patients can be accomplished by a number of ways.

Anthropometric measurements, biochemical testing, and skin antigen testing provide data which permit assessment of a patient's nutritional status [1]. Anthropometric studies found to be useful in the preoperative assessment for nutritional depletion include measurement of the triceps skinfold and arm circumference in addition to the height and weight of the patient. Biochemical testing should include the serum albumin, serum transfusion and serum transferrin, and serum creatinine concentrations in addition to the total peripheral lymphocyte count and nitrogen balance. When these data are analyzed and suggest nutritional depletion, surgery should be postponed until nutritional therapy can be instituted to correct the problem.

Preoperative evaluation

Preoperatively, each patient should be carefully examined for remote infections which could lead to haematogenous seeding of the postoperative wound with bacteria. The surgeon must inspect such sites as infected hair follicles or sebaceous glands of the skin, necessitating examination of skin of a disrobed patient. Infected toenails are often overlooked during the preoperative evaluation of patients unless the patient examined offer removal of clothes, including shoes and socks. Such infections should be treated before musculoskeletal surgery is performed. Asymptomatic urinary tract infections can usually be identified by the presence of bacteria on a routine preoperative urinalysis. They can then be confirmed with a Gram-stain and urine culture. Surgical intervention should be delayed until the infection has been treated and a sterile urine culture has been obtained with the patient off antibiotic therapy.

Occasionally, patients live symbiotically with chronic urinary infections which are resistant to treatment. The infection can be suppressed during the perioperative period, but the patient has an increased risk of developing postoperative sepsis. This is especially true if the contemplated reconstructive procedure includes the implantation of a foreign body such as an artificial knee or hip prosthesis. Under such circumstances the patient and surgeon must carefully individualize the risk–benefit ratios.

Another area of concern is the prostate in males over the age of 55 years. Such patients should be queried concerning nocturia and urinary frequency. Should the prostate gland feel enlarged to palpation, urological consultation is necessary. When transurethral prostate resection be necessary, it is more desirable to have such surgery performed prior to the surgical placement of orthopaedic implants than to request it postoperatively as urinary catheters are necessary following prostatic resection. Such circumstances certainly place the patient in a com-

promised position and increase the risk of haematogenous infection. If a trans-urethral prostatic resection is required, elective musculoskeletal surgery involving the implantation of foreign bodies should be delayed for 12 weeks to allow the resected portion of the prostate gland to re-epithelialize.

Orthopaedic surgeons can overlook the oral cavity during the preoperative evaluation of patients. Although it can be difficult to identify carious teeth, poor oral hygiene is usually apparent. When present, the patient should have appropriate dental examinations and treatment prior to musculoskeletal surgery.

Although such an extensive search for remote infections or potential causes of infection during the preoperative evaluation may seem excessive, it is surprising how often remote infections are responsible for septic complications of total joint arthroplasty. They are simple techniques requiring minimal time and provide both the surgeon and the patient with additional insurance against postoperative infections.

Prophylactic antimicrobial agents

The prophylactic administration of antimicrobial agent has become a well established principle for the reduction of postoperative sepsis. There is, however, some confusion over the application of this principle by surgeons. Should all patients having musculoskeletal surgery receive prophylactic antimicrobial? If not, which patient should and which patients should not? Which antimicrobial agents should be administered and when should they be administered?

All surgeons would agree that those procedures involving the implantation of large foreign bodies necessitate the prophylactic adminstration of antimicrobial agents [2]. The indications for operations involving the application of one or two screws or Steinmann pins are less clear. Certainly, any operation where a dead space which permits the formation of a haematoma should be associated with the administration of prophylactic antimicrobials. Operations requiring 2 or more hours would also justify the prophylactic administration of antimicrobial agents. In general, soft tissue operations, procedures implanting minimal metal devices, and those of short duration are not usually considered for administration of anti-microbial agents prophylactically. However, Henley and co-workers recently reported a statistically significant reduction in the incidence of postoperative sepsis in soft tissue and other musculoskeletal procedures not requiring a prosthetic device lasting 2 or more hours with the prophylactic administration of antimicrobials [3]. Procedures requiring less than 2 hours did not have an associated reduction in the incidence of sepsis. The application of these principles to musculoskeletal procedures must be left to the discretion of the individual surgeon, who is capable of making the wisest decision for each patient.

When the prophylactic administration of antimicrobial agents is thought to be indicated, the surgeon must select an agent that is bactericidal against the microorganisms associated with postoperative musculoskeletal sepsis in his or her hospital. Furthermore, the agent selected should be safe and inexpensive. In North America *Staphylococcus aureus* and *Staphylococcus epidermidis* remain the most common causal organisms isolated from postoperative infections of the musculoskeletal system. Streptococci are the third commonest isolates recovered. Gram-negative bacillary organisms are less common isolates. Thus, a first generation cephalosporin remains an ideal agent for the prophylactic administration to patients having musculoskeletal surgery.

Although some surgeons have advocated the use of a second or even a third generation of cephalosporin as the prophylactic agent of choice, there are few data to justify such recommendations. Occasionally, unique situations in some hospital environments may justify their use on a temporary basis. These agents are no more effective than a first generation cephalosporin against the usual causal organisms and they certainly are far more expensive.

The timing of the administration and the duration of prophylactic antimicrobials remain controversial. Although most surgeons initiate the administration of prophylactic antibiotics during surgery, the duration of administration varies widely. It would appear that most surgeons discontinue antimicrobials 48–72 hours after surgery. There is certainly no need to continue the administration of antibiotics for 5–7 days. In fact, such prolonged administration of antimicrobials appears to permit the development of remote infections. More recently some authorities have suggested that the antimicrobials may be discontinued after one to two doses administered during surgery and in the recovery room. Though such a brief period of administration may prove to be efficacious and cost effective, it has yet to be studied in depth.

Operating room environment

Ultraclean operating rooms, introduced to modern surgery by Sir John Charnley, have remained controversial. All surgeons would agree that if cleansing of the ambient environment can reduce the incidence of postoperative sepsis, it is worthwhile even if expensive [4]. Lidwell and co-workers have presented strong evidence to support the use of ultraclean operating rooms for total hip and total knee arthroplasty [5]. In their multicentre study of nineteen hospitals in which total joint procedures were randomized between a conventionally ventilated operating room and an operating room ventilated by an ultraclean-air system, a statistically significant reduction in the incidence of postoperative sepsis was found with those procedures performed in the ultraclean-air systems (63 of 4133 versus 23 of 3922; $P < 0.001$). Unfortunately, this elaborate and extensive study failed to control the use of prophylactic antimicrobials. The incidence of postoperative sepsis following total hip or knee arthroplasty performed with the prophylactic administration of antimicrobials in a conventional operating room was 24 of 2968 (0.8%). Similarly, the incidence of postoperative sepsis for these procedures performed in a room with an ultraclean-air system was 10 of 2863 (0.3); Chi^2 = 5.31, $P < 0.2$. Since the influence of the prophylactic administration of antimicrobial was not randomized, it is difficult to judge its impact on the study. It would appear, however, that total joint arthroplasty performed in a conventional operating room with adherence to strict aseptic techniques, including the administration of prophylactic antimicrobials, can be associated with postoperative infection rates which are statistically indistinguishable from those found in ultraclean operating rooms.

Hill and co-workers made similar observations in a multicentre study of the prophylactic administration of cefazolin. In this randomized, double-blind, placebo-controlled [6] study of ten centres in France, cefazolin statistically reduced ($P < 0.001$), the incidence of deep sepsis following total hip arthroplasty from 35 of 1067 (3.3%) in the control group to 10 of 1070 (0.9%). However, these investigators found 'the rate of hip infection was the same in a conventional theatre with prophylactic antibiotherapy as in a hyper-sterile theatre with or without antibiotherapy'.

Thus, it would appear that implant surgery must be performed in association with the prophylactic administration of antimicrobial therapy. The role of ultraclean operating rooms awaits clarification from other clinical studies which control the impact of antimicrobial therapy. In the interim, carefully performed implant procedures can be safely conducted in conventional operating rooms where there is strict adherence to aseptic technique and traffic control.

Osteomyelitis

Haematogenous osteomyelitis in the child is not only seen with less frequency than in the past, but is also more responsive to modern therapeutic modalities. Morrissy has demonstrated that minor trauma about the growth plate may be instrumental in the development of acute haematogenous osteomyelitis. The pathophysiological mechanism which is responsible for this 'locus minoris resistentiae' remains to be elucidated. Hobo, however, has suggested that there is limited phagocytic activity by the tissue-based mononuclear cells in and about the physeal plate. Traumatic injuries, although they may be minor in nature, may further compromise the phagocytic defences. The perceived reduction of patients with acute haematogenous osteomyelitis is difficult to explain. Certainly, the overall nutritional status of Western civilization has improved over the past 4 decades. The sophistication of patients and their parents has encouraged early medical evaluation and treatment. Without question, the availability of effective antimicrobials which physicians are willing to administer early have had a decidedly positive influence on the ultimate prognosis of acute haematogenous osteomyelitis. Most children can be cured without surgical intervention. Progres-

sion of this disease process into chronic osteomyelitis is distinctly uncommon in the absence of some major alteration of the immune system by a concomitant disease process.

Osteomyelitis in the adult patient is usually the sequelae of a traumatic injury. In contrast to acute haematogenous osteomyelitis where *S. aureus* and *B-haemolytic streptococcus* are recovered, Gram-negative bacillary organisms are recovered as pure or mixed isolates in almost half of the patients. Methicillin-resistant *S. aureus* is being recovered from clinical material from patients with musculoskeletal sepsis with increased frequency [7]. Essentially all adult patients with post-traumatic osteomyelitis will require a combination of surgical and medical therapy. Recovery of the causal organism(s) from deep tissue specimens and identification of the antimicrobial susceptibility pattern(s) are the first prerequisites of treatment. Surgical excision of foreign bodies, necrotic, and infected tissue must be meticulously performed. In recent years several new surgical modalities have permitted the modern orthopaedist, dramatically to help this group of patients.

The development of external fixator devices has permitted the management of the infected nonunion without introducing additional foreign material into the wound. The use of half-pins as well as transfixing pins permits the surgeon to construct external fixation apparatuses which will biomechanically enhance union. Sixty to 70% of infected non-unions will unite without supplemental bone grafting procedure with eradication of the septic process and the use of external fixation devices.

The availability of local muscle flaps, free microvascular flaps and cancellous bone grafting procedures have permitted the orthopaedist to aggressively treat osteomyelitic foci. Radical local resections, excising infected and poorly vascularized adjacent tissues back to healthy tissue, can now be performed as there are techniques which permit reconstruction of a functional extremity. A local muscle flap can be used in patients with a large defect of soft tissue and bone after debridement of an osteomyelitic lesion if the flap can be elevated and transposed into the defect without compromising its vascular supply [8]. The soleus or gastrocnemius muscle flap are the most frequently utilized flaps to achieve wound closure. The combination of radical

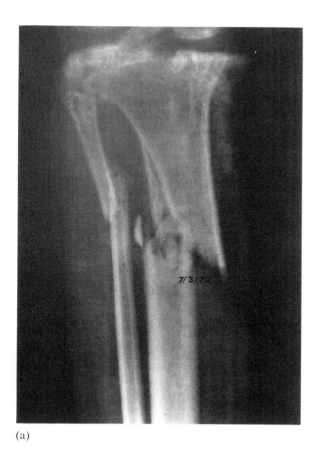

(a)

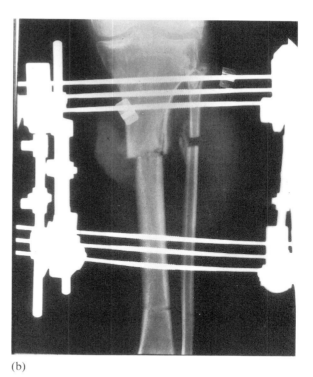

(b)

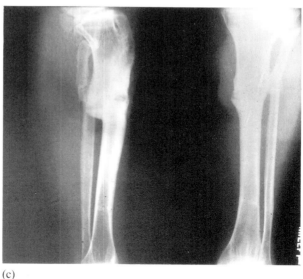

(c)

Fig. 28.1 Post-traumatic osteomyelitis 7 months following a crush injury to the tibia in a 26-year-old man. There is a 5 × 6 cm open draining wound.
(a) Anteroposterior roentgenogram of tibia 7 months following injury reveals malalignment with obvious non-union. (b) Following debridement the tibia was realigned, an external fixation device applied, and gastrocnemius muscle flap rotated into the soft tissue defect. Subsequently a split thickness skin graft was applied.
(c) Anteroposterior and lateral roentgenograms 18 months following treatment reveal healing with appropriate alignment. No further drainage has occurred 10 years following debridement.

debridement, wound closure with a local muscle flap, and specific antimicrobial therapy has successfully eradicated osteomyelitis in 93% of the patients treated.

When the infectious process, the radical local debridement, or the anatomic location precludes the use of a local muscle flap, a microvascular free flap composed of soft tissue alone, bone alone or a combination of both is possible. In general, wound closures with a free muscle flap should be the initial goal. If a major segmental, osseous defect exists, it can subsequently be managed with a free fibular flap (or a cancellous bone grafting procedure). Experience with a combined osseous and soft tissue one-staged free tissue transfer has not been as successful.

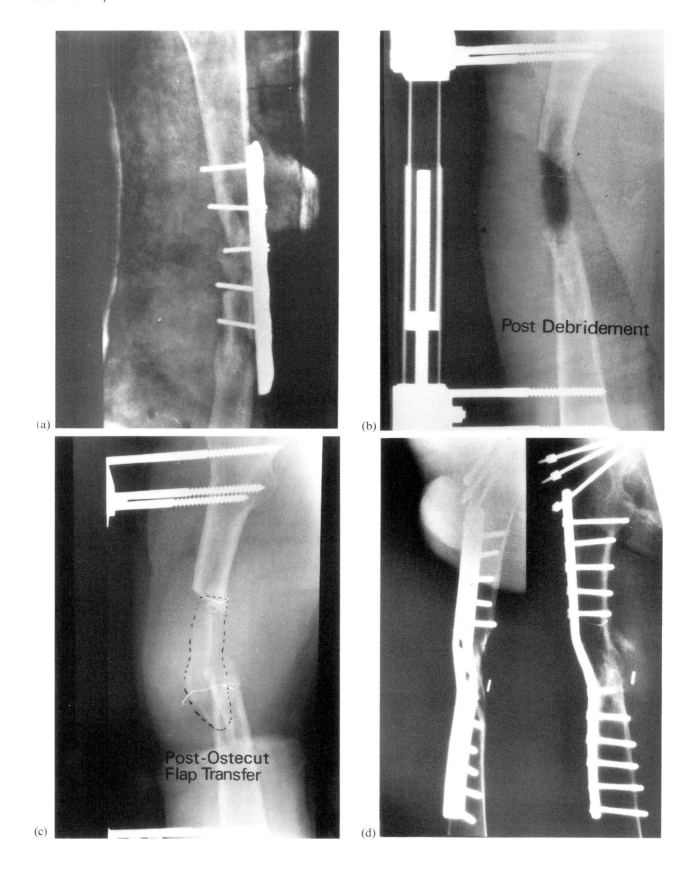

(a)

(b) Post Debridement

(c) Post-Ostecut Flap Transfer

(d)

Although such technically demanding procedures have not been as successful as the local muscle flaps, they have salvaged three-quarters of the patients so treated who in the past would have been relegated to abalative surgery.

Antimicrobial therapy for the adult patient with osteomyelitis should be specific for all of the causal organisms recovered from the deep tissue specimens obtained during debridement. The isolation of mixed aerobic–anaerobic organisms appears to adversely influence the prognosis [9]. The duration of parenteral therapy remains empiric, ranging from 3 to 6 weeks. Experience would dictate that 3 weeks of parenteral therapy followed by 4 weeks of oral therapy in patients with rapid wound healing is adequate. However, when wound healing is difficult to achieve and prolonged, parenteral therapy should be extended. Continuation of parenteral therapy, initiated in the hospital, at home with specialized catheters has proven to be effective [10].

The role of the depot administration of antibiotics utilizing antibiotic-impregnated polymethylmethacrylate beads is currently under clinical investigation. Preliminary studies by Klemm and others suggest that this technique is promising. However, it is disturbing to implant further foreign material into a wound, even temporarily, following a rigorous surgical excision of all necrotic bone, infected tissue, and foreign material. A biodegradable carrier would seem to be more appropriate. Nevertheless, orthopaedic surgeons look forward to the results of a prospective study currently in progress in North America.

Fig. 28.2 Infected non-union of femoral fracture in a 24-year-old medical student. A sinus tract from the lateral thigh incision extends deep to the fracture site.
(a) Anteroposterior roentgenogram reveals an intercalary fracture with non-union of the proximal fracture site.
(b) Anteroposterior roentgenogram following debridement and application of a Wagner apparatus. The intercalary fragment was united to the distal femur but was dead.
(c) Anteroposterior roentgenogram following wound closure with a free-vascularized osteocutaneous iliac crest flap. (d) Anteroposterior roentgenogram 3 months following the free flap. Further bone autogenous grafting and plate stabilization was performed. He is a practising physician without further drainage 7 years later.

Infections following total hip arthroplasty

The dramatic functional improvement following total knee or total hip arthroplasty can be significantly compromised should the procedure be complicated by postoperative wound sepsis. Fortunately, this dreaded complication occurs infrequently. When it does occur, aggressive surgical intervention is indicated in all but a minority of patients as antibiotics alone are ineffective.

Sepsis of a total hip arthroplasty occurs in one of three stages [11]. Stage I infections are those occurring during the immediate postoperative period and usually constitutes a colonized or infected haematoma. Such haematomas are best decompressed with aseptic techniques in the operating room prior to the development of spontaneous drainage. When the latter occurs, secondary bacterial invaders which are usually Gram-negative bacilli have access to the depths of the wound. Surgical decompression of the wound followed 2–3 weeks of specific antimicrobial therapy will eradicate the infectious process in the vast majority of patients.

Stage II infections are those which are associated with minimal symptomatology. Such infections are rarely associated with a febrile response, wound swelling or drainage. Characteristically, the patient will complain of pain, indicating that he or she has experienced pain since the immediate postoperative period. The paucity of symptoms usually delays the diagnosis of sepsis for 12–24 months following surgery. Imaging of the hip with In[111] labelled white blood cells has proven to be an effective diagnostic tool [12]. Patients with Stage II infections will require surgical extirpation of all foreign material to eradicate the infection [13].

Late haematogenous infections of the artificial joint compose Stage III infections. Usually the patient will be free of any symptoms referable to the total joint arthroplasty until the acute onset of pain associated with a febrile response. Infections in this group of patients should be treated with immediate aspiration of the joint. If microorganisms are seen with Gram stain of the aspirate or the aspirate has other features consistent with sepsis, prompt arthrotomy should be performed. Usually the prosthetic devices are found to be securely attached to bone. Treatment in-

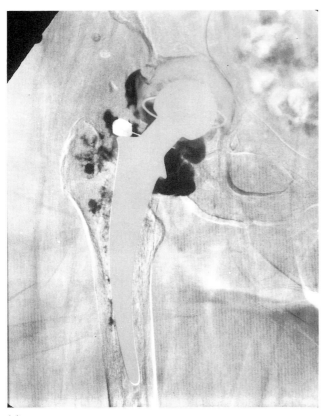

(a)

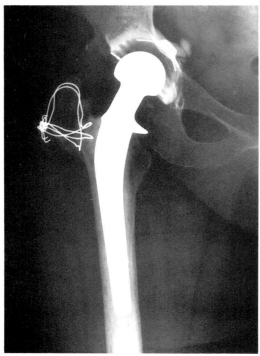

(b)

Fig. 28.3   Infected hip arthroplasty 18 months following
a total hip arthroplasty in a 58-year-old school teacher. A
two-staged procedure was used to reconstruct her hip.
(a) Anteroposterior roentgenogram following resection
arthroplasty. *Escherichia coli* was isolated from deep
tissue specimens. (b) Anteroposterior roentgenogram
following reconstruction of the hip in delayed fashion.
The hip was reconstructed 12 months following resection
arthroplasty. This roentgenogram was made 18 months
following reconstruction. She has a painless hip 5 years
following reconstruction.

cludes debridement without removal of the components followed by 4 weeks of parenteral antimicrobial therapy. Unfortunately, many patients with Stage III infection of an implant will experience recurrent infection. At this time, there are no methodologies to predict which patients will respond and which patients will experience recurrent sepsis. The varied clinical response may be related to the development of glycocalyx which is a glycoprotein permitting bacterial adherence to foreign bodies. Glycocalyx also appears to protect microorganisms from exposure to the host defence mechanisms. Unfortunately, there are no techniques which allow the clinician to differentiate those prostheses which have glycocalyx formation from those which do not.

Surgical reconstruction of the septic artificial joint requiring removal of the prosthetic components can be performed in a single stage, two stages or occasionally a three-staged procedure. The treatment of a patient with an infected total hip arthroplasty with surgical extirpation and reconstruction with another prosthesis during a single operation was introduced to the orthopaedic community by Buchholz [14]. This technique was based upon the principle of placing antibodies in polymethyl methacrylate [15]. Careful scrutiny of Buchholz's data suggests that he was more successful with this technique when treating infections which were associated with the isolation of less virulent microorganisms (Table 28.1). He was most successful in the treatment of

infections from which no bacteria could be recovered or those from which he recovered anaesthetic causal organisms. Recurrent sepsis occurred in half of the patients from which Gram-negative bacillary organisms were isolated. In a recent long-term follow-up of some 825 patients treated in Germany, Rüttger reported recurrent sepsis in 30% at 6 years and 50% at 11 years [6]. The preliminary results of a portion of a prospective study in North America suggest that this technique can be highly successful when the patients so treated are carefully selected. Ninety-six percent of 194 patients with an infected total hip or total knee arthroplasty treated at the Mayo Clinic or The Hospital for Special Surgery were free from recurrent sepsis 2 years following surgery.

Delayed reconstruction following surgical extirpation of the infected total joint arthroplasty is certainly a safer technique for the treatment of most deep infections of total joint arthroplasty. The timing of the reconstructive procedure is variable and empiric. Those patients with a less virulent causal organism (Table 28.2) can be reconstructed 3 months following resection arthroplasty, whereas those patients from whom a more virulent causal organism was recovered should have reconstruction of their hip delayed for a year. McDonald and Fitzgerald recently reported an overall success rate of 87% in the management of 84 infected total hip arthroplasties in 83 patients with a staged reconstruc-

Table 28.1 The relationship of treatment and the microbiology of the infection*

Microorganism	Percent with recurrent sepsis
Pseudomonas sp.	47
Proteus sp.	52
Klebsiella sp.	55
Escherichia coli	39
Group D streptococcus	47
Staphylococcus aureus	28
Peptococcus sp.	24
Propionibacterium acnes	16
Sterile	11

* Modified from Buchholz.

Table 28.2 The relationship of the microbiology to the timing of reconstruction

Less virulent causal organisms
Early reconstruction – 3 months

Methicillin-susceptible staphylococci
(*S. aureus* and *S. epidermidis*)
Anaerobic Gram-positive cocci
(*Peptococcus* sp. and *Peptostreptococcus* sp.)
Anaerobic Gram-positive bacilli
(*Propionibacterium acnes*)
Streptococci
(Excluding enterococci)

More virulent causal organisms
Late reconstruction – 12 months

Methicillin-resistant staphylocci
Gram-negative bacilli
Group D streptococcus (enterococcus)

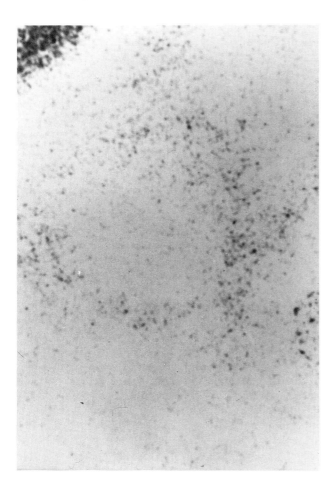

Fig. 28.4 An infected total hip arthroplasty in a 48-year-old woman 1 year following surgery. A one-staged procedure was utilized to reconstruct her hip. Indium image reveals increased uptake in the area of the greater trochanter. She remains pain free 4 years following reconstruction with antibiotic impregnated polymethyl methacrylate.

tive hip arthroplasty. When all of the polymethyl methacrylate was excised during the resection arthroplasty, reconstruction was delayed at least a year, systemic antimicrobials were administered for 28 days, and the causal organism was less virulent. The incidence of recurrent sepsis was significantly reduced ($P < 0.05$).

In the younger patient, a three-staged procedure may be indicated. The younger patient with an infected total hip arthroplasty would appear to be an ideal candidate for reconstruction with a biological ingrowth prosthesis. Frequently, there is insufficient bone stock, especially of the acetabulum following surgical extirpation and treatment of the infection to surgically implant a biological ingrowth prosthetic device. This group of patients can have partial reconstitution of the bony anatomy with the use of autogenous and allogenic bone grafts. Once incorporation of the bone graft has been accomplished, the hip can be reconstructed with ingrowth prosthetic devices. The timing of the bone grafting procedure and subsequent implantation of the prosthetic devices is empiric. Experience suggests the bone grafting procedure can be performed 3 months following surgical extirpation of the infected prosthesis in most patients. The bone graft is usually incorporated to such an extent to support an ingrowth prosthetic device 9 months later. Limited experience with this staged technique has been universally successful to date.

Spinal infections

Infections of the spinal column have historically been difficult diagnostic and therapeutic problems [16]. The diagnosis is frequently delayed, leading to increased morbidity and variable destruction of the osseous structures. Neurological deficits have been reported to occur in a variable percentage of the patients included in retrospective studies. Paralysis has been reported to occur in 5–50% of patients with vertebral osteomyelitis [17]. Hopefully, the introduction of imaging techniques exhibiting greater specificity and sensitivity for septic lesions will permit an earlier diagnosis eliminating or at least reducing the neurological sequelae.

Disc space infections following surgical intervention in the treatment of herniated nucleus pulposus are serious and debilitating complications [18]. Their clinical appearance is heralded by severe back pain with muscle spasms several weeks following discectomy. The surgical incision rarely indicates the sinister nature of the underlying pathology. Needle aspiration of the disc space and blood cultures will permit identification of the causal organism which is usually *S. aureus*. Application of a body cast or hip spica cast to immobilize the lumbar spine will afford the patient pain relief. Specific parenteral antimicrobial therapy should also be administered. Spontaneous fusion of adjacent vertebral bodies usually occurs, resolving the problem.

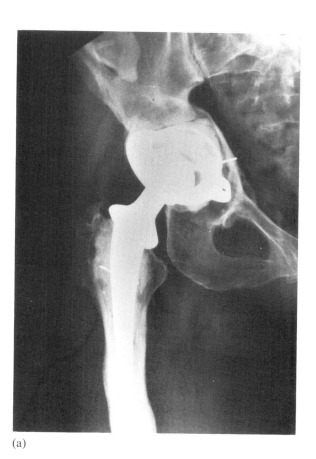

(a)

Fig. 28.5 Infected total hip arthroplasty in a 42-year-old woman who had post-traumatic arthrosis following a fracture dislocation. (a) Anteroposterior roentgenogram after three attempts with debridement to achieve an infected total hip arthroplasty. The acetabular component is obviously loose. *S. aureus* was isolated from a hip aspirate.
(b) Anteroposterior roentgenogram after bone grafts (autogenous iliac and allograft bone) were placed in the acetabulum and proximal femur 3 months following resection arthroplasty. (c) Nine months later an uncemented arthroplasty was performed. This anteroposterior roentgenogram was made 6 months following reconstruction. The hip remains painless 3 years following reconstruction.

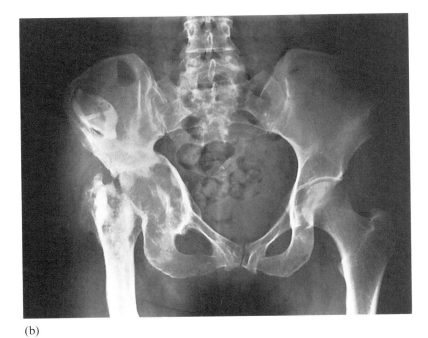

(b)

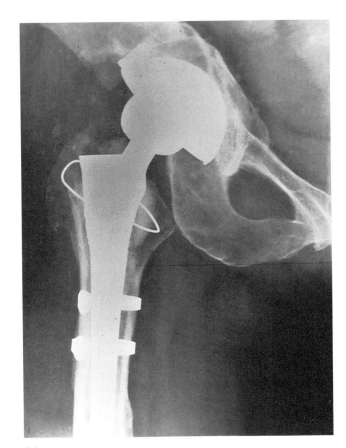

(c)

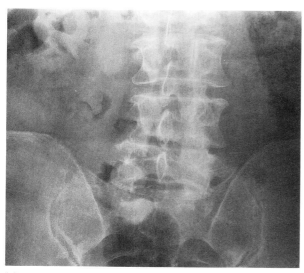

(a)

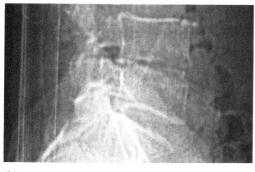

(b)

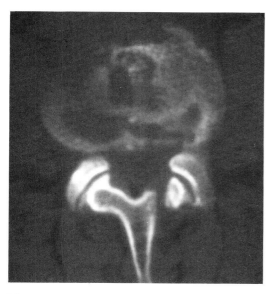

(c)

Fig. 28.6 Disc space infection following laminectomy and discectomy of the fourth lumber disc.
(a) Anteroposterior roentgenogram 8 weeks following surgery reveals asymmetrical collapse of the fourth lumbar disc space. (b) Lateral roentgenogram 9 weeks following discectomy. Narrowing of the fourth lumbar disc space with erosion of the end plates is evident. (c) CT through the fourth lumbar vertebra reveals erosion extending into the vertebral body. Spontaneous fusion of the fourth and fifth lumbar vertebral bodies occurred with cast immobilization.

References

1. Jensen, J. E., Smith, T. K., Jensen, T. G. *et al.* (1981) Nutritional assessment of orthopaedic patients undergoing total hip replacement surgery. In *The Hip*, Proceedings of the Ninth Open Scientific Meeting of The Hip Society (ed. E. A. Salvati), C. V. Mosby, St Louis, pp. 123–135.
2. Hill, C., Mazas, F., Flamont, R. and Eorard, J. (1981) Prophylactic cefazolin versus placebo in total hip replacement. *Lancet*, **April 11**, 795–797.
3. Henley, M. B., Jones, R. E., Wyatt, R. W. B. *et al.* (1986) Prophylaxis with cefamandole nafate in elective orthopedic surgery. *Clin. Orthop.*, **209**, 249–254.
4. Lidwell, O. M. (1983) Sepsis after total hip or knee joint replacement in relation to airborne contamination. *Philos. Trans. R. Soc. Lond. (Biol)*., **302**, 582–592.
5. Lidwell, O. M., Lowbury, E. J. L., Whyte, W. *et al.* (1982) Effect of ultraclean air in operating rooms on deep sepsis in the joint after total hip or knee replacement: a randomised study. *Br. Med. J.*, **285**, 10–14.
6. Nelson, C. L. (1986) Symposium: antibiotic-impregnated acrylic composites. *Contemp. Orthop.*, **12**, 85.
7. Bock, B. V., Pasiecznik, K. and Meyer, R. D. (1982) Clinical and laboratory studies of nosocomial *Staphylococcus aureus* resistant to methicillin and aminoglycosides. *Infect. Control*, **3**, 224–229.
8. Fitzgerald, R. H. Jr, Ruttle, P. E., Arnold, P. G. *et al.* (1985) Local muscle flaps in the treatment of chronic osteomyelitis. *J. Bone Joint Surg.*, **67(A)**, 175–185.
9. Hall, B. B., Fitzgerald, R. H. Jr and Rosenblatt, J. E. (1983) Anaerobic osteomyelitis. *J. Bone Joint Surg.*, **65(A)**, 30–35.
10. Poretz, D. M., Eron, L. J., Goldenberg, R. I. *et al.* (1982) Intravenous antibiotic therapy in an outpatient setting. *JAMA*, **248**, 336–339.
11. Fitzgerald, R. H. Jr (1986) Problems associated with the infected total hip arthroplasty. *Clin. Rheum. Dis.*, **12**, 537–554.
12. Merkel, K. D., Brown, M. L. and Dewanjee, M. K. (1985) Comparison of Indium-labeled-leukocyte imaging with sequential technetium-gallium scanning in the diagnosis of low-grade musculoskeletal sepsis. *J. Bone Joint Surg.*, **67(A)**, 465–476.
13. Fitzgerald, R. H. Jr and Jones, D. R. (1985) Hip implant infection. Treatment with resection arthroplasty and late total hip arthroplasty. *Am. J. Med.*, **78**, 225–228.
14. Buchholz, H. W., Elson, R. A., Engelbrocht, B. *et al.* (1981) Management of deep infection of total hip replacement. *J. Bone Joint Surg.*, **63B**, 353.
15. Wahlig, H. and Dingeldein, E. (1980) Antibiotics and bone cements. *Acta Orthop. Scand.*, **51**, 49–56.
16. Shitut, R. V., Goodpasture, H. C. and Marsh, H. O. (1987) Diagnosing hematogenous vertebral pyogenic osteomyelitis. *Complications in Orthopedics*, **2**, 32.
17. Eismont, F. J., Bohlman, H. H., Soni, P. L. *et al.* (1983) Pyogenic and fungal vertebral osteomyelitis with paralysis. *J. Bone Joint Surg.*, **65(A)**, 19–29.
18. Ford, L. T. (1977) Postoperative infection of lumbar intervertebral disk space. *South. Med. J.*, **69**, 1477.

29

Osteomalacia and osteoporosis

D. J. Baylink and M. R. Mariano-Menez

Metabolic diseases involving the skeleton usually result in either osteoporosis or osteomalacia. Of the two, osteopororis is much more common, yet osteomalacia is more readily cured. Osteoporosis is characterized by a reduced bone density, and osteomalacia is characterized by an increased amount of unmineralized bone matrix. Osteoporosis produces a structurally weakened bone, which increases the susceptibility to fractures and can lead to chronic morbidity and even mortality. The most common osteomalacia that is seen nowadays is that due to vitamin D deficiency. However, the bone pathology in vitamin D deficiency is complex in that mild vitamin D deficiency results in secondary hyperparathyroidism and bone loss, whereas severe vitamin D deficiency results in classical osteomalacia. Thus, the clinical presentation in mild vitamin D deficiency may be similar to that of osteoporosis, whereas the clinical presentation with severe vitamin D deficiency is that of classical osteomalacia, where the clinical presentation is bone pain, usually associated with stress fractures or pseudofractures. It is important to distinguish between osteoporosis and osteomalacia, because the treatment is very different for the two diseases.

Osteomalacia

Osteomalacia is a disorder characterized by defective mineralization of newly produced bone matrix. This leads to an accumulation of poorly mineralized or unmineralized matrix (osteoid). In growing children, impaired mineralization of the cartilaginous growth plates leads to the clinical picture of rickets. However, in adults where the epiphyseal growth plates have closed, only osteomalacia can occur. Recognition of the disease is important, since, in general, it can be successfully treated. The two most common causes of osteomalacia are: (1) vitamin D deficiency and (2) phosphate deficiency. The focus of this chapter will be on vitamin D deficiency, since it is the most common form. Not all vitamin D deficiency results in osteomalacia. Mild vitamin D deficiency results in osteoporosis. It is moderate to severe vitamin D deficiency that results in osteomalacia. In severe vitamin D deficiency, the predominant bone histologic picture is one of the accumulation of excess osteoid. In contrast, in mild vitamin D deficiency, laboratory and bone biopsy findings are indicative of secondary hyperparathyroidism with bone loss and only a modest impairment of mineralization. It is difficult to distinguish between mild vitamin D deficiency and severe vitamin D deficiency in terms of the predominant bone lesion without a bone biopsy. However, this is unnecessary in practical terms, since the management of mild and severe vitamin D deficiency is similar except that with severe deficiency, the treatment period is longer.

Aetiology and pathogenesis

The characteristic feature of osteomalacia is excess osteoid tissue on bone biopsy (Fig. 29.1).

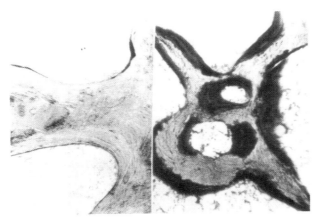

Fig. 29.1 Goldner's stained mineralized sections of bone from a normal subject (left) and from a patient with severe osteomalacia (right) Osteoid appears black and mineralized bone, gray. In the biopsy from the patient with osteomalacia, there is an increased amount of surface covered with osteoid and an increase in osteoid width.

Normally, osteoblasts elaborate new osteoid to replace the bone resorbed by osteoclasts. The osteoid then undergoes maturation before mineralization can proceed. In osteomalacia, the rate of osteoid deposition exceeds the rate of which mineral is deposited, resulting in increased osteoid width. The mineralization lag time (the time between onset of osteoid formation and its' mineralization) is prolonged [1]. The regulation of osteoid maturation and the onset of mineralization is not entirely clear, but both local mechanisms and systemic factors (1,25-dihydroxyvitamin D, [1,25-$(OH)_2$D] serum calcium and phosphate) are probably involved [2]. It is widely viewed that the defective mineralization is due to hypocalcemia and hypophosphatemia, from whatever cause, because a certain solubility product must be exceeded for calcium phosphate salts (hydroxyapatite) to form in the bone. It seems likely that, in addition to the physico-chemical effects, serum calcium and phosphorus also have an important local effect on osteoblasts to influence osteoid maturation [3].

Various metabolic perturbations can lead to osteomalacia (Table 29.1), but the most common cause is vitamin D deficiency [4,5]. Mild deficiency results in osteoporosis secondary to increased parathyroid hormone (PTH) secretion, whereas it is the severe deficiency of vitamin D that leads to osteomalacia. A schema of normal

Table 29.1   Causes of osteomalacia

I. Vitamin D deficiency
   1. Parent compound
      a) Dietary deficiency – vitamin D_2
      b) Gut malabsorption – vitamin D_2
         partial gastrectomy
         small bowel disease, resection, or bypass
         bile salt deficiency
         pancreatic insufficiency
      c) Inadequate sunlight exposure – vitamin D_3
   2. Vitamin D metabolite deficiencies
      a) Chronic liver disease – 25-ODH
      b) Anticonvulsant therapy – 25-ODH
      c) Chronic renal failure – 1,25-$(OH)_2$D

II. Phosphate depletion
   1. Phosphate binding antacids – aluminium hydroxide
   2. Renal phosphate leak
      a) Idiopathic
      b) Hereditary
         Vitamin D-resistant rickets
         Idiopathic hypercalciuria
      c) Vascular soft tissue tumour
      d) Metabolic acidosis
         Distal renal tubular acidosis

III. Inhibitors of mineralization
   Etidronate

vitamin D metabolism is shown in Fig. 29.2. The parent compounds are vitamin D_3 (cholecalciferol), which is synthesized in the skin from 7-dehydrocholesterol in response to ultraviolet irradiation, and vitamin D_2 (calciferol), which is found in fortified foods such as milk in the US but not in Europe. Thus, one must have inadequate sun exposure, as well as inadequate intestinal absorption of vitamin D, in order to become vitamin D deficient, as may occur in housebound or institutionalized elderly people [4]. Since vitamin D is stored in the body, and since these stores must be depleted before deficiency occurs, it may take several years before osteomalacia becomes symptomatic in malabsorptive syndromes; e.g. ten years or more after gastric or upper intestinal surgery [6,7]. With adequate exposure to sunlight, it may never become manifest. Other causes of vitamin D deficiency include: (1) chronic liver disease where

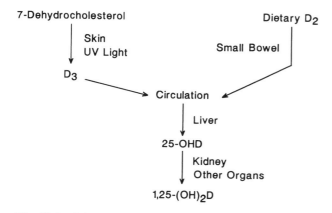

Fig. 29.2 Schema of normal vitamin D metabolism.

there may be impaired conversion of vitamin D_2 and vitamin D_3 to 25-hydroxyvitamin D (25-OHD) metabolite (the D_3 form of which is called calcifediol) [8,9]; (2) long-term anticonvulsant therapy where there may be hastened hepatic degradation of 25-OHD [10]; and (3) chronic renal failure where there may be impaired conversion of 25-OHD to the final, active metabolite $1,25\text{-}(OH)_2D_3$ [11].

Physiologic levels of vitamin D (the parent compound) or of 25-HD are inactive and, thus, it is only $1,25(OH)_2D$ that is the active form of this vitamin. Consequently, when we refer to vitamin D deficiency, we are referring to an absolute or relative deficiency of $1,25\text{-}(OH)_2D$. Early on during the course of vitamin D deficiency, the level of serum 25-OHD will drop to the point that there is now impaired conversion of 25-HD to $1,25\text{-}(OH)_2D$ [4]. This results in a slight decrease in serum calcium which, in turn, increases PTH which, in turn, increases the renal production of $1,25\text{-}(OH)_2D$. Thus, with mild vitamin D deficiency, we have a new steady state where the serum $1,25\text{-}(OH)_2D$ level is in the normal range but achieves this normal range only by virtue of secondary hyperparathyroidism. The excess PTH mobilizes calcium from the bone and increases renal tubular reabsorption of calcium [12]. At the same time, PTH reduces the renal tubular reabsorption of phosphate, leading to an increased excretion of phosphate by the kidney and a decreased serum phosphate. When the level of vitamin D deficiency becomes moderate to severe, it results in a low serum calcium, serum phosphate and serum calcium phosphate product, all of which impair mineralization [2].

The other major cause of osteomalacia, independent of vitamin D status, is hypophosphataemia [4,13,14] [Table 29.1]. Phosphate is ubiquitous in the diet and is so well absorbed that inadequate absorption is very rare unless phosphate binding antacids are used regularly [15]. Most cases of hypophosphataemia are not dietary but renal in origin. Thus, since serum phosphate is largely regulated by the renal tubular maximum for phosphorus (TmP), hypophosphataemia is usually attributable to a chronically depressed TmP resulting in a renal phosphate leak, either from an acquired or hereditary abnormality (Table 29.1).

As mentioned earlier, long term administration of either the bisphosphonate, etidronate, or fluoride has been found to be associated with inhibition of bone mineralization [16,17]. Awareness of this is important, since these agents are currently being used to treat other metabolic bone disorders; i.e. etidronate for Paget's disease of the bone and for osteoporosis and fluoride for osteoporosis. Etidronate is a synthetic analogue of pyrophosphate, which can inhibit resorption but, at the same time, can inhibit bone mineral deposition, particularly at doses exceeding 10 mg/kg per day [16]. Similarly, long term use of fluoride, particularly at high dosage, can also lead to accumulation of unmineralized matrix (osteoid), which is either partly or solely due to systemic calcium deficiency [18].

Clinical manifestations

The main symptoms in osteomalacia are progressive bone pain, proximal muscle weakness (except in vitamin D resistant rickets, where muscle weakness is not a feature), easy fatigability, and emotional depression [4,5,19]. As the disease progresses, bone pain and tenderness on pressure appear, particularly in the spine, ribs, shoulder girdle, pelvis, and extremities. The pain is aggravated by muscle strain, weight-bearing, and sudden movements. The skeletal pain is usually localized to sites of fractures or pseudofractures. Unless there is a high degree of suspicion, the condition can be mistaken for muscular rheumatism or arthritis. With advanced osteomalacia, skeletal deformities due to softening of the bone and microfractures can occur.

Diagnostic tests

In severe vitamin D deficiency, osteomalacia, serum calcium and phosphate are low, whereas in phosphate deficiency osteomalacia, only serum phosphate is low [20]. In most types of osteomalacia, serum alkaline phosphatase is elevated, although the mechanism for this is not known. In severe vitamin D deficiency osteomalacia, urinary calcium is almost always low because of impaired intestinal absorption of calcium and of the secondary hyperparathyroidism [20]. In contrast, osteomalacia due to idiopathic hypophosphataemia is associated with hypercalciuria [4]. In vitamin D resistant osteomalacia, urine calcium is frequently normal. In osteomalacia additional findings include a low serum 25-hydroxyvitamin D, a low 1,25-dihydroxyvitamin D, and a high serum PTH level.

Radiologically, osteomalacia may present as a nonspecific decrease in radiodensity of the bone due to the decreased mineral content. The trabecular pattern may appear blurred and fuzzy, particularly in severe cases. The distinguishing feature is the occurrence of painful or nonpainful pseudofractures (Looser's zone or Milkman's fractures), which are linear radiolucencies oriented more or less perpendicular to the cortex (Fig. 29.3.) Bone scans show increased activity at these sites. Pseudofractures usually occur symmetrically in the scapulae, ribs, pubic rami, proximal femur, or proximal ulnae [4]. They represent stress fractures in which the healing process is impaired by the mineralization defect but which heal promptly with appropriate therapy (Fig. 29.3).

In fully developed osteomalacia, the diagnosis can be made without difficulty from the clinical history, characteristic serum changes (see Diagnostic Tests), and appearance of pseudofractures on radiography. In subclinical osteomalacia, only a bone biopsy can definitively confirm the diagnosis [4]. However, it is usually not necessary to do an invasive bone biopsy in working up a patient suspected of having osteomalacia. The reason for this is that one can readily detect vitamin D deficiency even when mild by measurements of serum chemistry and, particularly, serum 25-HD. If a low serum 25-HD is found, one can treat this abnormal biochemical marker irrespective of whether or not the patient is known to have osteomalacia (see below) [20].

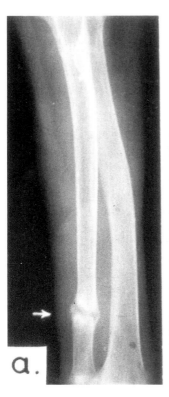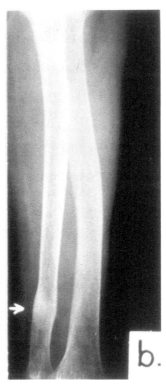

Fig. 29.3 Radiographs of pseudofracture of the ulna in the patient with severe osteomalacia. The pseudofracture before treatment is shown in (a), and the pseudofracture after 3 months of vitamin D therapy is shown in (b).

Thus, nowadays, bone biopsies are usually reserved for complex diagnostic problems [21].

The bone histological features of osteomalacia are increased osteoid width, decreased rate of osteoid maturation; i.e., a prolonged time between the deposition to subsequent mineralization of osteoid [1,22]. Under normal conditions, tetracycline is deposited at the mineralizing front (the interface between osteoid and mineralized bone), as a bright discrete label, whereas in osteomalacia, tetracycline labelling prior to bone biopsy shows widened, smudged tetracycline labels, if the rate of mineralization is significantly reduced, or no label at all if mineralization has ceased completely [21].

Treatment

Identification and treatment of the underlying cause of the vitamin or phosphate deficiency is essential to the management of osteomalacia. For example, maintenance on a gluten-free diet in patients with gluten enteropathy [4], surgical correction of intestinal fistulae or biliary obstruction [8,9], removal of a tumour that has caused osteomalacia (oncogenic osteomalacia) [23], are necessary for optimal patient management. In addition, some form of vitamin D, calcium or phosphate is usually required.

The logical choice for the treatment of the various forms of vitamin D deficiency would be: (1) the parent compound vitamin D (calciferol) for a nutritional deficiency where there is a deficiency of vitamin D_2/D_3; (2) 25-OHD3 (calciferol) for the low serum 25-hydroxyvitamin D seen in chronic liver disease or anticonvulsant therapy [8,9,10]; and (3) 1,25-$(OH)_2$D (calcitriol) for the 1,25-$(OH)_2$D deficiency seen in renal failure [24]. The parent compound, vitamin D, can also be used to treat a deficiency 25-OHD due to liver disease, because, even with liver disease (unless severe), a high dose of vitamin D will result in a normal serum level of 25-OHD [8,9]. In nutritional deficiency, vitamin D 1000 IU/day may be sufficient; but in liver disease, 5000-10 000 IU/day is usually required. The proper dose is determined by monitoring the serum 25-HD. In conclusion, vitamin D is used to treat nutritional vitamin D deficiency and also to treat a deficiency of 25-OHD due to liver disease, whereas 1,25-$(OH)_2$D is used to treat renal disease. Most abnormalities of vitamin D metabolism can be treated with either vitamin D or 1,25-$(OH)_2$D.

It is now appreciated that calcium deficiency per se can lead to osteomalacia and rickets [12,25]. For example, when fluoride stimulates a large increase in bone formation in elderly people who have limited ability to absorb calcium, there is a tendency for calcium deficiency. This calcium deficiency appears to be corrected by the addition of 1,25-$(OH)_2$D therapy [18].

It is important to monitor the patient during vitamin D or 1,25-$(OH)_2$D therapy for two reasons: (1) to make certain that the dose is adequate and (2) to avoid complications from excessive therapy, which, in the case of 1,25-$(OH)_2$D, can be hypercalcaemia. In nutritional vitamin D deficiency, we monitor vitamin D therapy, largely because we need to make certain the patient is adequately treated. Because the dose of vitamin D is usually only 1000 units or, perhaps, slightly more per day, and because this dose, even if continued for a long time, would not be toxic, we are less concerned about toxicity from vitamin D than we are about adequate responses. In patients with nutritional vitamin D deficiency given 1000 units of vitamin D per day, the serum 25-OHD level should return to the normal range within two to three months. This will be attended by a normalization of the low serum calcium and low serum phosphate. However, the elevated alkaline phosphatase may take several months of vitamin D therapy before it declines to the normal level, particularly if the vitamin D deficiency is severe [4,26]. The elevated serum PTH tends to decline as the serum calcium increases to normal. Pseudofractures can show definite evidence of healing within 3 months and are usually completely healed radiographically in less than one year (Fig. 29.3). In nutritional vitamin D deficiency, in addition to vitamin D supplementation, we also recommend at least 1500 mg/day of calcium, since, in order to cure the osteomalacia, the patient must deposit calcium in all of the excess unmineralized osteoid in the skeleton. There is sufficient phosphate in the diet, such that phosphate supplements are unnecessary in nutritional vitamin D deficiency.

Patients who have a low serum 25-OHD as a consequence of liver disease or of anticonvulsant therapy and who are treated with vitamin D are monitored in the same manner as that described above for vitamin D deficiency.

In patients with a deficiency of 1,25-(OH)$_2$D due to renal failure, it is well to start 1,25-(OH)$_2$D therapy early on during the course of renal disease in order to avoid some of the adverse effects on the skeleton of secondary hyperparathyroidism. The oral dose ranges from 0.25 to 1.0 μg per day, depending on the severity of the disease. As mentioned above, we are not only concerned about monitoring serum chemistries to be certain that the patient is having an optimal response, we are also concerned about excessive therapy, inasmuch as the side-effects of this medication can be significant and because it is impossible to predict, from the serum creatinine or from other measures of the degree of renal failure, the optimal dose of 1,25-(OH)$_2$D. The optimal dose is determined individually, based on biochemical monitoring. We routinely monitor serum calcium, PTH and alkaline phosphatase. If the patient has only early renal failure, urine calcium can also be monitored. The urine calcium will be low during the deficiency of 1,25-(OH)$_2$D and will increase into the normal range during 1,25-(OH)$_2$D therapy [20]. With a mild excess of 1,25-(OH)$_2$D therapy, there will be no change in serum calcium but an increase in urine calcium above the normal range of 250 mg/day in females and 300 mg/day in males; with a more severe excess, there will also be an increment in serum calcium. In patients with renal function, it is important not to administer thiazides with 1,25-(OH)$_2$D, because this further increases the risk for hypercalcaemia (thiazides decrease urine calcium excretion by increasing the renal tubular reabsorption of calcium.)

In patients with severe secondary hyperparathyroidism due to renal failure, i.v. injections of 1,25-(OH)$_2$D have been more effective than daily oral administration. Apparently, when 1,25-(OH)$_2$D is given by injection, the blood level of 1,25-(OH)$_2$D reaches a higher peak, as compared with oral administration, without causing hypercalcaemia [24]. The explanation for this is that when 1,25-(OH)$_2$D is given by mouth, it acts locally on the gut to increase calcium absorption, such that there is a preferential effect on calcium absorption over other target tissues such as the parathyroid gland, where it acts to decrease PTH secretion [24,27]. The increment in calcium absorption readily leads to hypercalcaemia, thus

limiting the dose of 1,25-(OH)$_2$D that can be given orally. In contrast, when 1,25-(OH)$_2$D is given i.v., it has equal effects to inhibit parathyroid hormone secretion and to increase calcium absorption, such that a relatively higher dose can be given without hypercalcaemia [24].

In phosphate deficiency states, neutral phosphate salts given at 2 or more grams per day in divided doses will improve bone mineralization. The most common adverse effect with oral phosphate is diarrhoea, especially at doses exceeding 2 g per day. In hypophosphatemic familial rickets (vitamin D resistant rickets), phosphate supplementation should be combined with 1,25-(OH)$_2$D for 3 reasons: (1) phosphate tends to lower serum calcium and increase PTH, which in turn will decrease the TmP for phosphate, thereby lowering the serum phosphate level, which is the main cause of osteomalacia in these patients; (2) these patients have not only an impaired renal tubular reabsorption of phosphate, but they also have impaired renal tubular synthesis of 1,25-(OH)$_2$D; (3) it is important that PTH not be elevated in these patients because PTH decreases serum phosphate and the cause of osteomalacia in these patients is a decreased serum phosphate. (Serum calcium and serum 1,25-(OH)$_2$D are the two major inhibitors of PTH secretion.) Thus, patients with vitamin D resistant rickets should receive large doses of neutral phosphate salts, 1,25-(OH)$_2$D therapy, which may range up to 2 μg per day, and, also, calcium supplements [13].

Hypophosphataemia seems to produce a mineralization defect regardless of the serum 1,25-(OH)$_2$D value. Accordingly, in hypophosphataemic vitamin D rickets and osteomalacia, one frequently sees a low 1,25-(OH)$_2$D serum value, whereas in hypercalciuric hypophosphataemia, there may be a low serum phosphate and a high serum 1,25-(OH)$_2$D. Both of these situations can result in osteomalacia. In practical therapeutic terms, it is important to know the serum level of 1,25-(OH)$_2$D in a given state of hypophosphataemia because, under certain conditions such as vitamin D resistant rickets, 1,25-(OH)$_2$D supplements will be required, whereas in others such as hypophosphataemic hypercalciuria, serum 1,25-(OH)$_2$D may be high and, thus, 1,25-(OH)$_2$D therapy would be contraindicated.

In general, if the patient is receiving 1,25-

(OH)$_2$D therapy and has normal renal function, the risk of hypercalcaemia can be reduced by limiting the total calcium intake to 1000 mg/daily. If larger amounts of calcium are given, it is essential to monitor the serum calcium at frequent intervals. The advantage of 1,25-(OH)$_2$D therapy is that all patients respond in some manner to 1,25-(OH)$_2$D therapy (with the exception of those rare individuals with mutant 1,25-(OH)$_2$D receptors). The disadvantage of 1,25-(OH)$_2$D is that it is such a potent drug that serious side-effects can occur.

Osteoporosis

In this chapter, we consider osteoporosis in both males and females, but, in our discussion of osteoporosis, we will focus more on female osteoporosis, because this disease is much more common in females than in males. Osteoporosis is defined as a reduction of bone density to a level that increases the risk of fracture with minimal or no trauma.

Osteoporosis is a common and costly disease. For example, it has been estimated that there are almost 20 million people in the US with osteoporosis at a health care cost of about $10 billion annually [28,29]. It is estimated that more than 25% of women over 65 years of age develop osteoporosis, and the prevalence increases further with age [30]. In men, osteoporosis usually becomes manifest in the 7th decade (senile osteoporosis), at which time the prevalence of this disease shows an overall female to male ratio of about 5:1 or greater.

Aetiology and pathogenesis

A variety of conditions can lead to osteoporosis (Table 29.2). Thus, in order to provide appropriate therapy, the underlying disorder must be recognized and corrected. Osteoporosis is classified as either primary, when the cause is not entirely established, or secondary, when the disease can be attributed to hereditary or acquired abnormalities. Primary osteoporosis is much more common than secondary osteoporosis. Of the various types of osteoporosis (Table 29.2), postmenopausal and senile osteoporosis are the most common forms, such that more than 90% of

Table 29.2   Classification of osteoporosis

I. Primary osteoporosis
  1. Idiopathic
    a) Juvenile
    b) Young adults

  2. Postmenopausal

  3. Senile (age 65+)

II. Secondary osteoporosis
  1. Associated with hereditable disorders of connective tissue
    a) Osteogenesis imperfecta
    b) Marfan's syndrome
    c) Morquio's syndrome
    d) Hurler's syndrome

  2. Endocrine disorders
    a) Cushing's disease
    b) Hyperthyroidism
    c) Acromegaly
    d) Hypogonadism
       i) oestrogen deficiency*
       ii) testosterone deficiency

  3. Drug induced
    a) Corticosteroids
    b) Anticonvulsants
    c) Heparin

  4. Immobilization

  5. Malignant states – multiple myeloma

  6. Others
    a) Lactase deficiency
    b) Malnutrition
    c) Renal calcium leak
    d) Cirrhosis
    e) Alcoholism

* Oestrogen deficiency before physiological menopause, i.e. oophorectomy, some athletes.

females presenting with a low bone density have postmenopausal or senile osteoporosis.

Postmenopausal osteoporosis

Bone loss occurs at the menopause because of the development of an imbalance in bone remodelling; both bone resorption and bone formation increase, but bone resorption increases more than bone formation, and the result is a net reduction of bone density. The skeletal sites at risk for fracture are those composed largely of trabecular bone: the vertebrae, ribs, distal radii and proximal femora, presumably because of the active remodelling in trabecular and endosteal cortical bone at these sites. Eventually, size and number of trabeculae are decreased and the cortices are thin, but the qualities of the bone produced appears morphologically normal (Fig. 29.4).

The dramatic decline in oestrogen production during the menopause is now known to play a predominant role in the postmenopausal acceleration of bone loss, and the mechanism of this oestrogen deficiency bone loss is being disclosed at the molecular level [31,32]. Because most nucleated cells have oestrogen receptors, it seems likely that the molecular mechanism whereby oestrogen affects bone probably includes a direct local action on bones cells, and, also secondary actions on other organs. Thus, oestrogen appears to have a direct action to decrease IL-1, IL-6 and TNFα and increase TGF-β production by osteoblasts, which, in turn, is thought to reduce osteo-

clastic resorption [31,32]. Thus, the increase in bone turnover which is typical of the postmenopausal state is thought to be, in part, a consequence of increased local production of IL-1, IL-6 and TNFα and decreased production of TGF-β. An example of the effect of oestrogen to decrease bone resorption through a secondary mechanism (endocrine) would be the effect of oestrogen to increase serum $1,25(OH)_2D$ and, thereby, improve calcium absorption, an effect which would tend to lower serum PTH and, thus, decrease bone resorption [33]. Despite these recent advances, postmenopausal osteoporosis is still traditionally considered a primary type, because oestrogen deficiency alone may not entirely account for the development of osteoporosis.

A number of factors other than oestrogen contribute to the development of osteoporosis. Genetic and environmental factors, for example, have been found to play a significant role in initiating and modifying the course of osteoporosis. Environmental factors include inadequate calcium intake, smoking, alcoholism and poor physical activity. As much as 70% of low bone density at the peak of skeletal maturity is thought to be genetically determined [34,35,36]. Accordingly, peak bone density is strongly influenced by heredity, race and sex, with males having more skeletal mass than females, and blacks more than whites [37,38].

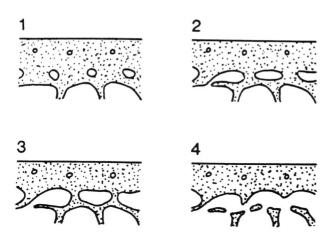

Fig. 29.4 Microscopic structural stages of cortical bone loss. Illustrated are the few successive stages in osteoclast-dependent thinning of cortical bone: (a) shows normal adult cortex; (b) shows enlargement of the subendosteal spaces and communication of these spaces with the marrow cavity; (c) shows further enlargement of these spaces and conversion of the inner third of the cortex to a structure that topographically resembles trabecular bone, with an attending expansion of the marrow cavity; (d) shows perforation and disconnection of the new trabecular structures. Loss of connectivity leads to a deterioration of mechanical performance of the corresponding bony structure. (Adapted with permission from Parfitt, AM, *Calcif Tissue Int* **36 (suppl.):** S123, 1984).

Senile osteoporosis

While oestrogen deficiency is known to play a dominant role in postmenopausal osteoporosis, the cause of senile osteoporosis (i.e. those presenting with osteoporosis after 65 years of age) is less certain. One of the major advances in understanding this type of osteoporosis is the recognition that the efficiency of calcium absorption declines with age and that this is attended by a progressive increase with age in serum PTH. Thus, it has been proposed that at least one of the causes of senile osteoporosis is secondary hyperparathyroidism [39]. This, however, only represents a subgroup of those patients presenting with osteoporosis who are more than 65 years of age. Some of these patients with secondary hyperparathyroidism will actually have mild vitamin D deficiency as manifested by a decrease in serum

25(OH)D. Mild vitamin D deficiency has been shown to occur in subjects residing at northerly latitudes [40]. Both of these abnormalities, namely, the decrease of calcium absorption with age and the deficiency of vitamin D, lead to decreased calcium absorption, are readily corrected, and, thus, are important to recognize. Not all patients with senile osteoporosis exhibit vitamin D deficiency or calcium malabsorption. Thus, it is clear that senile osteoporosis is a heterogeneous disease.

The classification of patients with primary osteoporosis into postmenopausal and senile is somewhat misleading [39]. For example, in order for a patient to exhibit fragility fractures in the first ten years after the menopause (i.e. postmenopausal osteoporosis), it seems likely that such a patient, in addition to postmenopausal bone loss, entered the postmenopausal period with a relatively low peak bone density. Thus, the pathogenesis of the osteoporosis in these patients would be more than merely oestrogen deficiency bone loss. Moreover, those patients presenting with fragility fractures after 65 years of age, and thus considered to have senile osteoporosis, could be patients who entered the menopause with a high peak bone density and, as a consequence, did not develop a low enough bone density during the postmenopausal years to develop fragility fractures until after 65 years of age. Thus, patients with primary osteoporosis may develop this skeletal disease as a consequence of the variable expression of several contributing factors which will include: (1) a low peak bone density; (2) a high bone loss rate at the menopause due to oestrogen deficiency; (3) poor calcium absorption; and (4) lifestyle factors (see above). In addition, it seems probable that there are a multitude of other factors that will eventually be disclosed to have a negative impact on bone density in patients over 65 years of age. One such potential factor could be the decline in serum IGF-I that occurs with age [41]. This is known to be an anabolic agent such that a deficiency of serum IGF-1 might lead to a decrease in bone formation.

Clinical manifestations

Osteoporosis is a chronic, progressive, debilitating disease that may remain silent until the patient suffers a fracture, often from minor trauma such as coughing, turning in bed, or bending. Back pain due to osteoporosis is typically aggravated by activity and relieved by rest. The spectrum of symptoms varies greatly, from the absence of pain to severe pain, depending largely on the extent and rapidity with which the fracture occurs and the pain threshold of the patient. For example, some patients have vague back pain without spinal fracture, whereas others have a spinal wedge fracture without a history of back pain.

In patients with osteoporosis, vertebral collapse with back pain is the most common presentation. The patient may complain of two types of pain: (1) there is an acute onset of pain in the area of the crushed vertebrae. This is sharp, severe, radiates laterally and is associated with paravertebral muscle spasm and percussion tenderness over the area. The severe pain may persist for 3–4 weeks and then gradually subside. Lack of improvement in the acute phase within 2–3 months should prompt a search for a possible pathologic cause of the fracture. (2) The other type of pain experienced in osteoporosis is mild, dull, usually described as an aching sensation or feeling of tiredness in the lower thoracic or lumbar area (especially after prolonged standing or activity), and is relieved by rest [42]. This type of pain tends to be chronic.

Progressive anterior wedging in the midthoracic spine produces the dowager's hump deformity (i.e. kyphosis), limits chest mobility, and results in loss of height and abdominal protuberance. In contrast, fractures in the lumbar vertebrae are usually collapse of the centrum resulting in a 'codfish' deformity. Hip and Colles' fractures, when they occur in the elderly, are most commonly related to osteoporosis. Hip fracture is by far the most serious complication of osteoporosis and can cause significant debilitation. Mortality from hip fracture exceeds 20% within 1 year [43] and, in those who survive, rehabilitation is often difficult and protracted.

Diagnostic tests

This section will largely deal with diagnostic tests for primary osteoporosis. It should be emphasized however, that the diagnosis of primary osteoporosis is made by excluding secondary causes of osteoporosis. This can usually be done by a history and physical examination and routine laboratory tests, although in some situations, extensive testing may be required in difficult cases to evaluate for secondary osteoporosis. Those diseases that should be considered in working up patients with osteoporosis are shown in Table 29.2 under secondary osteoporosis.

Bone densitometry

The first step in making the diagnosis of osteoporosis is to measure the bone density. This can be accomplished with either dual energy x-ray absorptiometry (DEXA) or by quantitative computerized tomography (QCT) [29,44]. Because osteoporosis is first seen in the spine, these density methods are generally applied to the spine. The other site of special clinical interest is the hip because of the serious clinical problem of hip fracture. The DEXA instrument is the only instrument that can measure hip bone density [45]. For individual patients, we routinely measure both QCT spinal bone density and DEXA hip bone density, because the correlation between spine and hip density is relatively poor. On the other hand, on a population basis, fracture risk can be predicted from a bone density measurement at any skeletal site [46].

The advantage of the QCT for measurement of bone density is that it can be applied to measure only trabecular bone, and, since trabecular bone is metabolically more active than cortical bone, more rapid changes are seen by QCT than by DEXA (measurement of) spinal bone density. The main disadvantages of the QCT approach are: (1) it does not have the high precision of the DEXA measurement; and (2) it is more expensive. The advantage of DEXA bone density measurements is that it is much more convenient than QCT measurements, because QCTs are only available at major medical centres. However, in elderly people (less so in younger subjects), there are frequently age related changes that compromise the validity of the DEXA measurement of the spine. For example there may be a considerable amount of osteophytosis and end-plate sclerosis (from degenerative disk disease) that spuriously increased the bone density value determined by DEXA. Furthermore, extraskeletal calcifications can also spuriously influence the

DEXA bone density. Thus, one can see patients with fragility fractures (spontaneous atraumatic fractures) who have normal bone density by DEXA but have low bone density by QCT. In any case, these potential diagnostic pitfalls with the DEXA instrument should be considered when the DEXA data are interpreted. Interpretation of bone density results is as follows:

1. Bone density that is above the fracture threshold and within 1 standard deviations of peak bone density. This is considered to be a normal bone density.
2. Bone density that is above the fracture threshold but is 1 standard deviations or more below the peak bone density. This is considered osteopenia.
3. Bone density that is below the fracture threshold or below 2.5 SD of young normal mean bone density. This is considered osteoporosis. The spinal fracture threshold for our QCT method is 100 mg/cc, though published fracture threshold values range from 70–110 mg/cc. The spinal fracture threshold for the hologic DEXA is 0.80 g/cm^2, for the lunar DEXA. 074 g/cm^2.

Calcium absorption

If the patient has a low bone density (either osteopenia or osteoporosis), the next step is to assess calcium absorption. Unfortunately, there is no commercially available validated test to make this assessment. None the less, we mention this parameter because we feel it is a key aspect of determining the cause of osteoporosis and because, in the future, this parameter will undoubtedly be routinely measured. We assess calcium absorption by determining the 24-hour urine calcium excretion in a patient on a total (diet plus supplements) calcium intake at 1500 mg for at least one week, which is the usual amount prescribed for osteoporotic patients [47]. In patients with either known primary hyperparathyroidism or a past history of kidney stones, this 24-hour urine should be collected while on a low calcium diet of 400 mg/day. The rationale for this test follows: when the patient is on a relatively high calcium intake (1500 mg/day), a 24-hour urine calcium of less than 100 mg/day suggests calcium malabsorption. This level of 100 mg/day is an arbitrary value based on the facts that: (1) urine excretion of

50 mg or less calcium per day while on a regular calcium diet is low, reflecting calcium deficiency or vitamin D deficiency; and (2) a urinary calcium level of 100 mg/day is substantially below the upper normal limit of 250 mg/day and, thus, would not be associated with an increased risk of renal stones. In addition, patients with secondary hyperparathyroidism (i.e. high serum PTH) due to calcium malabsorption seldom have 24-hour urine calcium volume above 100 mg. Therefore, we have defined 100 mg/day as a safe value to achieve with calcium and/or vitamin D or $1,25(OH)_2D$ therapy (see section on Treatment). It should be emphasized that this test to measure calcium absorption is a rational approach but is a test which has not been validated. The major reason for attempting to measure calcium absorption is that one can readily correct a deficiency of calcium absorption either by adding more calcium supplementation or, if this is ineffective, by adding vitamin D or calcitriol therapy.

Of the many serum chemistries that might be ordered during the workup of patients with osteoporosis (as determined by bone density evaluation), our focus is on only two parameters, serum PTH and serum 25(OH)D. We measure serum PTH because we have found high values in almost 20% of our clinic patients, either because of secondary or primary hyperparathyroidism. With respect to serum 25(OH)D measurement, the indication for this test depends upon where the patient resides. If the patient resides in northern Europe and is over 70 years of age, this test should be strongly considered because of a high prevalence of low serum 25(OH)D values in such patients [40]. However, patients living in southern California seldom exhibit low serum 25(OH)D. A low serum 25(OH)D in a patient with normal liver function indicates inadequate exposure to sunlight and, in addition, inadequate dietary intake of vitamin D. Figure 29.2 provides a schema of vitamin D metabolism.

Bone resorption

At the same time calcium absorption is estimated, bone resorption can be measured. This is assessed by 24-hour urine measurements of hydroxyproline/creatinine and is measured in the same urine sample that is used for the 24-hour calcium assessment. Because the diet normally contains hydroxyproline, the patient is placed on a hydroxyproline-free diet the meal prior to and the day of the 24-hour collection. The normal range for urine hydroxyproline/creatinine is quite broad, and there is no general agreement as to what values indicate high resorption. Since, in general, normal premenopausal women lose very little bone [30], we have arbitrarily selected the mean of the normal range for premenopausal women plus two standard deviations as the maximum upper normal limit of bone resorption. This value (in our laboratory) is equal to 25 mg hydroxyproline per gram creatinine. Thus, any postmenopausal patient with a value greater than 25 mg/gram is considered to have increased bone resorption and requires anti-resorptive therapy. If we wish to be more certain about preventing further bone loss, we attempt to achieve hydroxyproline/creatinine values at about 12.5 mg/gram of hydroxyproline/creatinine, which is the mean premenopausal level.

More than 80% of osteoporotic patients in our clinic have hydroxyproline/creatinine values greater than 12.5 mg per gram. Tests other than hydroxyproline can be used to assess bone resorption. These include measurements of urine crosslinks (i.e., pyridinoline/creatinine (PYR/CR) and deoxypyridinoline/creatinine (DPYR/CR) in urine) [48]. These tests are more accurate and are more specific indices of bone resorption than is hydroxyproline. Moreover, these measurements do not require a hydroxyproline-free diet. Normal values for the crosslinks are not as well established as for hydroxyproline. Our preliminary results suggest that the premenopausal mean plus or minus two standard deviations for pyridinoline/creatinine is about 44 ± 34 nM/mM and for DPYR/creatinine 10 ± 9 nm/mm. Because of the relatively large longitudinal variation of serum and urine assays for bone formation and bone resorption, we suggest that therapeutic decisions be made on more than an assay at one point in time.

Other tests that are sometimes used in the evaluation of patients with osteoporosis include radiographic evaluations to evaluate for the presence of fractures and for the possible presence of pathologic fractures. Radiographic features of osteoporosis include diffuse radiolucency, accentuation of vertical trabeculae (because of preferential loss of horizontally oriented trabeculae), cortical thinning, anterior wedging of thoracic vertebral bodies, and biconcavity or 'codfishing' of vertebral bodies [49]. In addition, the radionuclide bone scan is useful in determining whether a compression fracture is old or recent. Increased radionuclide activity at the site of a known fracture indicates ongoing healing (bone formation). The bone scan may also be valuable in detecting the presence of other bone disorders (i.e. metastatic bone lesions and degenerative or inflammatory changes).

Once the patient has had a bone density measurement, a calcium absorption assessment, and a bone resorption measurement, the patient is ready for application of a therapeutic regimen.

Treatment of osteoporosis

In this section, we will discuss the prevention and treatment of primary osteoporosis in females and males, but the focus will be on females because of the higher prevalence of osteoporosis in females. The therapeutic agents available for osteoporosis are shown in Table 29.3. The therapeutic principles that we describe below for the treatment of primary osteoporosis in females also apply, for the most part, to males and females with secondary osteoporosis. The therapeutic goals for osteoporosis are to decrease the pain associated with vertebral fractures and to prevent future fractures. The following are the therapeutic principles which we apply:

1. Patients with calcium malabsorption must be

Table 29.3   Classification of therapeutic agents for osteoporosis

I. Agents that decrease bone resorption
  1. Oestrogen
  2. Calcium
  3. Vitamin D
  4. Calcitonin
  5. Biphosphonates
  6. Testosterone
  7. $1,25(OH)_2D$ or $1\alpha D_3$

II. Agents that increase bone formation
  1. Fluoride
  2. Testosterone*
  3. Exercise* 4, PTH 1-34

* Increases bone formation, but increase in bone density is small.

treated with either vitamin D, larger amounts of calcium, or with either $1,25(OH)_2D$ (Calcitriol) or $1\alpha D_3$.
2. Patients with high urine calcium or a history of kidney stones should be given calcium supplements with caution.
3. All patients should be placed on an exercise program that should include walking, as well as upper body exercises (i.e., weight lifting) within the limits of the patient's disability.
4. Patients with a high bone resorption rate as determined by urine biochemical markers should be put on an antiresorptive therapy such as oestrogen replacement therapy, biphosphonate or calcitonin. (Only oral and i.v. etidronate and i.v. aredia are available in the US, whereas in some countries other bisphosphonates also are available.)
5. A patient who has a bone density below the fracture threshold should be referred to a treatment centre where the patient can be considered for fluoride therapy.
6. If a patient has severe bone pain from a recent spinal fracture, injectable calcitonin should be considered.

Low bone density is the major determinant of increased fracture risk in osteoporosis. It has

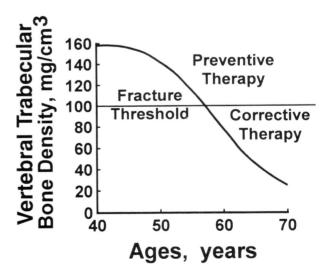

Fig. 29.5 This is a schema of the decline in bone density with age as determined by quantitative computer topography (QCT). The fracture threshold was shown to be 100 mg per cc [44]. In general, patients who have bone densities above the fracture threshold are placed on preventative therapy (see text), and patients who have densities below the fracture threshold are placed on corrective therapy, which includes preventative therapy plus a bone formation stimulator.

been demonstrated that the risk for fracturing in the spine is increased when the vertebral trabecular bone density measured by QCT is 100 mg/cc or less (defined here as the fracture threshold) [44]. A rational approach to therapy would, therefore, be prevention of bone loss when the bone density is above the fracture threshold (preventive therapy) and replacement of bone mass previously lost to a level above the fracture threshold when the bone density is below 100 mg/cc (corrective therapy) (Fig. 29.5). Table 29.3 lists the therapeutic agents (antiresorbers and bone formation stimulators) currently available for the preventive and corrective treatment of osteoporosis. A combination of agents (an inhibitor of bone resorption and a stimulator of bone formation) is usually employed in corrective therapeutic regimens in order to preserve trabecular architecture with antiresorptive therapy to increase bone mass above the fracture threshold and with a bone generation stimulator.

Preventive therapy

If the patient has normal bone density, we recommend preventive therapy using oestrogen, adequate calcium intake, and exercise. Preventive therapy is also recommended for patients with osteopenia and patients with osteoporosis. Patients with osteoporosis, in addition to preventive therapy, also require corrective therapy.

Exercise

It should be emphasized that inactivity can lead to bone loss. A 0.9% per week bone loss has been reported from the lumbar spine in patients on bed rest, and the bone loss was nearly restored with reintroduction of load bearing [50]. This emphasizes the deleterious effect of inactivity and the importance of an exercise program in the treatment of osteoporosis [51]. Based on recent studies, the exercise protocol we recommend includes walking two miles daily and engaging in some type of upper body exercise such as weight lifting (e.g. in an erect standing position – back extended – the patient holds a can of peas in each hand and lifts them over her head. Eventually, as strength improves, the patient should use 5 lb. weights in each hand for this type of exercise.) It

should be emphasized that all exercise should be designed to avoid injury.

Calcium, vitamin D, 1,25(OH)$_2$D and 1αD$_3$ therapy

Intestinal calcium absorption decreases with aging and is further reduced in osteoporotic patients when compared with controls [52]. This can lead to calcium deficiency which increases bone resorption by stimulation of parathyroid hormone secretion, whereas normal or high calcium absorption retards bone resorption. Heaney et al. [53] have shown that at least 1500 mg of calcium daily is required in order to overcome the negative calcium balance in postmenopausal women who are not oestrogen treated (Table 29.3). For those patients on oestrogen therapy, 1000 mg of calcium/day is recommended. Dietary calcium may be supplemented with calcium salts (e.g., calcium carbonate, phosphate, lactate, gluconate, or citrate) to meet the increased requirements. Absorption of calcium supplements can be estimated from the rise in urinary calcium (see section on Diagnostic tests).

If the patient has an appropriate urinary calcium excretion after consuming a diet containing a total 1500 mg/day, particularly if the patient also has a normal serum PTH and a normal serum 25(OH)D, this would constitute evidence of normal calcium absorption. The goal of administering calcium is to avoid bone loss and the high bone turnover that occurs with secondary hyperparathyroidism*. If the urine calcium were lower than 100 mg per 24 hours on a 1500 mg diet, the first diagnosis to be considered would be mild vitamin D deficiency which would be reflected by a low serum 25(OH)D. If this deficiency were found, the patient should be treated with at least vitamin D 1000 units daily for 2–3 months (Table 29.3). At this time, the serum 25(OH)D should be normal, and the calcium absorption test should be repeated to document that this has corrected the calcium malabsorption. If the serum 25(OH)D test is normal but the patient has an abnormal calcium absorption test, larger amounts of oral calcium, perhaps up to

---

* Recent evidence suggests that high bone turnover from any cause has an adverse effect on trabecular architecture (i.e. increases trabecular perforations([54].

2000–3000 mg/day, can be administered in an attempt to raise the urine calcium up to 100 mg per 24 hours. In addition, rather than using the most common forms of calcium supplements (i.e. calcium carbonates, or calcium phosphate), a more soluble form of calcium (i.e., calcium citrate) may be prescribed.

If increasing the dose of calcium and/or changing to a different calcium salt fails to increase urine calcium and decrease serum PTH (if evaluated) after three months of supplementation, calcitriol (Rocaltrol) 0.25 μg/day, or $1\alpha D_3$ 0.5 μg/day along with a total (diet plus supplements) calcium intake of 800–1000 mg/day, is prescribed (Table 29.3) [20]. (Higher calcium intakes increase the risk of hypercalcaemia). If after one week of this therapy the 24-hour urine remains below 100 mg/day, the dose of calcitriol is increased to 0.5 μg/day and the dose of $1\alpha D_3$ is increased to 1.0 μg/day. Larger doses of calcitriol or $1\alpha D_3$ are not recommended in elderly osteoporotic patients because of the risk of hypercalcaemia. To avoid the hypercalcaemia, patients on calcitriol or $1\alpha D_3$ therapy are monitored by measuring serum calcium one week after starting therapy (or changing the dose). Subsequently, serum and urine calcium are monitored every three to six months. Thiazides should not be prescribed with calcitriol or $1\alpha D_3$, inasmuch as the vitamin D analogue and thiazides together further increase the risk of hypercalcaemia (i.e. thiazides decrease urine calcium excretion and calcitriol increases calcium absorption, which together tend to promote an increase in serum calcium).

Antiresorptive therapy

If the patient has a high bone resorption rate, as determined by measurement of urine hydroxyproline/creatinine or urine pyridinoline/creatinine, the patient should be placed on antiresorptive therapy. It is important to detect a high bone resorption, because there are at least three different types of drugs to correct this abnormality; namely, oestrogen, bisphosphonates and calcitonin. On the other hand, if the patient has a bone resorption rate that is below the mean for premenopausal patients (see section on Diagnostic tests), these patients generally

show a poor response to antiresorptive therapy [55].

Oestrogen replacement therapy after oophorectomy or menopause has been shown to retard cortical and trabecular bone loss and reduce the risk of fracturing in the spine, hip, and wrist (Table 29.3) [56,57,58]. Unopposed oestrogen therapy increases the risk of endometrial cancer. To reduce this risk in a woman with an intact uterus, it is recommended that oestrogen be given cyclically (i.e., given on days 1–25 followed by 3-day free period) in combination with a progestational agent (Provera 5–10 mg/day) on the last 10–14 days of the cycle. This cyclic therapy allows sloughing of hyperplastic endometrium and, thus, is one means to reduce the risk of endometrial cancer. There is some evidence that oestrogen with or without progesterone therapy may increase the risk for breast cancer. We, therefore, recommend mammography examinations annually for all patients on oestrogen therapy.

This cyclic therapy usually causes withdrawal bleeding, a complication which is unacceptable to patients more than 65 to 70 years of age. In order to avoid withdrawal bleeding and, at the same time, prevent endometrial cancer, a current practice is to give the equivalent of Premarin 0.625 mg daily every day of the month and, in addition, a progestational agent such as Provera 2.5 mg daily every day of the month. After one year of this treatment, about 75% of patients will exhibit an atrophic endometrium (and thus have no increased risk of endometrial cancer) without withdrawal bleeding [59]. The lowest dose of oestrogen that has been found to be effective in preventing bone loss in postmenopausal women is 0.625 mg per day of conjugated oestrogen (Premarin) or its equivalent. Doses higher than 1.25 mg per day are associated with greater incidence of complications without deriving further benefit to the skeleton. The side effects reported with high dose oral oestrogens (including intravascular clotting, cholelithiasis, and hypertension) have been ascribed to the so called first pass effect in the liver. Ingested oestrogen undergoes partial metabolism to less active forms in the liver before delivery into the general circulation.

The transdermal dosage form of oestrogen, which delivers oestradiol (E2) through the skin into the systemic circulation in a constant controlled manner, bypasses the liver and reduces, if not eliminates, the complications attributed to enhanced hepatic effects [60,61].

Because the most rapid bone loss occurs in the early stages of menopause, the earlier oestrogen replacement therapy is initiated, the more effective it will be to prevent the development of osteoporosis. This also holds for other antiresorptive agents. Although oestrogen has its greatest effect to preserve bone density when it is given at the time of the menopause, even patients who are 70 years of age or older will benefit from the antiresorptive effects of oestrogen therapy. However, such patients are seldom inclined to tolerate the menses that occur in many women on oestrogen therapy with an intact uterus. Therefore, we frequently recommend etidronate or injectable calcitonin therapy to elderly osteoporotic patients with an intact uterus.

Although we employ a dose of 0.625 mg/day of conjugated oestrogens or its equivalent at the beginning of therapy, we have found that this dose is not adequate in all patients to reduce the bone resorption rate to the premenopausal value. With oestrogen replacement therapy, the nadir for the decrement in urine hydroxyproline/creatinine is at about 6 months [62]. At this time, if we do not find a normal (premenopausal) bone resorption level, we either increase the dose of oestrogen, or, if this is not tolerated, add another antiresorption agent at a low dose and re-evaluate the patient after another 6 months of therapy. It should be emphasized that, because the time-dependent variation in urine hydroxyproline/creatinine assay is large (i.e., the daily, weekly and monthly variation from unknown causes), the physician may not want to use a single value for therapeutic decision. Thus, the physician may wish to make therapeutic decisions on the basis of two or more similar lab results in sequence.

If a patient has osteoporosis or osteopenia and a normal resorption rate, the patient is still advised to take oestrogen replacement therapy because of the positive actions of oestrogen on the cardiovascular system. Moreover, if the patient has a normal bone density and a normal bone resorption rate, we still recommend oestrogen replacement therapy for the same reasons.

When oestrogen is contradicted or ineffective at the highest tolerated dose (for example, some patients complain of breast tenderness at even moderate doses of oestrogen), we use either etidronate or injectable calcitonin*. The recommended dose of etidronate is 400 mg/day for two weeks out of twelve weeks [63]. It has not yet been established that this dose is effective for all patients. While it is not known when the nadir for hydroxyproline/creatinine is reached on this therapeutic regimen, we suggest sampling at 6 month intervals after commencing therapy. It may be necessary to use higher doses (i.e., more continuous treatment) of etidronate to achieve a premenopausal urine hydroxyproline/creatinine. If so, higher doses should be given with some caution since larger doses of etidronate may cause osteomalacia. If higher doses are used, etidronate should be given intermittently to allow for the healing of the osteomalacia that could be caused by etidronate. It is also recommended that etidronate be given on an empty stomach (i.e., with no ingestion of food for 2 hours before or after, since any calcium in the GI tract will precipitate the etidronate and impair its absorption.) Side-effects to etidronate therapy are minor; we have observed only an occasional complaint of lower gastrointestinal discomfort.

The other agent for antiresorptive therapy is injectable salmon calcitonin (Miacalcin, Calcimar) (Table 29.3). The dose of calcitonin recommended in the PDR is 100 units daily. We are concerned that high daily injections may cause resistance [64]. Thus, we give lower doses (50 units subcutaneously daily), and we give the drug cyclically (3 months on and one month off). Some experts give even lower doses (i.e., 50 units three times weekly instead of daily). However, the theoretical advantage of these lower dose therapeutic regimens have not been experimentally validated. The nadir for the urine hydroxyproline/creatinine following daily calcitonin therapy is approximately three months, at which time the dose can be adjusted as necessary. The major problem with calcitonin therapy is that it must be given by injection. However, the nasal spray form of calcitonin is expected to be marketed sometime in 1995 in the US.

*Etidronate has been approved by the FDA for the treatment of Paget's disease. It has not, however, been approved by the FDA for the treatment of osteoporosis. Thus, the use of etidronate in the US is acknowledged as an off label use.

Corrective therapy

In those patients who have established osteoporosis (i.e., bone density below fracture
threshold with or without fragility fractures),
prevention of bone loss by antiresorptive
therapy, as described above, is insufficient to
eliminate the fracture risk (Fig. 29.5). For
example, with 12–18 months of antiresorptive
therapy, there is an increase in bone density of
about 3–5%, after which bone density stabilizes
while the patient continues to receive the drug. If
a patient has a spinal bone density as measured
by QCT of approximately 50 mg/cc and there is
only a 5% increase in bone density with antiresorptive therapy, the patient on this therapy will
continue to be over 48 density points (mg/cc)
below the fracture threshold of 100 mg/cc and,
thus, at severe risk for an osteoporotic fragility
fracture. In order to eliminate this risk for fracture or at least minimize the risk, corrective
therapy is required (Fig. 29.5). Two forms of
therapy have been shown to produce large increases in bone density: fluoride and PTH 1-34
(Table 29.3) [65,66,67]. Both agents stimulate
bone formation. Thus, bone formation agents
can produce large amounts in bone density,
whereas antiresorption agents produce small increases in bone density. Fluoride is an approved
therapy in some countries in Europe and in South
America but not in the US. PTH 1-34 is in
experimental human trials but is not approved
thus far in any country.

One might argue that it would be sufficient to
use a bone formation stimulator to replete skeletal losses without the addition of an anti-
resorber. In terms of the increment in bone
density produced, antiresorbers contribute only a
trivial amount to the combination of antiresorbers and bone formation stimulators to the
increase in bone density. However, antiresorbers
tend to decrease bone turnover, and recent
studies suggest the higher the bone turnover, the
greater the risk for fracture, independent of bone
density [68,69]. Thus, antiresorbers not only
cause a modest increase in bone density, but they
also preserve the trabecular architecture which is
important to bone strength. The goal of the
combination therapy would be to use bone
formation stimulators to increase overall density
and to use antiresorptive therapy: (1) to preserve
the trabecular architecture; and (2) to decrease

remodelling and, thus, decrease surface density
of remodelling excavations which serve as stress
concentrators on the trabecular surface (stress
concentrators would increase the risks of trabecular microfractures).

Fluoride is a strong bone formation stimulator, but its use for osteoporosis remains controversial. In the prospective clinical trial published
by the Mayo Clinic group in 1990, there was an
increase in spinal bone density but no significant
decrease in the spinal fracture rate [70]. On the
other hand, in a recent study by Pak, there was an
increase in spinal bone density and a significant
decrease in the spinal fracture rate [71]. In bone
biopsies from the Mayo Clinic study, many
patients exhibited highly significant morpho-
metric evidence of osteomalacia which we pre-
sume was, at least in part, due to calcium
deficiency [17,18]. It is conceivable that at least
part of the poor mechanical performance of the
bones in the patients in the Mayo Clinic trial was
a consequence of the calcium deficiency osteomalacia. One difference between the Mayo Clinic
study and the Pak study is that, in the Pak study,
the amount of fluoride given per unit time was
less; thus, the patients would be less likely to
develop osteomalacia.

The dose of fluoride used in those studies in
which a decrease in spinal fracture rate was seen
was about 20 mg of elemental fluoride a day,
usually given in two divided doses. One monitors
the serum fluoride levels after 2 months fluoride
therapy in order to achieve a serum level between
5–10 μM [72]. (The serum sample is obtained in
the morning before the dose of fluoride.) A serum
level of 5 μM or less is generally ineffective.
There is no evidence that serum levels between
10–20 μM have an adverse effect on the skeleton
or other tissues; however, serum fluoride levels
higher than 10 μM are more likely to be associated with side-effects from fluoride. The two
side-effects seen with fluoride are GI distress and
what is referred to as the peripheral pain syndrome. One only infrequently sees GI side-effects
with MFP fluoride or with time released sodium
fluoride. In past studies with plain sodium
fluoride, up to 50% of patients developed GI side-
effects. Thus, currently, the main side-effect of
fluoride is the peripheral pain syndrome (i.e.,
bone pain usually in weight bearing bones, particularly the feet). The cause of the peripheral
pain is unknown but probably reflects the stimu-

lation of periosteal bone formation [72,73]. Fluoride therapy may cause calcium deficiency, and this could aggravate the peripheral pain syndrome (see below). Withdrawing the fluoride for 1–3 weeks is usually sufficient to allow the pain to spontaneously resolve. Fluoride is then re-instituted at a lower dose.

All patients on fluoride therapy are monitored for the development of calcium deficiency. Recent evidence suggests that calcium deficiency can occur in fluoride treated patients even on 2000 mg calcium/day and that this can contribute to the osteomalacia seen with fluoride therapy [18]. Indeed, the increased prevalence of stress fractures reported in patients on fluoride therapy may have been due, in part, to the complication of calcium deficiency and osteomalacia. Thus, to avoid calcium deficiency, we monitor our patients for: (1) serum alkaline phosphatase (large increments of more than 100% of basal raise the possibility of calcium deficiency; (2) 24-hour urine calcium, which may drop below 50 mg per 24 hours; and (3) serum PTH, which increases above the basal level. When calcium deficiency occurs, as indicated by the above changes, the patient is treated with larger calcium supplements or with either $1,25(OH)_2D$ or $1\alpha D_3$ to increase calcium absorption [18].

Based on the above discussion, it is apparent that there are three main principles involved in fluoride therapy. First, the dose should be such that the patient has an approximate serum fluoride level of 5–10 μM. Serum fluoride values at 5 μM and below are ineffective. The appropriate serum level can be achieved by adjusting the dose of fluoride. Second, the patient must absorb adequate amounts of calcium either through calcium supplementation or through a combination of calcium supplementation and either $1,25(OH)_2D$ therapy or $1\alpha D_3$ therapy. Third, if the peripheral pain syndrome develops, and one has excluded calcium deficiency, the management of this problem is to discontinue the fluoride for one month and restart the patient at a lower dose, irrespective of the serum level. Even following these general principles there will be patients who do not respond adequately to fluoride with a rapid increase in bone density. We have found that even though there are patients who do not show dramatic increases in bone density early on, almost all patients will show some increase in bone density after several years of therapy.

Treatment of acute vertebral compression fractures

The primary symptom of osteoporosis is back pain, usually associated with a vertebral compression fracture. The acute pain is managed reasonably well with rest and analgesics. The biggest clinical problem that we see regarding acute fractures arises when the patient fails to immobilize herself, in which case, the pain is aggravated and fracture healing is impaired. Ambulatory patients experiencing unusual pain should be at bed rest with bathroom privileges for several days. In addition, particularly if the patient has severe pain, injectable salmon calcitonin at a dose of 100 units per day may substantially reduce the pain [74]. All patients are given a calcitonin skin test before therapy is initiated, and, if it is positive, the patient should not receive this medication. The potential side-effects of injectable calcitonin are flushing and nausea. If these side-effects occur, the dose of salmon calcitonin should be reduced to 50 units per day. If the lower dose is tolerated, then the dose can be gradually increased to 100 units a day, a dose which is necessary in order to control the pain attending acute vertebral fractures.

The above therapeutic management program is for the most part successful, though the physician must remember that osteoporosis is a chronic disease which, thus, requires long-term therapy along with appropriate monitoring of therapy and corresponding drug and dose adjustments.

The therapeutic principles presented above for female osteoporotic patients apply, for the most part, to males. For example, if calcium absorption is low, this is corrected as described above. Similarly, if the bone resorption rate is elevated, the patient is treated with antiresorptive therapy. Unfortunately, we do not have normal hydroxyproline/creatinine values in young male adults (i.e., at time when bone density should be stable), and, thus, we do not have a good estimate of the upper normal limit of bone resorption. Like the treatment of female osteoporotics, if the male osteoporotic has a bone density below the fracture threshold, the patient is treated with fluoride or referred to a centre for the evaluation of fluoride treatment.

In contrast to females, there is a subgroup of male osteoporosis patients who require testosterone therapy; namely, those elderly male patients who have a low serum testosterone (Table 29.3). In these patients, long acting testosterone preparations such as testosterone enanthate or cyprionate can be administered intramuscularly at a dose of about 100–200 mg every 2–3 weeks to correct the low serum testosterone. The optimal dose is one which maintains the serum testosterone in the normal range. We monitor serum testosterone one day after the injection and one day before the next injection.

Testosterone acts to decrease bone resorption and probably also increases bone formation [75,76]. An analogy exists between oestrogen therapy and breast cancer and testosterone therapy and prostate cancer. Accordingly, precaution must be exercised to exclude prostate cancer before testosterone therapy is initiated. Thus, the patient should receive a digital prostate examination as well as a serum PSA before initiating testosterone therapy. Moreover, such surveillance for prostate cancer is continued during the period of testosterone therapy. Testosterone therapy is discontinued if the patient develops evidence of prostate cancer.

To summarize, all patients with osteoporosis should routinely have an adequate calcium intake and an exercise programme. Any secondary causes of osteoporosis should be identified since they are usually treatable. Unless contraindicated, postmenopausal women should be placed on oestrogen to prevent or retard the accelerated bone loss that occurs in the postmenopausal period. Patients with evidence of increased bone resorption should receive antiresorptive therapy. Patients who have a bone density below the fracture threshold should be considered for fluoride therapy. This management programme is successful for the most part, though the physician must remember that osteoporosis is a chronic disease which requires a long period of time to correct the bone density deficit.

Acknowledgements

We thank Ms Jamie Lopez for typing the manuscript, Ms Carol Farrell and Ms Barbara Barr for editorial assistance, and Mr Jerry Bohn and the Medical Media staff for the figures. This work was supported, in part, by a VA Merit Review grant and funds from the National Institutes of Health (AR 31062), the Veterans Administration, and the Department of Medicine, Loma Linda University.

References

1. Baylink, D. J., Stauffer, M., Wergedal, J. *et al.* (1970) Formation, mineralization, and resorption of bone in vitamin D deficient rats. *J. Clin. Invest.*, **49**, 1122–1134.
2. Baylink, D. J., Morey, E. R., Ivey, J. L. *et al.* (1980) Vitamin D and bone. In: *Vitamin D; Molecular Biology and Clinical Nutrition* (ed. A. W. Norman) Marcel Dekker, Inc., New York, pp. 387–453.
3. Howard, G. and Baylink, D. J. (1980) Matrix formation and osteoid maturation in vitamin D deficient rats made normocalcemic by dietary means. *Miner. Electrolyte Metab.*, **3**, 44–50.
4. Baylink, D. J. (1994) Osteomalacia. In: *Principles of Geriatric Medicine and Gerontology, 3rd Edition*, (eds W. R. Hazzard, E. L. Bierman, J. P. Blass, W. H. Ettinger, J. B. Halter), McGraw Hill Inc. New York, chapter **77**, pp. 911–922.
5. Frame, B. and Parfitt, A. M. (1978) Osteomalacia: current concepts, *Ann. Int. Med.*, **89**, 966–982.
6. Morgan, D. B., Hunt, G. and Paterson, C. R. (1970) The osteomalacia syndrome after stomach operations. *Q. J. Med.*, **39**, 395.
7. Compston, J. E. *et al.* (1978) Osteomalacia after small-intestinal resection. *Lancet*, **1**, 9.
8. Herlong, H. F. *et al.* (1982) Bone disease in primary biliary cirrhosis: histological features and response to 25-hydroxyvitamin D. *Gastroenterology*, **83**, 103.
9. Compston, J. E. and Thompson, R. P. H. (1977) Intestinal adsorption of 25-hydroxyvitamin D and osteomalacia in primary biliary cirrhosis. *Lancet*, **1**, 721.
10. Davie, M. W. J. *et al.* (1983) Low plasma 25-hydroxyvitamin D and serum calcium levels in institutionalized epileptic subjects: associated risk factors, consequences and response to treatment and vitamin D. *Q. J. Med.*, **205**, 79.
11. Sherrard, D. J. *et al.* (1974) Quantitative histological studies on the pathogenesis of uremic bone disease. *J. Clin. Endocrinol. Metab.*, **39**. 119.
12. Stauffer, M., Baylink, D. J. and Wergedal, J. (1973) Decreased bone formation and mineralization and enhanced resorption in calcium deficient rats. *Am. J. Physiol.*, **225**, 269–276.
13. Drezner, M. K. *et al.* (1980) Evaluation of a role for 1,25 dihydroxy-vitamin D_3 in the pathogeneis and treatment of x-linked hypophophatemic

rickets and osteomalacia. *J. Clin. Invest.*, **60**, 1020.

14. Baylink, D. J., Wergedal, J. and Stauffer, M. (1971) Formation, mineralization, and resorption of bone in hypophosphatemic rats. *J. Clin. Invest.*, **50**, 2519–2530.

15. Carmichael, K. A. *et al.* (1984) Osteomalacia and osteitis fibrosa in a man ingesting aluminium hydroxide anatacid. *Am. J. Med.*, **76**, 1137.

16. Boyce, B. F. *et al.* (1984) Focal osteomalacia due to low-dose diphosphonate therapy in Paget's disease. *Lancet*, **1**, 821–824.

17. Lundy, M. W., Stauffer, M., Wergedal, J. E. *et al.* (1995) Histomorphometric analysis of iliac crest bone biopsies in placebo-treated versus fluoride-treated subjects. *Osteoporosis International*, **5**, 2–17.

18. Dure-Smith, B. A., Farley, S. M., Linkhart, S. G. *et al.* (1993) Fluoride treated patients become calcium deficient despite calcium supplements: correction with 1,25 vitamin D_3. *Fourth International Symposium on Osteoporosis and Consensus Development Conferences*, No. **79**, pp. 146.

19. Baylink, D. J. (1970) Metabolic bone disease. In: *Introduction to the Musculoskeletal System* (eds C. Rosse and D. K. Clawson). Harper and Row, New York, pp. 66–74.

20. Baylink, D. J. and Libanati, C. L. (1994) The actions and therapeutic applications of 1α-hydroxylated derivatives of vitamin D. *Akt. Rheumatol.*, **19** (suppl. 1) 10–18.

21. Gruber, H. E., Stauffer, M. E., Thomson, E. R. *et al.* (1981) Diagnosis of bone disease by core biopsies. *Semin. Hematol.*, **18**, 258–278.

22. Ivey, J. L., Gruber, H. E. and Baylink, D. J. (1980) Measurement and significance of rates of osteoid maturation and mineral accumulation. *Metab. Bone Dis. Rel. Res.*, **2**(S), 207–212.

23. McClure, J. and Smith, P. S., (1987) Oncogenic osteomalacia. *J. Clin. Pathol.*, **40**, 446.

24. Slatopolsky, E. *et al.* (1984) Marked suppression of secondary hyperparathyroidism by intravenous administration of 1,25 dihydroxycholecalciferol in uremic patients. *J. Clin. Invest.*, **74**, 2136.

25. Koo, W. W. K., and Tsang, R. (1984) Bone mineralization in infants. *Progress in Food and Nutrition Science*, **8**, 229–302.

26. Collins, N. *et al.* (1991) A progressive study to evaluate the dose of vitamin D required to correct low 25-hydroxyvitamin D levels, calcium, and alkaline phosphatase in patients at risk of developing antiepileptic drug-induced osteomalacia. *Q. J. Med., New Series*, **78**, 113.

27. Chertow, B. S., Baylink, D. J., Wergedal, J. E. *et al.* (1975) Decrease in serum immunoreactive parathyroid hormone in rats and in PTH secretion in vitro by 1,25 dihydroxycholecalciferol. *J. Clin. Invest.*, **56**(3), 668–678.

28. Peck, W. A., Riggs, B. L., Bell, N. H. *et al.* (1988) Research directions in osteoporosis. *Am. J. Med.*, **84**, 275–282.

29. Chesnut, C. H. III (1994) Osteoporosis. In: *Principles of Geriatric Medicine and Gerontology*. Third Edition. (eds Hazzard, W. R., Bierman, E. L., Blass, J. B., Ettinger, W. H., Halter). McGraw-Hill Inc., chapter **76**, pp. 897–909.

30. Mazess, R. B. (1982) On aging bone loss. *Clin. Orthop. Rel. Res.*, **165**, 238–252.

31. Gray, T. K., Lipes, B., Linkhart, T. *et al.* (1989) Transforming growth factor beta mediates the estrogen induced inhibition of UMR106 cell growth. *Connect. Tiss. Res.*, **20**(1–4), 23–32.

32. Girasole, G., Jilka, R. A., Passeri, G. *et al.* (1992) 17β Estrodial inhibits interleuken 6 production by bone marrow derived stromal cells and osteoblasts in vitro: A potential mechanism for the anti-osteoporotic effects of estrogens. *J. Clin. Invest.*, **89**, 883–891.

33. van Hoof, H. J. C., van der Mooren, M. J., Swinkels, L. M. J. W. *et al.* (1994) Hormone replacement therapy increases serum 1,25-dihydroxyvitamin D: a 2-year prospective study. *Calcif. Tissue Int.*, **55**, 417–419.

34. Smith, D. M. *et al.* (1973) Genetic factors in determining bone mass. *J. Clin. Invest.*, **52**, 2800.

35. Dequeker, J. *et al.* (1987) Genetic determinants of bone mineral content at the spine and radius: A twin study. *Bone*, **8**, 207.

36. Seeman, E. *et al.* (1989) Reduced bone mass in daughters of women with osteoporosis. *N. Engl. J. Med.*, **320**, 554.

37. Melton, L. J., III (1991) Differing patterns of osteoporosis across the world. In: *New dimensions in osteoporosis in the 1990's* (ed. Chesnut, C. H., III). *Hong Kong, Excerpta Medica Asia*, pp. 13–18.

38. Thomsen, K., Gotfredsen, A. and Christiansen, C. (1986) Is postmenopausal bone loss an age-related phenomenon? *Calcified Tissue International*, **39**, 123–127.

39. Riggs, B. L. and Melton, L. J., III (1986) Involutional osteoporosis. *N. Engl. J. Med.*, **314**, 1676–1686.

40. Chapuy, M. C., Arlot, M. E., Duboeuf, F. *et al.* (1992) Vitamin D_3 and calcium to prevent hip fractures in elderly women. *N. Engl. J. Med.*, **327**(23), 1637–1642.

41. Bennet, A. E., Wahner, H. W., Riggs, B. L. *et al.* (1984) Insulin-like growth factors I and II: Aging and bone density in women. *J. Clin. Endocrinol. Metab.*, **5**, 701–704.

42. Gruber, H. E. and Baylink, D. J. (1981) The diagnosis of osteoporosis. *J. Am. Geriatr. Soc.*, **29**, 490–497.

43. Lewinnek, G. E., Kelsey, J., White, A. A. *et al.* (1980) The significance and a comparative analysis of the epidemiology of hip fractures. *Clin. Orthop. Rel. Res.*, **152**, 35–43.

44. Odvina, C. V., Wergedal, J. R., Libanati, C. R. *et al.* (1988) Relationship between trabecular body density and fractures: A quantitative definition of spinal osteoporosis. *Metabolism*, **37(3)**, 221–228.

45. Dunn, W. L., Wahner, H. W. and Riggs, B. L. (1980) Measurement of bone mineral content in human vertebrae and hip by dual photon absorptiometry. *Radiology*, **136**, 485–487.

46. Melton, L. J. III, Atkinson, E. J., O'Fallon, W. M. *et al* (1993) Long-term fracture prediction by bone mineral assessed at different skeletal sites. *J. Bone Miner. Res.*, **8**, 1227–1233.

47. Heaney, R. P. *et al.* (1982) Calcium nutrition and bone health in the elderly. *Am. J. Clin. Nutrition*, **36**, 986–1013.

48. Bettica, P., Moro, L., Robins, S. P. *et al.* (1992) Bone-resorption markers galactosyl hydroxylysine, pyridinium crosslinks, and hydroxyproline compared. *Clin. Chem.*, **38(11)**, 2313–2318.

49. Pitt, M. (1983) Osteopenic bone disease. *Orthop. Clin. N. Am.*, **14**, 65–80.

50. Krolner, B. and Toft, B. (1983) Vertebral bone loss: An unheeded side-effect of therapeutic bed rest. *Clin. Sci.*, **64**, 537–540.

51. Eisman, J. A. *et al.* (1991) Exercise and its interaction with genetic influences in the determination of bone mineral density. *Am. J. Med.*, **5B (suppl.)**, 55–95.

52. Gallagher, J. C., Riggs, B. L., Eisman, J. *et al.* (1979) Intestinal calcium absorption and serum vitamin D metabolites in normal subjects and osteoporotic patients. *J. Clin. Invest.*, **64**, 729–736.

53. Heaney, R. P., Recker, R. R. and Saville, P. D. (1978) Menopausal changes in calcium balance performance. *J. Lab. Clin. Med.*, **92**, 953–963.

54. Parfitt, A. M. (1987) Trabecular bone architecture in the pathogenesis and prevention of fracture. *Am. J. Med.*, **82**, 68–72.

55. Civitelli, R., Gonnelli, S., Zacchei, F. *et al.* (1988) Bone Turnover in postmenopausal osteoporosis: Effect of calcitonin treatment. *J. Clin. Invest.*, **82**, 1268–1274.

56. Hutchinson, T. A., Polansky, S. M. and Feinstein, A. R. (1979) Postmenopausal oestrogens protect against fracture of hip and distal radius: A case control study. *Lancet*, **2**, 705–709.

57. Weis, N. S., Ure, C. L., Ballard, J. H. *et al.* (1980) Decreased risk of fractures of the hip and lower forearm with postmenopausal use of estrogen. *N. Engl. J. Med.*, **303**, 1195–1198.

58. Riggs, B. L., Seeman, E., Hodgson, S. F. *et al.* (1982) Effect of fluoride/calcium regimen on vertebral fracture occurrence in postmenopausal osteoporosis. *N. Engl. J. Med.*, **306**, 446–450.

59. Marshburn, P. B. and Carr, B. R. (1994) The menopause and hormone replacement therapy. In: *Principles of Geriatric Medicine and Gerontology, 3rd Edition.* (eds W. R. Hazzard, E. L. Biermman, J. B. Blass, W. H. Ettinger, J. B. Halter), McGraw-Hill Inc., chapter 74, pp. 867–878.

60. Chetkowski, R. J., Meldrum, D. R., Steingold, K. A. *et al.* (1986) Biologic effects of transdermal estradiol. *N. Engl. J. Med.*, **314**, 1615–1620.

61. Steingold, K. A., Cefalu, W., Pardridge, W. *et al.* (1986) Enhanced hepatic extraction of estrogens used for replacement therapy. *J. Clin. Endocrinol. Metab.*, **62**, 761–766.

62. Stephan, J. J., Pospichol, J., Schreiber, V. *et al.* (1989) The application of plasma tartrate-resistant acid phosphatase to assess changes in bone resorption in response to artificial menopause and its treatment with estrogen or norethisterone. *Calcified Tissue International*, **45**, 273–280.

63. Watts, N. B. *et al.* (1990) Intermittent cyclical etidronate treatment of postmenopausal osteoporosis. *N. Engl. J. Med.*, **323**, 73–79.

64. Gruber, H. E., Ivey, J. L., Baylink, D. J. *et al.* (1984) Long-term calcitonin therapy in postmenopausal osteoporosis. *Metabolism*, **33(4)**, 295–303.

65. Farley, S. M. G., Libanati, C. R., Mariano-Menez, M. R. *et al.* (1990) Fluoride therapy for osteoporosis promotes a progressive increase in spinal bone density. *J. Bone Min. Res.*, **5(1)**, S37–S42.

66. Farley, S. M., Wergedal, J. E., Farley, J. R. *et al.* (1990) Fluoride decreases spinal fracture rate: A study of over 500 patients. *3rd Intl. Symp. on Osteoporosis, Copenhagen, Denmark*, pp. 1330–1334.

67. Dempster, D. W., Cosman, F., Parisien, M. *et al.* (1993) Anabolic actions of parathyroid hormone on bone. *Endocrine Reviews*, **14(6)**, 690–709.

68. Parfitt, A. M. (1993) Pathophysiology of bone fragility. *Proceedings Fourth International Symposium on Osteoporosis and Consensus Development Conference*, Hong Kong, pp. 164–166.

69. Riggs, B. L., Melton, L. J. III, and O'Fallon, W. M. (1993) Toward optimal therapy of established osteoporosis: evidence that antiresorptive and formation-stimulating regimens decrease vertebral fracture rate by independent mechanisms. Proceedings *4th International Symposium on Osteoporosis and Consensus Development Conference*, Hong Kong, pp. 13–15.

70. Riggs, B. L. *et al.* (1990) Effect of fluoride treatment on the fracture rate in postmenopausal women with osteoporosis. *N. Engl. J. Med.*, **22**, 802–809.

71. Pak, C. Y. C., Sakhaee, K., Piziak, V. *et al.* (1994) Slow-release sodium fluoride in the management of postmenopausal osteoporosis: A randomized controlled trial. *Annals Internal Med.*, **120(8)**, 625–632.

72. Taves, D. R. (1970) New approach to the treatment of bone disease with fluoride. *Fed. Proc.*, **29**, 1185–1187.

73. Schulz, E. E., Engstrom, H., Sauser, D. D. *et al.* (1986) Osteoporosis: Radiographic detection of fluoride-induced extra-axial bone formation. *Radiology*, **159(2)**, 457–462.

74. Gennari, C. (1983) Clinical aspects of calcitonin in pain. *Triangle*, **22(2:3)**, 157–163.

75. Kasperk, C. H., Wergedal, J. E., Farley, J. R. *et al.* (1989) Androgens directly stimulate proliferation of bone cells in vitro. *Endocrinology*, **124(3)**, 1576–1578.

76. Riggs, B. L., Jowsey, J., Goldsmith, R. S. *et al.* (1972) Short and long-term effects of estrogen and synthetic anabolic hormone in post-menopausal osteoporosis. *J. Clin. Invest.*, **51**, 1659–1663.

30

Physics and technology of bone-mineral content measurements

R. R. Price and M. P. Sandler

Introduction

Aside from the conventional radiograph which is used for qualitative evaluation of bone status, there are three primary categories of instruments/methods which are currently being used for quantitative bone mineral content (BMC) assessment. These are: single photon absorptiometry (SPA), dual photon absorptiometry (DPA) and quantitative computed tomography (QCT) [1,2]. Both SPA and DPA are projection methods, and as such measure the sum of compact and cancellous bone at a specified site in the body. The SPA technique, usually applied to the distal ulna and radius, typically expresses BMC in terms of g/cm. This quantity is a 'linear density' which measures the grams of BMC per centimetre of length along the bone. The DPA technique is used to express BMC in terms of grams per projected cross-sectional area (g/cm^2) while QCT, a tomogaphic methodology, attempts to estimate bone density in terms of g/cm^3.

Each of the above methods is absorptiometric in nature, meaning that by using the known photon absorption properties of bone mineral, one estimates the 'amount of bone mineral' in a given unknown sample. The concepts of how and in what physical units the amount of bone should be expressed is still a matter of some discussion. Fortunately, there has been some degree of agreement in that bone density seems to be an important indicator of bone status. Bone density in this context has come to refer to that portion of the bone which remains when the specimen is ashed under extreme heat, commonly referred to as bone mineral. The rest of the bone is included under the component which demonstrates absorption properties of soft tissue. Thus, the bone density is expressed as a mass of bone mineral per unit of bone volume (g/cm^3). Since the bone matrix itself is a relatively random network of crystalline structure, estimates of bone density are usually quoted as the mean of many point density measurements over a specified bone site.

In each of the three techniques, bone mineral standards are commonly used for instrument calibration. The phantoms are generally calcium-hydroxyapatite crystals imbedded in a soft tissue equivalent material or dipotassium hydrogen phosphate (K_2HPO_4) solutions which have been cross-calibrated to actual bone ash weight.

SPA method

The SPA technique, introduced by Cameron and Sorenson in the early 1960s [3,4], has been produced commercially as a compact table-top device for measuring the linear density (g/cm) of bone mineral of the distal ulna and radius (Fig. 30.1). The SPA device typically employs an I-125 source (several hundred millicuries) which is narrowly collimated and rigidly coupled by means of a small C-arm to an opposed scintillation detector. The C-arm is scanned in a rectilinear motion over the region being examined. The transmitted intensity of the beam of mono-

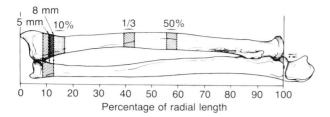

Fig. 30.1 Commonly used SPA sites in the radius and ulna. Distal sites for mixed trabecular/cortical and standard 1/3 from distal end for compact bone site (from [13]).

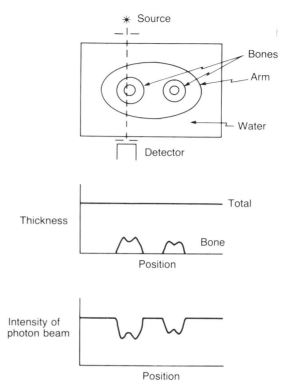

Fig. 30.2 Diagram of the SPA method.

chromatic photons from the source (28 keV) is recorded and used to calculate the average BMC of the region.

The SPA technique assumes (also assumed by DPA and QCT) that the body is composed of two components: soft tissue and bone mineral. If the beam of monochromatic photons of initial intensity I_o passes through 't' cm of soft-tissue and 'b' cm of bone mineral, the transmitted intensity, I, is given by:

$$I = I_o e^{-\mu_t t - \mu_b b}$$

where M_t and M_b are the linear attenuation coefficients of soft tissue and bone mineral, respectively, at the energy being used. In the SPA technique, I_o and I are measured at each point of the scan. The attenuation coefficients are constants which have been determined independently through calibration experiments. Calibration experiments usually measure a calibration set of bones which are then ashed to provide the actual BMC.

Since there are two unknowns in the above equation (t and b), the body part must be immersed in water or some other tissue equivalent material (Fig. 30.2) to yield a total thickness (T) which is constant. In this situation:

$$T = t + b,$$

This relationship is substituted into the original attenuation equation which is then solved for the bone content (b).

$$b = \frac{1}{\mu_b - \mu_t}\left(\ln\frac{I_o}{I} - \mu_t T\right)$$

$$b = \frac{1}{\mu_b - \mu_t}\left(\ln\frac{I'}{I}\right)$$

Where

$$I' = I_o e^{-\mu_t T}$$

In this case I' is a constant which is determined by measuring over a site which contains no bone.

Since the SPA method requires the use of an additional material to surround the body part under study, it can conveniently be used only for bones in the extremities.

In assessing bone disease, it is the density of the bone that is of interest instead of the total bone thickness. Total bone thickness is generally not a useful quantity because of its close dependence on the size of the person, i.e. large people have large bones with large thicknesses.

Bone density is determined by using the measuring mass attenuation coefficient (cm^2/g) instead of the linear attenuation coefficient (1/cm) which then in turn yields a mass thickness. Mass thickness has the units of g/cm^2 and is equal to the number of grams of bone mineral per square centimetre of projected areas through the bone. Cameron proposed a further normalization in SPA measurements of the wrist to minimize body size effects by dividing the BMC (g/cm²) by the diameter of the bone to yield a BMC linear density (g/cm). The result of this normalization is to yield a value which is equal to the number of grams of BMC per cm of distance along the axis of the bone.

DPA method

During the mid-1970s several laboratories began developing the DPA technique for assessing the bone mineral content of the lumbar spine [5–7]. During the past decade, this technique has been used to establish well defined values of normal spinal bone mineral mass. The dual photon absorptiometry technique now offers an accurate, inexpensive, and non-invasive test for the early detection of osteoporosis and other demineralizing diseases [8].

As the name implies, DPA utilizes two monoenergetic photon beams. With two beams, there are now two attenuation equations (one for each energy) which can be solved directly for the two unknowns (t and b) without additional material. With the DPA method, it now becomes convenient to examine any part of the body (Fig. 30.3) regardless of the overlying soft-tissue component.

$$I^L = I_o^L \, e^{-\mu_t^L t - \mu_b^L b}$$

$$I^H = I_o^H \, e^{-\mu_t^H t - \mu_b^H b}$$

In the DPA technique; it is possible to solve either for the bone mineral content or the soft tissue content. The solution for the bone mineral content is a follows:

$$b = \frac{\ln\left(\frac{I_o^L}{I^L}\right) - C_2 \ln\left(\frac{I_o^H}{I^H}\right)}{C_1}$$

where,

$$C_1 = \mu_b^L - \left(\frac{\mu_t^L}{\mu_t^H}\right)\mu_b^H$$

$$C_2 = \frac{\mu_t^L}{\mu_t^H}$$

where the superscripts L and H refer to the low and high energy beams, respectively, and C_2 (sometimes called the R-value) characterizes the

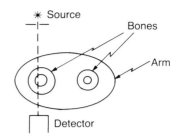

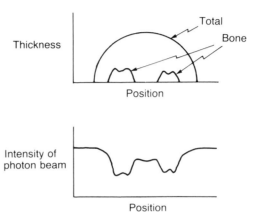

Fig. 30.3   Diagram of the DPA method.

attenuation of the two photon energies in soft tissue. In most DPA systems, the R-value is estimated independently for each patient by making measurements of a body site near to the bone of interest but which in fact contains no bone. (This is equivalent to setting b = 0 in the BMC equation and finding the best value for C_2.) For b = 0,

$$R = \ln\left(I_o^L/I^L\right)/\ln\left(I_o^H/I^H\right)$$

Errors in estimated BMC can result when R-values measured over soft tissue sites adjacent to bones are not representative of R-values of the bone soft tissue components. Specifically, this condition may arise in elderly osteoporotics where vertebral bone mineral may be replaced by fat rich yellow marrow. Since fat rich soft tissue is somewhat less attenuating than muscle based soft tissue, BMC estimates may be underestimated.

As with the SPA, mass absorption coefficients are used in place of the linear attenuation coefficients so that b is the measured mass per unit area (g/cm²), rather than thickness.

In the DPA method, an image of the BMC

(g/cm²) is created from a rectilinear scan of the region of interest in which the transmitted intensities of both energy beams are measured at each pixel location and then used to calculate the BMC.

DPA source

The most common source use for DPA systems is gadolinium-153. The Gd-153 energy spectrum (Fig. 30.4) is characterized by two primary photon groups. The low energy photon group is actually composed of a complex family of energies. The effective energy of the lower energy group is approximately 44 keV. The upper energy group consists of two energy lines, one at 97 keV and the other at 103 keV with a mean value of about 100 keV.

For *in vivo* applications, thin window NaI crystal is usually the detector of choice. Typical NaI systems will have energy resolutions of about 10% at 100 keV (FWHM) and produce an energy spectrum which does not resolve the internal structure of the two photon groups (Fig. 30.5).

The 44 and 100 keV energies of Gd-153 offer the almost ideal combination of energies in which the bone-soft tissue contrast is optimized with an acceptable beam attenuation.

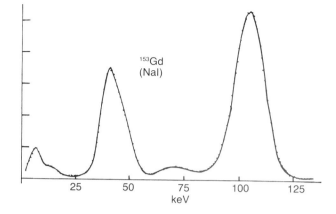

Fig. 30.5 NaI energy spectrum of ¹⁵³Gd.

Scanning apparatus

A computer-controlled rectilinear scanner is used to acquire the dual energy transmission images which are then used to create the intensity modulated BMC images. From the intensity modulated BMC imagers, regions of interest are selected, mean values of mass per unit area are calculated and then compared to the ranges of normal values.

In our laboratory, we have utilized a modified dual-probe nuclear medicine whole-body scanner for our DPA system (Fig. 30.6). This scanner allows great flexibility in the scanner format, making it possible to scan any portion of the body as well as the total body (Fig. 30.7).

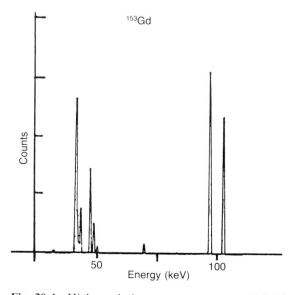

Fig. 30.4 High resolution energy spectrum of ¹⁵³Gd intrinsic germanium detector.

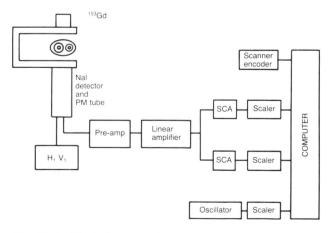

Fig. 30.6 Block diagram of a prototype DPA imaging system.

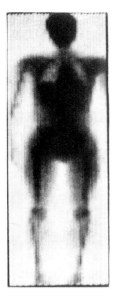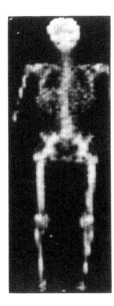

Fig. 30.7   Total body transmission scan at 40 keV (left) and the corresponding derived total body BMC image.

1. Corrections for scatter of 100 keV photons into the 44 keV channel.
2. Dead time corrections for count rate losses.
3. Beam hardening correction due to preferential attenuation of the low energy components of the energy subgroups.
4. Accurate methods for finding the bone edge for accurate calculations of mean values.

An error which has produced a great deal of discussion results from the basic assumption of the method. The basic assumption that the body consists of two absorptive components, bone and soft tissue, becomes a progressively poorer assumption as the fraction of fat increases. This error comes about because the attenuation coefficients which are assumed for soft tissue in the BMC calculation are no longer correct. Interactive corrections for fat contributions are useful in minimizing these uncertainties. Corrections for fat errors are more difficult in the QCT technique.

In our system, signals from the scanner's x and y position encoders, the single analyser pulses from the two photon groups and the pulses from a high frequency oscillator are all monitored and recorded simultaneously by the computer (PDP-11/55). The data are buffered in the computer's memory and then written to a disk at the end of each line. The recorded oscillator pulses make it possible to correct for scanner speed instabilities.

The horizontal sampling rate for our system is variable. Standard scans of the lumbar spine have 256 samples (pixels) per horizontal line (15 cm) and as many lines (3 mm steps) as necessary to accommodate the region of interest. The line stepping distances should be determined by the beam collimator. In our system, the beam is collimated to 6 mm. Commercial systems use beam diameters up to 13 mm. It is the beam diameter which determines the spatial resolution. Spatial resolution will be approximately equal to the beam diameter.

Corrections to the DPA method

In order to achieve a precision of the order of 2%, many corrections must be incorporated into the method. These include:

Imaging site

Early investigators attempted to assess skeletal status by measuring the bone mineral content of the distal ulna and radius and the os calcis. It was discovered that the primarily cortical bone of the ulna and radius was relatively insensitive to skeletal changes (Fig. 30.8). Os calcis measurements, though sensitive to weight-bearing changes, are not closely correlated with spine bone mineral. The lumbar spine or the proximal femur (composed primarily of trabecular bone) have generally been found to be more sensitive indicators of changes in bone metabolism and are currently

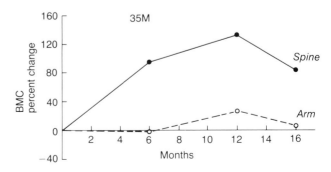

Fig. 30.8   Comparison of the relative change in BMC observed in the spine and wrist over a 16 month period.

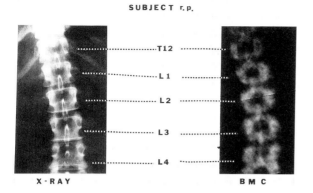

Fig. 30.9 Comparison of DPA image of the lumbar spine and a conventional X-ray in a normal volunteer.

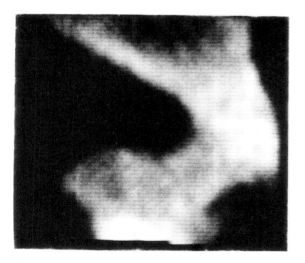

Fig. 30.10 DPA image of the proximal femur.

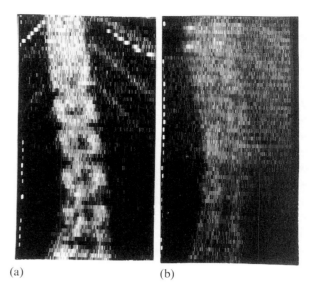

(a)   (b)

Fig. 30.11 (a) DPA spine image of a normal 28-year-old female, (b) DPA spine image of a 72-year-old female with known demineralizing disease.

30.11a is a scan of a 28-year-old female who was determined to have normal BMC for her age (Fig. 30.12a). The image in Fig. 30.11b is of a 72-year-old female with significant bone demineralization. The differences in the distinctness of the vertebral bodies and the reduction in overall image intensity are consistent with the measured bone mineral density values. When compared with expected values for normal women of the same general age group, the 72-year-old female was found to have a bone density value over two standard deviations below the mean for her age group (Fig. 30.12b). A value this low immediately identifies her as a member of a high risk group and requires immediate therapy.

Conditions which affect the measured bone mineral contact in DPA scans of the lumbar spine have been identified by Hahner [13].

Conditions which result in falsely high BMC include: significant aortic calcification, hypertrophic degenerative disease, bone grafts, lipoidal in the spinal canal, calcium-containing tablets in the GI tract and barium contrast material in the GI tract. Conditions which could lead to either high or low value of the BMC include: compression fracture, marked scoliosis, spinal deformities, post-traumatic vertebral changes and focal spinal bone lesions. Laminectomy can also lead to a falsely low value of BMC.

considered the sites of choice for bone measurements (Figs 30.9, 30.10).

The DPA image

An essential feature of the modern dual photon absorptiometry system is the creation of the bone mineral image. Because of the irregular structure of the vertebral column, it is essential to know what portion of the vertebral bodies are being measured. Figure 30.11 compares DPA images that demonstrate the visual differences between individuals of comparable ages but with quantitatively different BMC values. The image in Fig.

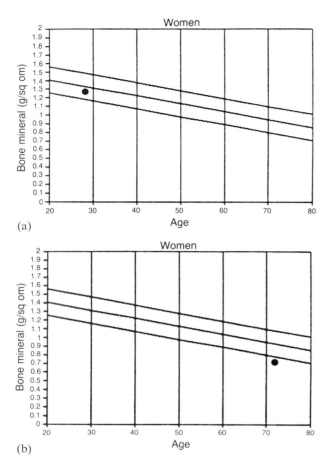

Fig. 30.12 Normal ranges of BMC as a function of age are used to assess those individuals at risk, i.e. those values falling outside the 2-SD limits. (a) BMC of 28-year-old female falls within the normal range of values. (b) BMC of the 72-year-old female falls outside the 2-SD limits and thus identifies this patient as being at risk for fractures.

QCT method

Quantitative computed tomography (QCT) is a method of BMC estimation which was developed as an adjunct to conventional CT scanning. Unlike both SPA and DPA, the QCT technique is inherently tomographic in nature. Because of its tomographic nature, BMC is expressed in terms of true density units (g/cm³) of small user selected regions of selected bones (typically the vertebral body). The tomographic aspect of QCT in principle) allows an estimate of trabecular bone independent of overlying cortical bone. Unfortunately, many factors effect the ability of the CT method to provide quantitative results and consequently the accuracy with which one corrects for these factors determines the final accuracy of the technique. The primary factor which contributes to the uncertainties in QCT values relates to beam-hardening artifacts. Since CT systems use filtered polyenergetic beams from X-ray tubes rather than monoenergetic beams for isotopic source, the effective energy at a point of the beam will vary depending upon what combination of tissue and bones the beam has passed through in getting to that point. QCT methods typically utilize a beam correction method which employs positioning a calibrated phantom near the bone of interest and forming a QCT scan with the phantom in place. For the lumbar spine, beam projection through other bones is avoided and if the phantom is positioned near the spine, it will be imaged with a beam quality approximately equal to the beam quality seen by the lumbar spine. Other factors affecting QCT measurements are partial volume effects, off-focal spot radiation, reconstruction algorithm variations and subject size and composition. QCT phantoms commonly consist of parallel cylinders filled with different concentrations of K_3HPO_4 which are placed beneath the patient.

A typical QCT scan will report a bone density based upon CT values (Hounsfield Units) from trabecular bone at the midplane of three to four lumbar vertebrae. The CT values are then used to 'look-up' the equivalent bone density using the CT numbers from the phantom cylinders and a calibration data set. The values are then averaged and reported in terms of equivalent g/cm³ of bone.

QCT may utilize either a single CT scan image (usually taken at a relatively low KVp value – 80 KVp) or two CT scan images (one at 80 KVp; the other a heavily filtered scan with KVp > 100 KVp). Dual-energy QCT has been shown to be generally more accurate but at the expense of higher radiation dose to the patient.

A significant uncertainty arises from the QCT method (whether single or dual photon) because of the basic measured quantity (CT number) being related to liner attenuation rather than mass attenuation and consequently being related to true density rather than mineral density. The difference between true density and mineral density being affected primarily by the fat-rich yellow marrow content. It has been shown that QCT measured spinal mineral values are reduced by about 7 mg per 10% of fat by volume at 80 KVp [2]. This effect can result in inaccuracies of 20–30% in elderly osteoporotics. It is estimated that dual-energy QCT may reduce this error to 5% if adequate scan time and radiation exposure are allowed.

Comparison of BMC modalities

The comparison of the three modalities (SPA, DPA and QCT) is usually expressed in terms of two quantities: precision and accuracy. Precision means the ability of the method to reproduce the same measured value. Precision is the factor of concern when the clinical question is whether or not the BMC of a patient is changing with time. Accuracy refers to whether or not the measured value is in fact the true correct value of BMC. Accuracy is important when the clinical question is whether this patient has a normal value of BMC or not.

The precision of SPA is approximately 1% [4]. It should be pointed out again, however, that SPA systems are generally only useful for peripheral sites. The precision of the DPA and single-energy QCT systems are approximately the same and range from 2 to 5%. Dual-energy QCT precision is approximately 4–10% [9–11].

Factors affecting the precision of SPA and DPA relate to the ability of the system or operator to locate the edges of the bones and the ability to carry out adequate corrections for source decay and counting system dead-time. The precision of the QCT method rests largely on the stability of the X-ray tube output and the ability of the operator to accurately reposition the patient and find the same midline region of interest location. The accuracy of repositioning must be within 1 mm in most cases.

The accuracy of each technique relates back to their ability to accurately make a measurement which will yield the value of the bones ash weight. Accuracy determinations are 6% for SPA [4], 5% for DPA [12] and 5–15% for QCT [11].

Radiation exposure

The radiation dose for the SPA method is approximately 10 mrem and approximately 10–20 mrem for the DPA method. QCT values range from 200 to 1000 mrem for single energy measurements to approximately twice these values for dual-energy measurements.

Conclusion

Each of these methods provides relatively accurate methods for measuring BMC status. DPA and QCT are both applicable to the axial skeleton and can be performed on an outpatient basis. Primarily because of its lower radiation burden, DPA may be used for frequent follow-up measurements and may also be a good candidate for a routine screening procedure, especially in those females who are at high risk for developing post-menopausal osteoporosis.

References

1. Price, R. R., Wagner, J., Larsen, K. L. *et al.* (1977) Techniques for measuring regional and total-body bone mineral mass to bone function ratios. IAEA-SM-210/164, *Medical Radionuclide Imaging*, Vol. II, Vienna.
2. Genant, H. K. (1985) Assessing osteoporosis: CT's quantitative advantage. *Diagnostic Imaging*, **August**, 52–57.
3. Cameron, J. R. and Sorensen, J. A. (1963) Measurement of bone mineral *in-vivo*: An improved method. *Science*, **142**, 230.
4. Cameron, J. R., Mazess, R. B. and Sorensen, J. A. (1968) Precision and accuracy of bone mineral determination by direct photon absorptiometry. *Invest. Rad.*, **3**, 141.
5. Price, R. R., Wagner, J., Larsen, K. *et al.* (1976) Regional and whole-body bone mineral content measurement with a rectilinear scanner. *Am. J. Roentgenol.*, **126**, 1277–1278.
6. Wilson, C. R. and Madsen, M. (1977) Dichromatic absorptiometry of vertebral bone mineral content. *Invest. Radiol.*, **12**, 180–184.
7. Madsen, M., Peppler, W. and Mazess, R. (1976) Vertebral and total body bone mineral by dual photon absorptiometry. In *Calcified Tissues* (eds S. Pors Nielsen and E. Hjorting-Hansen), FADL Publishing, Copenhagen.
8. Mazess, R. B., Peppler, W. W. *et al.* (1984) Does bone measurement on the radius indicate skeletal status? *J. Nucl. Med.*, **25(3)**, 281.
9. Dunn, W. L., Wahner, H. W. and Riggs, B. L. (1980) Measurement of bone mineral content in

human vertebrae and hip by dual photon absorptiometry. *Radiology*, **136**, 485–487.

10. LeBlance, A. D., Evans, H. J., March, C. *et al.* (1986) Precision of dual-photon absorptiometry measurements. *J. Nucl. Med.*, **27**, 1362–1363.

11. Genant, H. K., Cann, C. E., Ettinger, B. *et al.* (1985) Quantitative computed tomography for spinal mineral assessment. Current status. *J. Comp. Assist. Tomog.*, **9(3)**, 602–604.

12. Wahner, H. W., Dunn, W. L., Mazess, R. B. *et al.* (1985) Dual-photon Gd-153 absorptiometry of bone. *Radiology*, **156**, 203–206.

13. Wahner, H. W. (1986) Bone mineral measurements. In *Nuclear Medicine Annual* 1986 (eds L. M. Freeman and H. S. Weissmann), Raven Press, New York, pp. 195–225.

31

Limb salvage surgery for primary bone tumours

R. S. Sneath and R. J. Grimer

Introduction

Primary bone tumours are rare with an incidence of about 6 or 7 per million per year. In the past, treatment was limited to carrying out an appropriate amputation [1]. In the case of the most common tumour, osteosarcoma, metastases occurred in over 80% of patients within 18 months. Cade, in 1951 [2], appreciating the futility of many of these amputations for osteosarcoma and advocated the more humane approach of treating the primary tumour with radiotherapy followed by a period of careful follow-up. If the patient was free of any evidence of metastases 6 months after radiotherapy the affected bone was removed, usually by amputation. This treatment regime allowed many patients to keep their limbs for the few remaining months of their life, whilst some of the patients who had amputations were long-term survivors, around 20% at 5 years.

From 1970 onwards there was a steady increase in the conservation of limbs by reconstructive techniques for patients with chondrosarcomas, low-grade malignancies, and giant cell tumours [3]. In 1975 and 1976 the treatment of patients with osteosarcoma changed from radiotherapy and delayed amputation to chemotherapy and primary amputation. At this stage it became logical to consider limb salvage techniques for these patients. Late in the 1970s these techniques were also applied to Ewing's sarcoma and the malignant tumours of fibrous origin [4,5].

Over the last 15 years many centres in the world have taken a special interest in the treatment of primary malignant bone tumours. This interest has resulted in the development of teams with special expertise in radiology, pathology, chemotherapy, radiotherapy, bioengineering, physiotherapy and all aspects of orthopaedic surgery. Such a team will usually be led by an orthopaedic surgeon and the team will require at least 100 new cases per year to function efficiently, to gain experience and to have enough experience to develop the specialty through evaluation and research. Therefore, a team needs to serve a population of about 15 million or more to function efficiently, obviously this is not practical in some situations. On the other hand a population of about 100 million is required to be able to collect figures of statistical significance in a reasonable time. The answer lies in cooperation between centres in order that they may draw up protocols of treatment which they can all follow. This cooperation would both provide the necessary numbers for statistics and also stimulate advances in treatment due to the combined enthusiasm of the participants. In situations where the population treated by a team was lower than optimal that team could link into a bigger group in order to absorb the experience and receive the advice of that group.

We believe that it is most important not to encourage too many people to treat bone tumours themselves. We have therefore written this chapter as a source of information and not as a surgical manual, hoping that we may encourage the reader to refer cases to the appropriate centres.

Diagnosis

Diagnosing bone tumours is not straightforward. The presenting symptoms of pain followed by swelling are well known to all, but the rarity of these tumours coupled with the frequency of vague musculoskeletal aches and pains ensures that in many cases the diagnosis is overlooked for a considerable time. The symptoms which patients experience initially are remarkably consistent no matter what the tumour. The vast majority will start by noticing an ache in the involved part which gradually increases in severity and duration until there is significant pain. The pain may not be affected by activity and is often present at night. Whilst it will initially fluctuate in severity it eventually becomes constant and will only be partially alleviated by mild analgesics. In a few cases there will be no pain and swelling is the initial complaint. In half the cases, swelling and pain are the two presenting symptoms and when these are combined at the end of a long bone then a tumour must be high on the list of differential diagnoses.

A survey of recent cases referred to the Birmingham Bone Tumour Treatment Service has highlighted some of the problems in correctly diagnosing primary bone tumours at an early stage [6].

It surprised us how long patients put up with their symptoms before going to see a doctor, an average of 6 weeks for patients with osteosarcoma, 16 weeks for patients with Ewing's sarcoma and 21 weeks for patients with chondrosarcoma. What was even more concerning was the time after this for a diagnosis to be made and treatment instigated, a further 7 weeks for patients with osteosarcoma, 31 weeks for patients with Ewing's sarcoma and 30 weeks for patients with chondrosarcoma.

The cause of this delay was usually a low level of suspicion. When a tumour was suspected a radiograph was requested and this usually led to the correct diagnosis being made. When the diagnosis was not suspected a variety of treatments were instigated which were invariably of no bene-

fit and simply delayed the making of a correct diagnosis.

In all patients the plain radiograph alone invariably led to the correct diagnosis, eventually. In 13 out of 70 cases both the clinician and the radiologist failed to detect the tumour on the initial radiograph although evidence of the tumour was present on retrospective review of the films in all 13 cases.

Factors which led to the tumour being missed included poor quality radiographs and failure to demonstrate the whole of the lesion. Typical of this were the tumours of the distal femur of which 22% were missed on the initial radiograph. The changes which identify the presence of a tumour are well known but easily overlooked. They include ill-defined lysis or sclerosis, periosteal reaction and new bone formation, cortical destruction and localized soft tissue swelling.

The suspicion of any of these on a radiograph should alert the clinician to the possibility of a sarcoma and further investigations should be arranged. If in doubt, a radiograph of the opposite side for comparison is always helpful and readily obtainable. If the abnormality is still questioned a radioisotope bone scan is the investigation of choice. A normal scan will effectively rule out a primary sarcoma, but not necessarily a myeloma, whilst an abnormal scan should lead to further urgent investigation. By this stage a tumour will probably have entered the differential diagnosis but other possibilities such as infection, stress fractures and metastases must be kept in mind.

We found that delays allowed the tumour to increase in size, sometimes making limb salvage impossible. This was most marked with the group who had their initial radiograph reported as normal. This false sense of security resulted in delays of between 2 and 40 weeks before another radiograph was taken, all of which confirmed the correct diagnosis. In this group 58% required an amputation or were found to have inoperable tumours, compared with 15% of the patients who had their initial radiograph correctly interpreted. All the other patients underwent successful limb salvage surgery.

Once the possibility of a tumour is considered then the patient should be properly staged to assess the extent of the tumour both locally and distally [7]. The staging should include either CT or MRI scans of the tumour, CT scans of the chest and a bone scan. This staging process must be carried out before the biopsy.

The biopsy

The biopsy is a most important surgical procedure and should be carried out or supervised by the surgeon in charge of the case. The biopsy needs careful planning to ensure that the correct part of the tumour is sampled and also to ensure that as little normal tissue as possible is violated in order to reduce contamination by tumour cells to the smallest volume of tissue. Careful staging permits a choice of the biopsy route which will take the best sample of the tumour, avoid unnecessary contamination of normal tissues and lie in the operative route for any further surgery required [8].

Mankin *et al.* [9] found that biopsy-related problems occurred between 3–5 times more commonly when the biopsy was carried out in a referring centre. Our study has shown that problems are almost 10 times as common when biopsies are not carried out at a treatment centre. Cannon *et al.* [10] also found that the rate of local recurrence was increased from 7% to 38% in patients who did not have the biopsy track excised at the time of definitive surgery, usually in cases where the biopsy had been done prior to any planning by a surgeon who did not carry out the definitive procedure. At a National Institute of Health conference held in 1985 [11] the conclusion reached about the biopsy was that 'it should only be carried out by a surgeon if he is prepared to carry out definitive surgery also'. We wholeheartedly endorse this conclusion.

Nobody can be absolutely sure of the diagnosis prior to biopsy; therefore if all suspicious cases are referred to an orthopaedic oncology service some will be found to be benign. We accept this situation and consider it to be more preferable than the situation where cases are referred after poor staging and incorrect biopsies.

The surgeon who carries out the biopsy must adhere to the following criteria:

1. The biopsy track must be so placed and described that it can be subsequently readily identified and excised in continuity with the bulk of the tumour.
2. As far as possible no uninvolved compartments should be contaminated when performing the

biopsy. Obviously this is not always possible but the route should be as short as possible in normal tissues and avoid intramuscular planes, fatty spaces, neurovascular bundles, bursae and joints.
3. A representative sample of the tumour must be taken. Sampling of reactive tissue at the edge of the tumour and necrotic tumour are two of the reasons for a non-specific histopathological report.
4. There must be complete haemostasis and careful wound closure. A drain should not be used. Direct pressure will usually stop even the most haemorrhagic of tumours from bleeding; bleeding from inside a bone can be stopped by plugging the hole with Sterispon and a muscle plug.
5. Large amounts of normal or tumour bone should not be removed for fear of weakening the bone further. Where tumour tissue is extraosseous this tissue will be sufficient, where it is intraosseous either a core of bone can be removed or the cortex drilled and a medullary sample curetted out. A round hole weakens the bone much less than a square hole of similar dimensions.
6. The biopsy must be correctly labelled and despatched to the pathologist with a representative radiograph.
7. The pathologist must be familiar with bone pathology or be prepared to forward the samples to an expert at an early stage in any doubt about the diagnosis.

The above principles assume that an open biopsy is to be carried out. In specialist centres there may be a role for fine needle aspiration cytology or needle biopsy in selected cases. These techniques rely as much upon the expertise of the pathologist as the technical abilities of the surgeon.

Treatment

Once a diagnosis has been made a plan of treatment needs to be defined. This will involve both surgeon and oncologist in assessing the likely risks and benefits of immediate surgical resection of the tumour against other methods of controlling the tumour. These may consist of chemotherapy, which is particularly valuable for osteosarcoma, Ewing's sarcoma and malignant fibrous histiocytoma, or radiotherapy. Chondrosarcomas do not appear to respond to either chemotherapy or radiotherapy and require surgical resection alone.

The role of surgery is to remove completely the tumour with a surrounding cuff of normal tissue of sufficient dimensions to prevent any recurrence of the tumour. Any compromise of this principle jeopardizes the oncological success of the procedure and except in occasional circumstances cannot be justified.

Enneking [12] has defined four separate margins of resection which can be based on the surgical and pathological findings following a tumour resection. An intracapsular resection implies that dissection has actually occurred through the tumour (such as in curetting a giant cell tumour); a marginal resection has gone through the pseudocapsule around the tumour (as in shelling out a lipoma); a wide resection implies that there is a layer of normal tissue between the resection and the tumour and finally a radical resection is one in which the whole compartment containing the tumour has been removed (as in a disarticulation of the hip for a tumour of the distal femur). If the bulk of the resection conforms with one of the above margins but at one point there has been some tumour spill then this would be a contaminated resection and the risk of local recurrence would be similar to that following an intracapsular resection.

The level of transection of the bone must be planned in advance of the surgical procedure. If the bone is divided and found to contain tumour either macroscopically or on frozen section then it is too late as the surgical field has already been contaminated by tumour spill. Planning the level of transection needs careful assessment of all the staging modalities. Plane radiographs and bone scans are the least reliable two parameters whilst carefully performed CT scans or better still longitudinal MRI scans are the best. Even using these techniques it is still sometimes difficult to assess the end point of a permeative tumour such as Ewing's or central chondrosarcoma and in these situations we would recommend that a clearance biopsy be carried out at the proposed level of transection well before the time of definitive surgery – ideally at the same time as the initial biopsy.

Malignant tumours often form a pseudocapsule around themselves which may appear to be an inviting plane of surgical dissection to the inexperienced surgeon. The pseudocapsule is itself the outer rim of compressed tumour pressing against normal structures and there will always be tumour cells which have bridged across to the adjacent apparently normal tissues so that dissection through this plane will almost inevitably result in recurrence. To obtain a wide resection requires a layer of normal tissue between the plane of dissection and the tumour, and whilst this would ideally consist of a fascial layer many surgeons would consider a few mm of normal muscle tissue to be adequate.

The risk of local recurrence of the tumour is dependent not only on the margin of resection but also on the grade and type of the tumour. The grading of tumours has been standardized by Enneking [12]. The recurrence rate increases as the grade of the tumour increases and as the margin of resection gets less, as would be expected.

The majority of limb salvage resections will obtain either a marginal or wide resection and for high grade tumours there will be a consequent risk of local recurrence. Preoperative chemotherapy will usually result in some shrinkage of the tumour and in these cases the margins of the tumour will often become much better defined (Fig. 31.1) allowing the surgeon to leave more normal tissue intact whilst still achieving an adequate margin [13].

The limb salvage surgeon has to wear two hats – the first and most important is the oncological cap to ensure complete resection of the tumour – and the second is the orthopaedic hat to restore a functioning limb after. The two parts of the procedure are often intimately linked but the former must always take precedence over the surgeon's wishes to retain structures for reconstruction which may jeopardize the oncological resection.

Limb salvage surgery has developed in parallel with improved chemotherapy but the decision whether the limb can justifiably be saved is not only an oncological one. At the end of the day the patient has to be left with a useful functioning limb that is going to be of more use to him than an amputation. Strenuous efforts to preserve the foot following resection of a tumour of the distal tibia should be contrasted with the benefits of an immediate below knee amputation and early fitting of a prosthesis which will undoubtedly give a high level of satisfaction to the patient.

Unfortunately, the majority of tumours occur

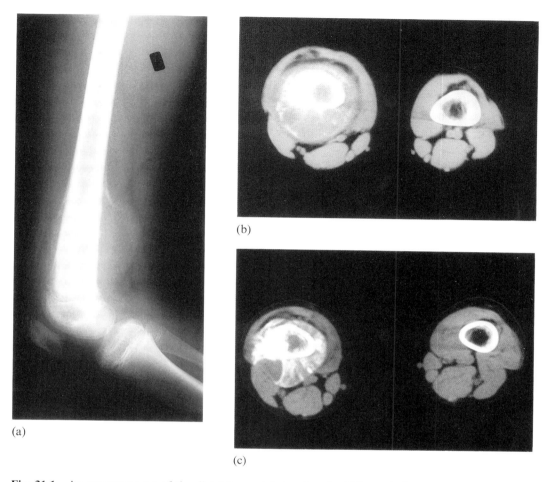

(a)

(b)

(c)

Fig. 31.1   An osteosarcoma of the distal femur (a) showing the CT scan before (b) and after chemotherapy (c) to demonstrate the slight decrease in size of the tumour but the increased mineralization and definition of the tumour.

more proximal than this and in these cases there is usually little doubt that a well executed limb salvage procedure will have considerable benefit over a high amputation. Sugarbarker *et al.* [14] reviewed a group of patients who had limb salvage surgery and compared them with a group who had had amputations. To their surprise there was remarkably little functional and psychological difference between the groups, although the patients who had limb salvage had also had radiotherapy which itself resulted in significant morbidity.

There are few specific contraindications to limb salvage surgery. Inability fully to resect the tumour and gross infection are the two most obvious ones. Occasionally a fulminating tumour can cause such systemic toxicity that an emer-gency amputation is needed to save the patient's life. In most other cases a planned decision can be made. Involvement of the joint by tumour means that an extra-articular resection is required and this may result in such a poor functional outcome that limb salvage is not justified. Involvement of the neurovascular bundle may often suggest that an amputation is required but it may be perfectly feasible to graft the involved vessels if the neural deficit is not likely to lead to too much disability. In the upper limb, particularly where exo-prostheses are of little functional value, every effort should be made to retain a functioning hand if at all possible.

The presence of metastases at diagnosis is a poor prognostic sign but is no contra-indication to limb salvage surgery as the retention of a functioning limb for what is left of the patient's life will enhance the quality of that life compared with an amputation.

Amputations

An amputation will be required if a tumour is found to be too extensive to remove without leaving an adequate margin of normal tissue. Ideally this decision should be made preoperatively but in some cases it can only be made at the time of surgery. All our patients undergoing limb salvage surgery are required to sign a consent form agreeing to an amputation, should it be found to be necessary during the course of the operation.

Limb salvage without reconstruction

There are several sites in the body where bones can be removed without causing serious functional loss. The ribs can be readily resected without much problem although the margins of resection may not be great. Parts of the tarsus and carpus can also be sacrificed. In the upper limb, the distal ulna can be removed with little problem as can the clavicle. The scapula can be removed in total or in part. A partial scapulectomy of the inferior pole leaves no functional disability but a total or even subtotal scapulectomy will result in almost complete loss of abduction of the arm and limit control of rotation of the arm. If the tumour involves the shoulder joint then it may still be possible to salvage the limb by carrying out a Tikhoff–Linberg procedure [15], that is an en bloc resection of both scapula and proximal humerus with the joint intact. This results in a flail shoulder but the hand and elbow still function normally [Fig. 31.2).

In the lower limb a surprisingly large amount of the fibula can be removed without causing disability (Fig. 31.3). Odd case reports also testify to the surprising stability of the knee following resection of a single tibial condyle but this will not usually provide an adequate margin for malignant tumours [16]. Various parts of the pelvis can be resected without recourse to reconstruction. The ischium and pubis can be resected separately or together and the breaking of the

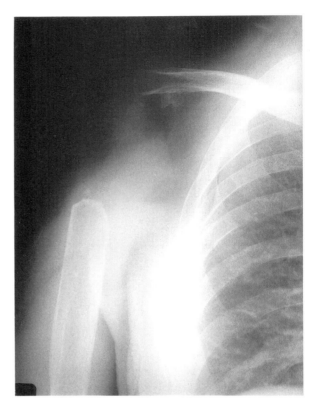

Fig. 31.2   Radiograph of the shoulder following a Tikhoff–Linberg resection for a tumour of the scapula and upper humerus.

pelvic ring in this manner rarely leads to problems (Fig. 31.4). The blade of the ilium can be removed but results in loss of abductor power. If the whole of the ilium is removed then the hip is unsupported and will be free to ride up and down with walking as in pseudarthrosis. A hemipelvectomy may be a better alternative.

Methods of reconstruction

Following resection of the majority of tumours some form of reconstruction will be required. The ingenuity of orthopaedic surgeons has resulted in a huge variety of techniques and has lead to several international symposia on limb salvage, at which attempts to standardize methods of assessment have been made [17]. The benefit of standardized assessment is that very different techniques can be compared to show the oncological success, the functional success and

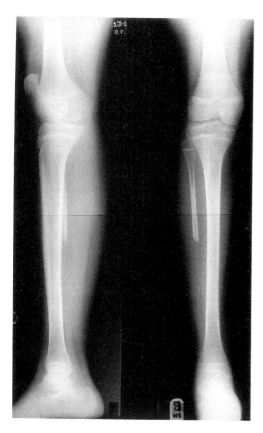

Fig. 31.3 Resection of the distal fibula for osteosarcoma: there was no functional deficit.

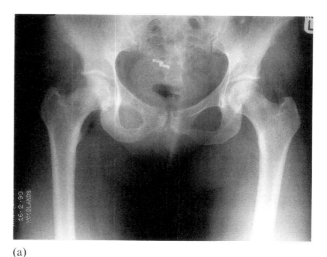

(a)

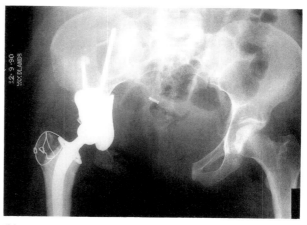

(b)

Fig. 31.4 Ewing's sarcoma of the right pubis and ischium involving the hip joint (a) treated with chemotherapy and resection with endoprosthetic replacement of the hemipelvis and hip joint (b).

the long term success of the procedure. As yet no one technique has been shown to be superior for any one site and thus many methods of reconstruction are practised in different centres.

The principal options available for reconstruction include:

endoprostheses;
allografts;
modified amputation (Van Nes
  rotationplasty);
autografts.

Endoprostheses

Endoprosthetic replacements for the reconstruction of defects left by resection of bone tumours have been carried out for many years [3]. Whilst endoprostheses were initially used for low grade tumours they have increasingly been used to bridge defects created by resection of malignant tumours.

These endoprostheses can either be custom built for the individual or alternatively a modular system can be used to fit the endoprosthesis to the gap created at the time of surgery [17]. The former method has the advantage that the endoprosthesis will definitely fit the patient and the level of resection of the tumour can be carefully planned in advance, but has the disadvantage of time required to manufacture the endoprosthesis (two to three weeks in most cases) and expense. With preoperative chemotherapy the time factor becomes less important as most chemotherapy regimes go on for between 7 and 12 weeks before there is an interval for surgery. Modular systems have the advantage of availability but the disadvantage that patients come in all shapes and sizes with the result that no system can hope to accommodate them all.

Endoprosthetic replacements for the distal femur, proximal tibia, proximal femur and proximal humerus are all available and have predictable results in terms of function and complications [17].

Endoprosthetic replacements about the knee of necessity require resection of the constraining ligaments of the knee and hence a constrained or semiconstrained type of knee joint will be required. These may then be either cemented in place or alternatively a non-cemented type of fixation can be employed.

The distal femur is one of the most satisfactory sites to replace, providing some part of the quadriceps mechanism can be left intact. Most patients will obtain an excellent range of flexion up to 130° with active extension and a normal gait. Many will be able to partake in limited exercise but should be advised against overactivity because of the risks of mechanical loosening [18].

The proximal tibia is a less gratifying site to replace, as there are often problems with retaining a functioning extensor mechanism and also with providing adequate soft tissue cover anteriorly. These problems have been largely overcome by the use of a gastrocnemius muscle flap for soft tissue cover and reconstruction of the extensor mechanism.

The proximal femoral replacement is really an extended hip replacement but without the muscle attachments of the abductors. These will usually be reattached to the fascia lata at the time of surgery and it is surprising how with time the majority of well motivated patients will lose their Trendelenburg gait and will obtain a very satisfactory functional result [19].

Tumours of the proximal humerus usually involve the deltoid and the insertion of the rotator cuff. In order to obtain an adequate margin of resection some if not all of these must be removed. Despite attempts to reconstruct the rotator cuff most replacements at this site will have limited flexion and little active abduction at the shoulder joint though there will still be ab-

duction at the scapulo-thoracic level. Extension is usually near normal. There will be some control of rotation, which may in fact be more than usual, but the main advantage of these endoprostheses is in providing a stable fulcrum for the elbow and hand to work about. There will undoubtedly be some limitation of the daily activites of living but this limitation pales in comparison with the disability of an amputation [20].

There are a large number of other endoprostheses which can be used to replace defects in the skeleton. These include replacements of the distal humerus, total humerus, proximal ulna and distal radius in the upper limb. In the lower limb it is possible to replace the whole of the femur with an almost imperceptible difference from normal, the mid-part of the femur and the hemipelvis for tumour about the acetabulum. These resections and the endoprostheses to reconstruct them are all infrequently required but in ex-

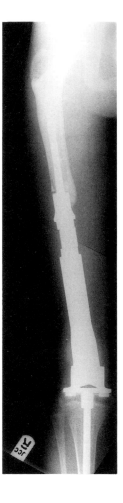

Fig. 31.5 Extendable endoprosthesis of the distal femur.

perienced hands will provide amazingly good functional results.

Endoprostheses can also be used for children for whom continued growth is expected by using passive or active lengthening prostheses. This work is still experimental but in our hands has proved reasonably satisfactory [21] (Fig 31.5).

Endoprostheses provide immediate stable replacements of bony defects with an acceptably low rate of early complications. In the longer term there are predictable complications such as mechanical loosening, infection, wear of the endoprosthesis and occasionally fracture of the endoprosthesis. Mechanical loosening is related to site being least common in the more proximal replacements. In our hands revision for mechanical loosening within 10 years has been necessary for 7% of the proximal femoral replacements, 32% of the distal femoral replacements and 45% of the proximal tibial replacements. Infection is also related to site with an initial 33% infection rate of the proximal tibial endoprostheses reduced to 6% following use of a medial head of gastrocnemius muscle flap to cover the implant.

Revision surgery for a failed implant is becoming increasingly common. Conservation of bone stock is all important and revision before bone stock is lost is becoming more essential, two stage revisions for infection have an 85% success in our hands.

Allografts

Allografts have been less widely used for reconstruction than endoprostheses, largely because of the need to have a large bone bank available for selecting the replacement grafts. The principles and ethical requirements of setting up a bone bank have been described by the American Association of Tissue Banks [22] and considerable experience is available from some centres [23,24]. The allograft types are osteoarticular when one side of the joint is replaced, intercalary when the joint surfaces are left intact and composite when the joint is replaced by a conventional prosthesis.

Intercalary grafts

Intercalary grafts tend to do well because they are relatively easy to fix securely and bone ingrowth will occur from both ends. The stresses on them are less than on osteoarticular grafts and whilst there is an incidence of delayed stress fracture these will usually unite following further fixation and bone grafting. These grafts find use for replacing diaphyseal tumours of the major long bones although tumours at these sites are rare.

Osteoarticular grafts

Osteoarticular grafts present significant problems of storage and preservation of the articular cartilage. They require rigid internal fixation to the remaining bone stock and following resection of a metaphyseal-diaphyseal tumour an extensive graft is usually required. Even though only a small part of these grafts will ever be revascularized there have been some impressive long term functional results [24,25].

Composite allografts

Composite allografts overcome some of the problems of joint stability and mobility that are encountered with osteoarticular grafts but still have the problems of fixation of the graft to the normal bone and also the problem of fixation of the joint prosthesis to the graft.

There have been few publications on the use of allografts for replacing defects created by the excision of high grade tumours. The postoperative chemotherapy that is required in most cases may possibly contribute to the high morbidity of this procedure. Dick *et al.* [26] reported on 27 patients who had chemotherapy and an allograft of some sort. There was a 51% rate of complications including skin necrosis, wound infections, allograft resorption, fractures and nonunions. Despite this, 60% of the survivors were judged to have a good or excellent result. These results are encouraging and certainly suggest the need for further research and experience with this technique.

One of the advantages of an allograft is that on the whole it tends to improve with time and has less likelihood of developing problems in comparison with an endoprosthesis where there tends to be an increased incidence of problems with time. Conversely, allografts require considerable protection for the first 2 years following surgery while union is taking place and in Dick's series they were all provided with a weight relieving caliper until union had occurred. Patients with endoprostheses are able to mobilize fully weight bearing within 6 weeks of the operation.

Modified amputation

The Van Nes rotationplasty was first described by Borggreve in 1930 [27] and subsequently by Van Nes in 1950 [28] for patients with proximal femoral focal deficiency. It can successfully be used to resect large and intraarticular tumours of the distal femur. The distal femur is resected in continuity with the joint and all the tissues of the lower two thirds of the thigh except for the sciatic nerve which is carefully filleted out of the back of the leg. This then leaves a proximal stump of the femur, attached to the lower leg from the top of the tibia down, held together only by the sciatic nerve and its branches. The tibia is rotated 180° and fixed to the proximal femur, and the femoral artery and vein are anastomosed to their respective partners in the lower leg. The length of the new limb is carefully adjusted so that the ankle joint is placed at the same level as the contralateral knee joint. Because the neurovascular bundle has been preserved the ankle will still work even though it is back to front (Fig. 31.6). The advantage of this procedure is that the rotated ankle will now work a prosthesis which can be fitted to the foot and will have both active flexion and extension and is thus more like a below knee prosthesis than an above knee one. After a period of walking re-education most patients will obtain function similar to that of a below knee amputee [29].

The advantages are that there will usually be a very wide margin of resection around the tumour with a low risk of recurrence and that the functional results are good. There can be problems with prosthesis fitting and the ankle/knee joint is subject to increased loading. This procedure can also be used in children where a considerable amount of growth is expected. The amount of growth expected in the resected femoral epiphysis can be calculated from the Anderson and Green [30] growth charts and the resected limb can be made longer by this amount less any growth anticipated in the distal tibial epiphysis (which is preserved). The opposite leg will continue to

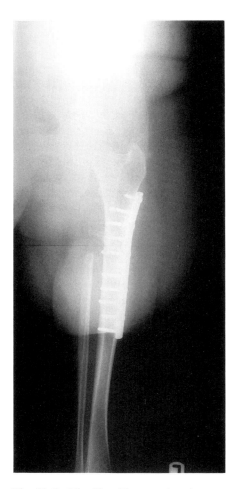

Fig. 31.6   The Van Nes rotationplasty.

grow and eventually the two knees should be at the same level.

Autografts

The role of autografts in limb preservation following tumour resections is really limited to bridging relatively short diaphyseal defects. The only bone which is both readily expendable and of sufficient versatility to be of any use is the fibula. This can be harvested either subperiosteally as a conventional graft or as a vascularized graft with a margin of muscle encasing the peroneal vessels [31].

The fibula has been used to bridge diaphyseal defects of the tibia (Fig. 31.7) and the humerus. It has been used to replace the lower end of the

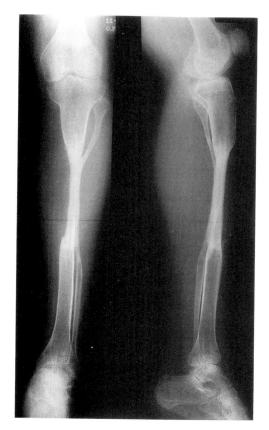

Fig. 31.7 Resection of a diaphyseal tumour of the tibia and replacement with a fibula autograft.

radius and we have used it to bridge defects of the sacroiliac region following resection of tumours there. Others have used it to replace defects in the femur but at this site it often requires supplementation with either internal fixation or another fibula. Once revascularized the fibula will slowly hypertrophy as it adapts to the stresses passing through it, an advantage which does not occur with allografts.

Conclusion

Recent advances in chemotherapy have prolonged survival for all the primary high grade malignant tumours of bone with most series quoting over 50% 5 year survival. This increased survival has meant that more than ever limb salvage procedures are justified in an attempt to maintain as normal a quality of life for this group of patients as possible. Amputations will still be necessary for tumour control and for the complications of limb salvage procedures but in the vast majority of cases a successful limb salvage procedure will provide a considerably better life style for the patient than a high amputation [32].

Limb salvage is a highly specialized field of work, combining complex oncological and reconstructive procedures in the same patient. It is not the sort of work to be embarked upon lightly and quite correctly the majority of this work is now carried out in specialized centres where the multidisciplinary teams are available. Early diagnosis and prompt referral to a specialist centre offers the patient the best chance of prolonged life and successful limb salvage.

References

1. Littlewood, H. (1922) Amputations at the shoulder and at the hip. *Br. Med. J.*, **1**, 381–383.
2. Cade, S. (1951) *Malignant Disease and its Treatment by Radium*, Vol 4. 2nd ed. Bristol, Wright.
3. Burrows, H. J., Wilson, J. N. and Scales, J. T. (1975) Excision of tumours of humerus and femur, with restoration by internal prostheses. *J. Bone Joint Surg.*, **57B**, 148–159.
4. Goorin, A. M., Abelson, H. T. and Frei, E. (1985) Osteosarcoma: fifteen years later. *N. Engl. J. Med.*, **313**, 1637–1645.
5. Sailer, S. L., Harmon, D. C., Mankin, H. J. *et al.* (1988) Ewing's sarcoma: surgical resection as a prognostic factor. *Int. J. Radiat. Oncol. Biol. Phys.*, **15**, 43–52.
6. Grimer, R. J. and Sneath, R. S. (1990) Diagnosing malignant bone tumours. *J. Bone Joint Surg.*, **72B**, 754–756.
7. Enneking, W. F., Spanier, S. S. and Goodman, M. A. (1980) A system for the surgical staging of musculoskeletal sarcoma. *Clin. Orthop.*, **153**, 106–120
8. Simon, M. A. (1982) Current concepts review: biopsy of musculoskeletal tumours. *J. Bone Joint Surg.*, **64A**, 1119–1120.
9. Mankin, H. J., Lange, T. A. and Spanier, S. S. (1982) The hazards of biopsy in patients with primary bone and soft tissue tumours. *J. Bone Joint Surg.*, **64A**, 1121–1127.
10. Cannon, S. R. and Dyson, P. H. P. (1986) Relationship of the site of open biopsy of malignant tumours to local recurrence following resection and prosthetic replacement. *J. Bone Joint Surg.*, **69B**, 492.
11. National Institute of Health (1985) Consensus

Conference on limb sparing treatment of adult soft-tissue sarcomas and osteosarcomas. *JAMA*, **254**, 1791–1794.

12. Enneking, W. F. (1983) *Musculoskeletal Surgery*. Churchill Livingstone, New York.

13. Simon, M. A. and Nachman, J. (1986) The clinical utility of preoperative chemotherapy for sarcomas. *J. Bone Joint Surg.*, **68A**, 1458–1463.

14. Sugarbaker, P. H., Barofsky, I., Rosenberg, S. A. and Gainola, F. J. (1982) Quality of life assessment of patients in extremity sarcoma clinical trials. *Surgery*, **91**, 17–23.

15. Linberg, B. E. (1928) Interscapulo-thoracic resection for malignant tumours of the shoulder joint region. *J. Bone Joint Surg.*, **10**, 344–349.

16. Sharif, D. T. and Braddock, G. T. F. (1988) Knee stability after partial excision of tibial plateau. *J. Bone Joint Surg.*, **71B**, 320.

17. Enneking, W. F. (1987) Modification of the system for functional evaluation of surgical management of musculoskeletal tumours. In *Limb Salvage in Musculoskeletal Oncology* (ed. W. F. Enneking), Churchill Livingstone, New York, pp. 626–639.

18. Roberts, P., Chan, D., Grimer, R. J. *et al.* (1991) Prosthetic replacement of the distal femur for primary bone tumours. *J. Bone Joint Surg.*, **73B**, 762–769.

19. Dobbs, H. S., Scales, J. T., Wislon, J. N. *et al.* (1981) Endoprosthetic replacement of the proximal femur and acetabulum. *J. Bone Joint Surg.*, **63B**, 219–224.

20. Ross, A. C., Sneath, R. S. and Scales, J. T. (1987) Endoprosthetic replacement of the humerus and elbow joint. *J. Bone Joint Surg.*, **69B**, 652–655.

21. Scales, J. T., Sneath, R. S. and Wright, K. W. J. (1987) Design and clinical use of extending prostheses. In *Limb Salvage in Musculoskeletal Oncology* (ed. W. F. Enneking), Churchill Livingstone, New York.

22. Friedlander, G. E. and Mankin, H. J. (1979) Guidelines for the banking of musculoskeletal tissues. *Newsletter, Am. Assn Tissue Banks*, **3**, 2–4.

23. Parrish, F. F. (1973) Allograft replacement of all or part of the end of a long bone following excision of a tumour: report of twenty-one cases. *J. Bone Joint Surg.*, **55A**, 1–22.

24. Mankin, H. J., Doppelt, S. and Tomford, W. (1983) Clinical experience with allograft implantation: the first ten years. *Clin. Orthop.*, **174**, 69–86.

25. Gebhardt, M. C., Roth, Y. F. and Mankin, H. J. (1990) Osteoarticular allografts for reconstruction in the proximal part of the humerus after excision of a musculoskeletal tumour. *J. Bone Joint Surg.*, **72A**, 334–345.

26. Dick, H. M., Malinin, T. I. and Mnaymneh, W. A. (1985) Massive allograft implantation following radical resection of high grade tumors requiring adjuvant chemotherapy treatment. *Clin. Orthop.*, **197**, 88–95.

27. Borggreve (1930) Kniegelenkseratz durch das in der Beinlangsachse um 180 gedrehte Fussgelenk. *Arch. Orthop. Unfall-chir.*, **28**, 175–178.

28. Van Nes, C. P. (1950) Rotation-plasty for congenital defects of the femur. *J. Bone Joint Surg.*, **32B**, 12–16.

29. Kotz, R. and Salzer, M. (1982) Rotation-plasty for childhood osteosarcoma of the distal part of the femur. *J. Bone Joint Surg.*, **64A**, 959–969.

30. Anderson, M. S., Messner, M. B. and Green, W. T. (1964) Distribution of lengths of the normal femur and tibia in children from 1 to 18 years of age. *J. Bone Joint Surg.*, **46A**, 1197–1202.

31. Gilbert, A. (1979) Vascular transfer of the fibula shaft. *Int. J. Microsurg.*, **1**, 100-102.

32. Harris, I. E., Leff, A. R. Gitelis, G. and Simon, M. A. (1990) Function after amputation, arthrodesis or arthroplasty for tumors about the knee. *J. Bone Joint Surg.*, **72A**, 1477–1485.

32

Chemotherapy and radiotherapy in sarcoma of bone and the musculoskeletal system

J. Bullimore

Malignant tumours of bone and the musculo-skeletal system are uncommon and exhibit a wide variety of histological types and clinical behaviour. The site of the tumour and the age of the patient profoundly influence the course of the disease. Treatment of this complex group of tumours requires the combined disciplines of surgery, radiotherapy and chemotherapy.

Radical treatment is preceded by careful clinical and radiological assessment to ascertain the extent of the local disease and to search for metastases. Conventional radiology and computed tomography (CT) scans of the primary site and the lungs, together with an isotope skeletal survey are undertaken. Magnetic resonance imaging, if available, is superior to CT imaging as scans in longitudinal as well as horizontal planes may be produced and the distinctions between tumour, normal tissue and scar tissue more easily delineated. Expert histological assessment of the original biopsy material and of the excised tumour are essential, as treatment is dictated by the histological classification and grading of the tumour and the assessment of the completeness of its excision.

Chemotherapy has become recognized as playing an essential role in the treatment of some malignant bone tumours, notably in patients with osteosarcoma, Ewing's sarcoma and primary lymphoma of bone. Other aggressive neoplasms with a propensity for early haematogenous spread, such as fibrosarcoma, malignant fibrous histiocytoma and haemangiopericytoma are also likely to benefit from its use.

Soft tissue sarcomas are, in general, treated according to their degree of histological differentiation, low grade tumours being treated by surgical excision with or without radiotherapy and high grade tumours having chemotherapy added to the other two modalities, but a uniform approach to their management is not yet agreed.

Management of chemotherapy and its toxicity

Chemotherapy for bone and soft tissue sarcomas utilizes drugs which, if they are to be given most effectively and their considerable toxicity minimized, must be administered only in hospitals where the expertise is available to deal with the complications which may arise. In addition, the timing of chemotherapy in relation to surgery and radiotherapy is critical and a large cancer centre where surgery, radiotherapy and cytotoxic therapy can all be carried out and where close collaboration between the clinicians can be obtained is the safest and best place for this type of treatment.

Prior to starting chemotherapy the haematological, renal and hepatic functions are assessed and rechecked before the start of each drug cycle. If there is failure of normal recovery treatment is delayed and, if necessary, drug dosage modified in subsequent cycles. Extravasation of chemotherapy agents may cause an acute local inflammatory reaction capable of progressing to tissue necrosis requiring skin grafting. For this reason cytotoxic drugs are usually given via a fast flowing intravenous drip either as an infusion or as a bolus injection. 'Long line' catheters inserted into the superior vena cava are increasingly used, especially in the treatment of children, and are kept in place throughout the cytotoxic therapy.

Toxic effects

Both acute and long term toxic effects arise. Of the acute effects, hair loss and gastrointestinal upset with nausea and vomiting are the most common, but more hazardous is the leucopenia which may result in the patient succumbing to overwhelming infection. Measles and chicken pox are life threatening in immunocompromised patients and *Herpes zoster* may become a generalized eruption. Oral moniliasis occurs frequently and may extend into the oesophagus and intestine. Infections with *Pneumocystis carinii* and cytomegalovirus, rarely seen in other branches of clinical practice, are not uncommon in immunosuppressed patients.

Thrombocytopenia may lead to bruising, spontaneous haemorrhage and anaemia. A number of drugs cause cardiac, renal, pulmonary and hepatic damage and cytotoxic therapy must be properly monitored if severe toxicity is to be avoided. Some agents, notably vincristine, are neurotoxic and may give rise to paraesthesia, paralytic ileus and, rarely, palsies of peripheral and cranial nerves.

Late toxicity may include reduced fertility or sterility and permanent impairment of cardiac, pulmonary, renal and hepatic function. There may be impairment of growth and normal development in children and such defects must be monitored in order to correct them as far as possible. The psychological effects of unpleasant treatment require experienced and expert management if both acute and long term disturbance are to be avoided.

Cytotoxic drugs and ionizing radiation are known to be carcinogenic. The study of children with second malignancies has revealed that the risk of developing cancer is 10–20 times greater in patients who have been cured of a neoplasm than that of age-matched individuals from the normal population [1]. Genetic factors have a greater influence in paediatric than in adult malignancy, but there is little doubt that survivors of one tumour are at increased risk of developing a new primary cancer irrespective of age.

The principles of chemotherapy

The rationale of adjuvant chemotherapy is based on the hypothesis that at the time of presentation many patients have micrometastases undetectable by currently available diagnostic means. Cytotoxic treatment given soon after surgery when the residual tumour burden is at a minimum should have the greatest chance of eradicating the disease.

Cell kinetics

Normal and malignant tissues are composed of cells some of which are actively proliferating, some which may be recruited into the proliferating portion and the remainder which are incapable of division. The proliferating portion is termed the growth fraction.

The rate of growth of a tissue depends on the balance between cell production and cell loss. Cell production varies with the size of the growth fraction and the cell cycle time, i.e. the time it takes for a cell to replicate. The cell cycle is a series of events through which a cell passes in order to duplicate, it is divided into phases; G_1, (standing for gap 1), is a short period of preparing to enter the synthetic phase, S. During S phase, purine and pyrimidine nucleotides are built up into DNA using the DNA of the cell as a template. At the end of S, when the DNA and other cell constituents have been doubled, the cell enters G_2 (gap 2), for a short time before dividing in mitosis (M). Following M, the daughter cells may enter a resting phase G_0 or go straight into another cell cycle via G_1.

Cell loss increases as a tumour enlarges and the blood supply becomes inadequate leading to cell death and necrosis. Cells are also lost to the growth potential of the tumour if they become so differentiated that they can no longer divide.

A single dose of a cytotoxic drug kills a fraction of the tumour cells and a similar dose given

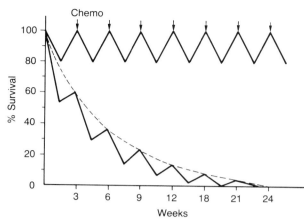

Fig. 32.1 Diagrammatic graph showing the effect of repeated cycles of chemotherapy on normal tissues (e.g. marrow, reflected in the peripheral blood count) upper line, and malignant tissues, lower line.

after an interval will kill the same fraction of the surviving cells, i.e. the diminution is exponential. Similar kinetics apply to normal tissues but normal cells are capable of more rapid repair of cytotoxic damage than malignant. A tumour 1 cm in diameter contains 10^9 cells and the tumour burden, even after surgery, may be many times this number. If a tumour is to be eradicated, chemotherapy must be given repeatedly. The difference in speed of repair of normal and malignant tissues is exploited by using repeated cycles of chemotherapy. Second and subsequent doses of chemotherapy must be given as soon as normal tissue repair has taken place, failure to do so would allow time for recovery of the cancer cells and completely negate the benefit of the

previous cycles. The bone marrow is one of the tissues most sensitive to chemotherapy, and its state is reflected in the peripheral blood. For this reason the return of the blood count to normal levels is taken as an indicator that the other tissues have recovered, and that the next cycle of drugs may be safely given. The optimum interval between chemotherapy cycles is usually 3 weeks (Fig. 32.1).

Chemotherapy drugs

Cytotoxic drugs are most damaging to tissues which contain a large proportion of actively dividing cells. The bone marrow, gut endothelium and hair follicle cells are for this reason particularly vulnerable. Most chemotherapy agents act only on cells in the cell cycle and are termed cycle specific, e.g. cyclophosphamide and doxorubicin. Some drugs act only on cells in a particular phase of the cell cycle and are called phase specific drugs, e.g. methotrexate which affects cells in S phase, and vincristine those in mitosis. There are a small number of agents which damage both resting cells and those in cell cycle. These are termed non-cycle specific drugs, but the damage they inflict is not uniform, being more severe on cells that are in cycle than those that are not; these agents include mustine, the nitrosoureas and ionizing radiation (Fig. 32.2). The cell killing effect of phase specific drugs used over a short time interval increases with dose only until all the cells in the relevant phase have been affected. Thereafter increasing the dose will

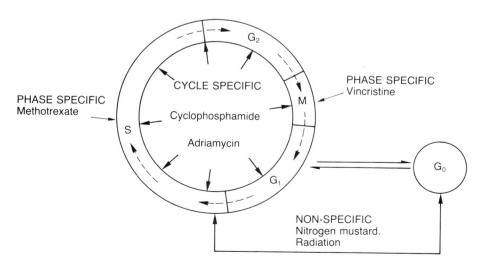

Fig. 32.2 The cell cycle and site of action of some cytotoxic drugs.

not kill more cells. If, however, an S phase specific drug, such as methotrexate, is allowed to act over several days, as cells enter S they are killed. The toxicity of phase specific drugs, therefore, increases with the length of exposure time.

Mechanism of action

Cytotoxic drugs kill cells by inflicting chemical damage and by interfering with their ability to duplicate. Therapeutic cytotoxic drugs fall into the following categories:

Alkylating agents, e.g. nitrogen mustard, cyclophosphamide, melphalan

These form alkyl bonds between the strands of DNA, so that when the two strands are required to split in mitosis they are unable to do so. Abnormal chromosomal breaks occur and the daughter cells produced are non-viable. Nitrosoureas such as BCNU and CCNU have similar properties to alkylating agents.

Antimetabolites, e.g. methotrexate, cytosine arabinoside, 5-fluorouracil

These combine with the building blocks used to construct DNA and interfere with enzyme pathways. Methotrexate is an antimetabolite which interferes with the folic acid cycle; by inhibiting dihydrofolate reductase it stops the production of tetrahydrofolic acid, interrupting DNA and RNA production. The biochemical block may be bypassed by giving calcium leukovorin (folinic acid rescue). Normal tissues more readily utilize the leukovorin than the tumour cells and can be selectively rescued.

Antibiotics, e.g. actinomycin D, doxorubicin

These bind with DNA blocking replication.

Alkaloids, e.g. vincristine, vinblastine, VP16 (etoposide)

Their actions like those of the other groups are not fully understood but it is known that vincristine exerts its action by preventing the formation of the spindle in mitosis.

Others

There are a number of synthetic agents which have been discovered in the course of screening substances with likely formulae for anti-cancer activity, e.g. cis-platinum, DTIC (imidazole carboxamide). These act in complex ways, but frequently include some alkylating activity.

Treatment of malignant bone tumours

Primary malignant tumours of bone account for 1–1.5% of deaths from cancer. Bone cancer occurs at all ages, but is seen most often in young adults and children, comprising 7% of childhood neoplasms. A characteristic of malignant bone tumours is that they metastasize early to lung and later, to other bones and elsewhere. Since the early 1970s there has been an improvement in survival of patients due to the development of treatment which employs the long established disciplines of surgery and radiotherapy together with cytotoxic drugs. Not only have cure rates improved but, encouraged by the local response of the tumours to chemotherapy, surgeons have undertaken limb preserving operations using endoprostheses, thus improving the quality of life both for those patients who survive and those who do not.

Osteosarcoma

The incidence of this aggressive tumour is approximately 3 per million population per year, and although it occurs at any age, it is most common in adolescence. There is a second peak of incidence in the older age group mainly due to the association with Paget's disease of bone. It may affect any bone but is most commonly seen in long bones, 90% occurring in the region of the knee.

Before the advent of adjuvant chemotherapy the cure rate, taken from several historical series, was in the order of 20% [2]. The treatments available were amputation or radiotherapy followed by delayed amputation at 6 months, if no metastases had appeared. The first indication that the cure rate might be improved occurred in the early 1970s, when reports of temporary shrinkage of lung metastases, brought about by chemotherapy appeared. The drugs found to be effective were high dose methotrexate (HDMTX), doxorubicin (adriamycin), and cyclophosphamide. Methotrexate was given at dosages ranging from 1 g/M² to 10 g/M² or more. An intravenous infusion usually over 6 hours was given, followed by folinic acid rescue. Other drugs used included bleomycin, actinomycin D, and vincristine, but of the early drugs high dose methotrexate and doxorubicin were the most effective.

Following the demonstration of the response of metastases to chemotherapy, it was but a short step to attempt to prevent their appearance by using cytotoxic drugs in prophylaxis. Improved survival of patients treated with adjuvant doxorubicin [3] and high dose methotrexate with vincristine and doxorubicin [4] were reported. There followed a rash of reports on various drugs and drug combinations used as adjuvant therapy claiming projected cure rates in the region of 70%. The reports suffered the criticism of small numbers of patients studied and too short periods of observation. This led to scepticism, as the prophesized major improvements were not realized and five year disease-free survival rates in the order at 30–40% were being achieved. The need for properly conducted controlled studies which would include large numbers of patients was recognized and multicentre trials of adjuvant chemotherapy in non-metastatic osteosarcoma were started.

The Medical Research Council (MRC), in a controlled trial of adjuvant chemotherapy, compared the use of low dose methotrexate (200 mg/M²) and vincristine versus low dose methotrexate, vincristine and doxorubicin. Although the appearance of metastases was delayed compared with historical controls, the five year survival was 27% with no significant difference between the two arms [5]. It was not until 1982, when Rosen published the results of his 'T10' regime that hope was rekindled that cure rates in excess of 80% might be obtained [6]. The protocol consisted of preoperative chemotherapy using HDMTX with doxorubicin and bleomycin, cyclophosphamide and actinomycin D (BCD). If on histological examination of the excised tumour 90% was necrotic, the same chemotherapy was used postoperatively. If less than

90% necrosis had been achieved cis-platinum was substituted for methotrexate. Using the histopathological findings to direct postoperative chemotherapy resulted in an actuarially assessed disease-free survival of 92% at 2 years. Other groups have attempted to repeat Rosen's work but although such good results have not been achieved there is little doubt that the T10 regime was more successful than any previous protocol.

A report from the Mayo Clinic that adjuvant chemotherapy had not influenced the survival of patients between 1963 and 1974 [7] gave rise to claims that the improvements in long term survival were brought about by changes in the natural history of the disease rather than by chemotherapy. To test this hypothesis, in 1978 the Paediatric Oncology Group in the United States, started a controlled trial of adjuvant chemotherapy of T10 type given at the time of initial therapy versus chemotherapy delayed until the appearance of metastatic disease. In a short time the delayed chemotherapy group were faring so badly that the trial was terminated [8].

Preoperative (neo adjuvant) chemotherapy is now accepted, based on the results of numerous single arm and randomized controlled trials. Intra-arterial chemotherapy may also prove to have a place. High dose methotrexate intravenously, followed by intra-arterial cisplatin combined with intravenous doxorubicin, was used in the treatment of 164 patients and resulted in a 66% disease free survival at an average follow up time of 54 months [9].

Neutropenia due to chemotherapy limits the dose of drug that may be given safely. The discovery of granulocyte colony stimulating factor (G-CSF) has led to its successful use in preventing or reducing life threatening neutropenia and more speedy recovery of the neutrophil count following cytotoxic chemotherapy. Dose escalation studies are being undertaken to establish if more intensive chemotherapy supported by G-CSF will improve survival. The Medical Research Council (MRC) and the European Organisation for Research on the Treatment of Cancer (EORTC) have undertaken a randomized controlled trial of cisplatin and doxorubicin 3 weekly preoperatively and postoperatively compared with the same doses of the drugs given 2 weekly, with the addition of G-CSF given on days 4 to 13 of each cycle.

Treatment of pulmonary metastases

At the same time as expertise was being gained in adjuvant chemotherapy for patients with no overt metastases, interest was growing in attempts to rescue those patients with lung involvement. The surgical removal of solitary lung

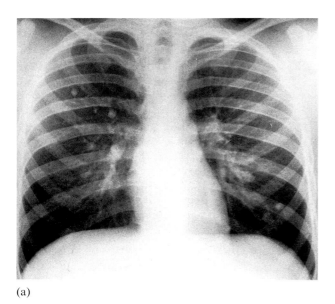

(a)

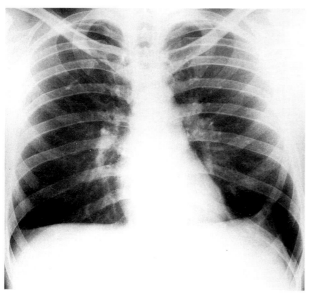

(b)

Fig. 32.3 (a) Radiograph of chest showing multiple bilateral metastases from osteosarcoma. (b) Radiograph of the same patient 12 years from resection of six metastases from each lung.

metastases had had some success, and with the addition of chemotherapy it was hoped that the cure rate would improve. Patients surviving their primary tumour are kept under close surveillance for the appearance of secondary tumours. Regular chest radiographs and CT scans enable metastases to be identified early and many are deemed suitable for resection. Techniques of multiple local resections have been developed so that several lesions may be removed without seriously compromising the respiratory function of the patient. In some reported series, 3 year disease-free survival rates of 40% have been achieved [9]. All patients with pulmonary metastases, and no other evidence of disease should be considered for metastatectomy. One or more cycles of chemotherapy precede resection, using drugs to which the patient has not previously been exposed. Postoperatively chemotherapy is continued for a further 6 months. Patients found to have involvement of the visceral or parietal pleura fare badly and those in whom further lung metastases appear within a year of a previous thoracotomy have a poor outlook [10].

Multiple or bilateral metastases need not be a contraindication to resection. This can be illustrated by two patients of the author. The first, a 15-year-old boy who had six metastases removed from each lung in planned sequential thoracotomies, has remained disease free for 17 years. He leads an active life and has two children (Fig. 32.3). The second, a nurse, who at the age of 17 years had a thoracotomy for removal of the first of a series of 'solitary' lung metastases, is disease free 7 years from her fourth thoracotomy, having survived more than 13 years from the initial appearance of secondary lung tumours. Her nursing training was commenced after the first thoracotomy and in spite of repeated surgery she has returned to normal working duties.

Limb preservation (see chapter 31)

The observation that in some patients extensive necrosis of tumour followed preoperative chemotherapy led to attempts to preserve the limb. Currently pre- and postoperative chemotherapy are used and the tumour resected with the insertion of an endoprosthesis. The majority of limb tumours are suitable for local resection and all patients should be considered for limb preservation. Even when metastases are known to be present the opinion of a surgeon, expert in this operative procedure, should be sought as endo-prosthetic insertion is often the best palliative therapy.

Ewing's sarcoma

Ewing's sarcoma was until as recently as the 1960s a tumour with an appalling prognosis. Less than 15% of patients survived 5 years, most of them succumbing to metastatic disease in the lungs and in other bones. Ewing recognized the tumour as an entity in its own right when he first described it in 1921. It is principally a neoplasm of children and young people, 90% occurring under the age of 30 years. Any bone may be involved but the most common sites are the femur and the pelvis. Factors that adversely affect prognosis are the size and site of the tumour and the presence of metastatic disease, the axial skeleton being the most unfavourable primary site [11].

Treatment

Before Ewing recognized the radiosensitivity of the tumour, surgical resection or amputation was the usual therapy. Local recurrence and meta-static disease were almost universal and in sub-sequent years, radiotherapy became the more common choice of treatment in order to spare the patient mutilating surgery. Radiotherapy tech-niques improved after 1964, when Phillips and Higinbothom [12] reported higher cure rates and higher local control rates where the entire bone as well as the local tumour and soft tissues extension were included in the treated volume. This change was brought about by the observation that on histological examination of amputated speci-mens malignant cells often extended throughout the marrow cavity.

In the 1960s more effective cytotoxic drugs were developed and metastatic disease was found to be responsive to them. The agents used in-cluded mustine, cyclophosphamide, vincristine and actinomycin D. The encouraging responses led to patients without overt metastatic disease receiving vincristine and cyclophosphamide after completion of radiotherapy and the disease-free

survival increased. Other drug combinations were studied, most of which included vincristine, cyclophosphamide and adriamycin in con-junction with a variety of agents such as actino-mycin D, methotrexate and BCNU. Survival rates showed further improvement and the US Intergroup Ewing's Sarcoma Study reported, in 1980, a 3-year disease-free survival rate of 56% [13]; Ewing's sarcoma has a tendency for late relapse and the 6-year disease-free survival rate of 49% reported from the Institut Gustave-Roussy using similar chemotherapy is probably a more reliable indication of the cure rate [14]. The combination of ifosfamide and etoposide has been shown to be effective both as initial therapy and in those patients in whom previous chemo-therapy has failed.

Chemotherapy is given initially, and provided there is satisfactory tumour reduction, continued for up to four cycles, surgical resection is then undertaken. In the case of limb tumours tech-niques of limb preservation with endoprosthetic bone replacement may be used. Radiotherapy is only employed if histological examination of the surgical specimen reveals incomplete excision, if the tumour is too bulky for treatment by means of an endoprosthesis or if it is in an unsuitable site for surgical removal. Following irradiation of initially inoperable tumours, when the tumour bulk has been reduced, surgical resection is once more considered. Chemotherapy is continued to complete 1 year. Increasingly, surgical removal and limb preservation in tumours which pre-viously would have been judged irresectable has become possible.

Radiotherapy

Techniques have been designed to reduce the undesirable long term effects of irradiation. Megavoltage external beam irradiation is em-ployed, and when treating a limb tumour care is taken that a length of skin and subcutaneous tissue is left untreated, in order to provide lym-phatic drainage, and to prevent the later develop-ment of distal oedema. Chemotherapy allows techniques of radiotherapy to be safely modified and when treating children it is now possible to avoid irradiating the epiphysis furthest from the tumour, thus allowing some growth of the limb to continue. Irradiation in the order of 40 Gy in 4 weeks is employed using large fields which include most of the bone. The fields are then reduced to cover the local extent of the tumour and a further 20 Gy in two weeks given (Fig. 32.4). The observation that patients in whom the primary tumour is treated surgically develop less local recurrence but more systemic metastases than those in whom primary tumour is treated by radiotherapy has led to further studies of the use of preoperative radiotherapy.

Tumours of the pelvis present particular problems; both the local recurrence rate and the metastatic rate are high. The tumours are frequently large and the administration of high doses of radiation is rendered difficult due to their proximity to the gut. The radiation fields necessary may compromise the marrow and delay the administration of chemotherapy. When, in spite of preoperative chemotherapy the tumour remains too large to remove, irradiation to a dose of

40 Gy in 4 weeks may enable resection to be undertaken. The case of a 20-year-old girl treated by the author illustrates this policy. She was found to have a Ewing's sarcoma of the right iliac bone. There were no detectable metastases, but a large soft tissue component was present. Primary surgery other than hemi-pelvectomy was considered impossible. Following two cycles of chemotherapy consisting of vincristine, cyclophosphamide, doxorubicin and cis-platinum, tumour reduction was insufficient to permit surgery. She received radiotherapy to 40 Gy in 4 weeks using 8 MeV photons, and there followed considerable regression of the lesion (Figs 32.5a, b). Surgery was undertaken 4 weeks from the end of radiotherapy, and chemotherapy was continued postoperatively to complete a year. The patient had no local recurrence (Fig 32.5c) and the cosmetic appearance was good enough to enable her to wear a bikini. She died of metastatic disease 6 years from presentation.

Treatment of metastatic disease

Radiotherapy may result in useful palliation of symptomatic metastatic disease. Localized treatment of metastases or half body irradiation for widespread disease may be effective for several months.

Marrow ablative treatment with chemotherapy or whole body irradiation combined with autologous bone marrow transplantation or the reinfusion of stem cells, previously harvested from the patient's peripheral blood, may result in more prolonged remissions. This type of therapy is now beginning to be used in the treatment of patients who present with poor prognosis disease.

Soft tissue sarcoma

Malignant tumours which arise from the mesenchymal supportive tissues of the body, together make up less than 1% of cancer. They comprise a collection of rare tumours with variable clinical courses and their treatment is far from uniform. As they usually present as a painless lump often on an extremity and noted for some months, their serious nature is frequently overlooked. Malig-

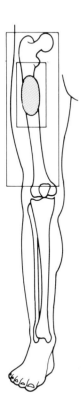

Fig. 32.4 Radiotherapy treatment volumes used in Ewing's sarcoma of the femur, showing the larger volume treated to 40 Gy in 4 weeks and the smaller volume which receives a further 20 Gy. Note the epiphysis which is furthest from the lesion and the strip of tissue medially which are excluded from treatment.

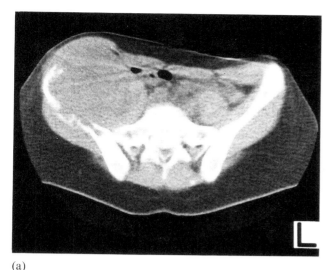

(a)

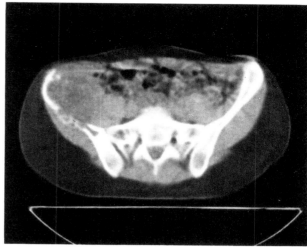

(b)

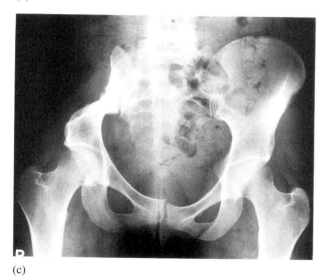

(c)

Fig. 32.5 (a) CT scan of the pelvis showing a Ewing's sarcoma of the right ilium following two cycles of chemotherapy. The oblique line represents the medial edge of the planned irradiated volume. (b) CT scan following 40 Gy in 4 weeks megavoltage irradiation showing tumour reduction. (c) Radiograph of pelvis 2 years from radical resection of the tumour.

nancy may not be suspected and inadequate excision performed.

Malignant fibrous histiocytoma, fibrosarcoma and liposarcoma are equally common and together account for about 50% of soft tissue sarcomas. Synovial sarcoma, leiomyosarcoma, angiosarcoma, and a number of very rare tumours make up the remainder. Soft tissue sarcomas arise most commonly in the buttocks or thighs and may develop in sites of previous injury or old operation scars. They are most common in older age groups, 35% arising in patients over 55 years of age. The commonest paediatric soft tissue sarcoma is rhabdomyosarcoma which accounts for 5% of cancer in children. Rarely, soft tissue sarcoma occurs in patients belonging to families with a predisposition to certain types of cancer. This has been described as the SBLA cancer syndrome and consists of a familial grouping of sarcoma (S), breast, brain and bone (B), leukaemia, lung and laryngeal cancer (L) and adrenal cortical carcinoma (A) [15].

Importance of histological classification and grading

Expert pathology is of great importance in the management of soft tissue sarcomas. A comprehensive study of 1215 sarcomas was carried

Table 32.1 Staging system for soft tissue sarcoma (from Russell *et al.*, 1977)

	Stage	GTNM parameters
Key	Stage IA	$G_1\ T_1\ N_0\ M_0$
G: histopathological grade (1, 2 or 3)	IB	$G_1\ T_2\ N_0\ M_0$
	Stage IIA	$G_2\ T_1\ N_0\ M_0$
T: tumour size	IIB	$G_2\ T_2\ N_0\ M_0$
T_1, tumour < 5 cm in diameter	Stage IIIA	$G_3\ T_1\ N_0\ M_0$
T_2, tumour > 5 cm in diameter	IIIB	$G_3\ T_2\ N_0\ M_0$
T_3, invasion of major vessels, nerves or bones	IIIC	$G_{1-3}\ T_{1-2}\ N_1\ M_0$
N_1: biopsy proven metastases to regional lymph node(s)	Stage IVA	$G_{1-3}\ T_3\ N_{0-1}\ M_0$
M_1: clinically evident distant metastases	IVB	$G_{1-3}\ T_{1-3}\ N_{0-1}\ M_1$

out by the Task Force for Sarcoma of the Soft Tissues of the American Joint Commission for Cancer Staging and End Result Reporting [16]. An analysis of the natural history of the different sarcomas was made from which a staging system has been derived which can be used as a guide to appropriate management. It combines international TNM staging with histological grading to create a staging system which has relevance to this varied group of tumours (Table 32.1). The tumours are placed in grades 1, 2 or 3 according to the degree of differentiation, grade 3 being the least differentiated. The TNM staging is based on clinical and radiological assessment. The importance of this type of combined staging is that it allows unfavourable histology to outweigh the importance of tumour size when planning therapy.

Radiotherapy

The high rate of local recurrence both of well differentiated and poorly differentiated tumours led to more extensive surgical procedures being undertaken as initial therapy. A marked improvement in local control resulted, being achieved in 70–95% of patients [17]. The cure rate in patients with low grade tumours improved, but not in those with high grade tumours who continued to die from metastatic disease.

Cure resulting from radiotherapy alone in some inoperable low grade tumours led to oper-

able tumours of the extremities being treated by less mutilating surgery combined with radiotherapy. In order to eradicate residual tumour external beam megavoltage irradiation to 60–65 Gy in 6 to $6\frac{1}{2}$ weeks is necessary. There are, however, other types of ionizing radiation which can be used alone or in conjunction with megavoltage photon irradiation. Electron beam and interstitial therapy using radioactive materials such as iridium wire allow locally high doses to be given. It has been argued [18] that if radiotherapy is planned as part of initial therapy there are advantages to it being given preoperatively. The treatment volume may be smaller and the risk of spillage of viable cells at operation lessened. In addition, radiotherapy is not delayed by postoperative complications, and as the tumour frequently diminishes in volume, removal with less extensive surgery is facilitated. Anoxic tissue is known to be radioresistant and a blood supply undisturbed by surgery is an advantage. Histological examination of the excised tumour will confirm the extent of tumour necrosis achieved by the therapy and aid in deciding if a further postoperative boost is needed.

Delayed healing is not a problem if 40 Gy in 4 weeks is not exceeded and surgery carried out within 4–6 weeks of finishing radiotherapy. In this short interval the changes associated with long term radiation damage which may result in impaired healing will not have had time to develop.

Conversely, the use of postoperative radiotherapy has the advantage of immediate surgery, histological information from the whole tumour before it has been altered by therapy, and no anxiety about wound healing. The advantages of preoperative radiation probably outweigh those of postoperative but this is a matter which would be difficult to prove without a controlled clinical trial.

Chemotherapy

Treatment of children with rhabdomyosarcoma now achieves a cure rate in the order of 70% [20]. Preoperative chemotherapy, using vincristine, actinomycin D and cyclophosphamide have been the mainstay of treatment. Doxorubicin and ifosfamide may also be used. If the tumour is then operable, surgical resection is undertaken and if complete excision has not been achieved, postoperative radiotherapy is given. In some sites, such as the orbit or nasopharynx, radiotherapy is the treatment of choice following initial chemotherapy.

The favourable response to chemotherapy seen in rhabdomyosarcoma is not repeated in most other soft tissue sarcomas.

Grade 1 soft tissue tumours virtually never metastasize and do not require chemotherapy. Grade 3 tumours have a high risk of metastatic spread and studies have indicated that this spread is reduced if chemotherapy is given [19]. Drugs such a cis-platinum, doxorubicin and ifosfamide have been shown to be effective in high grade tumours and it is hoped that further evaluation of their role as adjuvant therapy in controlled clinical trials will lead to improved cure rates. To date no clear evidence of benefit has been produced.

Some unsolved problems of therapy

The choice of drugs, the best drug combinations, the duration of cytotoxic therapy and the optimum timing of chemotherapy in relation to surgery and radiotherapy is not yet known. There is now a tendency for protocols to consist of shorter periods of more intensive chemotherapy and it has become usual to give at least part of the chemotherapy preoperatively.

Newer drugs include carboplatin which is better tolerated than cis-platinum, and epirubicin which is less cardiotoxic than its analog doxorubicin. Confirmation is awaited that they are as effective as their forerunners.

Further assessment of intra-arterial chemotherapy preoperatively or in combination with radiotherapy may prove it to be beneficial in limb preservation and in the treatment of tumours in unfavourable sites. Encouraging reports of the use of doxorubicin and cis-platinum intra-arterially have been published [20].

The way forward to successful therapy for malignant bone tumours probably lies in the direction clinicians are already taking. Integrated therapy using surgery, radiotherapy and chemotherapy is complex and sometimes hazardous, and if the potential benefits are to be reaped, treatment should be carried out in specialized centres where the necessary expertise is available.

References

1. Meadows, A. T. and Hobbie, W. L. (1986) The medical consequences of cure. *Cancer*, **58**, 524–528.
2. Dahlin, D. C. and Coventry, M. B. (1967) Osteogenic sarcoma – a study of six hundred cases. *J. Bone Joint Surg.*, **49A**, 101.
3. Cortes, E. P., Holland, J. F., Wang, J. J. and Glidewell, O. (1977) Amputation and Adriamycin (ADM) in primary osteogenic sarcoma (OS), 5 year report. *Proc. AACR ASCO*, **18**, 297.
4. Jaffe, N., Traggis, D., Frei, E. III *et al.* (1977) Survival in osteogenic sarcoma: impact of multidisciplinary treatment. *Proc. AACR ASCO*, **18**, 279.
5. Report of the Working Party On Bone Sarcoma to the Medical Research Council (1986) A trial of chemotherapy in patients with osteosarcoma. *Br. J. Cancer*, **6**, 513–518.
6. Rosen, G., Capparos, B., Huvos, A. G. *et al.* (1982) Preoperative chemotherapy for osteogenic sarcoma: selection of post-operative adjuvant chemotherapy based on the response to pre-operative chemotherapy. *Cancer*, **40**, 1221.
7. Taylor, W. F., Ivins, J. C., Dahlin, D. C. and Pritchard, D. J. (1978) Osteogenic sarcoma experience at the Mayo Clinic, 1963–1974. In *Immunotherapy of Cancer: Present Status of Trials in Man* (eds W. D. Terry and D. Windhurst), Raven Press, New York, pp. 257–268.
8. Link, M., Gorrin, A., Miser, A. *et al.* (1986) The role of adjuvant chemotherapy in the treatment of osteosarcoma of the extremity. Preliminary

results of the multi-institutional osteosarcoma study. (Proceedings of the American Society of Clinical Oncology, Houston, May 1985). *New Eng. J. of Med.*, **314(25)**, 1600–1606.

9 Bacci, G., Picci, P., Ferrari, S. *et al.* (1993) Primary chemotherapy and delayed surgery for non-metastatic osteosarcoma of the extremities. *Cancer*, **72**, 3227–3238.

10. Putnam, J. B., Roth, J. A., Wesley, M. N. *et al.* (1983) Survival following aggressive resection of pulmonary metastases from osteogenic sarcoma: Analysis of prognostic factors. *Ann. Thorac. Surg.*, **36**, 516–523.

11. Al-Jilaihawi, A. N., Bullimore, J. A., Mott, M. G. and Wisheart, J. D. (1988) Combined chemotherapy and surgery for pulmonary metastases from osteogenic sarcoma: results of 10 years experience. *Eur. J. Cardio-Thorac. Surg.*, **2**, 37–42.

12. Pomeroy, T. C. and Johnson, R. E. (1975) Combined modality therapy of Ewing's sarcoma. *Cancer*, **36**, 47.

13. Phillips, R. F. and Higinbothom, N. L. (1967) The curability of Ewing's endothelioma of bone in children. *J. Pediatr.*, **70**, 391.

14. Razek, A., Peres, C. A., Tefft, M. *et al.* (1980) Intergroup Ewing's Sarcoma Study: local control related to radiation dose, volume and site of primary lesion in Ewing's sarcoma. *Cancer*, **46**, 516.

15. Zucker, J. M., Henry-Amar, M., Sarrazin, D. *et al.* (1983) Intensive systemic chemotherapy in localised Ewing's sarcoma in childhood. *Cancer*, **52**, 415–423.

16. Lynch, H. T., Mulcahy, G. M., Harris, R. E. *et al.* (1978) Genetic and pathological findings in a kindred with hereditary sarcoma, breast cancer, brain tumours, leukemia, lung and adrenal cortical carcinoma. *Cancer*, **41**, 2055.

17. Russell, W. O., Cohen, J., Enzinger, F. *et al.* (1977) A clinical and pathological staging system for soft tissue sarcomas. *Cancer*, **40**, 1562–1570.

18. Cantin, J., McNeer, G. P., Chu, F. C. *et al.* (1968) The problem of local recurrence after treatment of soft tissue sarcoma. *Ann. Surg.*, **68**, 47–53.

19. Suit, H. D., Proppe, K. H. and Bramwell, V. H. C. (1982) Soft tissue. In *Treatment of Cancer* (eds K. E. Halnan, J. L. Boak, D. Crowther *et al.*), Chapman and Hall, London, pp. 607–623.

20. Ragab, A., Gehan, E., Maurer, H. *et al.* (1992) Intergroup Rhabdomyosarcoma Study (IRS) 111: Preliminary report of the major results. (Abstract). *Proc. Am. Soc. Clin. Oncol.*, **11**, 363.

21. Rosenberg, S. A., Tepper, J., Galtstein, E. *et al.* (1963) Prospective randomised evaluation of adjuvant chemotherapy in adults with soft tissue sarcomas of the extremities. *Cancer*, **52**, 424–434.

22. Stephens, F. O., Tattersall, M. H. N., Marsden, V. *et al.* (1987) Regional chemotherapy with the use of cis-platin and doxorubicin as primary treatment for advanced sarcomas in shoulder, pelvis, and thigh. *Cancer*, **10**, 724–735.

Index